HANDBOOK *of*
SEXUALITY-RELATED
MEASURES

HANDBOOK *of* SEXUALITY-RELATED MEASURES

Edited by

Clive M. Davis

William L. Yarber

Robert Bauserman

George Schreer

Sandra L. Davis

SAGE Publications
International Educational and Professional Publisher
Thousand Oaks   London   New Delhi

For information:

SAGE Publications, Inc.
2455 Teller Road
Thousand Oaks, California 91320
E-mail: order@sagepub.com

SAGE Publications Ltd.
6 Bonhill Street
London EC2A 4PU
United Kingdom

SAGE Publications India Pvt. Ltd.
M-32 Market
Greater Kailash I
New Delhi 110 048 India

Printed in the United States of America

Library of Congress Cataloging-in-Publication Data

Main entry under title:

Handbook of sexuality-related measures / edited by Clive M. Davis ... [et al.].
   p. cm.
  Includes bibliographical references and index.
  ISBN 1-4129-1336-5 (pbk)
  1. Sexology—Research—Handbooks, manuals, etc. 2. Birth control—
Research—Handbooks, manuals, etc. 3. Hygiene, Sexual—Research—Handbooks, manuals, etc.
4. Sexual behavior surveys—Handbooks, manuals, etc. 5. Questionnaires. I. Davis, Clive M., 1940-
  HQ60 .H36 1997
  306.7'07'2—ddc21   98-19732

     00 01 02 03 04 10 9 8 7 6 5 4 3 2

Acquiring Editor:	Jim Nageotte
Production Editor:	Astrid Virding
Editorial Assistant:	Karen Wiley
Copy Editor:	Kate Peterson
Typesetter/Designer:	Marion Warren
Indexer:	Paul Corrington
Cover Designer:	Candice Harman

Contents

Aging

AIDS (see HIV/AIDS)

Anxiety (also see Guilt)

Arousal/Arousability

Assault (see Aggression, Rape)

Assertiveness (also see Initiative/Initiation)

Attitudes (also see Behavior, Beliefs, Emotions, Ideology, and Knowledge; also see specific attitude topics)

Awareness

Behavior

Beliefs

Birth Control (see Contraception)

Bisexuality (see Homosexualities)

Body-Centered Sexuality (see Body Image)

Body Image

HIV/AIDS

Homophobia

Homosexualities

Identity (see Experience, Gender Identity, and Homosexualities)

Ideology (also see Attitudes, Knowledge)

Illness (see Diabetes, Disability, Medical, Ostomy)

Influence

Preface to the First Edition

Fundamental to increasing the understanding of individual and societal sexual expression is research. Fundamental to sound research is reliable and valid measurement. Although there have been many questionnaires, scales, inventories, interview schedules, etc. developed to measure a myriad of sexuality-related states and traits, attitudes and behaviors, variations, and deviations, only a few of these have been used sufficiently for their reliability and validity to have been firmly established.

For an instrument to be used, it must be available to the community of professionals in the field. Unfortunately, most of the instruments developed in the emerging field of sexual science have not been easily accessible. The few published in their entirety in the professional literature are those that have been most widely used. Most instruments, however, have been described only briefly in articles reporting the results of research involving their use. Many of these have been difficult to obtain because it has been necessary to trace the author(s) to request a copy of the instrument and the required additional information about it. Often, this difficulty has led to the next researcher or practitioner abandoning the search and developing his or her own instrument.

Although adding additional measures to the arsenal of resources available is desirable, reinventing the wheel, rather than improving on the available models, can also inhibit progress. Thus, with this volume, we are addressing this problem of availability. We believe researchers and practitioners working in the diverse areas of human sexuality will find it useful to have at their fingertips descriptions and, in most cases, complete reproductions of many of the most promising measurement tools.

In an effort to produce this volume, we searched the published literature and a good deal of the unpublished literature we could obtain. We also sought suggestions from our colleagues. To produce the manuscripts, we solicited brief papers from the original authors. The overwhelming majority happily answered our request, and most of those papers are included here. Because we found no commercial publisher sufficiently interested in the project to support it, we are publishing it ourselves. Given that fact, some limitations were necessary. We could not include every submission. In those areas where one or two instruments met the psychometric criteria of minimal reliability and construct validity, we occasionally omitted other available papers. In a few cases, we have included a brief description of such an instrument. In many other areas, however, we have included more complete descriptions of instruments that have not been adequately tested, simply because they were the only ones available.

Not all of even the fairly well-known instruments are included. In some cases, it was not possible to obtain the necessary copyright permissions. In others, we simply could not get a reply from the author. In a few cases, we have also presented a brief description of these instruments.

There are fewer papers dealing with assessment in the applied setting than we would like and had hoped. In large part, this failing is the result of the difficulty we had in finding such resources. Although we are confident that those working in the applied settings of education, counseling, and therapy are doing evaluation and outcome research, we had greater difficulty tracing the assessment instruments used in these areas than we did in tracing those used in more basic research. We will continue our efforts in these areas in the hope that more of these can be included in a later edition.

We hope that this volume will stimulate more and better research by making the task of measurement or assessment easier. We also hope that this volume will be the first step in a process whereby those who develop new instruments in our field and those who gather data concerning the instruments published here will have a mechanism for communicating their work to others. Thus, we encourage those using these measures and developing others to communicate with us concerning contributions to a second edition, hopefully, larger and better than this one.

Preface to the Second Edition

In the first edition of this compendium, we published approximately 100 brief chapters describing a wide variety of instruments useful to measuring sexuality-related constructs. In this edition, we have reproduced most of those chapters (with some additional editing, either by the authors or by us), and we have added more than 100 new instruments. As with the first edition, there are some instruments that are described only briefly, primarily because the author of the instrument was not able to provide us with a more complete paper. In some instances, we have been able to include only a sampling of items from the instrument. In most cases, this is because the instrument is sold commercially and restricted by copyright regulations. In these instances, details about how to obtain the instrument are included. Also, there are a number of instruments that will be known to many readers that are not mentioned at all. These are not included, unfortunately, because we were unable to obtain a response from the author(s) to our request for a paper or the necessary information. We will continue to work on these and to include more of them in the next edition. We also welcome suggestions from readers about other instruments to include in future editions, and we invite authors to submit material without invitation. As this project grows, it has become increasingly difficult to identify all the available instruments and to track down the authors, so assistance from the community of sexual scientists and practitioners is most welcome.

ACKNOWLEDGMENTS

We wish to thank all of those who have contributed to the second edition of this compendium. Most important are the authors of the more than 200 separate chapters contained herein. Without them, this edition simply could not have been produced. We also want to thank the many people who reported to us that they had found the first edition very useful and encouraged us to undertake the revision. Without that support, it is unlikely we would have taken on the task again. We want to single out for special thanks Sharon Lewis for retyping most of the chapters that were in the first edition. It was a tedious job that she completed efficiently and without complaint. Also, we want to acknowledge the support of Syracuse University and Indiana University for the various forms of support each offered during the years that we have worked on this project, both in the first and second editions. Finally, we want to thank all of those at Sage Publications who have provided support and assistance in completing this project.

CLIVE M. DAVIS
Syracuse, New York
WILLIAM L. YARBER
Bloomington, Indiana
ROBERT BAUSERMAN
Ann Arbor, Michigan
GEORGE SCHREER
Plymouth, New Hampshire
SANDRA L. DAVIS
Syracuse, New York

Abortion Attitude Scale

Linda A. S. Berne,[1] *University of North Carolina at Charlotte*

This scale measures attitude toward therapeutic abortion. Combined with assessments of attitudes toward adoption and keeping the child, results may assist a professional in counseling toward positive resolution of an unintended pregnancy.

Description

This is a 14-item Likert-type scale (6-point) with response options labeled from *strongly agree* to *strongly disagree*. There is no neutral or *no opinion* category. It is designed for high school and college students. Readability level is 8.1 (Fry Formula). Tested samples include high school seniors, rural and urban college students, Right-to-Life members and abortion clinic employees.

Response Mode and Timing

Respondents circle the number indicating their agreement/disagreement with each statement. The scale requires 6-8 minutes to complete.

[1]Address correspondence to Linda A. S. Berne, Department of Health Promotion and Kinesiology, University of North Carolina at Charlotte, Charlotte, NC 28223.

Scoring

Step 1--Reverse the point scale for Items 1, 3, 4, 7, 9, 12, 14.
Step 2--Total point responses for all items.
Step 3--Use the following scoring scale to interpret results.

> 70-56 Strong pro-abortion
> 55-44 Moderate pro-abortion
> 43-27 Unsure
> 26-16 Moderate pro-life
> 15-0 Strong pro-life

Reliability

Sloan (1983) reported the total estimate of reliability to be .92. A factor analysis to determine the unidimensionality of the scale produced correlations above .64 for each item and a mean item correlation of .74.

Validity

Sloan reported high construct validity with five supported hypotheses predicting differences between Right-to-Life members and abortion services personnel, and between pro-choice and pro-life students.

Reference

Sloan, L. A. (1983). Abortion attitude scale. *Health Education, 14*(3), 41-42.

Exhibit

Abortion Attitude Scale

Directions: This is not a test. There are no wrong or right answers to any of the statements, so just answer as honestly as you can. The statements ask you to tell how you feel about legal abortion (the voluntary removal of a human fetus from the mother during the first three months of pregnancy by a qualified medical person). Tell how you feel about each statement by circling one of the choices beside each sentence. Here is a practice statement:

    SA   A   SLA   SLD   D   SD   Abortion should be legalized
(SA = strongly agree; A = agree; SLA = slightly agree; SLD = slightly disagree; D = disagree; SD = strongly disagree)

Please respond to each statement and circle only one response. No one else will see your responses without your permission.

1. The Supreme Court should strike down legal abortions in the United States.[a]
2. Abortion is a good way of solving an unwanted pregnancy.
3. A mother should feel obligated to bear a child she has conceived.
4. Abortion is wrong no matter what the circumstances are.
5. A fetus is not a person until it can live outside its mother's body.
6. The decision to have an abortion should be the pregnant mother's.
7. Every conceived child has the right to be born.
8. A pregnant female not wanting to have a child should be encouraged to have an abortion.
9. Abortion should be considered killing a person.
10. People should not look down on those who choose to have abortions.

11. Abortion should be an available alternative for un-married, pregnant teenagers.
12. Persons should not have the power over the life or death of a fetus.

13. Unwanted children should not be brought into the world.
14. A fetus should be considered a person at the moment of conception.

Source. This scale is reprinted with permission of the author.
a. Each item is preceded by the 6-point scale.

Scale of Favorability Toward Abortion

Barbara Finlay,[1] *Texas A&M University*

This scale measures the degree of favorability toward abortion by determining the number and kinds of situations the respondent finds acceptable as justification for abortion.

Description

The scale is an eight-item Guttman scale. Each item suggests one possible circumstance in which a woman might desire an abortion. The circumstances range from a health-threatening pregnancy to an unwanted pregnancy, and they include a variety of other factors such as the age and marital status of the woman. The respondent indicates which circumstances, in his or her opinion, justify a woman's desire to have an abortion.

Response Mode and Timing

Respondents are presented with the list of nine items and are instructed to indicate, by circling the appropriate letters, which circumstances they think justify a woman's desire to have an abortion. Those items describing circumstances not believed to justify abortion are left blank. The scale is very simple to complete and usually takes less than a minute.

Scoring

A score of 1 is assigned to circled items, and a 0 is given to those left uncircled. Items a through h are then summed to get the overall score. The score ranges from 0 to 8, with a higher score indicating greater favorability toward abortion. A score of 0 generally indicates strong opposition to abortion, as even abortion to protect the life of the mother

is rejected. A ninth item is not added to the score but is used to check the validity of the answers (see below).

Reliability

Guttman scale analysis was applied to this scale, with satisfactory results. The coefficient of reproducibility was .92, and the coefficient of scalability was .74 (Finlay, 1981). Thus, the scale qualifies for most respondents as a cumulative scale, in which one's total score represents one's entire pattern of scores on these items.

Validity

A validity check is built into the questionnaire to ensure that respondents are actually reading the items and answering in a meaningful way. A ninth item reads, "No circumstances *ever* justify abortion." If this item is circled, and all others are left blank, the score of 0 is accepted as valid. However, if all nine items are blank, then it is probable that the individual skipped over the items without reading them, because all blanks on the first eight should almost always be associated with a circled ninth item. This response pattern is coded as missing data. Similarly, if all nine items are circled, a logical inconsistency exists, and the case is not taken as valid.

In a second validity test, the score was correlated with another item about abortion appearing in a different section of a larger questionnaire. This item asked one's opinion on "legalized abortion," with five response categories ranging from *strongly oppose* to *strongly favor*. The correlation between the two scores was .77 (Finlay, 1981).

Reference

Finlay, B. A. (1981). Sex differences in correlates of abortion attitudes among college students. *Journal of Marriage and the Family, 43,* 571-582.

[1]Address correspondence to Barbara Finlay, Department of Sociology, Texas A&M University, College Station, TX 77843-4351; email: b-finlay@tamu.edu.

Exhibit

Scale of Favorability Toward Abortion

Which of the following circumstances, in your opinion, justify a woman's desire to have an abortion? (Circle all that apply.)

a. The pregnancy is a result of rape.
b. The "woman" is an unmarried 14-year-old.
c. The woman is an unmarried 25-year-old.
d. The woman's life may be endangered by the pregnancy.
e. The woman feels she cannot afford another baby.

f. The woman simply does not want another baby now.
g. The woman wants an abortion; her husband disapproves.
h. The woman had German measles, and she fears the baby may have been harmed.
i. No circumstances *ever* justify abortion.

Source. This scale is reprinted with permission of the author.

Abortion Delay Questionnaire

John Lynxwiler,[1] *University of Central Florida*
Michele Wilson, *University of Alabama at Birmingham*

The Abortion Delay Questionnaire (ADQ) was developed to examine aspects of women's decisions to terminate unwanted pregnancies. In particular, we were interested in features of the decision-making process that contributed to delays in seeking abortion for nonhealth reasons (Lynxwiler, 1994; Lynxwiler & Wilson, 1994). Extant research has shown that decisional delays increase the social, psychological, and medical costs of the abortion procedure (Franz & Reardon, 1992; Speckhard & Rue, 1992). However, the majority of previous researchers have relied on demographic surveys of secondary data or follow-up interviews with women who have undergone abortions (Dagg, 1991). The ADQ examines features of the decisional process prior to the abortion procedure, and thereby, it overcomes problems associated with information recon-structed from past experiences. This research strategy provides data on the decision-making process as it unfolds for women. In addition, the data have proven useful for clinic personnel who are interested in tailoring the pre- and postabortion counseling services of their programs.

Description

The ADQ consists of a six-page, self-administered survey that is completed by women who have undergone preabortion counseling and scheduled an abortion procedure. The survey requires the cooperation of abortion clinic personnel who administer the instrument, provide additional information on the respondent's actual gestation period from sonogram tests, and indicate whether the procedure was completed as scheduled.

A total of 52 items are included in the questionnaire. The items include fixed and open-ended questions that provide data on several aspects of the respondent's lifestyle and abortion decision. Demographic information includes respondent's age, race, marital status, education, income,

[1]Address correspondence to John Lynxwiler, Department of Sociology and Anthropology, P.O. Box 25000, University of Central Florida, Orlando, FL 32816-1360; email: jlynx-wil@pegasus.cc.ucf.edu.

employment, residence, and religious and political orientations. The instrument also taps information on respondent's sexual history and contraceptive use. Commitment to the abortion decision is measured through several questions that assess abortion attitudes, whether the woman would seek an abortion if it were not legal, whether she would have another abortion, and the impact of clinic protesters on her decision to seek an abortion. Finally, a number of questions examine aspects of the decision-making process. These items ask respondents to indicate why they are seeking an abortion, what factors caused them to delay their decision, with whom they discussed their decision, the other's response to their decision, and the impact of other's response on their decision to have an abortion.

Response Mode and Timing

The self-administered questionnaire is given to respondents by clinic staff in a packet that includes other clinic forms. A cover letter notes the purpose of the survey and a request for anonymity. The questionnaire combines closed-ended and open-ended questions. It requires about 20 minutes to complete. The response rate has been very high: Over 90% complete the survey.

Reliability and Validity

The questionnaire represents a unique effort to gain information on the decision-making process prior to the abortion procedure. It was designed as an exploratory instrument to collect descriptive data on decisional delays. As a result, the reliability and validity of the instrument may be problematic and more research is needed to assess its utility. However, when data collected from clinic populations using the questionnaire are compared with extant research on abortion delays and state- and national-level data on abortion patients, the instrument reveals a high level of consistency in patient profiles on comparable questions (Lynxwiler & Gay, 1994).

References

Dagg, P. K. B. (1991). The psychological sequelae of therapeutic abortion-denied and completed. *American Journal of Psychiatry, 48,* 578-585.

Franz, W., & Reardon, D. (1992). Differential impact of abortion on adolescents and adults. *Adolescence, 27,* 161-172.

Lynxwiler, J. (1994). Facing an unwanted pregnancy: Women who abort and those who change their minds. *Free Inquiry Into Creative Sociology, 22,* 125-137.

Lynxwiler, J., & Gay, D. (1994). Reconsidering race differences in support for legal abortion. *Social Sciences Quarterly, 75,* 67-84.

Lynxwiler, J., & Wilson, M. (1994). A case study of race differences among late abortion patients. *Women & Health, 21,* 43-56.

Speckhard, A. C., & Rue, V. M. (1992). Postabortion syndrome: An emerging public health concern. *Journal of Social Issues, 48*(3), 95-120.

Exhibit

Abortion Delay Questionnaire

Clinic Form _____ Date _____

This form asks for information about you, your pregnancy, and your situation. Your responses will help other patients in the future. We appreciate your cooperation in giving us the information. Feel free to add comments if you wish.

Instructions: Please answer the following questions as honestly as possible. *Do not write your name on this survey.*

1. Date of birth
2. Please circle your race.
   a. Black
   b. White
   c. Other _____
3. What is your religious preference?_____
4. Number of years of school completed? _____
5. If you are a student, what grade are you in? _____
6. Please circle your current marital status.
   a. Single
   b. Married
   c. Divorced
   d. Widowed
   e. Separated
7. Have you ever had a child?
   a. Yes   b. No
8. If yes, how many? _____
9. What are their ages? _____
10. If you have children, with who do they currently live?_____

11. In what city or town do you live? _____
12. Why are you getting an abortion? _____
_____
_____
_____
_____

13. Are you currently employed?
    a. Yes   b. No
14. How many hours a week do you work? _____
15. What is your occupation? _____
16. Who do you live with? Please *circle all that apply.*
    a. Mother   d. Husband/boyfriend   g. Friend/roommate
    b. Father   e. Grandmother/grandfather   h. By yourself
    c. Sister/brother f. Uncle/aunt   i. Other _____
17. Do you use any type of birth control?
    a. Yes   b. No
18. If you do, what kind do you use most often?
    a. Pills   c. Diaphragm   e. Foam
    b. Condom   d. Sponge   f. Other_____
19. If you use a birth control device, do you use it regularly?
    a. Yes   b. No
20. At what age did you first have intercourse? _____
21. On the average, how often do you have intercourse?
    a. More than once a week
    b. Once a week
    c. Two-three times a month
    d. Once a month
    e. Rarely
22. How many WEEKS pregnant do you think you are at this time? _____
23. What caused you to believe you are pregnant? _____
_____
24. Did anyone come to the clinic with you today?
    a. Yes   b. No
25. Who came with you to the clinic today? _____
26. Why did you delay making the decision about whether or not to have an abortion until now? Choose the ONE answer which best fits your situation.
    a. I didn't know or was unsure that I was pregnant.
    b. I didn't realize how far along I was.
    c. I was scared of having an abortion.
    d. I haven't had time or the opportunity to get to the clinic.
    e. I didn't have the money before now.
    f. I just hoped it would go away.
    g. I just couldn't make up my mind.
    h. I really didn't want an abortion.
    i. I was afraid to tell anyone that I was pregnant.
    j. Other _____
27. For each of the following situations, circle the answer which best fits your opinion.

    Do you think it should be possible for a pregnant woman to get a legal abortion . . .

	Strongly agree	Agree	Unsure	Disagree	Strongly disagree
If there is a strong chance of serious defect in the baby.	1	2	3	4	5
If she does not want anymore children.	1	2	3	4	5
If her health is at risk because she is pregnant.	1	2	3	4	5
If she is too young to care for a baby.	1	2	3	4	5
If she became pregnant as a result of rape.	1	2	3	4	5
If she cannot afford a child.	1	2	3	4	5
If she is not married.	1	2	3	4	5
If she wants an abortion for any reason.	1	2	3	4	5

28. Have you ever had an abortion?
    a. Yes   b. No

29. If you have had an abortion, how many? _____
30. How far along were you with each previous abortion? _____
   _____

31. How many of your friends or relatives have had abortions?
   a. None that I know of
   b. One or two
   c. Three to five
   d. Five or more
32. Who have you talked to about the possibility of an abortion?
   Please circle all that apply.
   a. Mother   f. Husband/boyfriend   k. Roommate/friend
   b. Father   g. Grandmother/grandfather   l. Other _____
   c. Sister/brother h. Uncle/aunt _____   m. No one
   d. My children   i. Cousin
   e. Doctor or nurse j. An anti-abortion group
33. Who, if anyone, tried to *discourage* you from seeking an abortion? _____
34. What impact did their discouragement have on your decision? _____
   _____

35. If no one had supported your decision, would you still have decided to have an abortion?
   a. Definitely yes
   b. Probably yes
   c. Probably not
   d. Definitely not
36. Where did you get the money to pay for your abortion? _____
   _____

37. Would you ever have another abortion?
   a. Yes
   b. Yes, but only if the circumstances were the same
   c. Probably not
   d. Definitely not
38. If abortions were not legally available, would you have sought an illegal abortion?
   a. Definitely yes
   b. Probably yes
   c. Probably not
   d. Definitely not
39. Did you consider carrying this pregnancy to term and keeping the baby?
   a. Yes, it was a serious consideration
   b. I thought about it, but not seriously
   c. No, it was not a serious consideration
40. Did you consider adoption as an alternative to abortion?
   a. Yes, it was a serious consideration
   b. I thought about it, but not seriously
   c. No, it was not a serious consideration
41. Under different circumstances, would you have carried this pregnancy to term?
   a. Definitely yes
   b. Probably yes
   c. Probably not
   d. Definitely not
42. Before you became pregnant, did you think abortion was:
   a. Wrong under all circumstances
   b. Okay under certain circumstances
   c. Okay under all circumstances
43. Would you tell anyone that you have had an abortion?
   a. Definitely yes
   b. Probably yes
   c. Probably not
   d. Definitely not

44. If a friend were experiencing an unwanted pregnancy, would you encourage her to have an abortion?
    a. Definitely yes
    b. Probably yes
    c. Probably not
    d. Definitely not
45. Besides church and school, how many community organizations do you belong to? _____
46. How often do you attend religious services?
    a. Once a week or more
    b. About once a month
    c. A few times a year
    d. Never
47. Compared to most people you know, how religious are you?
    a. Very religious
    b. Fairly religious
    c. Only slightly religious
    d. Not at all religious
48. Politically, do you consider yourself:
    a. Very conservative
    b. Conservative
    c. Moderate
    d. Liberal
    e. Very liberal
49. Which of the following categories does your household income fit into?
    a. Less than $10,000 per year
    b. $10,000 to $15,000 per year
    c. $15,000 to $20,000 per year
    d. $20,000 to $30,000 per year
    e. $30,000 to $40,000 per year
    f. $40,000 or more per year
50. Were there any protesters or picketers outside the clinic when you arrived?
    a. Yes   b. No
51. If so, did their presence affect you in any way? _____
52. In what way did they affect you? _____

Thank you for your help.

If you have any additional comments, please use the space below.

Perceptions of Shared Responsibility: An Attitude Survey About Abortion Decision Making

Ione J. Ryan and Patricia C. Dunn,[1] *East Carolina University*

This 19-item questionnaire is designed to obtain data on the following questions:

1. To what extent do college men and women feel the male should share in the responsibility for abortion decision making in cases of unplanned pregnancy?

2. Are there significant differences between college students' attitudes toward extent of shared responsibility in abortion decision making with respect to sex, religious preference, level of religious activity, marital status, and ethnic background?

A secondary purpose for the questionnaire is to obtain data on college students' attitudes toward various reasons for abortion: to avoid genetic defects, as a method of birth control, to protect the mother's health, or on demand (for any reason).

Description

Brief descriptions of seven situations, based on actual counseling cases, of unplanned pregnancy among college students are presented: when a couple is married, engaged, dating steadily, dating casually, involved in a single sexual encounter, considering a repeat abortion, and no longer in a relationship. Using a scale of 1 to 5, in descending order of involvement, respondents rank the extent to which they perceive males should share in the abortion decision in each of the seven situations described. Willingness for males to assume financial as well as emotional support for an abortion decision is used as the gauge of involvement. The scale consists of the following:

1. *Completely involved* (male should be informed of pregnancy and abortion should take place only with his complete agreement).
2. *Very much involved* (male should be informed of pregnancy and should support emotionally and financially the female's decision to abort even is he disagrees with the decision).
3. *Moderately involved* (male should be informed of pregnancy and should support the decision financially even if he disagrees).
4. *Slightly involved* (male should be informed of pregnancy but should not support the decision financially unless he chooses).
5. *No involvement* (male should be informed—female should assume complete responsibility for decision).

Demographic data also are included in the questionnaire (age, sex, marital status, ethnic background, class level, religious preference, and level of religious activity), as well as information on students' attitudes toward reasons for abortion.

Response Mode and Timing

Administration of the questionnaire takes approximately 30 minutes. Respondents fill in an answer sheet distributed with the questionnaire, both of which are returned to the administrator within the time allotted. Respondents check the appropriate response on the demographic items (1-7) and on the items relative to attitudes toward reasons for abortion (8-11). In responses to the extent of perceived male participation in abortion decision making relative to unplanned pregnancy, respondents will fill in the appropriate response number using the 5-point scale. Responses are made anonymously.

Scoring

Attitude toward abortion is scored as the algebraic sum of the scores on Items 8-11. A higher score indicates a more negative attitude toward abortion.

Attitude toward involvement of the male partner in abortion decision making is scored as the algebraic sum of the scores on Items 12-18. A higher score indicates a more negative attitude toward the involvement of the male partner.

Reliability

Test-retest reliability over a 2-week period was .76 using the Pearson product-moment formula. A class of 16 students in an upper-division health education course was used as the sample.

Validity

No external validity has been established. The assumption is that the items that an individual checks have validity for that individual.

Reference

Ryan, I. J., & Dunn, P. C. (1983). College students' attitudes toward shared responsibility in decisions about abortions: Implications for counseling. *Journal of American College Health, 31,* 231-235.

[1]Address correspondence to Patricia C. Dunn, Department of Health Education, East Carolina University, Greenville, NC 27858; email: dunnp@mail.ecu.edu.

Exhibit

Perceptions of Shared Responsibility: An Attitude Survey About Abortion Decision Making

Record all answers for this survey on this sheet. Please do not make marks on the survey. DO NOT SIGN YOUR NAME.

Background information: Please complete the following by checking the appropriate space(s).

1. Marital status
   _____ 1. Single   _____ 3. Divorced   _____ 5. Widowed
   _____ 2. Married   _____ 4. Separated
2. Sex
   _____ 1. Male   _____ 2. Female
3. Age
   _____ 1. 18   _____ 4. 21   _____ 7. 24
   _____ 2. 19   _____ 5. 22   _____ 8. Over 24
   _____ 3. 20   _____ 6. 23
4. Ethnic background
   _____ 1. Black   _____ 2. White   _____ 3. Other
5. Classification
   _____ 1. Freshman   _____ 3. Junior   _____ 5. Other
   _____ 2. Sophomore   _____ 4. Senior
6. Religious preference
   _____ 1. Catholic   _____ 3. Jewish   _____ 5. None
   _____ 2. Protestant   _____ 4. Other
7. Level of religious activity
   _____ 1. Very active   _____ 3. Slightly active
   _____ 2. Moderately active _____ 4. Not active
8. Your attitude toward abortion on demand (for any reason)
   _____ 1. Favorable   _____ 2. Uncertain   _____ 3. Unfavorable
9. Your attitude on abortion for birth control method
   _____ 1. Favorable   _____ 2. Uncertain   _____ 3. Unfavorable
10. Your attitude on abortion to protect the mother's health
    _____ 1. Favorable   _____ 2. Uncertain   _____ 3. Unfavorable
11. Your attitude toward abortion to avoid genetic defects
    _____ 1. Favorable   _____ 2. Uncertain   _____ 3. Unfavorable

DIRECTIONS: Please read each of the situations described below and respond to each by recording the corresponding number in the space provided on your Answer Sheet. PLEASE DO NOT MAKE ANY MARKS ON THIS SURVEY.[a]

12. John and Mary are both college seniors, engaged to be married in June after graduation. In mid-February, Mary learns she is pregnant (approximately 6 weeks). She decides to have an abortion. To what extent do you feel John should be involved?

    1. Completely involved (John should be informed of pregnancy and abortion should take place only with his complete agreement.)
    2. Very much involved (John should be informed of pregnancy and should support, emotionally and financially, Mary's decision to abort even if he disagrees with the decision.)
    3. Moderately involved (John should be informed of pregnancy and should support the decision financially even if he disagrees.)
    4. Slightly involved (John should be informed of pregnancy but should not support decision financially unless he chooses.)
    5. No involvement (John should not be informed. Mary should assume complete responsibility for decision.)

13. David and Jane have been married for four years when she becomes pregnant. She decides to have an abortion. To what extent should David be involved?[b]
14. Steve and Judy have been dating steadily for two years. Judy becomes pregnant. Steve wants to marry her but she wants an abortion. To what extent should Steve be involved?

15. After a casual date with Jake two months earlier, Susan learns that she is pregnant. She and Jake have not dated since that time, although they see each other occasionally in passing on campus and are friendly. Susan decides she wants to have an abortion. To what extent should Jake be involved?

16. Elsa and Paul have started seeing each other again after having broken off their engagement five months ago. Elsa becomes pregnant. Elsa decides to have an abortion. To what extent should Paul be involved?

17. June and Dick dated for two years. Six months ago June had an abortion with Dick's knowledge and support. She runs out of birth control pills and becomes pregnant again. She decides to have a second abortion. To what extent should Dick be involved?

18. Rick and Rachel both date someone else steadily, but one night at a party they end up with each other. Rachel becomes pregnant as a result. She decides to have an abortion. To what extent should Rick be involved?

19. Should Rick's and Rachel's steadies be informed of the situation?
    1.   Yes
    2.   No
State your reasons on the answer sheet in the space provided for your reasons for your response to number 19 above.

a. A separate answer sheet is provided for Items 12-19. Respondents are also given space for additional comments.
b. The five-choice scale above is reproduced for each item (12-18), with appropriate name changes.

Abortion Attitude Scale and Abortion Knowledge Inventory

Stanley Snegroff,[1] *Adelphi University*

The Abortion Attitude Scale (AAS) is designed to determine each respondent's position or negative attitude toward abortion as a method of birth control. The Abortion Knowledge Inventory (AKI) is designed to determine each respondent's knowledge about abortion. The results from the use of these instruments can be used to understand, counsel, educate, and communicate with individuals and groups concerning abortion. Insight can be gained into how abortion attitudes and knowledge relate and possibly affect each other. In addition, the instruments may be used independently for examining various demographic data as they relate to abortion attitudes and/or knowledge.

Description

Abortion Attitude Scale. The AAS is a 30-item, Likert-type, 5-point, summated rating scale with response options labeled from *strongly agree* to *strongly disagree*. There is an *undecided* category. The population used for development of the scale was undergraduate students from the City University of New York. Initially, the items for the scale were developed from a review of the literature in relevant content areas, as well as consulting 12 professionals involved in abortion and sexuality education programs. The content areas are moral and social, birth control/family planning, legal, women's rights, rights of the unborn, and health.

Initially, 300 items were generated. These were reduced by eliminating all statements that appeared to be factual. The remaining items were submitted to 12 authorities in the fields of abortion and sexuality education for the purpose of judging relevance and clarity. Following this, the feasibility of the items as scale items was ascertained by administering the statements to 60 students, who were

[1]Address correspondence to Stanley Snegroff, Health Studies Department, Adelphi University, Garden City, NY 11530; email: snegroff@adlibv.adelphi.edu.

asked to comment on their clarity. The above procedures reduced the number of statements to 52. The 30 attitude statements that comprise the final instrument were determined by conducting an item analysis explained below. The final 30 statements were then placed in random order.

Abortion Knowledge Inventory. The AKI is a 30-item test with a four-option, multiple-choice format. The population used for development of the inventory consisted of undergraduate students from the City University of New York. Initially, the items for the inventory were developed from a review of the literature in content areas relevant to abortion knowledge, as well as consulting with 12 professionals in abortion and sexuality education programs. The content areas are abortion methods and procedures, legal issues, abortion statistics, birth control (general and abortion as), prenatal development, female reproductive system, and psychological and physical effects of abortion.

Initially, 80 items were generated. They were reduced in number by submitting them to 12 authorities in the fields of abortion and sexuality education, who were asked to rate and comment on each question as to its relevance as abortion knowledge. Questions were rechecked by having the authorities answer them, providing jury validation (Goode & Hatt, 1952). Following this, the feasibility of the remaining 56 questions was ascertained by administering them to 60 students from the target population, who were asked to comment on their clarity. The 30 questions that comprise the final inventory were determined by doing an internal consistency item analysis, explained below. To eliminate response set, the correct options were arranged so that there would be an approximately equal number of each option (a, b, c, d). When using the AKI, certain questions should be updated and certain answer options should be changed depending on the most recent abortion laws, procedures, and restrictions. In addition, the geographic locality referred to in certain questions may be changed.

The AAS and AKI are best applied to populations similar to those involved in the initial development: undergraduate college students. Both instruments may be adapted for use with other populations.

Response Mode and Timing

The AAS should take no longer than 15 minutes and the AKI no longer than 30 minutes. There are printed instructions on each instrument (see exhibits). If both instruments are to be used, then the AAS should precede the AKI.

Scoring

Abortion Attitude Scale. The attitude scale continuum range is as follows: 150 = favorable; 120 = midpoint, favorable; 90 = undecided; 60 = midpoint, unfavorable; 30 = unfavorable. Weights assigned for scoring are as follows: *strongly agree* (5), *agree* (4), *undecided* (3), *disagree* (2), *strongly disagree* (1), for the favorable attitude statements and the reverse for the unfavorable statements. Favorable statements are 3, 4, 6, 9, 11, 12, 14, 15, 17, 20, 22, 25, 27, 28, 30.

Abortion Knowledge Inventory. Correct answers are assigned a value of (1), incorrect (0). A percentage score is obtained by dividing the number of correct answers by 30. Correct answers are identified in the exhibit. (The instrument packet includes scoring sheets for the AAS and the AKI.)

Reliability

Abortion Attitude Scale. Reliability coefficient by the split-half method was .91 (Garrett, 1966).

Abortion Knowledge Inventory. Reliability coefficient by the split-half method was .79 (Garrett, 1966).

Validity

Abortion Attitude Scale. In addition to content validity, an item analysis, *t* test for independent groups (Edwards, 1957) was performed by administering 52 acceptable statements to 121 individuals from the target population to obtain their scores. The *t* values were calculated and rank ordered, and the 30 most differentiating statements, *t* value 1.75 or greater, were selected for the final attitude scale.

Abortion Knowledge Inventory. In addition to content validity and jury validation, an internal consistency item analysis, point biserial *r* (Garrett, 1966) was performed by administering 56 acceptable questions to 127 individuals from the target population to obtain their scores. The *r* values were calculated and rank ordered, and the 30 most discriminating questions, *r* value .20 or greater, were selected. Secondary considerations for choosing the final 30 questions were the percentage of respondents choosing the correct option and the percentage answering each of the four options (Thorndike & Hagen, 1961).

Other Information

These scales were copyrighted (1978) by Stanley Snegroff. They are reproduced here by permission of Snegroff and Family Life Publications, distributor of the package. The instrument may not be reproduced or used without permission. It is a violation of the copyright laws to do so. The package of instruments is available from Family Life Publications, 219 Henderson Street, P.O. Box 427, Saluda, NC 28733.

References

Edwards, A. L. (1957). *Techniques of attitude scale construction.* New York: Appleton-Century-Crofts.

Garrett, H. E. (1966). *Statistics in psychology and education.* New York: David McKay.

Goode, W. T., & Hatt, P. K. (1952). *Research methods.* New York: McGraw-Hill.

Kerlinger, F. N. (1964). *Foundations of behavioral research.* New York: Holt, Rinehart & Winston.

Shaw, M., & Wright, J. (1967). *Scales for the measurement of attitudes.* New York: McGraw-Hill.

Thorndike, R. L., & Hagen, E. (1961). *Measurement and evaluation in psychology and education.* New York: Wiley.

Exhibit

Abortion Attitude Scale

Instructions

Following are thirty (30) statements about abortion. They have been arranged in such a manner as to permit you to indicate the extent to which you agree or disagree with each statement. *Remember,* there are no correct or incorrect answers. Be sure to respond with your own feelings, and not as to how someone else would expect or want you to answer.

Read each statement carefully and proceed as rapidly as possible, indicating the extent to which you agree or disagree according to the following scale.

SA = strongly agree, A = agree, U = undecided, D = disagree, SD = strongly disagree

Place an X through the response that most closely corresponds to your own feelings about each statement.

If instructed to do so, you may indicate topics you wish to discuss further on the last page of this instrument.

1. Abortion penalizes the unborn for the mother's mistake.   sa a u d sd
2. Abortion places human life at a very low point on a scale of values.   sa a u d sd
3. A woman's desire to have an abortion should be considered sufficient reason to do so.   sa a u d sd
4. I approve of the legalization of abortion so that a woman can obtain one with proper
   medical attention.   sa a u d sd
5. Abortion ought to be prohibited because it is an unnatural act.   sa a u d sd
6. Having an abortion is not something that one should be ashamed of.   sa a u d sd
7. Abortion is a threat to our society.   sa a u d sd
8. Abortion is the destruction of one life to serve the convenience of another.   sa a u d sd
9. A woman should have no regrets if she eliminates the burden of an unwanted child with
   an abortion.   sa a u d sd
10. The unborn should be legally protected against abortion since it cannot protect itself.   sa a u d sd
11. Abortion should be an alternative when there is contraceptive failure.   sa a u d sd
12. Abortions should be allowed since the unborn is only a potential human being and not an
    actual human being.   sa a u d sd
13. Any person that has an abortion is probably selfish and unconcerned about others.   sa a u d sd
14. Abortion should be available as a method of improving community socioeconomic
    conditions.   sa a u d sd
15. Many more people would favor abortion if they knew more about it.   sa a u d sd
16. A woman should have an illegitimate child rather than an abortion.   sa a u d sd
17. Liberalization of abortion laws should be viewed as a positive step.   sa a u d sd
18. Abortion should be illegal, for the Fourteenth Amendment to the Constitution holds that no
    state shall "deprive any person of life, liberty or property without due process of law."   sa a u d sd
19. The unborn should never be aborted no matter how detrimental the possible effects
    on the family.   sa a u d sd
20. The social evils involved in forcing a pregnant woman to have a child are worse than any
    evils in destroying the unborn.   sa a u d sd
21. Decency forbids having an abortion.   sa a u d sd
22. A pregnancy that is not wanted and not planned for should not be considered a pregnancy
    but merely a condition for which there is a medical cure, abortion.   sa a u d sd
23. Abortion is the equivalent of murder.   sa a u d sd
24. Easily accessible abortions will probably cause people to become unconcerned and careless
    with their contraceptive practices.   sa a u d sd
25. Abortion ought to be considered a legitimate health measure.   sa a u d sd
26. The unborn ought to have the same rights as the potential mother.   sa a u d sd
27. Any outlawing of abortion is oppressive to women.   sa a u d sd
28. Abortion should be accepted as a method of population control.   sa a u d sd
29. Abortion violates the fundamental right to life.   sa a u d sd
30. If a woman feels that a child might ruin her life she should have an abortion.   sa a u d sd

Exhibit

Abortion Knowledge Inventory

Instructions

This test is a measure of what you know about abortion. Decide which choice (a, b, c, or d) best completes each statement or answers each question and circle that letter in the column to the right of the questions.
Example:

1. Abortions are performed on   a ⓑc d
    a. men
    b. women
    c. plants
    d. birds

The circle around the b in the response column indicates the answer.

1. After the twelfth week of pregnancy which method of abortion would most likely be used?   a b ⓒd
    a. x-ray radiation   c. "salting out"
    b. dilation and curettage ("D & C")   d. suction
2. An abortion performed during the first ten weeks of pregnancy, in which there are
   no complications, usually requires a hospital or clinic stay of   ⓐb c d
    a. a few hours   c. 3 days
    b. 1 day (24 hours)   d. 4 days to a week
3. An advantage of the suction method of abortion is that   a b cⓓ
    a. a woman can regulate the process herself   c. an anesthetic is usually unnecessary
    b. a woman can delay having an abortion as   d. it has the lowest complication rate
       long as is legally possible
4. The unborn is aborted from within the   a b cⓓ
    a. vagina   c. ovaries
    b. fallopian tubes   d. uterus
5. In many abortion facilities it is common practice to combine the suction method of abortion with
   which of the following methods?   a bⓒd
    a. x-ray radiation   c. dilation and curettage ("D & C")
    b. "salting out"   d. hysterotomy
6. Which of the following abortion methods requires the least time to remove the unborn?   a b cⓓ
    a. hysterotomy   c. dilation and curettage ("D & C")
    b. x-ray radiation   d. suction
7. When an abortion is performed by the "salting out" method, the entire process generally takes about   a b cⓓ
    a. 1-2 hours   c. 12-18 hours
    b. 6-10 hours   d. 24-48 hours
8. The medical specialist who is most qualified to perform an abortion is a (an)   a bⓒd
    a. urologist   c. gynecologist
    b. pediatrician   d. internist
9. Which of the following is not a method of contraception?   a bⓒd
    a. withdrawal   c. abortion
    b. vasectomy   d. rhythm
10. Which of the following is the most efficient method of birth control?   aⓑc d
    a. condom   c. IUD (intrauterine device)
    b. abortion   d. vaginal diaphragm
11. A recommendation of the U.S. Commission on Population Growth and the American Future
    was to   a bⓒd
    a. place greater restrictions on abortions   c. liberalize access to abortion services
       for married women   d. permit abortions only to save the
    b. popularize safe abortions as a primary   life of the mother
       means of population control
12. Which of the following do most experts agree to be the most widely used method of
    birth control in the world?   aⓑc d
    a. oral contraceptive ("the pill")   c. abortion
    b. condom   d. IUD (intrauterine device)

13. A spontaneous abortion is one in which   a b c(d)
    a. the offspring lives for a short period of time   c. the woman self-induces the abortion
       after being aborted
    b. the physician introduces a drug orally and this   d. the abortion takes place naturally
       brings on the abortion

14. Generally, at what time in the menstrual cycle are women fertile?   a(b)c d
    a. at the beginning   c. at the end
    b. around the midpoint   d. a few times during each cycle

15. Which of the following is the most reliable early symptom of pregnancy?   (a)b c d
    a. missing a menstrual period   c. slight blood loss just before the end
                                                              of the menstrual cycle
    b. feeling sick in the morning   d. cramps and a heavy feeling in
                                                              the abdominal area

16. Beginning externally and proceeding internally, the structures of the female reproductive system are   a(b)c d
    a. ovaries, vagina, vulva,   c. uterus, vagina, fallopian tubes,
       fallopian tubes   vulva, ovaries
    b. vulva, vagina, uterus,   d. vagina, fallopian tubes, uterus,
       fallopian tubes   ovaries, vulva

17. It is extremely difficult to harm the unborn by striking the outer surface of a woman's
    abdomen because   a(b)c d
    a. a woman develops a protective layer of fat   c. the unborn is emersed in fluid that is
       around the unborn   housed in a sack
    b. the muscles of the abdomen become stronger   d. the surface of the abdomen develops
       during pregnancy   a natural reflexive resistance to
                                                              physical damage

18. During which months of pregnancy is infection with German measles (rubella) most likely
    to cause an abnormality in the unborn?   (a)b c d
    a. 1-3   c. 7-9
    b. 4-6   d. the danger is equally great all the time

19. If a birth takes place during the fifth month of pregnancy, the chances of survival for the offspring
    are most likely   (a)b c d
    a. 0 percent   c. 20 percent (1 in 5)
    b. 10 percent (1 in 10)   d. 30 percent (1 in 3)

20. When a woman attempts to self-induce an abortion by physical means such as running or lifting
    a heavy object, she will probably   a b c(d)
    a. cause an abortion to take place   c. cause an abnormality in the unborn
    b. cause stress and strain on the unborn   d. have little or no effect on the unborn

21. Most women who have abortions   a b(c)d
    a. have severe guilt feelings   c. require some psychiatric care
    b. become severely depressed   d. have minor or no adverse feelings

22. After the legal limit for abortion on request runs out, a woman in (*Your State*)   a b c d*
    a. cannot receive a legal abortion   c. can receive a legal abortion if
    b. can receive a legal abortion if it is necessary   she has been raped
       to save her life   d. can receive a legal abortion if it is
                                                              discovered that the child will be
                                                              severely deformed or retarded

23. The (*Your City*) Health Code requires that all abortion facilities   a b c d*
    a. not perform more than two abortions on the   c. inform women that if they need a
       same person   second abortion the cost would be
    b. give contraceptive counseling as part of   greater
       their services   d. inform women that abortion takes
                                                              the life of a potential human being

24. In a (*Your City*) municipal hospital, which of the following applies to a woman between the ages of
    17 and 21 who desires an abortion?   a b c d*
    a. consent from both parents or both guardians   c. consent from any related adult
    b. consent from one parent or guardian   d. consent from anyone other than the
                                                              woman is unnecessary

25. The woman most likely to obtain a legal abortion in the United States is   (a)b c d
    a. single and white   c. single and black
    b. married and white   d. married and black

26. According to a recent nationwide poll, the percentage of people favoring full liberalization of
abortion laws in the United States is approximately   a b(c)d
   - a. 20 percent   c. 65 percent
   - b. 45 percent   d. 80 percent

27. A nationwide poll conducted in 1969 indicated that most physicians take the following stand
regarding abortion on request?   (a)b c d
   - a. favorable   c. undecided
   - b. opposed   d. refused to get involved in the controversy

28. Most legal abortions in the United States are performed on women in which of the following
age groups?   a(b)c d
   - a. 19 years or less   c. 25-29 years
   - b. 20-24 years   d. 30-34 years

29. In the United States the percentage of legal abortion performed on married women
is approximately   a b(c)d
   - a. 10 percent   c. 30 percent
   - b. 20 percent   d. 40 percent

30. Shortly after New York State's new abortion law took effect, it was found that in New York City   a b(c)d
   - a. there was less chance of dying from legal abortion than from giving birth   c. women became less concerned about becoming pregnant
   - b. legal abortions led to a greater amount of non-marital sexual activity   d. most women waited as long as legally possible before deciding on an abortion

*The correct answer will vary according to local or state law for Item 22. The correct answer may vary according to local ordinance for Items 23 and 24.

Heterosexual Molestation of Boys Inventory

Sylvia R. Condy, *Anchorage, Alaska*
Donald I. Templer,[1] *California School of Professional Psychology–Fresno*

The purpose of the two instruments, Heterosexual Molestation of Boys–Male Subjects, and Heterosexual Molestation of Boys–Female Subjects, is to assess molestation of boys by older females. The research employing the instrument was based on the serendipitous findings of Petrovich and Templer (1984) that 49 (59%) of 83 convicted rapists incarcerated in a medium security prison reported a history of having been molested by a woman. The instruments were constructed for research in which we systematically investigated the nature, parameters, and correlates of

women molesting boys (Condy, 1985; Condy, Templer, Brown, & Veaco, 1987).

Description

These self-report instruments are not psychometric tools insofar as they do not quantify molestation and provide a continuous variable with a molestation score or scores. We regard them as historical information inventories. The one for males contains eight continuous variables, two bivariates, and four multiple-answer option questions. The inventory for females contains 10 continuous variables, two bivariates, and five multiple-answer option questions. In both inventories molestation is operationally defined as sexual contact with a boy under the age of 16 by a female over the age of 16 and at least 5 years older than the boy.

[1]Address correspondence to Donald I. Templer, California School of Professional Psychology, 1350 M Street, Fresno, CA 93721-1881.

Response Mode and Timing

The instruments take less than 10 minutes to complete because the responses of the subjects are given by a check in most instances.

Reliability

No studies of reliability have been conducted. Rather, reliability is assumed from the construct validity data.

Validity

The instruments have construct validity insofar as the network of variable interrelationships, in addition to the correspondence of information provided by the reports of males and females, provides a meaningful pattern. The mean age of the molested boy is ordinarily around 12 years and the molesting female is typically in her early or mid-20s. In the overwhelming majority of cases, sexual intercourse takes place. (Such occurs much less than when males molest female children.) The preponderance of the molesting females are friends of the family, neighbors, and baby-sitters.

References

Condy, S. R. (1985). *Parameters of heterosexual molestation of boys.* Unpublished doctoral dissertation, California School of Professional Psychology–Fresno.

Condy, S. R., Templer, D. I., Brown, R., & Veaco, L. (1987). Parameters of sexual contact of boys with women. *Archives of Sexual Behavior, 87,* 379-394.

Petrovich, M., & Templer, D. I. (1984). Heterosexual molestation of children who later became rapists. *Psychological Reports, 54,* 810.

Exhibit

Heterosexual Molestation of Boys Inventory–Male Subjects

Questionnaire–Male Subjects

1. Age _____   2.   Education _____
3. Race (check one):
   - _____ a. Asian
   - _____ b. Black
   - _____ c. Hispanic
   - _____ d. American Indian
   - _____ e. White
   - _____ f. Other _____
4. How far did your father go in school? (Circle the grade)
   0   1   2   3   4   5   6   7   8   9   10   11
   12   13   14   15   16   17   18   19   20 or more
5. How far did your mother go in school? (Circle the grade)
   0   1   2   3   4   5   6   7   8   9   10   11
   12   13   14   15   16   17   18   19   20 or more
6. Before you were 16 years old, did you ever have sexual contact with a woman or girl who was 5 years or more older than yourself?
   - _____ a. yes
   - _____ b. no
7. If yes, how many times did you have such an experience? _____
8. If yes, with how many different women? _____
9. If yes, how old were you at the time or times? _____
10. If yes, how old was the woman or girl (women or girls)? _____
11. If yes, what type of sexual activity occurred? (check more than one if more than one activity occurred)
    - _____ a. intercourse
    - _____ b. oral sex upon you
    - _____ c. oral sex upon her
    - _____ d. her touching your penis
    - _____ e. your touching her genitals
    - _____ f. your touching her breasts
    - _____ g. other _____
12. If yes, what was your relationship to the woman or girl (women or girls)?
    - _____ a. mother
    - _____ b. aunt
    - _____ c. cousin
    - _____ d. sister
    - _____ e. grandmother
    - _____ f. friend
    - _____ g. neighbor
    - _____ h. teacher
    - _____ i. baby-sitter
    - _____ j. stranger
    - _____ k. other

13. If yes, how did it happen?
    _____ a. I wanted to do it and she agreed
    _____ b. she wanted to do it and I agreed
    _____ c. I forced her
    _____ d. she forced me
    _____ e. other _____
14. If yes, did the woman or girl (women or girls) have alcohol or drug abuse problems?
    _____ a. yes
    _____ b. no
    _____ c. don't know
15. If yes, did the woman or girl (women or girls) have mental or emotional problems?
    _____ a. yes
    _____ b. no
    _____ c. don't know
16. If yes, did you feel good or bad about the experience or experiences?
    _____ a. good
    _____ b. bad
17. If yes, what sort of effect did this experience or experiences have on your adult sex life?
    _____ a. a good effect
    _____ b. a bad effect
    _____ c. no effect

Exhibit

Heterosexual Molestation of Boys Inventory–Female Subjects

Questionnaire–Female Subjects

1. Age _____ 2. Education _____
3. Race (check one):
    _____ a. Asian   _____ d. American Indian
    _____ b. Black   _____ e. White
    _____ c. Hispanic   _____ f. Other _____
4. How far did your father go in school? (Circle the grade)
    0   1   2   3   4   5   6   7   8   9   10   11
    12   13   14   15   16   17   18   19   20 or more
5. How far did your mother go in school? (Circle the grade)
    0   1   2   3   4   5   6   7   8   9   10   11
    12   13   14   15   16   17   18   19   20 or more
6. Did you ever have sexual contact with a boy before he was 16 years old, when you were 5 years or
    more older than he?
    _____ a. yes   _____ b. no
7. If yes, how many times did you have such an experience? _____
8. If yes, with how many different boys? _____
9. If yes, how old were you at the time or times? _____
10. If yes, how old was the boy or boys? _____
11. If yes, what type of sexual activity occurred?
    (check more than one if more than one activity occurred)
    _____ a. intercourse
    _____ b. oral sex upon you
    _____ c. oral sex upon him
    _____ d. your touching his penis
    _____ e. his touching your genitals
    _____ f. his touching your breasts
    _____ g. other _____

12. If yes, what was your relationship to the boy or boys?
     _____ a. father   _____ g. neighbor
     _____ b. uncle   _____ h. teacher
     _____ c. cousin   _____ i. baby-sitter
     _____ d. brother   _____ j. stranger
     _____ e. grandfather   _____ k. other _____
     _____ f. friend

13. If yes, how did it happen?
     _____ a. I wanted to do it and he agreed   _____ d. he forced me
     _____ b. he wanted to do it and I agreed   _____ e. other _____
     _____ c. I forced him

14. Did you have sex with a man or boy at least 5 years older than you before you were 16?
     _____ a. yes   _____ b. no

15. If yes, what was the relationship of the man or boy to you?
     _____ a. father   _____ g. neighbor
     _____ b. uncle   _____ h. teacher
     _____ c. cousin   _____ i. baby-sitter
     _____ d. brother   _____ j. stranger
     _____ e. grandfather   _____ k. other _____
     _____ f. friend

16. If yes, how old were you at the time or times? _____
17. If yes, how old was he at the time or times? _____

Trauma-Related Beliefs Questionnaire

Ann Hazzard,[1] *Emory University School of Medicine*

The Trauma-Related Beliefs questionnaire (TRB; Hazzard, 1993) was developed to assess beliefs reflective of Finkelhor and Browne's (1986) model of traumagenic dynamics among sexual abuse survivors. Sexual abuse is postulated to alter a child's cognitive and affective orientations to the world along four dimensions: self-blame/stigmatization, betrayal, powerlessness, and traumatic sexualization. Many abused children blame themselves for the abuse and feel isolated and different from others. They generally feel betrayed, certainly by the offender and perhaps by other adults who were unable to protect them. Sexually abused children often view themselves as powerless. Because they were unable to control access to their bodies, they may

believe they are unable to control other aspects of their lives. Finally, sexually abused children have been introduced to sexuality at a developmentally inappropriate time, often in a confusing or threatening manner, leading to negative beliefs and feelings about sexuality. Finkelhor and Browne postulated that traumagenic beliefs along these four dimensions underlie other common psychological/behavioral problems in adult survivors. The scale was developed to allow testing of this conceptual model of trauma sequelae in survivors and may also be useful in treatment planning or evaluation.

Description

The TRB consists of 56 items, each rated on a 5-point Likert-type scale ranging from 0 (*absolutely untrue*) to 4

[1]Address correspondence to Ann Hazzard, Box 26065, Grady Hospital, 80 Butler Street, Atlanta, GA 30335.

(*absolutely true*). The scale was derived from an original pool of 87 items that were piloted on a sample of 56 female adult sexual abuse survivors. The measure includes four subscales: Self-Blame/Stigmatization (29 items), Betrayal (10 items), Powerlessness (10 items), and Traumatic Sexualization (7 items).

Response Mode and Timing

Respondents circle one number to represent how true each statement is of them. The questionnaire takes approximately 10 minutes to complete.

Scoring

Some items are reversed so that higher scores on each item reflect stronger, maladaptive trauma-related beliefs. For each subscale, the mean of all subscale items, which can range from 0 to 4, is computed. Subscale items (with R reflecting items that are reverse scored) are as follows: Self-Blame/Stigmatization (3, 4, 5, 8, 12, 13, 18R, 19R, 23, 24, 25R, 30, 31, 32, 33, 34, 35, 36, 38, 39R, 43R, 44, 46, 47, 48, 49, 50, 55R, 56); Betrayal (1, 14, 20, 26R, 37, 40, 45R, 51, 52, 54); Powerlessness (6, 7, 9, 15, 17R, 21, 27, 28R, 41, 53); and Traumatic Sexualization (2, 10, 11, 16, 22, 29R, 42). A total TRB score is also computed, which represents the mean of all items.

Reliability

In a sample of 56 adult female sexual abuse survivors, the total TRB scale had an internal reliability coefficient alpha of .93. Coefficient alphas for the subscales were as follows: Self-Blame/Stigmatization .89; Betrayal .86; Powerlessness .78; and Traumatic Sexualization .87.

Validity

Validity of the measure, as well as a preliminary test of Finkelhor and Browne's (1986) conceptual model, was assessed by entering TRB subscale scores into multiple regression equations predicting other questionnaire measures of psychological and behavioral symptomatology. As predicted, self-blaming attitudes predicted lower self-esteem (42% of variance), more interpersonal problems (46% of variance), more depression (7% of variance), and greater overall psychological distress (38% of variance). Betrayal beliefs were related to interpersonal problems as predicted (6% of variance), were also related to an external locus of control (8% of variance), but were not related to depression as predicted by the model. Unexpectedly, betrayal beliefs were also associated with sexual problems (16% of variance). Powerlessness beliefs predicted an external locus of control (30% of the variance) and, as predicted, depression (38% of the variance). Finally, beliefs reflective of sex-related anxiety predicted anxiety in general (10% of the variance) and avoidance of sexuality (23% of the variance). Overall, findings supported 8 of 11 hypotheses concerning the relationship between trauma-related beliefs and other psychological/behavioral outcomes, based on Finkelhor and Browne's model of traumagenic dynamics in sexual abuse victims.

References

Finkelhor, D., & Browne, A. (1986). Initial and long-term effects: A conceptual framework. In D. Finkelhor (Ed.), *A sourcebook on child sexual abuse* (pp. 143-179). Beverly Hills, CA: Sage.

Hazzard, A. (1993). Trauma-related beliefs as mediators of sexual abuse impact in adult women survivors: A pilot study. *Journal of Child Sexual Abuse, 2*(3), 55-69.

Exhibit

Trauma-Related Beliefs Questionnaire

Directions: Below are some statements of different thoughts and feelings. Some statements are about what happened in the past, in other words, your experience(s) of sexual abuse. Other statements are about your current views concerning various issues. For each statement, please circle one number to indicate how untrue or true the statement is to you. The rating scale is as follows:

0 = Absolutely untrue
1 = Mostly untrue
2 = Partly true, partly untrue
3 = Mostly true
4 = Absolutely true

There are no right or wrong answers. Please circle the number that indicates how you *really* think or feel.

	Absolutely untrue	Mostly untrue	Partly true, Partly untrue	Mostly true	Absolutely true
1. People often take advantage of others.	0	1	2	3	4
2. Thinking about sex upsets me.	0	1	2	3	4
3. I was to blame for what happened.	0	1	2	3	4
4. I often wonder "why me?"	0	1	2	3	4

	Absolutely untrue	Mostly untrue	Partly true, Partly untrue	Mostly true	Absolutely true
5. I feel I should be punished for what I did.	0	1	2	3	4
6. Most things in life can't be controlled.	0	1	2	3	4
7. Something like this might happen to me again.	0	1	2	3	4
8. The abuse happened to me because I was not smart enough to stop it from happening.	0	1	2	3	4
9. No matter what I do, I can't stop bad things from happening.	0	1	2	3	4
10. I get frightened when I think about sex.	0	1	2	3	4
11. I wish there was no such thing as sex.	0	1	2	3	4
12. The abuse was my fault because I used sexual activities to obtain attention or rewards from the abuser.	0	1	2	3	4
13. Most other abuse victims are coping better than I am.	0	1	2	3	4
14. If you love someone, sooner or later that person will let you down.	0	1	2	3	4
15. I often worry that I will be abused again.	0	1	2	3	4
16. Sex is dirty.	0	1	2	3	4
17. I can protect myself in the future.	0	1	2	3	4
18. The person who abused me was to blame for what happened.	0	1	2	3	4
19. I did what most children would do in similar circumstances.	0	1	2	3	4
20. Nobody really cares about anyone but themselves.	0	1	2	3	4
21. I can't control what happens to me.	0	1	2	3	4
22. Sex is disgusting.	0	1	2	3	4
23. I feel guilty about what happened.	0	1	2	3	4
24. I am inferior to other people because I did not have normal experiences.	0	1	2	3	4
25. I believe something positive has come out of my abuse.	0	1	2	3	4
26. I can depend on close friends to help me.	0	1	2	3	4
27. More bad things happen to me than to other people.	0	1	2	3	4
28. I can usually achieve what I want in most situations.	0	1	2	3	4
29. Sex is beautiful.	0	1	2	3	4
30. This happened to me because I always have bad luck.	0	1	2	3	4
31. I must have permitted sexual activities because I wasn't forced into it.	0	1	2	3	4
32. I just don't understand why this happened.	0	1	2	3	4
33. I should be handling this better than I am.	0	1	2	3	4
34. This happened to me because I am a bad person.	0	1	2	3	4
35. I should have been able to prevent the abuse.	0	1	2	3	4
36. I am ashamed about what happened.	0	1	2	3	4
37. I have to know people for a long time before I can trust them.	0	1	2	3	4
38. I am embarrassed when I see people who know what happened.	0	1	2	3	4
39. I have found a way to make sense of what happened.	0	1	2	3	4
40. People always expect something in return for being nice.	0	1	2	3	4
41. It doesn't pay to try hard because things never turn out right anyway.	0	1	2	3	4
42. I hate sex.	0	1	2	3	4
43. I was too young to stop this from happening.	0	1	2	3	4
44. It is unnatural to feel any pleasure during sexual abuse.	0	1	2	3	4
45. Most men are trustworthy.	0	1	2	3	4
46. I was tricked into the abuse.	0	1	2	3	4
47. My passivity encouraged the abuse to continue.	0	1	2	3	4
48. I will never be able to lead a normal life.	0	1	2	3	4
49. I feel I have caused trouble for many people.	0	1	2	3	4
50. I am different than other people.	0	1	2	3	4

	Absolutely untrue	Mostly untrue	Partly true, Partly untrue	Mostly true	Absolutely true
51. It is dangerous to get close to anyone because they always betray you.	0	1	2	3	4
52. You can't depend on women.	0	1	2	3	4
53. People don't have much influence over the way things turn out.	0	1	2	3	4
54. It is hard to tell the difference between affection and sexual touching.	0	1	2	3	4
55. There were good reasons for the choices I made as a child.	0	1	2	3	4
56. This happened to me because I am not a strong person.	0	1	2	3	4

The Battered Woman Scale

Christine Mattley and Martin D. Schwartz,[1] *Ohio University*

This scale was developed to test the proposition that battered women, and in particular women who are in shelter houses, develop particular gender role trait ascriptions that are predicted in the more theoretical literature. Because this scale shows that battered women test differently than similarly situated nonbattered women, the scale may be of some use to measure shelter house programming on the self-concepts of battered women. Gender role trait ascriptions are mutable.

Although the self-esteem and personality of battered women have been extensively studied, research on gender role trait ascriptions has been virtually absent from the literature. One reason for this absence is a too common assumption that batterers are narrowly masculine and survivors are narrowly feminine (Pagelow, 1981; Walker, 1979). The Battered Woman Scale (BWS) was developed to measure the extent to which survivors' gender role trait ascriptions have been affected by battering contexts. The supposition behind the scale is not that there is something about the gender role identities of women that *causes* them to be battered. Rather, battering contexts consist of interactions that lead women to see themselves in particular ways. So, for example, whereas others (e.g., Burke, Stets,

& Pirog-Good, 1988) have conceptualized gender identity as the independent variable, the BWS is premised on the assumption that survivors' gender role identity is the dependent variable; it is caused by the battering.

Description

Measuring gender role trait ascriptions is not new. For more than 20 years, Bem's Sex Role Inventory (Bem, 1974) and Spence and Helmreich's Personal Attributes Questionnaire (PAQ; Spence, Helmreich, & Stapp, 1974) have been widely used on a variety of samples of men and women. Our interest in a new scale came from a realization that although the PAQ has been extensively tested on college students and can be easily used with a wide variety of women, only some of the questions are particularly relevant for battered women. Specifically, the literature on battered women suggests that some attributes are more likely to be particularly salient to battered women than others. Consequently, we constructed the BWS using seven questions from the PAQ that match the attributes suggested in the literature. These questions not only come from the masculine and feminine scales widely used in scoring the PAQ but also from the undifferentiated scale, which is very rarely used in scoring the PAQ. We administered the entire PAQ to provide distracter questions, but used only the seven chosen questions for the BWS.

---
[1]Address correspondence to Martin D. Schwartz, Department of Sociology and Anthropology, Lindley Hall, Ohio University, Athens, OH 45701-2979; email: mschwartz1@ohiou.edu.

In a pretest, women residing at shelters found the semantic differential format and some of the wording of the PAQ to be confusing and cumbersome. Based on their comments, we modified it to a Likert-type scale format and changed some of the wording to make it more understandable to high school graduates and nongraduates. A validation split sample drawn from several college classes was given either the original version or the newer Likert-type version, yielding virtually identical results on each item.

Response Mode and Timing

Respondents can use either a machine-scorable answer sheet or just circle the number from 0 to 4 that indicates how strongly they agree or disagree with each of the 24 statements as descriptions of themselves. The scores range from 0 for *strongly agree* to 4 for *strongly disagree*. The instrument takes approximately 10 minutes to complete.

Scoring

The seven questions from the PAQ used to construct the BWS were Questions 1, 4, 6, 7, 13, 23, and 24. Each was coded so that scores in the predicted direction received the maximum score using a 0-4 Likert-type system. To make the scoring consistent with other questions, when the theoretical literature suggested that battered women would score low rather than high, the question was reverse scored. This required reverse coding on Questions 1, 4, 6, 7, 13, and 23 (see Schwartz & Mattley, 1993) and creates a scale with scores ranging (in theory) from 0 to 28. A high score indicates a strong endorsement of those gender role traits predicted in the literature on battered women.

Validity

Mattley and Schwartz (1990) found a significant difference in comparing women from both rural and urban shelter houses for battered women with a control group of women with nearly identical social class characteristics (but claiming no history of abuse) seeking help from social service agencies. Using discriminant function analysis to differentiate statistically between the two groups, they found that the two predictor variables of the BWS score and race produced an eigenvalue of .59, with group membership explaining 37% of the variance. Although African American women score somewhat differently than European American women, the *relationship* described above holds: African American women emerging from violent relationships score significantly higher than other African American women.

References

Bem, S. L. (1974). The measurement of psychological androgyny. *Journal of Consulting and Clinical Psychology 42*, 155-162.

Burke, P., Stets, J., & Pirog-Good, M. (1988). Gender identity, self-esteem and physical and sexual abuse in dating relationships. *Social Psychology Quarterly, 51*, 272-283.

Mattley, C. L., & Schwartz, M. D. (1990). Emerging from tyranny. *Symbolic Interaction, 13*, 281-289.

Pagelow, M. D. (1981). *Woman battering*. Beverly Hills, CA: Sage.

Schwartz, M. D., & Mattley, C. L. (1993). The Battered Woman Scale and gender identities. *Journal of Family Violence, 8*, 277-287.

Spence, J. T., Helmreich, R. L., & Stapp, J. (1974). The Personal Attributes Questionnaire. *JSAS Catalog of Selected Documents in Psychology, 4*, 43.

Spence, J. T., & Helmreich, R. L. (1978). *Masculinity and femininity*. Austin: University of Texas Press.

Walker, L. E. (1979). *The battered woman*. New York: Harper & Row.

Exhibit

The Battered Woman Scale

The statements below ask about what kind of person you think you are. Each statement is followed by several numbers you should use to describe yourself by agreeing or disagreeing with the statement. 0 = Strongly agree, 1 = Agree, 2 = Don't know, 3 = Disagree, 4 = Strongly disagree. For example:

I am artistic.   0   1   2   3   4

If you think you are very artistic you would circle 0, if you think you are somewhat artistic you would circle 1, if you don't know you would circle 2, if you are not very artistic you would circle 3, and if you are not at all artistic you would circle 4. Please use the above scale to describe yourself according to the following statements.

1. I am aggressive.	0	1	2	3	4
2. I am independent, I can take care of myself.	0	1	2	3	4
3. I am emotional.	0	1	2	3	4
4. I am dominant.	0	1	2	3	4
5. I panic under pressure.	0	1	2	3	4
6. I am easily influenced.	0	1	2	3	4
7. I am able to devote myself completely to others.	0	1	2	3	4
8. I am a gentle person.	0	1	2	3	4
9. I am not at all helpful to others.	0	1	2	3	4
10. I am competitive.	0	1	2	3	4

11. I am sophisticated or worldly.	0	1	2	3	4
12. I am kind.	0	1	2	3	4
13. I don't care what other people think of me.	0	1	2	3	4
14. My feelings are easily hurt.	0	1	2	3	4
15. I am aware of the feelings of others.	0	1	2	3	4
16. I can make decisions easily.	0	1	2	3	4
17. I never give up easily.	0	1	2	3	4
18. I cry easily.	0	1	2	3	4
19. I am very self-confident.	0	1	2	3	4
20. I think I am better than other people.	0	1	2	3	4
21. I am not very understanding of other people.	0	1	2	3	4
22. I am cold in my relations with other people.	0	1	2	3	4
23. I need security.	0	1	2	3	4
24. I go to pieces under pressure.	0	1	2	3	4

Source. This scale is reprinted with permission of the authors.

Early Sexual Experiences Checklist

Rowland S. Miller and James A. Johnson,[1] *Sam Houston State University*

Self-report biases and definitional problems have plagued studies of sexual abuse of children. Various investigators have forced respondents to label themselves as "sexually abused" (e.g., Kercher & McShane, 1984) or to make subtle distinctions among vague categories (e.g., "kissing or hugging in a sexual way"; Kilpatrick, 1986) to be counted as victims of deleterious, unwanted childhood sexual experiences. Miller, Johnson, and Johnson (1991) created the Early Sexual Experiences Checklist (ESEC) to provide an efficient, accessible procedure for detecting such experiences that avoids these methodological and conceptual problems. The ESEC merely asks respondents to check any specific, overt sexual behaviors that occurred when the respondents did not want them to. Coupled with reports of (a) the respondent's age during the events, (b) the age of the person who initiated the events, or (c) any coercion, the ESEC allows diverse operationalizations of unwanted sexual experience that span the existing literature on sexual abuse (Kendall-Tackett, Williams, & Finkelhor, 1993). The straightforward, mechanical checklist method eschews evaluative, pejorative terminology and is thus rela-

tively noninvasive. It is also simple and direct and very inexpensive, making it practical for use with large, heterogeneous populations.

Description

The ESEC contains nine items listing explicit sexual behaviors and two additional items that allow respondents either to describe a further sexual event or to pick *none of the above*. The checklist ordinarily includes additional questions—which may vary according to investigators' needs—that obtain (a) the respondent's sex, (b) the respondent's age at the time of the most bothersome event, (c) the age of the other person involved, (d) the identity (e.g., "stranger") of the other person, (e) the frequency and duration of the most bothersome experience, and (f) the presence and type of any coercion. Items using a 1 (*not at all*) to 7 (*extremely*) Likert-type format also obtain various ratings of the most bothersome event (e.g., "How much did it bother you then?" "How much does it bother you now?").

Response Mode and Timing

Respondents are ordinarily instructed to indicate with a check any sexual behaviors that were unwanted and that occurred before they were 16 years old. (This age limit may

[1]Address correspondence to Rowland S. Miller, Division of Psychology and Philosophy, Sam Houston State University, Huntsville, TX 77341-2447; email: psy_rsm@shsu.edu.

be changed for different applications of the checklist.) Thereafter, because many respondents will have encountered more than one type of sexual experience, respondents are typically asked to circle the experience that bothered them the most and to answer any further questions with regard to that specific event. The checklist and any additional questions usually fit on two sheets that take only 4 or 5 minutes to complete.

Scoring

Respondents who report unwanted sexual experiences can readily be distinguished from those who do not, and the percentage of the sample reporting each type of unwanted experience is easily calculated. A useful distinction can also be made between those who have encountered relatively severe events, such as oral-genital contact or anal or vaginal intercourse, and those who have encountered less severe events, such as the exhibition of, or fondling of, sexual organs. Miller et al. (1991) showed that such distinctions are made by lay judges, and Anderson, Miller, and Miller (1995) demonstrated that the two different types of experiences are linked to different adult outcomes.

The results obtained by the ESEC resemble those obtained by the laborious, much costlier face-to-face interviews often advocated by methodologists (Wyatt & Peters, 1986); Anderson et al. (1995) found that 9% of the women and 3% of the men in a heterogeneous college sample reported a youthful history of severe victimization by another person 5 or more years older than themselves. An additional 15% of the women and 6% of the men reported less severe experiences that were initiated by substantially older partners. Remarkably, if all such experiences are counted—regardless of the age of the partner—nearly half of the sample (48%) had some unwanted sexual experience during childhood or young adolescence.

Reliability

Using Cohen's kappa, a conservative statistic that corrects for chance agreement among diverse categories, the average 1-month test-retest reliability of the ESEC is .92 (Miller & Johnson, 1997).

Validity

Importantly, the ESEC captures reports of childhood sexual abuse that escape other paper-and-pencil techniques.

Using the ESEC, Miller and Johnson (1997) found that 56% of a college sample who reported abuse in the form of unwanted, bothersome childhood experiences with partners 5 or more years older than themselves nevertheless specifically reported that they had *not* been "sexually abused." Thus, fewer than half of those who had encountered sexual abuse actually labeled themselves as "abused." Nonetheless, their experiences were detected by the ESEC. Anderson et al. (1995) have also found that adult respondents reporting any unwanted experiences on the ESEC evidenced more depression and neuroticism, and lower self-esteem, than did those who had encountered no such experiences. Furthermore, those reporting relatively severe experiences (i.e., unwanted oral-genital contact or anal or vaginal intercourse) were more impulsive, used more alcohol and other drugs, and were less secure and more anxious and avoidant in their interpersonal relations than were those who had not had such severe experiences. The ESEC methodology thus replicated the findings of other techniques for assessing abuse, but also extended those findings by allowing comparison of the sequelae of different types of abuse experiences.

References

Anderson, J. H., Miller, R. S., & Miller, G. A. (1995, August). *Adult sequelae of unwanted childhood sexual experiences*. Paper presented at the meeting of the American Psychological Association, New York.

Kendall-Tackett, K. A., Williams, L. M., & Finkelhor, D. (1993). Impact of sexual abuse on children: A review and synthesis of recent empirical studies. *Psychological Bulletin, 113,* 164-180.

Kercher, G., & McShane, M. (1984). Prevalence of child sexual abuse victimization in an adult sample of Texas residents. *Child Abuse & Neglect, 8,* 495-501.

Kilpatrick, A. (1986). Some correlates of women's childhood sexual experiences: A retrospective study. *The Journal of Sex Research, 22,* 221-242.

Miller, R. S., & Johnson, J. A. (1997). *Abuse victims don't always feel "abused": Using checklists to detect childhood sexual abuse.* Unpublished manuscript.

Miller, R. S., Johnson, J. A., & Johnson J. K. (1991). Assessing the prevalence of unwanted childhood sexual experiences. *Journal of Psychology & Human Sexuality, 4,* 43-54.

Wyatt, G. E., & Peters, S. D. (1986). Methodological considerations in research on the prevalence of child sexual abuse. *Child Abuse & Neglect, 10,* 241-251.

Exhibit

Early Sexual Experiences Checklist

Your sex:_____ Male_____ Female

Early Sexual Experiences

When you were under the age of sixteen (16), did any of these incidents ever happen to you *when you did not want them to?*

Please check those that occurred:

_____ Another person showed his or her sex organs to you.
_____ You showed your sex organs to another person at his or her request.
_____ Someone touched or fondled your sexual organs.
_____ You touched or fondled another person's sex organs at his or her request.
_____ Another person had sexual intercourse with you.
_____ Another person performed oral sex on you.
_____ You performed oral sex on another person.
_____ Someone told you to engage in sexual activity so that he or she could watch.
_____ You engaged in anal sex with another person.
_____ Other (please specify): _____
_____ None of these events ever occurred.

If any of these incidents ever happened to you, please answer the following questions by *thinking about the one behavior that bothered you the most.*

In addition, please *circle* the behavior above that bothered you the most.

1. How old were you when it happened? _____
2. Approximately how old was the other person involved? _____
3. Who was the other person involved?
   _____ relative _____ friend or acquaintance _____ stranger
4. If the other person was a relative, how were they related to you? (i.e., cousin, father, sister, etc.) _____
5. How many times did this behavior occur?
   _____ just once _____ twice _____ 3 or 4 times _____ 5 times or more
6. Over how long a period did this behavior occur?
   _____ just once _____ a month or less _____ several months _____ a year or more
7. How much did the experience *bother* you at the time?

1	2	3	4	5	6	7
Not at all			Moderately			Extremely

8. How much does the experience *bother* you *now?*

1	2	3	4	5	6	7
Not at all			Moderately			Extremely

9. What kind of psychological pressure or physical force did the person use, if any? *Please check all that apply:*
   _____ They tried to talk you into it.
   _____ They scared you because they were bigger or stronger.
   _____ They said they would hurt you.
   _____ They bribed you.
   _____ They pushed, hit, or physically restrained you.
   _____ You were afraid they wouldn't like or love you.
   _____ They physically harmed or injured you.
   _____ They threatened you with a weapon.
   _____ They drugged you or got you drunk.
   _____ Other (please specify): _____
   _____ None of these occurred.

Source. This checklist is reprinted with permission of the authors.

What-If-Situations-Test

Alan G. Nemerofsky,[1] *Essex Community College*
Deborah T. Carran, *Johns Hopkins University*

The What-If-Situations-Test (WIST; Nemerofsky, 1986) was developed to measure performance of preschool-age children in sexual abuse prevention programs. The WIST is constructed from the learning objectives of the Children's Primary Prevention Training Program (Nemerofsky, Sanford, Baer, Cage, & Wood, 1986) and is composed of situations that require the child to determine how he or she would respond. The test items measure both the skills and concepts taught in the prevention program, as well as addressing skills and concepts thought to be essential in reducing the risk of sexual victimization (Conte, Rosen, & Saperstein, 1986; Wurtele, 1987). The WIST can be used as a pretest measure, as well as a measure of performance in sexual abuse prevention programs.

Description

The WIST consists of 29 items addressing (a) the names and location of the child's "private parts," (b) appropriate requests to touch or to examine the child's genitals by physicians, (c) requests for touching of the child's genitals by others, (d) requests for the child to touch another individual's genitals, (e) the child's right to refuse to be touched, (f) appropriate requests to touch (hug/kiss) the child by others, (g) requests to keep secrets, (h) requests to keep secrets about genital touching, (i) attempts to provide gifts/bribes/presents/incentives to touch the child's genitals or have the child touch the genitals of another person, (j) actions to be taken if the child was afraid and/or uncomfortable, and (k) the child's role in potential abuse situations.

Eleven items require the child to make a determination about the appropriateness of an action or situation (e.g., If someone touches a child's private parts, should the child tell?). Seventeen items deal with actions that a child could take in abuse situations (e.g., What would you do if someone touched your private parts?). One item addresses the names and location of the child's private parts.

Response Mode and Timing

The WIST is administered, on an individual basis, by the child's teacher. The child's responses are written down verbatim and scored by comparison to a key. The test requires approximately 15 minutes to complete.

Scoring

Scores can range from 0 to 64, with higher scores indicating greater understanding of child sexual abuse prevention skills and concepts. WIST items are differently keyed according to the nature of the item. The 11 WIST items requiring the child to make a determination about the appropriateness of an action or situation are scored 0 points for a wrong answer and 1 point for a correct response. The 17 items addressing actions a child could take in abuse situations receive 1 point for an assertive or motoric answer, 2 points for disclosure, and 3 points for both an assertive and disclosure response. The WIST item that requires the child to name and locate his or her private parts receives 0 points for a wrong answer, 1 point for a partial answer (e.g., child names only one private part), and 2 points for a complete correct answer (e.g., a girl's private parts are her vagina, buttocks, and breasts).

Reliability

In a sample of 1,044 3- to 6-year-old children (Nemerofsky, 1991), the Cronbach's alpha for the WIST was .83, indicating good reliability.

Validity

In a study using the WIST pretest mean score as the covariate, WIST posttest mean scores of children who had completed a sexual abuse prevention training program were compared to the control group of children who had not received the training. A significant difference was found between groups, with the experimental group of children scoring significantly higher on the WIST posttest following participation in the sexual abuse prevention training program than the control group of children who had not received the training (Nemerofsky, Carran, & Rosenberg, 1994).

References

Conte, J. R., Rosen, C., & Saperstein, L. (1986). An analysis of programs to prevent the sexual victimization of children. *Journal of Primary Prevention, 6,* 141-155.

Nemerofsky, A. G. (1986). *The What-If-Situations-Test.* Baltimore, MD: Author.

Nemerofsky, A. G. (1991). *Child sexual abuse prevention: Teacher and child variables affecting the learning of skills and concepts in sexual abuse prevention programs.* Unpublished doctoral dissertation, Johns Hopkins University, Baltimore, MD.

Nemerofsky, A. G., Carran, D. T., & Rosenberg, L. A. (1994). Age variation in performance among preschool age children in a sexual abuse prevention program. *Journal of Child Sexual Abuse, 3,* 85-102.

[1]Address all correspondence to Alan G. Nemerofsky, Director, MH/HS Program, Essex Community College, 7301 Rossville Boulevard, Baltimore, MD 21237; email: windance 42@aol.com

Nemerofsky, A. G., Sanford, H. J., Baer, B., Cage, M., & Wood, D. (1986). *The children's primary prevention training program*. Baltimore, MD: Author.

Wurtele, S. K. (1987). School-based sexual abuse prevention programs: A review. *Child Abuse & Neglect, 11*, 483-495.

Exhibit

What-If-Situations-Test

Child Code Number:

Circle: Pretest   Posttest

1. Tell me the names of your private parts:
2. What would you do if someone touched you in a way you did not like?
3. What would you do if someone touched you in a way that you liked?
4. What would you do if someone asked you to keep a secret?
5. What would you do if someone tried to touch your private parts?
6. What would you do if someone touched you in a way that made you feel uncomfortable?
7. Is it OK for a mom or dad to give you a hug if you want one?   (Circle)   Yes   No
8. Do you have to let anyone touch you on your private parts?   (Circle)   Yes   No
9. What would you do if someone touched your private parts?
10. What would you do if someone said they would give you a present if you would keep a secret?
11. If someone makes a child touch their private parts:
    a. Did the child do anything wrong? Yes   No
    b. Is it the child's fault?   Yes   No
    c. Should the child tell?   Yes   No
    d. Should the child ask for help?   Yes   No
12. What would you do if someone asked you to touch their private parts?
13. What would you do if someone asked you to keep a secret about touching private parts?
14. What would you do if someone said they would give you a present if you would touch their private parts?
15. What would you do if someone made you touch their private parts?
16. If someone touches a child's private parts:
    a. Did the child do anything wrong? Yes   No
    b. Is it the child's fault?   Yes   No
    c. Should the child tell someone?   Yes   No
    d. Should the child ask for help?   Yes   No
17. Would it be OK for your doctor to look at your private parts if you were hurt there?   Yes   No
18. What would you do if you were scared or confused or felt uncomfortable?
19. What would you say if someone asked you to touch their private parts?
20. What should a child do if someone touched his/her private parts and promised not to do it again?
21. If someone touched your private parts:
    a. What would you say?
    b. What would you do?
    c. Who would you tell?

Unwanted Childhood Sexual Experiences Questionnaire

Michael R. Stevenson,[1] *Ball State University*

The Unwanted Childhood Sexual Experiences Questionnaire can be used to document the age and extent of respondents' unwanted childhood sexual experiences with adults. Instructions intentionally refer to unwanted childhood sexual experiences rather than abusive sexual experiences or experiences of sexual victimization in an attempt to avoid unintended bias in reporting. It defines an adult as someone who is at least 5 years older than the respondent.

Description

Each of the 13 items refers to a different set of behaviors that can be categorized as minimal contact (Items 1-3), moderate contact (Items 4-8), or maximal contact (Items 9-13). Items were drawn from a larger questionnaire designed by Finkelhor (1979) and have been used in other studies (e.g., Fromuth, 1986; Stevenson & Gajarsky, 1992).

Response Mode and Timing

Respondents simply indicate in the space provided the age or ages at which any of the unwanted sexual behaviors occurred. The scale can be completed in less than 5 minutes.

Scoring

The questionnaire allows for the reporting of the frequency with which each of the behaviors occur in the sample, and the ages at which the behaviors occurred.

[1]Address correspondence to Michael R. Stevenson, Department of Psychological Science, Ball State University, Muncie, IN 47306; email: 00mrstevenso@bsuvc.bsu.edu.

Reliability

The intention of this questionnaire is to document whether specific unwanted behaviors have occurred, and the items are not intended to constitute a scale. Reliability has not been assessed directly.

Validity

Using this measure, Stevenson and Gajarsky's (1992) sample of college students reported frequencies of unwanted sexual experiences that were consistent with earlier reports (e.g., Finkelhor, 1979, 1984; Groth, 1979). Although the percentage of men reporting unwanted sexual experiences was somewhat higher than some previous estimates, it was quite consistent with others (e.g., Popen & Segal, 1988).

References

Finkelhor, D. (1979). *Sexually victimized children.* New York: Free Press.

Finkelhor, D. (1984). *Child sexual abuse: New theory and research.* New York: Free Press.

Fromuth, M. E. (1986). The relationship of childhood sexual abuse with later psychological and sexual adjustment in a sample of college women. *Child Abuse & Neglect, 10,* 5-15.

Groth, N. A. (1979). Sexual trauma in the life histories of rapists and child molesters. *Victimology: An International Journal, 4*(1), 10-16.

Popen, P. J., & Segal, H. J. (1988). The influence of sex and sex-role orientation on sexual coercion. *Sex Roles, 19,* 689-701.

Stevenson, M. R., & Gajarsky, W. M. (1992). Unwanted childhood sexual experiences relate to later revictimization and male perpetration. *Journal of Psychology & Human Sexuality, 4,* 57-70.

Exhibit

Unwanted Childhood Sexual Experiences Questionnaire

It is now generally realized that most people have sexual experiences as children and while growing up. By "sexual" it is meant any behavior or event that might seem "sexual" to you. Please try to remember the unwanted, that is, sexual experiences that were forced on you or done against your will by an adult (someone at least five or more years older than you), while growing up. Indicate if you had any of the following experiences *before* the age of 16.

1. An invitation or request to do something sexual.   Age(s) _____
2. Kissing and hugging in a sexual way.   Age(s) _____
3. An adult showing his/her sex organs to you.   Age(s) _____

 4. You showing your sex organs to an adult.   Age(s) _____
 5. An adult fondling you in a sexual way.   Age(s) _____
 6. You fondling an adult in a sexual way.   Age(s) _____
 7. An adult touching your sex organs.   Age(s) _____
 8. You touching an adult person's sex organs.   Age(s) _____
 9. An adult orally touching your sex organs.   Age(s) _____
10. You orally touching an adult person's sex organs.   Age(s) _____
11. Intercourse, but without attempting penetration of the vagina.   Age(s) _____
12. Intercourse (penile-vaginal penetration).   Age(s) _____
13. Anal intercourse (penile-anal penetration).   Age(s) _____

Sexual History and Adjustment Questionnaire

Robin J. Lewis and Louis H. Janda,[1] *Old Dominion University*

This measure was developed to assess participants' retrospective reports of (a) frequency of sleeping in the bed with parents between the ages of 0-5 and 6-11 years; (b) frequency of seeing parents, as well as others, naked between 0-5 years and 6-11 years; (c) parental attitudes toward sexuality; (d) participants' level of comfort in discussing sexuality with parents; and (e) perceptions of parental discomfort regarding sexuality. Information on current adjustment and sexual behavior was also obtained.

Description

This instrument would be appropriate for populations of older adolescents and adults. Items 1-10 assess retrospective reports of childhood experiences with nudity and sleeping in the parental bed. Items 11-19 assess the participant's perceptions of parental attitudes toward sex and discussion of sexuality, as well as how often there was demonstration of physical affection in the family. Items 20-29 assess the participant's current sexual behavior and attitudes toward himself or herself. Item 30 addresses feelings of discomfort about the physical contact and affection displayed in one's family.

[1]Address correspondence to Robin J. Lewis, Department of Psychology, Old Dominion University, Norfolk, VA 23529-0267; email: rjl100f@viper.mgb.odu.edu.

Response Mode, Timing, and Scoring

Respondents are asked to indicate their response to each item by circling the number that best reflects their answer to a question using a 5-point Likert-type scale. The anchors of the scale vary by section. Investigators may be interested in individual responses, such as frequency of seeing one particular parent naked, and may wish to sum responses across ages (e.g., index for maternal nudity would be sum of response for nudity at ages 0-5 plus nudity at ages 6-11). Or investigators may wish to sum for a total parental nudity index (cf. Lewis & Janda, 1988) by summing all responses for mother and father across ages.

A similar approach is used with the items about parental attitudes. Investigators may combine items for maternal attitudes (e.g., comfort discussing sexual matters; positive vs. negative attitude), as well as similar items for paternal attitudes. Alternatively, a global measure of attitudes may be generated. In our previous research (Lewis & Janda, 1988), however, we found some differences in maternal and paternal attitudes. Thus, investigators are urged to be cautious in this regard.

In our previous research (Lewis & Janda, 1988), we examined the sexual adjustment items separately. Interested investigators might wish to combine items to generate a more global measure of adjustment.

Reliability

A number of subscales for this measure can be constructed, depending on researchers' interests. Internal consistency was demonstrated for the following subscales using coefficient alpha:

1. Parental Nudity subscale (sum Items 1, 2, 3, 4): .74
2. Overall Nudity subscale (sum Items 1-8): .77
3. Parental Bed subscale (sum Items 9-10): .80
4. Maternal Attitudes subscale (sum Items 11, 13, 15): .77
5. Paternal Attitudes subscale (sum Items 12, 14, 16): .78
6. Overall Attitudes subscale (sum Items 11-16): .78

No test-retest reliability has been obtained for this measure.

Validity

No formal validation of this measure has been reported. It would be appropriate to demonstrate validity by correlating subscales of this measure with established measures of sexual adjustment and perhaps global attitudes about one's family. The items on this measure clearly demonstrate face validity. It would also be helpful to examine the degree to which a socially desirable response set might influence responses. To that end, examination of the correlation between these items and a measure of social desirability (e.g., Reynolds, 1982) would provide useful information.

References

Lewis, R. J., & Janda, L. H. (1988). The relationship between adult sexual adjustment and childhood experiences regarding exposure to nudity, sleeping in the parental bed, and parental attitudes toward sexuality. *Archives of Sexual Behavior, 17,* 349-362.

Reynolds, W. M. (1982). Development of reliable and valid short forms of the Marlowe-Crowne Social Desirability Scale. *Journal of Clinical Psychology, 38,* 119-125.

Exhibit

Sexual History and Adjustment Questionnaire

Retrospective Reports of Childhood Experiences With Nudity and Sleeping in the Parental Bed

Please use the following scale for Questions 1-10:

1	2	3	4	5
Almost never	Rarely	Sometimes	Often	Very often

1. When you were between the ages of 0-5, how often do you remember seeing your mother naked?
2. When you were between the ages of 6-11, how often do you remember seeing your mother naked?
3. When you were between the ages of 0-5, how often do you remember seeing your father naked?
4. When you were between the ages of 6-11, how often do you remember seeing your father naked?
5. When you were between the ages of 0-5, how often do you remember seeing your same-sex siblings or friends naked?
6. When you were between the ages of 6-11, how often do you remember seeing your same-sex siblings or friends naked?
7. When you were between the ages of 0-5, how often do you remember seeing your opposite-sex siblings or friends naked?
8. When you were between the ages of 6-11, how often do you remember seeing your opposite-sex siblings or friends naked?
9. When you were between the ages of 0-5, how often do you remember sleeping in the same bed as your parents?
10. When you were between the ages of 6-11, how often do you remember sleeping in the same bed as your parents?

Parental Attitudes Items

Please use the following scale for Questions 11-14:

1	2	3	4	5
Extreme discomfort	Moderate discomfort	neither comfort nor discomfort	moderate comfort	extreme comfort

11. In general, over the course of your childhood, please rate the degree of comfort you felt in talking about sexual matters with your mother:
12. In general, over the course of your childhood, please rate the degree of comfort you felt in talking about sexual matters with your father:
13. While you were growing up, please rate the degree of comfort you think your mother felt when talking about sexuality:

14. While you were growing up, please rate the degree of comfort you think your father felt when talking about sexuality:

15. How would you characterize your mother's attitude toward sexuality when you were growing up?

1	2	3	4	5
extremely negative	moderately negative	neither positive nor negative	moderately positive	extremely positive

16. How would you characterize your father's attitude toward sexuality when you were growing up?

1	2	3	4	5
extremely negative	moderately negative	neither positive nor negative	moderately positive	extremely positive

17. Overall, how well do you feel that your upbringing prepared you to deal with issues of sexuality and sexual relationships?

1	2	3	4	5
not at all	poorly	adequately	pretty well	very well

18. How often do you remember issues of sexuality being discussed in your home when you were growing up?

1	2	3	4	5
almost never	rarely	sometimes	often	very ofen

19. In general, how often was physical contact/affection displayed in your family?

1	2	3	4	5
almost never	rarely	sometimes	often	very often

Sexual Adjustment Items

Please use the following scale for Questions 20-29:

1	2	3	4	5
strongly disagree	somewhat disagree	neither agree nor disagree	somewhat agree	strongly agree

20. I feel good about myself.
21. I experience guilt or anxiety when it comes to my sex life.
22. I am happy with my sex life.
23. I am heterosexual.
24. I have sex more often than most people of my age and situation (e.g., married versus single).
25. I tend to engage in casual sexual relationships.
26. I have experienced sexual problems.
27. I would like my sex life to be more active than it is.
28. I am very consistent in making certain that birth control is a part of my sexual encounters.
29. I am knowledgeable about sex.
30. Regarding physical contact and affection in your family how often do you remember having feelings of discomfort about this contact?

1	2	3	4	5
Almost never	Rarely	Sometimes	Often	Very often

Attitudes Toward Sexuality Scale

Terri D. Fisher,[1] *Ohio State University at Mansfield*
Richard G. Hall, *Mansfield, Ohio*

The Attitudes Toward Sexuality Scale (ATSS) was developed to allow the comparison of the sexual attitudes of adolescents between the ages of 12 and 20 and their parents. An instrument was needed that was brief, simplistic, and nonoffensive to facilitate its use with younger adolescents and yet still be valid for adults. To this end, items from calderwood's (1971) Checklist of Attitudes Toward Human Sexuality were modified and an objective scoring system was added.

Description

The ATSS consists of 13 statements related to topics such as nudity, abortion, contraception, premarital sex, pornography, prostitution, homosexuality, and sexually transmitted diseases. The 5-point Likert-type response format ranges from *strongly disagree* to *strongly agree*. The original scale contained 14 items, but one of the items contributed so little to the total score variance that it was dropped from the scale. This measure is appropriate for adolescents aged 12 and older as well as adults.

Response Mode and Timing

Respondents simply indicate the degree of their agreement or disagreement with the statement by circling the number on the response scale that most closely reflects their reaction. The ATSS requires no more than 5 minutes to complete.

Scoring

Items 1, 4, 5, 7, 8, 11, and 13 are reverse scored by assigning a score of 1 if 5 was marked, a score of 2 if 4 was marked, and so forth. Then the number of points is totaled. Scores can range from 13 to 65 with lower scores indicating greater conservatism about sexual matters and higher scores indicating greater permissiveness about sexual matters.

Reliability

For a sample of 35 early adolescents (ages 12-14), the Cronbach alpha coefficient was .76. Among 47 middle

adolescents (ages 15-17), the alpha was .65, and for a group of 59 late adolescents (18-20 years old), the alpha was .80. The alpha for the total group of adolescents was .75. Among 141 parents (ages 31-66), the alpha was .84. The test-retest reliability coefficient, using an independent sample of 22 persons ages 18 to 28 over a 1-month time period, was .90.

Validity

In a sample of college students between the ages of 18 and 28, the ATSS correlated highly with the Heterosexual Relations (Liberalism) scale of the Sex Knowledge and Attitude Test (SKAT; Lief & Reed, 1972), $r(42) = .83$. The ATSS was also correlated with the Abortion scale, $r(42) = .70$, the Autoeroticism scale $r(42) = .54$, and the Sexual Myths scale, $r(42) = .59$.

In a study of adolescents and their parents, age was negatively correlated with the ATSS score, $r(280) = -.18$, although for the young and middle adolescents combined, age was positively related to the ATSS score, $r(82) = .37$. Amount of education was found to be significantly correlated with the total scale score for the adult subjects, $r(139) = .20$. Religiosity, as measured by church attendance, was significantly correlated to ATSS scores for the middle adolescents, $r(45) = -.32$; the older adolescents, $r(57) = -.44$; and the adults, $r(139) = -.41$, such that people who regularly attended church tended to be more conservative in their sexual attitudes. As has been found on other measures of sexual attitudes, males indicated more permissive sexual attitudes than females, $F(1, 274) = 4.1$.

References

calderwood, d. (1971). *About your sexuality*. Boston: Beacon.

Fisher, T. D. (1986). An exploratory study of parent-child communication about sex and the sexual attitudes of early, middle, and late adolescents. *Journal of Genetic Psychology, 147,* 543-557.

Fisher, T. D. (1987). Family communication and the behavior and attitudes of college students. *Journal of Youth and Adolescence, 16,* 481-495.

Fisher, T. D., & Hall, R. G. (1988). A scale for the comparison of the sexual attitudes of adolescents and their parents. *The Journal of Sex Research, 24,* 90-100.

Lief, H. I., & Reed, D. M. (1972). *Sex Knowledge and Attitude Test.* Philadelphia: University of Pennsylvania, Center for the Study of Sex Education in Medicine.

[1]Address correspondence to Terri D. Fisher, Ohio State University at Mansfield, 1680 University Drive, Mansfield, OH 44906; email: fisher.16@osu.edu.

Exhibit

Attitudes Toward Sexuality Scale

For each of the following statements, please circle the response that best reflects your reaction to that statement.

1	2	3	4	5
strongly disagree	somewhat disagree	neutral	somewhat agree	strongly agree

1. Nudist camps should be made completely illegal.

| | 1 | 2 | 3 | 4 | 5 |

2. Abortion should be made available whenever a woman feels it would be the best decision.[a]
3. Information and advice about contraception (birth control) should be given to any individual who intends to have intercourse.
4. Parents should be informed if their children under the age of eighteen have visited a clinic to obtain a contraceptive device.
5. Our government should try harder to prevent the distribution of pornography.
6. Prostitution should be legalized.
7. Petting (a stimulating caress of any or all parts of the body) is immoral behavior unless the couple is married.
8. Premarital sexual intercourse for young people is unacceptable to me.
9. Sexual intercourse for unmarried young people is acceptable without affection existing if both partners agree.
10. Homosexual behavior is an acceptable variation in sexual preference.
11. A person who catches a sexually transmitted (venereal) disease is probably getting exactly what he/she deserves.
12. A person's sexual behavior is his/her own business, and nobody should make value judgments about it.
13. Sexual intercourse should only occur between two people who are married to each other.

Source. This scale was originally published in "A Scale for the Comparison of the Sexual Attitudes of Adolescents and Their Parents," by T. D. Fisher and R. G. Hall, 1988, *The Journal of Sex Research, 24,* 90-100. Reprinted with permission.

a. The 5-point scale is repeated after each item.

The Sexual Knowledge and Attitude Test for Adolescents

William Fullard[1] and Dennis A. Johnston, *Temple University*
Harold I. Lief, *University of Pennsylvania*

The Sexual Knowledge and Attitude Test for Adolescents (SKAT-A) was developed to assess knowledge and attitudes about sexuality, the relationships between them, and to ex-

[1]Address correspondence to William Fullard, Department of Psychological Studies in Education, Ritter Annex 207, Temple University (004-00), Philadelphia, PA 19122; email: wfullard@vm.temple.edu.

amine and correlate demographic characteristics and sexual behaviors in adolescents and young adults. The scale described here represents a significant revision from the initial version described in Lief, Fullard, and Devlin (1990). The SKAT-A was based on Lief and Reed's (1972) Sex Knowledge and Attitude Test (SKAT). The original SKAT (see page 32) was developed primarily to assess sexual information among health professionals. The need for an instrument appropriate for adolescents and young adults continues. Thus, the current SKAT-A addresses this need.

Description

The original (1990) version provided information about demographics, attitudes, knowledge, and behavior relating to sexuality. The Demographics section was designed to collect information on socioeconomic status (SES), residence, school experience, and so forth. The Attitude section consisted of 43 statements using a 5-point, Likert-type format (1 = *strongly agree, 5 = strongly disagree*). The Knowledge section contained 61 items with the format varying between true/false (40 items) and multiple-choice items (21 items). An extensive Behavior Inventory was included to attempt to gather data on a variety of sexual behaviors, for previously reported normative information on behavior that had not been related specifically to knowledge and attitude factors.

The current version of the Demographics section requests basic information on age, school experience, and SES. It can be modified to meet the needs of individual investigators.

The Attitude section contains 40 items designed to address the content areas of the original SKAT-A, again using a 5-point, Likert-type response format. These items have been reworded based on information acquired from previous administrations of the test. In an attempt to reduce response bias, 11 items are reverse scored. The current Attitude scale contains five specific content subscales: masturbation (8 items), homosexuality (4 items), pornography (4 items), premarital sex (6 items), and abortion (4 items). High scores on the Attitude scale indicate a more liberal attitude.

The Knowledge section reflects considerable revision based on psychometric analyses using data from the earlier version. It consists of 40 items employing a true/false/not sure format. Twenty-four items are reverse scored. The multiple-choice format was eliminated to improve the psychometric integrity of the scale. In addition, item analyses supported the reduction of the scale to 40 items. Information covers topics including pregnancy, contraception, rape, masturbation, and sex education.

The Behavior Inventory was constructed to serve a variety of investigative purposes. Questions include items examining onset of sexual activity, number of partners, and specific behaviors (dating, contraceptive use, sexual practices, etc.). As an inventory, this instrument can be modified to meet the needs of individual researchers.

Over 1,000 individuals have taken the SKAT-A in its current version. However, the psychometrics presented here are derived from a subsample consisting of 385 undergraduate students from two universities in the Northeast. Two hundred eighty four (74%) were female. The mean age was 19.6 years (range 17 to 22 years). Working-through upper-middle-class individuals were represented, typical of the students at the respective universities. The sample was 73% Caucasian, 18% Black, and the remainder Asian or Hispanic individuals. This sample has one obvious bias,

namely, the lack of an adolescent group. Recognizing this, we have administered the SKAT-A to 700 high school adolescents.

Response Mode and Timing

The SKAT-A is primarily a forced-choice, paper-and-pencil instrument. As such, participants are required to respond directly to options provided on the instrument. There are, however, instances within the Behavior Inventory requiring participants to supply responses (e.g., age at first intercourse). The administration of the SKAT-A requires about 30 minutes. Administration time includes all four sections (Demographics, Attitude, Knowledge, and Behavior).

Scoring

The Attitude section for the SKAT-A uses a 5-point Likert-type scale. Scores are obtained by adding the responses to each of the 40 items. Of the 40 items, 11 items are reversed in an attempt to offset response bias. The Knowledge section is scored by adding the total number correct on the scale. A trichotomized (true/false/not sure) response format is used. Twenty-four items are reverse scored. Correct responses earn 1 point. Incorrect or *not sure* responses earn no points. Although a separate scoring key is not available currently, a machine-scorable version is under development.

Reliability and Validity

Internal consistency estimates were computed for each of the five subscales within the Attitude scale. They were masturbation, .87; homosexuality, .83; pornography, .73; premarital sex, .77; and abortion, .73. The full 40-item alpha coefficient was .89. Temporal stability was calculated over a 2-week period on 50 participants. A test-retest coefficient of .89 was obtained for the full-scale Attitude scores. Thus, the Attitude scale demonstrates adequate reliability.

Internal consistency for the Knowledge scale was .74. Although acceptable, this coefficient may be depressed as a result of the content heterogeneity within the scale. Test-retest reliability for the Knowledge scale is .80 over a 2-week period.

Evidence for the construct validity of the Attitude and Knowledge scales was obtained using correlational analyses with items from these scales and selected behavior items. Each of the five subscales within the Attitude scale was shown to be correlated with other SKAT-A responses in such a way that supports the meaning and interpretation of the scales. For example, liberal attitudes about masturbation are associated with greater frequency of masturbatory behavior ($r = .38$). Liberal attitudes toward homosexuality were significantly related to sexual knowledge ($r = .32$), such that the more knowledge about sexuality, the more liberal the attitude. Individuals who hold more liberal attitudes toward premarital sex are more likely to have engaged in sexual intercourse ($r = .22$). In contrast, conservative attitudes toward abortion are associated with greater church attendance ($r = -.24$) and religious importance ($r = -.28$). A more liberal attitude toward pornography predicts both viewing of pornographic material ($r = .31$) and the reading of pornographic material ($r = .32$). A one-item self-rating of sexual attitudes (1 = *very conservative* to 10 = *very liberal*) was correlated with full-scale Attitude scores ($r = .49$) supporting the construct validity of the scale. All correlations were significant at the .01 level.

Evidence for the validity of the Knowledge scale was demonstrated through the correlation of Knowledge scale scores and logically related items from the Attitude scale and Behavior Inventory. Sexual knowledge and sexual attitude scores were related ($r = .44$). More knowledgeable individuals were more likely to hold liberal attitudes. Sexual behaviors are also related to sexual knowledge such that more knowledgeable individuals are more likely to have engaged in sexual intercourse ($r = .13$). An additional finding was that more knowledgeable individuals used contraception more frequently ($r = .19$). All correlations are significant at the .01 level. The strength of these correlations is affected by the fact that the decision to engage in sexual activity is a multifaceted construct difficult to capture in univariate analyses.

The SKAT-A represents our attempt to provide a well-standardized instrument to assess some important aspects of sexuality. It should prove useful in both teaching and research settings. The instrument is not meant to be used for individual diagnostics but should provide general information about group performance. The addition of the adolescent group described earlier will increase the age range of the instrument as well as provide an important database for this group. Information about obtaining the SKAT-A and scoring procedures may be secured from the authors.

References

Lief, H. I., Fullard, W., & Devlin, S. J. (1990). A new measure of adolescent sexuality: SKAT-A. *Journal of Sex Education and Therapy, 16,* 79-91.

Lief, H. I., & Reed, D. M. (1972). *Sex Knowledge and Attitude Test.* Philadelphia: University of Pennsylvania, Center for the Study of Sex Education in Medicine.

Mathtech Questionnaires:
Sexuality Questionnaires for Adolescents

Douglas Kirby,[1] *ETR Associates*

The questionnaires have two purposes: first, to measure the most important knowledge areas, attitudes, values, skills, and behaviors that either facilitate a positive and fulfilling sexuality or reduce unintended pregnancy among adolescents; and second, to measure important possible outcomes of sexuality education programs.

The Centers for Disease Control funded Mathtech, a private research firm, to develop methods of evaluating sexuality education programs. Mathtech reviewed existing questionnaires for adolescents and determined that it was necessary to develop new questionnaires. With the help of about 20 professionals in the field of adolescent sexuality and pregnancy, Mathtech identified more than 100 possible outcomes of sexuality education programs and then had

100 professionals rate (anonymously) each of those outcomes according to its importance in reducing unintended pregnancy and facilitating a positive and fulfilling sexuality. Mathtech then calculated the mean ratings of those outcomes and developed questionnaires to measure many of the most important outcomes. The questionnaires that measure these important outcomes include the Knowledge Test, the Attitude and Value Inventory, and the Behavior Inventory.

KNOWLEDGE TEST

Description

The Knowledge Test is a 34-item multiple-choice test. It includes questions in the following areas: adolescent physical development, adolescent relationships, adolescent sexual activity, adolescent pregnancy, adolescent marriage, the

[1]Address correspondence to Douglas Kirby, ETR Associates, P.O. Box 1830, Santa Cruz, CA 95061-1830.

probability of pregnancy, birth control, and sexually transmitted disease. It has been used successfully with both junior and senior high school students.

To develop the questionnaires, we completed the following steps: (a) generated between 5 and 20 items in each of the content areas that the 100 professionals indicated as important; (b) pretested the questionnaire with small groups of adolescents and adults, and clarified many items; (c) administered the questionnaire to 729 adolescents, analyzed their answers, removed items that were too easy or too difficult, and also removed items not positively related to the overall test score; (d) removed questions from content domains that had too many questions; and (e) made numerous refinements following subsequent administrations of the questionnaires and reviews by other professionals.

Response Mode and Timing

Respondents circle the single best answer to each question. Bright students commonly take about 15 to 20 minutes; slower students may take as long as 45 minutes to complete the questionnaire.

Scoring

The answers to the test are included at the end of the test (see the exhibit). To obtain the percentage correct, count the number of correct answers and divide by 34. No special provisions are made for students who do not answer questions.

Reliability

The test was administered to 58 adolescents on one occasion, and then again 2 weeks later. The test-retest reliability coefficient was 89.

Validity

Older students obtained higher scores than younger students, and students with overall higher grade point averages had higher scores than students with lower grade point averages. Content validity was determined by experts who selected both the domains and the items for the domains.

ATTITUDE AND VALUE INVENTORY

Description

The Attitude and Value Inventory includes 14 different scales, each consisting of five, 5-point Likert-type items. The responses were *strongly disagree, disagree, neutral, agree,* and *strongly agree.* The scales are identified in Table 1.

To develop the questionnaires, we completed the following steps: (a) generated 5 to 10 items for each of the psychological outcomes rated important by the 100 experts; (b) had the items reviewed by small groups of both adults and adolescents, who made suggestions for changes; (c) had two psychologists trained in questionnaire design and scale construction examine each item for unidimensionality and clarity; and (d) had more than 200 adolescents complete the questionnaire, removing those items that had

Table 1 Reliability Coefficients for the Scales in the Attitude and Value Inventory

Cronbach's alpha	Scale
.89	Clarity of long-term goals
.73	Clarity of personal sexual values
.81	Understanding of emotional needs
.78	Understanding of personal social behavior
.80	Understanding of personal sexual response
.66	Attitude toward gender roles
.75	Attitude toward sexuality in life
.72	Attitude toward the importance of birth control
.94	Attitude toward premarital sex
.58	Attitude toward the use of force and pressure in sexual activity
.70	Recognition of the importance of the family
.73	Self-esteem
.85	Satisfaction with personal sexuality
.81	Satisfaction with social relationships

a correlation coefficient greater than .30 with the Crowne and Marlowe (1964) Social Desirability Scale, which had the lowest scale loadings on each scale and which had mean scores near the minimum or maximum possible score.

Response Mode and Timing

Respondents should circle the number indicating their agreement or disagreement with each item. Bright adolescents complete the questionnaire in about 10 minutes; slower students may take a half hour.

Scoring

Following the Attitude and Value Inventory are all the scales, with the items grouped by scale. In front of each item is a plus sign or a minus sign, indicating whether the item should be positively scored or reverse scored. The mean score for each scale should be determined by adding the responses and dividing by 5. Higher scores represent more favorable attitudes.

Reliability

Reliability was determined by administering the questionnaire to 990 students and calculating Cronbach's alpha. These are included in Table 1.

BEHAVIOR INVENTORY

Description

Many behaviors have at least three important components or aspects to them: the skill with which the behavior is completed, the comfort experienced during that behavior, and the frequency of that behavior. The Behavior Inventory measures these three aspects of several kinds of behavior. The actual measures are identified in Tables 2 and 3.

The questions measuring skills use 5-point scales with answers ranging from *almost always* to *almost never;* those

Table 2 Reliability Coefficients for the Scales in the Behavior Inventory

Test-retest r[a]	n	Alpha[b]	n	Scale
.84	39	.58	541	Social decision-making skills
.65	36	.61	464	Sexual decision-making skills
.57	41	.75	529	Communication skills
.68	32	.62	409	Assertiveness skills
.88	17	.58	243	Birth control assertiveness skills
.69	40	.81	517	Comfort engaging in social activities
.66	36	.66	461	Comfort talking with friends, girl/boyfriend, and parents about sex
.40	33	.63	133	Comfort talking with friends, girl/boyfriend, and parents about birth control
.62	39	.73	156	Comfort talking with parents about sex and birth control
.44	41	NA[c]	NA	Comfort expressing concern and caring
.68	35	.68	455	Comfort being sexually assertive (saying no)
.70	37	NA	NA	Comfort having current sex life, whatever it may be
.38	14	.86	449	Comfort getting and using birth control

a. The test-retest coefficient is the correlation coefficient based on two administrations of the same questionnaire 2 weeks apart.

b. Alpha is Cronbach's alpha based on all the intercorrelations within each scale.

c. NA means not applicable because alpha requires two or more items, and these scales had only one item.

Table 3 Test-Retest Reliability Coefficients for the Behavior Questions in the Behavior Inventory

r[a]	Question
1.00	Q43: Ever had sexual intercourse
.78	Q44: Had intercourse last month
.88	Q45: Frequency of intercourse last month
.97	Q46: Frequency of intercourse last month with no birth control
.89	Q47: Frequency of intercourse last month using diaphragm, withdrawal, rhythm, or foam (without condoms)
.97	Q48: Frequency of intercourse last month using pill, condoms, or IUD
.80	Q49: Frequency of conversations with parents about sex last month
.81	Q50: Frequency of conversations with friends about sex last month
.83	Q51: Frequency of conversations with boy/girlfriend about sex last month
.71	Q52: Frequency of conversations with parents about birth control last month
.69	Q53: Frequency of conversations with friends about birth control last month
.75	Q54: Frequency of conversations with boy/girlfriend about birth control last month

Note. N = 41.

a. The measure of reliability is the correlation coefficient between the two administrations of the questionnaire given 2 weeks apart.

measuring comfort use 4-point scales ranging from *comfortable* to *very uncomfortable;* those measuring sexual activity, use of birth control, and frequency of communication ask how many times during the previous month the respondent engaged in the specified activity.

It is important to realize that the questions measuring skill do not try to assess skill in the classroom but, instead, measure the frequency with which respondents actually use important skills in everyday life.

The panel of 100 experts rated most highly most of the skills, areas of comfort, and behaviors for which we developed measures. We tried many different ways of measuring skills, and after a variety of attempts and pretests with small groups of adolescents, we settled on the current approach in which we identified key behaviors in various skills and simply asked what proportion of the time respondents engage in those behaviors.

The scales measuring comfort and behaviors flowed directly from the outcomes specified by the experts. We conducted minitests with both adults and adolescents to determine for how many months they could accurately measure their communication and sexual behavior. Nearly all adolescents could remember their behavior for the previous month.

The entire inventory was reviewed by psychologists, who examined each item for clarity, unidimensionality, and comprehensibility. More than 100 adolescents completed the questionnaire; their responses indicated that most data were reliable.

Because of the great sensitivity of these questions, the researcher should (a) get appropriate approval to administer the questionnaire, (b) emphasize to the students that completing the questionnaire is voluntary, and (c) take every reasonable measure to assure that the answers remain absolutely anonymous. Remember, if students learn that some particular girl (or boy) has experienced (or not experienced) sex, that person's reputation can be greatly damaged.

Response Mode and Timing

Respondents should circle the number indicating their agreement or disagreement with each item. The questionnaire takes adolescents between 20 and 45 minutes to complete. Adolescents who are brighter or not sexually active complete it more quickly.

Scoring

Most of the questions measuring skills or comfort should be combined into scales. Following the inventory are the items grouped into scales. In front of each item measuring a skill or area of comfort is a plus sign or a minus sign, indicating whether the item should be positively scored or reverse scored. The mean score for these scales should be determined by adding the responses and dividing by the number of items. Higher scores represent more favorable attitudes.

The questions measuring the existence and frequency of sexual behavior should not be combined into scales. Moreover, higher scores do not commonly represent more favorable behaviors.

Reliability

For all items, test-retest reliability was determined by administering the questionnaire twice, 2 weeks apart. However, because some students were not sexually active, the sample sizes are unreasonably low for some items. Moreover, the test-retest reliability coefficients are artificially low for some items because the sexual activities of teenagers change from one 2-week period to the next. Consequently, Cronbach's alpha is also given for those scales having two or more items. All of these coefficients are presented in Tables 2 and 3.

Validity

The most sensitive of the behavior questions had other questions that should have been consistent. For example, 10 different questions provide information about whether the respondent had had sex. Specifically written computer programs indicated that more than 95% of the questionnaires had answers that were consistent.

Other Information

Appropriate citation of the scales (Kirby, 1984) is requested.

References

Crowne, D. P., & Marlowe, D. (1964). *The approval motive: Studies in evaluative dependence.* New York: Wiley.

Kirby, D. (1984). *Sexuality education: An evaluation of programs and their effects.* Santa Cruz, CA: Network.

Exhibit

Knowledge Test

We are trying to find out if this program is successful. You can help us by completing this questionnaire.

To keep your answers confidential and private, do *not* put your name anywhere on this questionnaire. Please use a regular pen or pencil so that all questionnaires will look about the same and no one will know which is yours.

Because this study is important, your answers are also important. Please answer each question carefully.
Thank you for your help.

Name of school or organization where course was taken: _____

Teacher's name: _____

Your birth date: Month _____   Day _____

Your sex (Check one): Male _____   Female _____

Your grade level in school (Check one): 9 _____   10 _____   11 _____   12 _____

Please circle the one best answer to each of the questions below.

1. By the time teenagers graduate from high schools in the United States:
    a. only a few have had sex (sexual intercourse).
    b. about half have had sex.
    c. about 80% have had sex.
2. During their menstrual periods, girls:
    a. are too weak to participate in sports or exercise.
    b. have a normal, monthly release of blood from the uterus.
    c. cannot possibly become pregnant.
    d. should not shower or bathe.
    e. all of the above.

3. It is harmful for a woman to have sex (sexual intercourse) when she:
    a. is pregnant.
    b. is menstruating.
    c. has a cold.
    d. has a sexual partner with syphilis.
    e. none of the above.

4. Some contraceptives:
    a. can be obtained only with a doctor's prescription.
    b. are available at family planning clinics.
    c. can be bought over the counter at drug stores.
    d. can be obtained by people under 18 without their parents' permission.
    e. all of the above.

5. If 10 couples have sexual intercourse regularly without using any kind of birth control, the number of couples who become pregnant by the end of 1 year is about:
    a. one.
    b. three.
    c. six
    d. nine.
    e. none of the above.

6. When unmarried teenage girls learn they are pregnant, the largest group of them decide:
    a. to have an abortion.
    b. to put the child up for adoption.
    c. to raise the child at home.
    d. to marry and raise the child with the husband.
    e. none of the above.

7. People having sexual intercourse can best prevent getting a sexually transmitted disease (VD or STD) by using:
    a. condoms (rubbers).
    b. contraceptive foam.
    c. the pill.
    d. withdrawal (pulling out).

8. When boys go through puberty:
    a. they lose their "baby fat" and become slimmer.
    b. their penises become larger.
    c. they produce sperm.
    d. their voices become lower.
    e. all of the above.

9. Married teenagers:
    a. have the same social lives as their unmarried friends.
    b. avoid pressure from friends and family.
    c. still fit in easily with their old friends.
    d. usually support themselves without help from their parents.
    e. none of the above.

10. If a couple has sexual intercourse and uses no birth control, the woman might get pregnant:
    a. anytime during the month.
    b. only 1 week before menstruation begins.
    c. only during menstruation.
    d. only 1 week after menstruation begins.
    e. only 2 weeks after menstruation begins.

11. The method of birth control that is *least* effective is:
    a. a condom with foam.
    b. the diaphragm with spermicidal jelly.
    c. withdrawal (pulling out).
    d. the pill.
    e. abstinence (not having intercourse).

12. It is possible for a woman to become pregnant:
    a. the first time she has sex (sexual intercourse).
    b. if she has sexual intercourse during her menstrual period.
    c. if she has sexual intercourse standing up.
    d. if sperm get near the opening of the vagina, even though the man's penis does not enter her body.
    e. all of the above.

13. Physically:
     a. girls usually mature earlier than boys.
     b. most boys mature earlier than most girls.
     c. all boys and girls are fully mature by age 16.
     d. all boys and girls are fully mature by age 18.

14. It is impossible now to cure:
     a. syphilis.
     b. gonorrhea.
     c. herpes virus #2.
     d. vaginitis.
     e. all of the above.

15. When men and women are physically mature:
     a. each female ovary releases two eggs each month.
     b. each female ovary releases millions of eggs each month.
     c. male testes produce one sperm for each ejaculation (climax).
     d. male testes produce millions of sperm for each ejaculation (climax).
     e. none of the above.

16. Teenagers who choose to have sexual intercourse may possibly:
     a. have to deal with a pregnancy.
     b. feel guilty.
     c. become more close to their sexual partners.
     d. become less close to their sexual partners.
     e. all of the above.

17. As they enter puberty, teenagers become more interested in sexual activities because:
     a. their sex hormones are changing.
     b. the media (TV, movies, magazines, records) push sex for teenagers.
     c. some of their friends have sex and expect them to have sex also.
     d. all of the above.

18. To use a condom the correct way, a person must:
     a. leave some space at the tip for the guy's fluid.
     b. use a new one every time sexual intercourse occurs.
     c. hold it on the penis while pulling out of the vagina.
     d. all of the above.

19. The proportion of American girls who become pregnant before turning 20 is:
     a. 1 out of 3.
     b. 1 out of 11.
     c. 1 out of 43.
     d. 1 out of 90.

20. In general, children born to young teenage parents:
     a. have few problems because their parents are emotionally mature.
     b. have a greater chance of being abused by their parents.
     c. have normal birth weight.
     d. have a greater chance of being healthy.
     e. none of the above.

21. Treatment for venereal disease is best if:
     a. both partners are treated at the same time.
     b. only the partner with the symptoms sees a doctor.
     c. the person takes the medicine only until the symptoms disappear.
     d. the partners continue having sex (sexual intercourse).
     e. all of the above.

22. Most teenagers:
     a. have crushes or infatuations that last a short time.
     b. feel shy or awkward when first dating.
     c. feel jealous sometimes.
     d. worry a lot about their looks.
     e. all of the above.

23. Most unmarried girls who have children while still in high school:
     a. depend upon their parents for support.
     b. finish high school and graduate with their class.
     c. never have to be on public welfare.

      d. have the same social lives as their peers.

      e. all of the above.

24. Syphilis:

      a. is one of the most dangerous of the venereal diseases.

      b. is known to cause blindness, insanity, and death if untreated.

      c. is first detected as a chancre sore on the genitals.

      d. all of the above.

25. For a boy, nocturnal emissions (wet dreams) means he:

      a. has a sexual illness.

      b. is fully mature physically.

      c. is experiencing a normal part of growing up.

      d. is different from most other boys.

26. If people have sexual intercourse, the advantage of using condoms is that they:

      a. help prevent getting or giving VD.

      b. can be bought in drug stores by either sex.

      c. do not have dangerous side effects.

      d. do not require a prescription.

      e. all of the above.

27. If two people want to have a close relationship, it is important that they:

      a. trust each other and are honest and open with each other.

      b. date other people.

      c. always think of the other person first.

      d. always think of their own needs first.

      e. all of the above.

28. The physical changes of puberty:

      a. happen in a week or two.

      b. happen to different teenagers at different ages.

      c. happen quickly for girls and slowly for boys.

      d. happen quickly for boys and slowly for girls.

29. For most teenagers, their emotions (feelings):

      a. are pretty stable.

      b. seem to change frequently.

      c. don't concern them very much.

      d. are easy to put into words.

      e. are ruled by their thinking.

30. Teenagers who marry, compared to those who do not:

      a. are equally likely to finish high school.

      b. are equally likely to have children.

      c. are equally likely to get divorced.

      d. are equally likely to have successful work careers.

      e. none of the above.

31. The rhythm method (natural family planning):

      a. means couples *cannot* have intercourse during certain days of the woman's menstrual cycle.

      b. requires the woman to keep a record of when she has her period.

      c. is effective less than 80% of the time.

      d. is recommended by the Catholic church.

      e. all of the above.

32. The pill:

      a. can be used by any woman.

      b. is a good birth control method for women who smoke.

      c. usually makes menstrual cramping worse.

      d. must be taken for 21 or 28 days in order to the effective.

      e. all of the above.

33. Gonorrhea:

      a. is 10 times more common than syphilis.

      b. is a disease that can be passed from mothers to their children during birth.

      c. makes many men and women sterile (unable to have babies).

      d. is often difficult to detect in women.

      e. all of the above.

34. People choosing a birth control method:
    a. should think only about the cost of the method.
    b. should choose whatever method their friends are using.
    c. should learn about all the methods before choosing the one that's best for them.
    d. should get the method that's easiest to get.
    e. all of the above.

Answers to the Knowledge Questionnaire

Question	Answer	Question	Answer
1	b	18	d
2	b	19	a
3	d	20	b
4	e	21	a
5	d	22	e
6	a	23	a
7	a	24	d
8	e	25	c
9	e	26	e
10	a	27	a
11	c	28	b
12	e	29	b
13	a	30	e
14	c	31	e
15	d	32	d
16	e	33	e
17	d	34	c

Attitude and Value Inventory

The questions below are not a test of how much you know. We are interested in what you believe about some important issues. Please rate each statement according to how much you agree or disagree with it. Everyone will have different answers. Your answer is correct if it describes you very well.

Circle: 1 = if you Strongly Disagree with the statement.
                2 = if you Somewhat Disagree with the statement.
                3 = if you feel Neutral about the statement.
                4 = if you Somewhat Agree with the statement.
                5 = if you Strongly Agree with the statement.

1. I am very happy with my friendships.[a]
2. Unmarried people should not have sex (sexual intercourse).
3. Overall, I am satisfied with myself.
4. Two people having sex should use some form of birth control if they aren't ready for a child.
5. I'm confused about my personal sexual values and beliefs.
6. I often find myself acting in ways I don't understand.
7. I am not happy with my sex life.
8. Men should not hold jobs traditionally held by women.
9. People should never take "no" for an answer when they want to have sex.
10. I don't know what I want out of life.
11. Families do very little for their children.
12. Sexual relationships create more problems than they're worth.
13. I'm confused about what I should and should not do sexually.
14. I know what I want and need emotionally.
15. No one should pressure another person into sexual activity.
16. Birth control is not very important.
17. I know what I need to be happy.
18. I am not satisfied with my sexual behavior (sex life).

19. I usually understand the way I act.
20. People should not have sex before marriage.
21. I do not know much about my own physical and emotional sexual responses.
22. It is all right for two people to have sex before marriage if they are in love.
23. I have a good idea of where I'm headed in the future.
24. Family relationships are not important.
25. I have trouble knowing what my beliefs and values are about my personal sexual behavior.
26. I feel I do not have much to be proud of.
27. I understand how I behave around others.
28. Women should behave differently from men most of the time.
29. People should have sex only if they are married.
30. I know what I want out of life.
31. I have a good understanding of my own personal feelings and reactions.
32. I don't have enough friends.
33. I'm happy with my sexual behavior now.
34. I don't understand why I behave with my friends as I do.
35. At times I think I'm no good at all.
36. I know how I react in different sexual situations.
34. I have a clear picture of what I'd like to be doing in the future.
38. My friendships are not as good as I would like them to be.
39. Sexually, I feel like a failure.
40. More people should be aware of the importance of birth control.
41. At work and at home, women should not have to behave differently from men, when they are equally capable.
42. Sexual relationships make life too difficult.
43. I wish my friendships were better.
44. I feel that I have many good personal qualities.
45. I am confused about my reactions in sexual situations.
46. It is all right to pressure someone into sexual activity.
47. People should not pressure others to have sex with them.
48. Most of the time my emotional feelings are clear to me.
49. I have my own set of rules to guide my sexual behavior (sex life).
50. Women and men should be able to have the same jobs, when they are equally capable.
51. I don't know what my long-range goals are.
52. When I'm in a sexual situation, I get confused about my feelings.
53. Families are very important.
54. It is all right to demand sex from a girlfriend or boyfriend.
55. A sexual relationship is one of the best things a person can have.
56. Most of the time I have a clear understanding of my feelings and emotions.
57. I am very satisfied with my sexual activities just the way they are.
58. Sexual relationships only bring trouble to people.
59. Birth control is not as important as some people say.
60. Family relationships cause more trouble than they're worth.
61. If two people have sex and aren't ready to have a child, it is very important they use birth control.
62. I'm confused about what I need emotionally.
63. It is all right for two people to have sex before marriage.
64. Sexual relationships provide an important and fulfilling part of life.
65. People should be expected to behave in certain ways just because they are male or female.
66. Most of the time I know why I behave the way I do.
67. I feel good having as many friends as I have.
68. I wish I had more respect for myself.
69. Family relationships can be very valuable.
70. I know for sure what is right and wrong sexually for me.

a. The five response options are repeated following each item.

Scales in the Attitude and Value Inventory

Clarity of Long-Term Goals: –Q10, +Q23, +Q30, +Q37, +Q51.
Clarity of Personal Sexual Values: –Q5, –Q13, –Q25, +Q49, +70.
Understanding of Emotional Needs: +Q14, +Q17, +Q48, +Q56, –Q62.
Understanding of Personal Social Behavior: –Q6, +Q19, +Q27, –Q34, +Q66.
Understanding of Personal Sexual Responses: –Q21, +Q31, +Q36, –Q45, –Q52.
Attitude Toward Various Gender Role Behaviors: –Q8, –Q28, +Q41, +Q50, +Q65.
Attitude Toward Sexuality in Life: –Q12, –Q42, +Q55, –Q58, +64.
Attitude Toward the Importance of Birth Control: +Q4, –Q16, +Q40, –Q59, +Q61.
Attitude Toward Premarital Intercourse: +Q2, +Q20, –Q22, +Q29, –Q63.
Attitude Toward the Use of Pressure and Force in Sexual Activity: –Q9, +Q15, –Q46, +Q47, +Q54.
Recognition of the Importance of the Family: –Q11, –Q24, +Q53, –Q60, +Q69.
Self-Esteem: +Q3, –Q26, –Q35, +Q44, –Q68.
Satisfaction With Personal Sexuality: –Q7, –Q18, +Q33, –Q39, +Q57.
Satisfaction With Social Relationships: +Q1, –Q32, –Q38, –Q43, +Q67.

Note. + means the item is positive; – means the item is negative and should be reverse scored. On some scales, people will have different views about whether larger scores represent socially desirable or undesirable scores.

Behavior Inventory

Part 1

The questions below ask how often you have done some things. Some of the questions are personal and ask about your social life and sex life. Some questions will not apply to you. Please do not conclude from the questions that you should have had all of the experiences the questions ask about. Instead, just mark whatever answer describes you best.

Circle: 1 = if you do it *almost never,* which means about 5% of the time or less.
  2 = if you do it *sometimes,* which means about 25% of the time.
  3 = if you do if *half the time,* which means about 50% of the time.
  4 = if you do it *usually,* which means about 75% of the time.
  5 = if you do it *almost always,* which means about 95% of the time or more.
  DNA = if the question *does not apply* to you.

1. When things you've done turn out poorly, how often do you take responsibility for your behavior and its consequences?[a]
2. When things you've done turn out poorly, how often do you blame others?
3. When you are faced with a decision, how often do you take responsibility for making a decision about it?
4. When you have to make a decision, how often do you think hard about the consequences of each possible choice?
5. When you have to make a decision, how often do you get as much information as you can before making the decision?
6. When you have to make a decision, how often do you first discuss it with others?
7. When you have to make a decision about your sexual behavior (for example, going out on a date, holding hands, kissing, petting, or having sex), how often do you take responsibility for the consequences?
8. When you have to make a decision about your sexual behavior, how often do you think hard about the consequences of each possible choice?
9. When you have to make a decision about your sexual behavior, how often do you first get as much information as you can?
10. When you have to make a decision about your sexual behavior, how often do you first discuss it with others?
11. When you have to make a decision about your sexual behavior, how often do you make it on the spot without worrying about the consequences?
12. When a friend wants to talk with you, how often are you able to clear your mind and really listen to what your friend has to say?
13. When a friend is talking with you, how often do you ask questions if you don't understand what your friend is saying?
14. When a friend is talking with you, how often do you nod your head and say "yes" or something else to show that you are interested?
15. When you want to talk with a friend, how often are you able to get your friend to really listen to you?

16. When you talk with a friend, how often do you ask for your friend's reaction to what you've said?
17. When you talk with a friend, how often do you let your feelings show?
18. When you are with a friend you care about, how often do you let that friend know you care?
19. When you talk with a friend, how often do you include statements like "my feelings are . . . ," "the way I think is . . . ," or "it seems to me"?
20. When you are alone with a date or boy/girlfriend, how often can you tell him/her your feelings about what you want to do and do not want to do sexually? (If you are a boy, boy/girlfriend means girlfriend; if you are a girl, it means boyfriend.)
21. If a boy/girl puts pressure on you to be involved sexually and you don't want to be involved, how often do you say "no"? (If you are a boy, boy/girl means girl; if you are a girl, it means boy.)
22. If a boy/girl puts pressure on you to be involved sexually and you don't want to be involved, how often do you succeed in stopping it?
23. If you have sexual intercourse with your boy/girlfriend, how often can you talk with him/her about birth control?
24. If you have sexual intercourse and want to use birth control, how often do you insist on using birth control?

Part 2

In this section, we want to know how uncomfortable you are doing different things. Being "uncomfortable" means that it is difficult for you and it makes you nervous and uptight. For each item, circle the number that describes you best, but if the item doesn't apply to you, circle DNA.

Circle: 1 = if you are *comfortable.*
2 = if you are *a little uncomfortable.*
3 = if you are *somewhat uncomfortable.*
4 = if you are *very uncomfortable.*
DNA = if the question *does not apply* to you.

25. Getting together with a group of friends of the opposite sex.[b]
26. Going to a party.
27. Talking with teenagers of the opposite sex.
28. Going out on a date.
29. Talking with friends about sex.
30. Talking with a date or boy/girlfriend about sex. (If you are a boy, boy/girlfriend means girlfriend; if you are a girl, it means boyfriend.)
31. Talking with parents about sex.
32. Talking with friends about birth control.
33. Talking with a date or boy/girlfriend about birth control. (If you are a boy, boy/girlfriend means girlfriend; if you are a girl, it means boyfriend.)
34. Talking with parents about birth control.
35. Expressing concern and caring for others.
36. Telling a date or boy/girlfriend what you want to do and do not want to do sexually.
37. Saying "no" to a sexual come-on.
38. Having your current sex life, whatever it may be (it may be doing nothing, kissing, petting, or having intercourse).

If you are not having sexual intercourse, circle DNA in the four questions below.

39. Insisting on using some form of birth control, if you are having sex.
40. Buying contraceptives at a drug store, if you are having sex.
41. Going to a doctor or clinic for contraception, if you are having sex.
42. Using some form of birth control, if you are having sex.

Part 3

Circle the correct answer to the following two questions.

43. Have you ever had sex (sexual intercourse)? yes no
44. Have you had sex (sexual intercourse) during the last month? yes no

Part 4

The following questions ask how many times you did some things during the last month. Put a number in the right hand space to show the number of times you engaged in that activity. If you did not do that during the last month, put a "0" in the space.

Think *carefully* about the times that you have had sex during the last month. Think also about the number of times you did not use birth control and the number of times you used different types of birth control.

45. Last month, how many times did you have sex (sexual intercourse)   _____ times in the last month
46. Last month, how many times did you have sex when you or your partner
     did not use any form of birth control?   _____ times in the last month
47. Last month, how many times did you have sex when you or your partner
     used a diaphragm, withdrawal (pulling out before releasing fluid), rhythm
     (not having sex on fertile days), or foam without condoms?   _____ times in the last month
48. Last month, how many times did you have sex when you or your partner
     used the pill, condoms (rubbers), or an IUD?   _____ times in the last month

If you add your answers to Questions 46, 47, and 48, the total number should equal your answer to Question 45. (If it does not, please correct your answers.)

49. During the last month, how many times have you had a conversation or
     discussion about sex with your parents?   _____ times in the last month
50. During the last month, how many times have you had a conversation or
     discussion about sex with your friends?   _____ times in the last month
51. During the last month, how many times have you had a conversation
     or discussion about sex with a date or boy/girlfriend? (If you are a boy,
     boy/girlfriend means girlfriend; if you are a girl, it means boyfriend.)   _____ times in the last month
52. During the last month, how many times have you had a conversation or
     discussion about birth control with your parents?   _____ times in the last month
53. During the last month, how many times have you had a conversation
     or discussion about birth control with your friends?   _____ times in the last month
54. During the last month, how many times have you had a conversation
     or discussion about birth control with a date or boy/girlfriend?   _____ times in the last month

Thank you for completing this questionnaire.

a. The six response options are repeated following Items 1-24.
b. The five response options are repeated following Items 25-42.

Scales in the Behavior Inventory

Social decision-making skills

+Q1
−Q2
+Q3
+Q4
+Q5
+Q6

Sexual decision-making skills

+Q7
+Q8
+Q9
+Q10
−Q11

Communication skills

+Q12
+Q13
+Q14
+Q15
+Q16
+Q17
+Q18
+Q19

Assertiveness skills

+Q20
+Q21
+Q22

Birth control assertiveness skills

+Q23
+Q24

Comfort engaging in social activities

–Q25
–Q26
–Q27
–Q28

Comfort talking with friends, girl/boyfriend, and parents about sex

–Q29
–Q30
–Q31

Comfort talking with friends, girl/boyfriend, and parents about birth control

–Q32
–Q33
–Q34

Comfort talking with parents about sex and birth control

–Q31
–Q34

Comfort expressing concern and caring

–Q35

Comfort being sexually assertive (saying "no")

–Q36
–Q37

Comfort having current sex life, whatever it may be

–Q38

Comfort getting and using birth control

–Q39
–Q40
–Q41
–Q42

Note. + means the item is positive; – means the item is negative and should be reverse scored.

Assessing Adolescents' Perceptions of the Costs and Benefits of Engaging in Sexual Intercourse

Stephen A. Small,[1] *University of Wisconsin–Madison*

The Adolescent Perceived Costs and Benefits Scale for Sexual Intercourse (Small, Silverberg, & Kerns, 1993) was developed to measure the costs and benefits that adolescents perceive for engaging in nonmarital sexual intercourse. Adolescent sexual activity is often viewed as problematic because of its potential risk to the adolescent's health and life prospects, as well as the possible negative consequences for the broader society. The present measure considers the adolescent as a decision maker and is based on the assumption that if we wish to understand why adolescents become sexually active, it is important to understand the positive and negative consequences adolescents associate with engaging in the behavior.

[1]Address correspondence to Stephen A. Small, Department of Child and Family Studies, School of Human Ecology, University of Wisconsin–Madison, 1300 Linden Drive, Room 120, Madison, WI 53706; email: sasmall@ facstaff.wisc.edu.

Description

The Adolescent Perceived Costs and Benefits Scale for Sexual Intercourse consists of two independent subscales of 10 items each. The Perceived Costs subscale assesses the perceived costs associated with engaging in sexual intercourse; the Perceived Benefits subscale assesses the perceived benefits of sexual activity. Each item is responded to using a 4-point Likert-type format. Responses range from 0 (*strongly disagree*) to 3 (*strongly agree*). The scale is based on current research and theory on adolescent development, which views the adolescent as a decision maker and recognizes the importance of understanding the meanings that adolescents ascribe to behavior.

The scale was developed over a multiyear period and involved extensive interviews with a diverse sample of adolescents. It underwent a number of refinements as a result of pilot testing. A parallel measure for assessing adolescents' perceptions of the costs and benefits of using alcohol is also available (see Philipp, 1993; Small et al., 1993).

Response Mode and Timing

Respondents are asked to indicate the number corresponding to their degree of agreement or disagreement with each of the items. This can be done by circling the appropriate response or filling it in on a machine-scorable answer sheet. Each subscale takes approximately 3-5 minutes to complete.

Scoring

For each subscale a total perceived costs or benefits score is obtained by summing the 10 individual items. Scores can range from 0 to 30 with a higher score reflecting higher perceived costs or benefits. Individual items can also be examined to gain insight into the primary or modal reasons particular groups of adolescents perceive for engaging or not engaging in sexual intercourse.

Reliability

Internal reliability, as determined by Cronbach's alpha, was .86 for both the Perceived Costs and the Perceived Benefits subscales based on a sample of 2,444 male and female adolescents. Based on a sample of 124 male and female adolescents the subscales had a test-retest reliability over a 2-week period of .70 and .65 for the cost and benefits scales, respectively.

Validity

As expected, Small et al. (1993) found that adolescents who were not sexually active perceived significantly more costs for engaging in sexual intercourse than their sexually active peers. The correlation between sexual intercourse status and perceived costs was $r = .32$. Females perceived more costs ($M = 17.30$) for engaging in sexual intercourse than their male counterparts ($M = 14.80$).

Small et al. (1993) reported that adolescent females perceived fewer significant benefits ($M = 17.68$) for engaging in sexual intercourse than their male peers ($M = 18.22$). The correlation between sexual activity status and the Perceived Benefits subscale was small but significant ($r = .11$). Overall, sexually active teens perceived more benefits than adolescents who were not sexually active. However, although the perceived benefits scores for the non-sexually active teens remained stable across grade levels, after the ninth grade there was a decrease in the perceived benefits scores of teens who were sexually active. Small et al. suggested two possible explanations for this finding. First, with experience sexually active teens may come to realize that many of their beliefs regarding the benefits of sexual intercourse do not hold true. Second, at younger ages, when sexual intercourse is generally less acceptable, teens must first believe there are many benefits for sexual intercourse before becoming sexually active. At older ages, when sexual activity is more acceptable, there is less of a need to be convinced of the value of the behavior before engaging in it.

In unpublished data, Small (1996) found that the regularity of birth control use among sexually active teens was positively correlated ($r = .24$) with the Perceived Costs subscale and but was not correlated with the Perceived Benefits subscale. In addition, adolescents who reported more supportive and positive relations with their parents perceived more costs for engaging in sexual intercourse than adolescents who had a poorer relationship with their parents.

Small (1991) found that adolescents who intended to go on to college were more likely than their non-college-bound peers to report that fear of pregnancy was a primary reason for not having sexual intercourse. Consistent with the literature on adolescent peer influence, as the age of the adolescent increased, fewer agreed that peer pressure was a major reason why a teen would engage in sexual intercourse. Similarly, older teens were much more likely than younger teens to report that curiosity (i.e., "Teens have sex to see what it's like") was a reason for having sexual intercourse.

References

Philipp, M. (1993). *From the adolescent's perspective: Understanding the costs and benefits of using alcohol.* Unpublished doctoral dissertation, University of Wisconsin–Madison.

Small, S. A. (1991, October). *Understanding the reasons underlying adolescent sexual activity.* Paper presented at the symposium, Teen Sexuality Challenge . . . Bridging the Gap Between Research and Action, University of Wisconsin–Green Bay.

Small, S. A. (1996). [Teen Assessment Project findings]. Unpublished data, Department of Child and Family Studies, University of Wisconsin–Madison.

Small, S. A., Silverberg, S. B., & Kerns, D. (1993). Adolescents' perceptions of the costs and benefits of engaging in health-compromising behaviors. *Journal of Youth and Adolescence, 22,* 73-87.

Exhibit

Adolescent Perceived Costs and Benefits Scale for Sexual Intercourse

Perceived Costs Subscale

Why Teenagers Don't Have Sexual Intercourse

Instructions: Below are some of the reasons that teens give for NOT having sexual intercourse. Please indicate how much you agree or disagree with each reason. If you're not sure, give your best guess.

1. Teenagers don't have sex because they think it is morally wrong or against their religion.
2. Teenagers don't have sex because they don't want to get a sexually transmitted disease (STD) or a disease like AIDS.
3. Teenagers don't have sex because their parent(s) don't approve.
4. Teenagers don't have sex because they don't feel old enough to handle it.
5. Teenagers don't have sex because their friends won't approve.
6. Teenagers don't have sex because they or their partner might get pregnant.
7. Teenagers don't have sex because they aren't in love with anyone yet.
8. Teenagers don't have sex because they don't need it to make them happy.
9. Teenagers don't have sex because they would feel guilty.
10. Teenagers don't have sex because they or their partner might get pregnant, which might mess up their future plans for college, school, or a career.

   Responses: 0 = Strongly agree   1 = Agree   2 = Disagree   3 = Strongly disagree

Perceived Benefits Subscale

Why Teenagers Have Sexual Intercourse

Instructions: Below are some of the reasons that teens give for having sexual intercourse. Please indicate how much you agree or disagree with each reason. If you're not sure, give your best guess.

1. Teenagers have sex because it helps them forget their problems.
2. Teenagers have sex because it makes them feel grown up.
3. Teenagers have sex because they *want* to get pregnant or become a parent.
4. Teenagers have sex as a way to get or keep a boyfriend or girlfriend.
5. Teenagers have sex because it makes them feel good.
6. Teenagers have sex because it makes them feel loved.
7. Teenagers have sex because they want to fit in with their friends.
8. Teenagers have sex because they want to see what it's like.
9. Teenagers have sex because it makes them feel more confident and sure of themselves.
10. Teenagers have sex because people they admire or look up to make it seem like a "cool" thing to do.

   Responses: 0 = Strongly agree   1 = Agree   2 = Disagree   3 = Strongly disagree

The Feelings Scale: Positive and Negative Affective Responses

George Smeaton and Donn Byrne,[1] *State University of New York at Albany*

An important precursor of behavioral responses to sexual stimuli (or any other stimuli) is the affective responses they elicit (Byrne, 1983; Byrne & Kelley, 1981). Through associative learning, pairing positive affect with neutral stimuli can result in positive affect being elicited by such stimuli, as well as subsequent approach responses. In the same manner, pairing stimuli with negative affect can result in those stimuli eliciting negative affect and avoidance responses. Additionally, affective responses are transformed into enduring attitudinal responses and cognitive justifications of such responses (Byrne, Fisher, Lamberth, & Mitchell, 1974; Byrne & Kelley, 1989). Thus, the ability to assess affective responses would greatly facilitate the prediction of a wide variety of behavioral, attitudinal, and cognitive responses to sexual stimuli. For this reason, the Feelings Scale (Byrne et al., 1974) was constructed to provide a means for individuals to report the degree to which they are currently experiencing 11 emotional states.

Description

Introduced in a study by Byrne and Sheffield (1965), the original version of the Feelings Scale required self-ratings of the following affective states, each represented by a 5-point rating scale: sexually aroused, disgusted, entertained, anxious, bored, and angry. Each state was represented by a 5-point rating scale anchored by the presence and absence of the emotion (e.g., *angry-not angry*) and containing three unlabeled intermediate points. A later variation of this scale, titled the Effectance Arousal Scale (Byrne & Clore, 1974), added two states—uneasy and confused—to the original set of affective states, and it included items requesting respondents to assess their desire to know what others are currently thinking and to rate the similarity of their current feelings to those they experience while dreaming. In the final version of the Feelings Scale (Byrne et al., 1974), the following five additional emotional states were added to the Byrne and Sheffield (1965) set: afraid, curious, nauseated, depressed, and excited. The scale is appropriate for use with any respondent possessing the level of verbal skill required to comprehend the terminology.

Response Mode and Timing

Respondents circle the point on each scale corresponding to their assessment of the degree to which they are experiencing each of the 11 emotional states. The scale requires less than 5 minutes to complete.

Scoring

A factor analysis of the enlarged final version of the scale conducted by Byrne et al. (1974) revealed that the scale contained two orthogonal factors accounting for 90% of the total variance. The first factor, labeled Positive Affect, consists of the items excited, entertained, sexually aroused, anxious, curious, and (with negative loading) bored. The second factor, Negative Affect, consists of the items disgusted, nauseated, angry, and depressed. A cross-validation of this factor loading by Griffitt, using respondents from a different university, revealed it to be very stable across samples. On the basis of these findings, indexes of positive and negative affect were calculated by summing each of the responses of the positive and negative factors, using reverse scores for the item bored. The item afraid was omitted because its loading was not above .30 on either factor.

Reliability

Because the emotional states assessed by the Feelings Scale are very transient, test-retest coefficients of reliability would not be appropriate for this measure. Using data from a study employing 166 males and females (Smeaton & Byrne, 1986), however, we have assessed the scale's internal consistency using Cronbach's alpha. Given the factor loadings obtained by Byrne et al. (1974), an alpha coefficient of .65 was obtained for the positive factor and .72 for the negative factor. Because these alpha levels are somewhat low, we examined the interitem correlations from this recent data set and concluded that the original factor loadings may no longer be accurate. When the item bored is excluded, the positive factor alpha increases to .73, and when the item afraid is included in the negative factors, its alpha increases to .83.

Validity

The validity of the self-reports of affective states obtained using the Feelings Scale is well documented by the findings of studies that have used them in conjunction with measures of individual differences known to affect responses to erotic material. High negative affect scores following exposure to sexual stimuli have been found to be positively correlated with sex guilt (Griffitt & Kaiser, 1978), erotophobia (Becker & Byrne, 1985; Fisher & Byrne, 1978), and the restrictiveness of an individual's sexual socialization (Fisher & Byrne, 1978). Moreover,

[1]Address correspondence to Donn Byrne, Department of Psychology, State University of New York at Albany, 1400 Albany Ave., Albany, NY 12222; email: db034@cnsibm.albany.edu.

positive affect scores have been found to be positively correlated with the frequency of past intercourse and masturbation (Griffitt, 1975) and erotophilia (Becker & Byrne, 1985; Kelley, 1985; Kelley, Byrne, Greendlinger, & Murnen, 1997), and negatively correlated with sex guilt and authoritarianism (Kelley, 1977; Kelley et al., 1997). Finally, consistent with the frequently reported finding that males react more positively to erotic material than females (Abelson, Cohen, Heaton, & Suder, 1971; Becker & Byrne, 1985; Griffitt, 1973; Kenrick, Springfield, Wagenhals, Dahl, & Ransdell, 1980; Schmidt & Sigusch, 1970), several researchers have reported higher positive affect scores among males than females following exposure to heterosexual erotic material (Becker & Byrne 1985; Griffitt & Kaiser, 1978; Kelley, 1977; Kelley et al., 1997).

Support for the validity of the Feelings Scale can also be derived from studies that have used it to predict behavioral and attitudinal responses. Positive affect levels have been found to be correlated with response accuracy in a learning task when correct responses were reinforced with presentations of erotic slides (Griffitt & Kaiser, 1978). Moreover, reports of negative affect in response to erotic materials have been found to be positively correlated with the labeling of such material as pornographic (Byrne et al., 1974; Fisher & Byrne, 1978). In addition to evaluations of erotic material, Feelings Scale responses have been found to be predictive of attraction to other persons. Consistent with the reinforcement-affect theory of attraction (Clore & Byrne, 1974), reports of high levels of positive affect while in the presence of a novel stimulus person is predictive of a high level of attraction to that person (Kelley, 1982). Finally, Griffitt, May, and Veitch (1974) found that among individuals whose affective response to sexual stimuli are primarily positive, sexual arousal led to more visual contact, closer physical proximity, and more positive evaluations of opposite-sex strangers than same-sex strangers.

References

Abelson, H., Cohen, R., Heaton, E., & Suder, C. (1971). National survey of public attitudes toward and experience with erotic materials. In *Technical report of the Commission on Obscenity and Pornography* (Vol. 6, pp. 1-137). Washington, DC: Government Printing Office.

Becker, M. A., & Byrne, D. (1985). Self-regulated exposure to erotica, recall errors and subjective reactions as a function of erotophobia and type a coronary-prone behavior. *Journal of Personality and Social Psychology, 48,* 760-767.

Byrne, D. (1983). Sex without contraception. In D. Byrne & W. A. Fisher (Eds.), *Adolescents, sex, and contraception* (pp. 3-31). Hillsdale, NJ: Lawrence Erlbaum.

Byrne, D., & Clore, G. A. (1974). Effectance arousal and attraction. *Journal of Personality and Social Psychology, 6* (4, Whole No. 638).

Byrne, D., Fisher, J. D., Lamberth, J., & Mitchell, H. E. (1974). Evaluations of erotica: Facts or feelings? *Journal of Personality and Social Psychology, 29,* 111-119.

Byrne, D., & Kelley, K. (1981). *An introduction to personality* (3rd ed.). Englewood Cliffs, NJ: Prentice Hall.

Byrne, D., & Kelley, K. (1989). Basing legislative action on research data: Prejudice, prudence, and empirical limitations. In D. Zillmann & J. Bryant (Eds.), *Pornography: Recent research, interpretations, and policies considerations* (pp. 363-385). Hillsdale, NJ: Lawrence Erlbaum.

Byrne, D., & Sheffield, J. (1965). Response to sexually arousing stimuli as a function of repressing and sensitizing defenses. *Journal of Abnormal Psychology, 70,* 114-118.

Clore, G. L., & Byrne, D. (1974). A reinforcement-affect model of attraction. In T. L. Huston (Ed.), *Perspectives on interpersonal attraction* (pp. 41-67). New York: Academic Press.

Fisher, W. A., & Byrne, D. (1978). Individual differences in affective, evaluative, and behavioral responses to erotica. *Journal of Applied Social Psychology, 8,* 355-365.

Griffitt, W. (1973). Response to erotica and the projection of response to erotica in the opposite sex. *Journal of Experimental Research in Personality, 6,* 330-338.

Griffitt, W. (1975). Sexual experience and sexual responsiveness: Sex differences. *Archives of Sexual Behavior, 4,* 529-540.

Griffitt, W., & Kaiser, D. L. (1978). Affect, sex guilt, gender, and the rewarding-punishing effects of erotic stimuli. *Journal of Personality and Social Psychology, 8,* 830-858.

Griffitt, W., May, J., & Veitch, R. (1974). Sexual stimulation and interpersonal behavior: Heterosexual evaluative responses, visual behavior, and physical proximity. *Journal of Personality and Social Psychology, 30,* 367-377.

Kelley, K. (1977). *Affective predictors of sexual attitudes.* Unpublished doctoral dissertation, Purdue University, West Lafayette, IN.

Kelley, K. (1985). The effects of sexual and/or aggressive film exposure on helping, hostility, and attitudes about the sexes. *Journal of Research in Personality, 19,* 472-483.

Kelley, K. (1982). Predicting attraction to the novel stimulus person: Affect and concern. *Journal of Research in Personality, 16,* 32-40.

Kelley, K., Byrne, D., Greendlinger, V., & Murnen, S. K. (1997). Content, sex of viewer, and dispositional variables as predictors of affective and evaluative responses to erotic films. *Journal of Psychology & Human Sexuality, 9,* 53-71.

Kenrick, D. T., Springfield, D. O., Wagenhals, W. L., Dahl, R. H., & Ransdell, H. J. (1980). Sex differences, androgyny, and approach responses to erotica: A new variation on the old volunteer problem. *Journal of Personality and Social Psychology, 38,* 517-524.

Schmidt, G., & Sigusch, V. (1970). Sex differences in responses to psychosexual stimulation by films and slides. *The Journal of Sex Research, 6,* 10-24.

Smeaton, G., & Byrne, D. (1986). *The effects of fear-arousing, sexual, romantic, and humorous appeals on the effectiveness of contraceptive advertisements.* Unpublished manuscript, State University of New York at Albany.

Exhibit

The Feelings Scale

At this point in time I feel:

Sexually aroused　　　　　　　　　　　　　　　　　　　　Not aroused

A　　　　　　B　　　　　　C　　　　　　D　　　　　　E[a]

Disgusted	Not disgusted
Entertained	Not entertained
Anxious	Not anxious
Bored	Not bored
Angry	Not angry
Afraid	Not afraid
Curious	Not curious
Nauseated	Not nauseated
Depressed	Not depressed
Excited	Not excited

a. The response options follow each emotion.

Revised Attraction to Sexual Aggression Scale

The Editors

This instrument was developed by Malamuth (1989a, 1989b) to measure attraction to sexual aggression.

References

Malamuth, N. M. (1989a). The Attraction to Sexual Aggression Scale: Part one. *The Journal of Sex Research, 26,* 26-49.
Malamuth, N. M. (1989b). The Attraction to Sexual Aggression Scale: Part two. *The Journal of Sex Research, 26,* 324-354.

Exhibit

Social Relationships Research

Instructions: On the following pages there are a variety of different questions. Please answer all the questions to the best of your ability. If you are unsure of the answer to a question, please give your best guess. It is important that all of the questions be answered. There are no right or wrong answers, and no "trick" questions. Please answer the question by placing a tick in the box you choose, like this: ✓. Please work quickly and be *as honest* as possible. Your responses will be kept completely confidential. Thank you for your cooperation.

1. People frequently think about different activities even if they never do them. For each kind of activity listed, please indicate how often you have thought of trying it:

　　　　　　　　　　　　　　　　　Never　　　　Sometimes　　　　Often
　　a.　Necking (deep kissing)[a]
　　b.　Petting

	Never	Sometimes	Often

c. Oral sex
d. Heterosexual intercourse
e. Anal intercourse
f. Homosexual acts
g. Group sex
h. Bondage sex
i. Whipping, spanking sex
j. Robbing a bank
k. Raping a woman
l. Forcing a female to do something sexual she didn't want to do
m. Being forced to do something sexual you didn't want to do
n. Transvestism (wearing women's clothes)
o. Sex with children
p. Killing someone
q. Selling illegal drugs

2. Whether or not you have ever thought of it, do you find the idea of:

	Very Unattractive	Somewhat Unattractive	Somewhat Attractive	Very Attractive

a. Necking (deep kissing)[b]

3. What percentage of *males* do you think would find the following activities sexually arousing?
a. Anal intercourse[c]
b. Group sex
c. Homosexual acts
d. Armed robbery
e. Bondage sex
f. Whipping, spanking sex
g. Rape
h. Robbing a bank
i. Forcing a female to do something sexual she really didn't want to do
j. Killing someone
k. Transvestism
l. Sex with a child
m. Being forced to do something sexual they didn't want to do

4. What percentage of *females* do think would find the following activities sexually arousing?
a. Anal intercourse[d]

5. How sexually arousing do you think you would find the following activities if you engaged in them (even if you have never actually engaged in them and never would)?

	Not arousing at all	Very arousing

a. Oral sex[e]
b. Heterosexual intercourse
c. Anal intercourse
d. Homosexual acts
e. Group sex
f. Bondage sex
g. Whipping, spanking sex
h. Robbing a bank
i. Raping a female
j. Forcing a female to do something sexual she didn't want to do
k. Transvestism (wearing women's clothes)
l. Being forced to do something sexual you didn't want to do
m. Sex with children
n. Killing someone

6. If you were sure that no one would ever find out and that you'd never be punished for it, how likely would you be to do the following?

                                        Very unlikely   Very likely
   a. Oral sex[f]
   b. Heterosexual intercourse
   c. Anal intercourse
   d. Homosexual acts
   e. Group sex
   f. Bondage sex
   g. Whipping, spanking sex
   h. Robbing a bank
   i. Raping a female
   j. Forcing a female to do something sexual she didn't want to do
   k. Transvestism (wearing women's clothes)
   l. Sex with children
   m. Killing someone
   n. Selling illegal drugs

7. If your best male friend were assured that no one would find out and that he'd never be punished for it, how likely do you think he would be to do the following:

                                        Very unlikely   Very likely
   a. Oral sex[g]

8. Approximately what percentage of your male friends, would you estimate, have done the following:
   a. Anal intercourse[h]
   b. Group sex
   c. Homosexual acts
   d. Armed robbery
   e. Bondage sex
   f. Whipping, spanking sex
   g. Rape
   h. Robbing a bank
   i. Forcing a female to do something sexual she didn't want to do
   j. Killing someone
   k. Transvestism
   l. Sex with a child
   m. Being forced to do something sexual they didn't want to do
   n. Selling illegal drugs

9. How likely do you think it is that at some point in the future you might try the following activities?

                                        Very unlikely   Very likely
   a. Oral sex[i]

End of questionnaire

Thanks for your responses

Source. This scale is reprinted with permission of the author.

a. These items are followed by boxes under each of the response options, providing a place for the respondent to mark with a check (✓) the option chosen.

b. The same response options as shown for Item 1 are repeated, with boxes under each of the four response options.

c. The response options are indicated by 11 boxes identified from 0% to 100%.

d. The same response options as shown for Item 3 are repeated.

e. Seven boxes between the two anchors are provided for responses.

f. The same response options as shown for Item 5 are repeated.

g. The same response options as shown for Item 5 are repeated.

h. The response options are indicated by 11 boxes identified from 0% to 100%.

i. The same response options as shown for Item 5 are repeated.

Aggressive Sexual Behavior Inventory

Donald L. Mosher,[1] *University of Connecticut*

The Aggressive Sexual Behavior Inventory (ASBI; Mosher & Anderson, 1986) was developed to measure sexual aggression by men against women that occurs in dating or other heterosocial-heterosexual situations. College men, but particularly college men with a macho personality constellation that includes callous sexual attitudes toward women, frequently use these tactics (Mosher & Anderson, 1986). In studies of sexual aggression, answers to a single question about the occurrence of date rape or to a hypothetical question asking about the likelihood of rape if one were not going to be caught suffer from problems of unreliability and false reporting. Although men might also under- or overreport on these 20 items, the summed score, when anonymous, is a better estimate of each man's history of aggressive sexual behavior. The ASBI can be treated as an individual-differences measure of sexual aggression or as a dependent variable when studying predictive correlates of aggressive sexual behavior.

Description

The ASBI consists of 20 items (or a 10-item short form) arranged in a 7-point Likert-type format to rate frequency of occurrence from 1 (*never*) to 7 (*extremely frequently*). From the responses of a sample of 125 college men to 33 items, a varimax factor analysis with an orthogonal rotation extracted six factors that were named sexual force, drugs and alcohol, verbal manipulation, angry rejection, anger expression, and threat.

Response Mode and Timing

Respondents can circle the number from 1 to 7 corresponding to their frequency of using the tactic, but the more common scoring is to mark the answers on machine-scorable answer sheets. The inventory requires approximately 5 minutes to complete.

Scoring

All 20 items are keyed in the same direction with a higher score indicating a greater frequency of aggressive sexual behavior. Scores can range from 20 to 140 or from 10 to 70 on the short form. For each specific factor, the percentage of 125 University of Connecticut college men who endorsed one of more items in the factor and the numbers of the items loading most highly on specific factors follows: sexual force, 28%, 3, 9, 11, 14, 17, 19; drugs and alcohol, 75%, 2, 6, and 15; verbal manipulation, 64%, 1, 4, 7, and 20; angry rejection, 43%, 10 and 13; anger expression,

46%, 8, 16, and 18; and threat, 13%, 5 and 12. The 10-item short form includes Items 1, 4, 5, 6, 11, 12, 13, 15, 18, and 19.

Reliability

In a sample of 125 college men (Mosher & Anderson, 1986), the Cronbach alpha for the summed scores from the 20 items was .94. It is recommended that the summed score of the 20 items be regarded as a homogeneous measure of aggressive sexual behavior. The short form of 10 items had a Cronbach alpha of .87 in a sample of 55 male rock musicians (Zaitchik, 1986).

Validity

As expected, Mosher and Anderson (1986) found that the summed score of the ASBI was significantly correlated with macho personality, $r = .33$; callous sexual attitudes, $r = .53$; violence as manly, $r = .23$; and danger as exciting, $r = .26$, as measured by the Hypermasculinity Inventory (Mosher & Sirkin, 1984). As expected, aggressive sexual behavior (Anderson, 1983) was significantly negatively correlated with sex-guilt, $r = -.53$, and hostility-guilt, $r = -.49$, as measured by the Mosher Forced-Choice Guilt Inventory (Mosher, 1966). When 125 college men imagined themselves in the role of rapist during guided imagery of a realistic-violent and nonerotic-rape, men scoring higher on aggressive sexual behavior, in comparison to men scoring lower, reported significantly more subjective sexual arousal, as hypothesized, but they also, contrary to expectations, experienced more affective anger, distress, fear, shame, and guilt (Mosher & Anderson, 1986). These results were interpreted as consistent with the revivification by the guided imagery of rape of the sexually aggressive men's mood-congruent, state-memories (Bower, 1981) of their own previous acts of sexual aggression. In a sample of rock musicians, Zaitchik (1986) found that the ASBI was correlated .75 with macho personality, .72 with cocaine use, .70 with amphetamine use, .50 with marijuana use, and −.35 with life satisfaction.

References

Anderson, R. D. (1983). *Hyper-masculine attitudes, aggressive sexual behaviors, and the reactions of college men to a guided imagery presentation of realistic rape.* Unpublished master's thesis, University of Connecticut, Storrs.

Bower, G. H. (1981). Mood and mercy. *American Psychologist, 36,* 129-148.

Mosher, D. L. (1966). The development and multitrait-multimethod matrix analysis of three measures of guilt. *Journal of Consulting Psychology, 30,* 25-29.

Mosher, D. L., & Anderson, R. D. (1986). Macho personality, sexual aggression, and reactions to guided imagery of realistic rape. *Journal of Research in Personality, 20*(2), 77-94.

[1]Address correspondence to Donald L. Mosher, 5051 North A1a, PH1-1, North Hutchinson Island, FL 34949; email: dlmosher@aol.com

Mosher, D. L., & Sirkin, M. (1984). Measuring a macho personality constellation. *Journal of Research in Personality, 18,* 150-163.

Zaitchik, M. (1986). *Macho personality and life satisfaction in rock musicians.* Unpublished master's thesis, University of Connecticut, Storrs.

Exhibit

Aggressive Sexual Behavior Inventory

Instructions: The following 20 items sample behavior that sometimes occurs in dating or man-woman sociosexual interactions. The items describe various techniques, which may or may not be successful, for gaining increased sexual access to women. Some of the behaviors are acceptable to some men and others are not. Because you are an anonymous subject in a psychological study, you are asked to be as truthful as you can be. Each item is to be rated on a 7-point scale of the frequency of past use of the tactic in which 1 means *never* and 7 means *extremely frequently.* If, for example, an item said, "I shave with an electric razor," you would mark the item with a 1, if you never shave with an electric razor, with a 7, if you shaved extremely frequently with an electric razor, and with a number between 2-6 to represent the relative frequency with which you shaved with an electric razor. Record your answers on the separate answer sheet.

1. I have threatened to leave or to end a relationship if a woman wouldn't have sex with me.
2. I have gotten a woman drunk in order to have sex with her.
3. I have waited my turn in line with some other guys who were sharing a "party girl."
4. I have told a woman that I wanted to come into her apartment so I could get her where I wanted.
5. I have warned a woman that she could get hurt if she resisted me, so she should relax and enjoy it.
6. I have gotten a woman high on marijuana or pills so she would be less able to resist my advances.
7. I have told a woman I was petting with that she couldn't stop and leave me with "blue balls."
8. I have blown my top and sworn or broken something to show a woman that she shouldn't get me angry.
9. I have brought a woman to my place after a date and forced her to have sex with me.
10. I have told a woman I was going out with that I could find someone else to give me sex if she wouldn't.
11. I have calmed a woman down with a good slap or two when she got hysterical over my advances.
12. I have promised a woman that I wouldn't harm her if she did everything that I told her to do.
13. I have called a woman an angry name and pushed her away when she would not surrender to my need for sex.
14. I have forced a woman to have sex with me and some of my pals.
15. I have turned a woman on to some expensive drugs so that she would feel obligated to do me a sexual favor.
16. I have roughed a woman up a little so that she would understand that I meant business.
17. I have pushed a woman down and made her undress or torn her clothes off if she wouldn't cooperate.
18. I have gripped a woman tightly and given her an angry look when she was not giving me the sexual response I wanted.
19. I have gotten a little drunk and forced a woman that I'm with to have sex with me.
20. I have told a woman that her refusal to have sex with me was changing the way I felt about her.

Perceived Attitudes Toward Sexuality of the Elderly Among Socially Related Reference Groups

John B. Bond, Jr.,[1] *University of Manitoba*
Richard R. Tramer, *Winnipeg, Manitoba*

This instrument attempts to measure older adults' views of various individual and group (reference group) attitudes toward sexual activity among elderly persons. Whereas a number of researchers have examined the attitudes of various respondents toward sexuality among elderly persons, our approach focuses on the beliefs of older adults with respect to attitudes held by these reference groups and individuals. The assumption is that an individual's perception of attitudes of others is more likely to influence his or her behavior than the actual attitudes held by others.

Description

This scale is part of a larger questionnaire administered to 273 married, older adults (ages 56-75) in a study investigating the relationships between sexual behavior and attitudes, locus of control, beliefs, life and marital satisfaction, and self-image. A portion of the results from this study relating to this scale were reported by Bond and Tramer (1983).

The scale consists of 11 items, identifying reference groups or individuals and asking respondents to indicate whether they believe each group or individual would respond favorably or unfavorably to elderly individuals being active sexually. In addition to determining the respondent's views of perceptions of others' attitudes toward sex among elderly persons, respondents' own attitudes are tapped. For married couples, discrepancies in perceived or actual attitudes can be calculated, discussed, and perhaps serve to stimulate the therapeutic process regarding sexual difficulties. Appropriate or inappropriate sexual counselors might also be identified, based on attitudes perceived as similar to self-reports of respondents. Other reference groups might be added to this measure, as appropriate.

Response Mode and Timing

In this self-administered scale, respondents are asked to circle the appropriate choice on a 5-point Likert-type scale—(1) *unfavorable*, (2) *somewhat favorable*, (3) *indifferent*, (4) *somewhat favorable*, (5) *favorable*—how they think various individuals and groups felt toward sex among elderly persons. The 11 identified groups and individuals

include five age-related reference groups: young people (16-20), adults (21-45), middle aged (45-64), elderly males, and elderly females. The six socially related reference groups are your clergyman, your doctor, your spouse, your friends, your children, and yourself. The selected reference groups are based on the reports of significant others obtained through interviews.

The scale requires an average of 12 minutes for completion. Item scores range from 1 (*unfavorable*) to 5 (*favorable*). The scale yields a total perceived attitude score (sum of all items minus Item 9 [yourself]); scores grouped in a particular manner (e.g., age-related or socially related reference groups); or individual scale items.

Scoring

All 11 items are scored in the same direction. The total attitude score may range from 11 to 55. Two subscales may be created using the (a) five items including age (Age-Related Reference Groups) with scores ranging from 5 to 25, or (b) six remaining items (Socially Related Reference Groups) ranging from 6 to 30.

Reliability

No reliability/stability information is available.

Validity

Correlations (N = 273) of .30 (p < .001) and .36 (p < .001) between the respondents' sexual behavior and perceived attitude (yourself) and perceived spouses' attitudes (your spouse), respectively, were obtained. Correlations (N = 273) of .09 (p = .21) and .09 (p = .21) between perceived total attitude score and Crowne and Marlowe's (1964) Social Desirability Scale and between total attitude score and Edwards's (1957) Social Desirability Scale were obtained. Bond and Tramer (1983), using the concept of age homophyly, hypothesized that perceived attitudes toward sex among elderly persons would be ordered by age of the reference group. The results supported the concept, indicating that older adults believe that the younger the age of the person the less favorable the perceived attitudes of that person toward sexual relations among elderly persons. Although the lack of relationship to the Crowne and Marlowe and the Edwards measures suggests a confidence in the validity of the instrument, stability has yet to be demonstrated.

[1]Address correspondence to John B. Bond, Jr., Department of Family Studies, University of Manitoba, Winnipeg, Manitoba R3T 2N2, Canada; email: bond@bldghumec.lan1.umanitoba.ca.

References

Bond, J. B., & Tramer, R. (1983). Older adult perceptions of attitudes toward sex among the elderly. *Canadian Journal on Aging, 2,* 63-70.

Crowne, D. P., & Marlowe, D. (1964). *The approval motive: Studies in evaluative dependence.* New York: Wiley.
Edwards, A. (1957). *The social desirability variable in personality assessment and research.* New York: Dryden.

Exhibit

Perceived Attitudes Toward Sexuality of the Elderly

Considerable differences in attitudes exist toward sex in the elderly. Some individuals view it favorably (i.e., sex is good, important, etc.). Others view it unfavorably (i.e., sex in the elderly is dirty, wrong, unhealthy, etc.).

Following is a list of individuals and groups. Please rate on a 5-point scale of favorable vs. unfavorable individuals' or groups' attitudes toward sex in the elderly as you see it. For example, if you feel that a group's attitude toward sex in the elderly is favorable, you circle 5; if it is indifferent, circle 3; if it is somewhat unfavorable, circle 2, etc.

Young people (16-20)[a]   Your clergyman
Adults (21-45)   Your doctor
Middle aged (46-64)   Yourself
Elderly males   Your spouse
Elderly females   Your friends
Your children

a. The 5-point scale is provided for each of the 11 items.

Aging and Sexuality Questionnaire

Norma L. McCoy,[1] *San Francisco State University*
Judy G. Bretschneider, *Atherton, California*

The Aging and Sexuality Questionnaire (ASQ) was designed to study sexual interest and behavior, both past and present, in samples of older adults.

Description

The ASQ has a total of 88 questions and consists of two parts: a demographics section and a sexual attitudes and behaviors section. The demographics section consists of a

total of 26 questions. The first 20 questions request information on respondent's age, marital status, ethnicity, religion, education, present income, and income before retirement. The final six questions ask for health-related information, including current physical health, change in health, current mental health, maintaining health, and present medication usage. The sexual attitudes and behaviors section consists of 62 questions (to save space, the numbers in the exhibit do not conform exactly to the numbering described here). A total of 45 questions are answered on 7-point scales. Endpoints range from *never, do not (did not) perform, do not (did not) enjoy, not at all important,* and *extremely unhappy* to *several times a day, perform (per-*

[1]Address correspondence to Norma L. McCoy, Department of Psychology, San Francisco State University, 1600 Holloway Avenue, San Francisco, CA 94132; email: mccoy@sfsu.edu.

formed) regularly, enjoy (enjoyed) very much, very important, and *extremely happy.* The remaining questions ask for age at first intercourse; age at first masturbation; age at first sexual fantasy; and the number, type, duration, and quality of any current sexual relationships.

The ASQ can be used with a wide age range of older adults, both male and female.

Response Mode and Timing

Respondents mark a printed form made up of Likert-type scale alternatives and other shorter lists of categories, choosing one in each case, or they write ages or enter time intervals for relationship length(s). In addition, there are comment fields for respondents to volunteer extra information. Experience suggests that a relatively educated and healthy older adult can complete the ASQ in 20-30 minutes.

Scoring

No norm-based scoring procedures exist for the ASQ. Ratings on comparable item subsets may be summarized

and understood to represent a single construct of greater or lesser sexual activity and enjoyment.

Reliability

No reliability analyses exist for the ASQ.

Validity

Published research (Bretschneider & McCoy, 1988) shows that the ASQ samples a wide range of important questions relating to aging and sexuality, and, thus, possesses good content validity.

Reference

Bretschneider, J. G., & McCoy, N. L. (1988). Sexual interest and behavior in healthy 80- to 102-year-olds. *Archives of Sexual Behavior, 17,* 109-129.

Exhibit

Aging and Sexuality Questionnaire

Sexual Attitudes and Behavior

1. Do you ever think or daydream about being close, affectionate and intimate with the opposite sex (sexual partner)?[a]
   (*never* to *several times a day*)
2. At what age did you first experience this type of daydreaming?
3. Who usually initiated a sexual encounter in your younger years (18-50 yrs.), yourself or your partner?
   (*almost always my partner* to *almost always me*)
4. Who usually initiates a sexual encounter now, yourself or your partner?
   (*almost always my partner* to *almost always me*)
5. How important would you say that the sexual part of your life was to you in your younger years?
   (*not at all important* to *very important*)
6. How important would you say that the sexual part of your life is to you now?
   (*not at all important* to *very important*)
7. How often did you engage in touching and caressing with a partner (without having sexual intercourse) in your younger years?
   (*never* to *several times a day*)
8. How often do you engage in touching and caressing with a partner (without having sexual intercourse) now?
   (*never* to *several times a day*)
9. How much did you "enjoy" touching and caressing with a partner (without having sexual intercourse) in your younger years?
   (*did not enjoy* to *enjoyed very much*)
10. How much do you "enjoy" touching and caressing with a partner (without having sexual intercourse) now?
    (*do not enjoy* to *enjoy very much*)

Assuming appropriate circumstances and partner(s) for each of the activities below, circle the number that best describes your current attitude.

11. Reading erotic (sexy) literature.
    (*do not perform* to *perform regularly*)
    (*do not enjoy* to *enjoy very much*)
12. Looking at erotic (sexy) pictures.
    (*do not perform* to *perform regularly*)
    (*do not enjoy* to *enjoy very much*)

13. Attending erotic films or watching erotic (cable) television.
(*do not perform* to *perform regularly*)
(*do not enjoy* to *enjoy very much*)
14. Breast petting.
(*do not perform* to *perform regularly*)
(*do not enjoy* to *enjoy very much*)
15. (Male) sucking partner's breast; (female) having breast sucked.
(*do not perform* to *perform regularly*)
(*do not enjoy* to *enjoy very much*)
16. Petting partner's genitals (sex organs).
(*do not perform* to *perform regularly*)
(*do not enjoy* to *enjoy very much*)
17. Petting of your genitals (sex organs) by partner.
(*do not perform* to *perform regularly*)
(*do not enjoy* to *enjoy very much*)
18. Stimulating partner's genitals (sex organs) with your mouth.
(*do not perform* to *perform regularly*)
(*do not enjoy* to *enjoy very much*)
19. Mouth stimulation of your genitals (sex organs) by partner.
(*do not perform* to *perform regularly*)
(*do not enjoy* to *enjoy very much*)
20. Sexual activity with someone of your own sex.
(*do not perform* to *perform regularly*)
(*do not enjoy* to *enjoy very much*)
21. At what age did you have your first sexual experience (intercourse) with a partner?
22. How often did you have sexual intercourse with a partner in your younger years (18-50)?
(*never* and *several times a day*)
23. How often do you have sexual intercourse with a partner now?
(*never* to *several times a day*)
24. How much did you "enjoy" having sexual intercourse with a partner in your younger years?
(*did not enjoy* to *enjoyed very much*)
25. How much do you "enjoy" having sexual intercourse with a partner now?
(*do not enjoy* to *enjoy very much*)
26. Are you satisfied with your partner(s) as lover(s)?
(*extremely unhappy* to *extremely happy*)
27. Are you satisfied with your partner(s) as human being(s)/friend(s)?
(*extremely unhappy* to *extremely happy*)
28. Masturbation: at what age did you first have a sexual experience with self-stimulation of your genitals?
29. How often did you masturbate in your younger years?
(*never* to *several times a day*)
30. How often do you masturbate now?
(*never* to *several times a day*)
31. How much did you "enjoy" masturbating in your younger years?
(*did not enjoy* to *enjoyed very much*)
32. How much do you "enjoy" masturbating now?
(*do not enjoy* to *enjoy very much*)

If you live in a retirement home, please answer Questions 33-35, then continue to Question 41.

If you do not live in a retirement home, please answer Questions 36-40, then continue to Question 41.

33. Do you now have a regular sexual partner?
(*none* to *more than one*)
34. If you answered "yes" to Question 33, please fill in the following chart. Specify how long you have been involved in each relationship.
35. How would you rate your relationship with each partner? Please fill in the chart by circling the appropriate number that best describes how you feel.
(*very unhappy* to *very happy* for each relationship)
36a. Are you now living with a sexual partner?
36b. If yes: how long have you been living with this partner?

36c. How old is this partner?

37. How would you rate your relationship with this partner?
(*very happy* to *very unhappy*)

38. Are you presently having sexual intercourse with this partner?

39a. Are you presently having sexual intercourse with a partner who is not living with you?

39b. If yes: how long have you had a relationship with this partner?

39c. How old is this partner?

40. How would you rate your relationship with this partner?
(*very unhappy* to *very happy*)

41. In your younger years, did you have sexual intercourse outside your marriage?
(*never* to *very often*)

42. Do you feel that living in your present environment prevents you from engaging in sexual activity?
(*no, never* to *yes, all the time*)

43. Do you feel that living in your present environment increases your chances for engaging in sexual activity?
(*no, never* to *yes, all the time*)

44. Did you experience guilt, inhibition, and discomfort over sexual feelings and behavior as a result of the way you were raised in your younger years?
(*no, never* to *yes, all the time*)
    A. Is this still true now?
(*no, never* to *yes, all the time*)
    B. Do you have any comments?

45. During the past six months, how frequently have you experienced each of the following sexual problems? Please complete the chart on the following page.
    Low drive, lack of interest[b]
    Reaching orgasm (coming) sooner than desired
    Inability to have an orgasm
    Orgasms do not occur often enough
    Loss of interest in partner
    Sexual dissatisfaction with partner
    No partner
    Not enough opportunity for sexual encounters
    Fear of poor performance
    Partner's loss of interest in sex
    Worry about non-sexual problems

For men only

    Inability to get an erection
    Inability to hold an erection
    Partner's vaginal pain or lack of lubrication

For women only

    Lack of vaginal lubrication (wetness)
    Vaginal pain during intercourse
    Partner's inability to achieve or maintain erection

Other

46. Have you found it difficult to be honest in answering this questionnaire?
47. Are there any comments you wish to make concerning this questionnaire or the topic covered?

---

a. Each item is followed by a 7-point scale, anchored as shown. In most cases, intermediate points on the scale are identified with labels as well.
b. The four response alternatives provided are *never, rarely, occasionally,* and *usually.*

Senior Adult Sexuality Scales

Estelle Weinstein,[1] *Hofstra University*

The SASS (Senior Adult Sexuality Scales) is a multidimensional measurement instrument suitable for assessing senior adult (60+) sexual attitudes, sexual interests, and a specific set of sexual activities.

Description

The SASS consists of five parts. Part I, the first Biographical Information section, includes 14 questions that gather general descriptive information (see the exhibit).

Part II, the Sexual Attitude Scale, consists of 16 items that address approval or disapproval of various sexually related activities or concepts (e.g., premarital and extramarital sexual activity, abortion, contraception, and masturbation). It is intended to measure the extent to which the sexual orientation of an individual is liberal or conservative.

Part III, the Sexual Interest Scale, refers to a concept of "interest," encompassing a feeling of concern for, desire for, or preference for particular set of sexual activities, whether or not one is a participant. The interest subscales (Experimental and Traditional) were developed as a quantitative measure of the degree of interest in a fairly comprehensive set of sexual activities. The items were selected from a taxonomy of items that represent the range of sexual activities commonly practiced or of interest to middle-aged to older adults.

The Experimental subscale consists of 10 items covering sexual behaviors involving partner choices (e.g., group sex, sex with considerably younger partners, nonmarital sex). The Traditional subscale consists of seven items covering intimate sexual behaviors such as kissing, petting, intercourse, orgasm, and so forth. Interest levels are based on desire for a specific activity if it was readily available whenever one wanted it.

Part IV, the Sexual Activities Scale, was designed to assess the construct *sexual activity*. Sexual activity refers to the wide range of activities or behaviors involved in sexual expression and interaction. This scale was developed to measure a limited range of specific sexual activities such as sexual intercourse, cuddling, petting, sexual initiation, orgasm, and so on.

Part V, Biographical Information II, asks the respondents the degree to which their participation in athletic, social, and sexual activities has changed from their 30s or 40s as compared to now. Also included here are questions that will allow for an identification of the sexual orientation of the sample and/or individual, as well as space for the respondents to comment on the total instrument.

The 68-item preliminary questionnaire was developed from an initial pool of 100 items selected from extant measures applicable to other subpopulations and from colleagues' suggestions. Face validity, clarity, and applicability to the desired constructs were determined by five professionals and five senior adults, who assigned the items to three hypothesized underlying factors (attitudes, interests, activities).

To substantiate that the scales representing the hypothesized factors were psychometrically sound, data from 314 respondents were subjected to a principal axis factor analysis with squared multiple correlation coefficients as initial estimates of communality. The criteria used to determine the number of factors included an examination of the proportion of variance (POV) accounted for, the number of factors with eigenvalues greater than 1, and an assessment of the substantive interpretability of the factors. Solutions were explored with one to six factors. The best solution found was a four-factor solution, accounting for 51% of the common factor variance.

The result of factor analyses performed on the three preliminary scales separately—to determine if any interpretable pattern was being masked by an overall solution—further substantiated acceptance of the combined solution. The existence of the hypothesized constructs was strongly substantiated in that each factor emerged separately. The only modification to the initial expectation is that two factors explaining sexual interest emerged rather than one, hence, the Traditional and Experimental subscales.

The retained solution was rotated orthogonally and obliquely. The oblique solution revealed no meaningful correlations among the factors; thus, the orthogonal solution was used to interpret the factors and to select the final items to be included in the scales and subscales.

Because a minimum criterion of .4 on the factor loadings was considered meaningful or substantial, the items included in the final scales had factor loadings of .4 or more on one factor and less than .4 on all other factors. If two items were redundant, then other theoretical criteria were applied. Each final scale consisted on a homogeneous set of items influenced by one major factor (Alan & Yen, 1979).

Response Mode and Timing

Respondents are instructed to answer the questions by circling an appropriate number or placing a check in a space provided. On the average, 30-40 minutes are required to complete the entire questionnaire.

---
[1]Address correspondence to Estelle Weinstein, Department of Health Studies, Sport Sciences, and Physical Education, Hofstra University, Hempstead, Long Island, NY 11550; email: hprlzs@vaxc.hofstra.edu.

Scoring

Each item on the Sexual Attitude Scale (Part II) is scored on a 7-point scale where 1 = *strongly agree* and 7 = *strongly disagree*. When the entire scale is summed, low scores will represent a more conservative sexual attitude orientation and high scores a more liberal sexual attitude orientation. A liberal or conservative attitude of the group toward a particular item can also be assessed.

Each item on the Sexual Interest Scale (Part III, both Experimental and Traditional subscales) is scored on a 7-point scale where 7 = *very interested* and 1 = *not interested*. All items are worded so that a high score represents a high degree of interest, and a low score represents a low degree of interest. To check for consistency of responses, some items were worded differently, although addressing the same concerns. The items on each subscale can be added and comparisons made between groups. The subscales should be administered as one scale but scored separately because collapsing them into one scale may result in invalid and inappropriate conclusions.

The items on the Sexual Activities Scale (Part IV) are rated in a somewhat new format successfully tested in a major study of teen behavior by the Centers for Disease Control (Kirby, Alter, & Scales, 1979). The question format is, "How often do you . . . ?" The respondent is instructed to fill in the correct number on the line provided as follows:

___ times   ___ times   ___ times   ___ times   ___ never
per day   per week   per month   per year

Applying statistical procedures to the raw data to arrive at the common denominator of weekly, monthly, or yearly participation is necessary for comparisons. When this is completed, the scores can be added. A high number reflects more frequent sexual activity and a low number less frequent sexual activity. Individual items can be examined separately, describing frequency for a particular activity. The total frequency for any one individual or one item is best discussed as a relative comparison to some group or individual. The Sexual Activities Scale should be used by researchers interested only in the quantity of activity.

Reliability

Cronbach's alpha reliability coefficients were calculated for each of the scales of the SASS (Nunnally, 1978). The Sexual Attitude Scale and the Sexual Interest subscales have respectable reliabilities of .87, .90, and .84, respectively. The Sexual Activities Scale has a somewhat lower reliability coefficient of .66.

Validity

Face validity and content validity was substantiated by a professional and senior adult review. Construct validity is strongly confirmed by the results of the factor analysis, as the items in each scale and subscale intercorrelated and loaded separately on the respective factor, with no overlap. The orthogonal solution, as the most appropriate solution to explain the data, showed the distinctness of the factors, which acts as further confirmation of construct validity.

The SASS was used in a study of age-segregated and age-integrated living arrangements of senior adults as they relate to their sexual attitudes, interest, and activities. The data across scales were collected on the SASS and subjected to a discriminant function analysis where significant differences were detected between the groups (Weinstein, 1984). Research of this nature serves to support the construct validity of the scales.

Other Information

The full SASS (preliminary and final versions) is available from Estelle Weinstein.

References

Allen, M. J., & Yen, W. M. (1979). *Introduction to measurement theory*. Monterey, CA: Brooks/Cole.

Kirby, D., Alter, J., & Scales, P. (1979). *An analysis of U.S. sex education programs and evaluation methods*. Springfield, VA: National Technical Information Service.

Nunnally, J. (1978). *Psychometric theory*. New York: McGraw-Hill.

Weinstein, E. (1984). Senior adult sexuality-community living styles. *Dissertation Abstracts International*. (University Microfilms No. 1015, 3)

Weinstein, E., & Rosen, E. (1988). Senior adult sexuality in age-segregated and age-integrated living styles. *International Journal of Aging & Human Development, 27*, 261-270.

Exhibit

Senior Adult Sexuality Scales

Biographical Information I (Part I)

Instructions: Please answer all questions by placing a check or a statement in the appropriate space provided.

1. Marital status:
   Married _____   Remarried _____   Single _____
   Divorced _____   Widowed _____   Separated _____
   Unmarried (living together) _____   Other (specify) _____

2. If remarried:
   More than 10 years _____   Less than 10 years _____
3. How many children do you have?
   None _____   One _____   Two _____   Three _____   Four or more _____
4. Education:
   Completed elementary school _____   Some high school _____
   College graduate _____   Some college _____
   Other (specify) _____   Graduate school _____
5. Religious affiliation:
   Catholic _____   Protestant _____   Jewish _____   Other (specify) _____
6. How religious do you consider yourself?
   Very religious _____   Moderately religious _____
   Somewhat religious _____   Not religious _____
7. State of retirement:
   Fully retired _____   Partially retired _____   Full-time employed _____
8. How would you rate your present state of health?
   Excellent _____   Good _____   Fair _____   Poor _____
9. Lifetime occupation: _____
   (i.e., homemaker, salesperson, executive, lawyer, etc.)
10. Current income from all sources:
    Under $15,000 _____   Between $15-25,000 _____   Between $25-35,000 _____
    Between $35-50,000 _____   Above $50,000 _____
11. Type of community in which you are living more than half of each year:
    Small town _____   Small city _____   Large city _____
    Retirement community _____   Suburban community _____
12. If you checked retirement type community in Question 11, where was the original residence in which you spent the major portion of your working life?
    Small town _____   Small city _____   Large city _____
    Suburban community _____   Other (specify) _____
13. What is your age? _____ years
14. What is your sex? _____ Female _____ Male

Senior Adult Sexuality Scales (SASS) (Part II)

Attitudes–Scale I

1. I think there is too much sexual freedom today.[a]
2. Abortion is a greater evil than bringing an unwanted child into the world.
3. Sexual activity among older single senior citizens is not acceptable behavior.
4. Premarital sexual intercourse is morally wrong.
5. Women should not initiate sexual activity as often as men.
6. Stronger laws should be passed to curb homosexuality.
7. Frequent desire for oral-genital sex is an indicator of an excessive sex drive.
8. Sexual intercourse should only occur between married partners.
9. Masturbation is generally an unhealthy practice.
10. Sexual activity between young adults simply for enjoyment is unacceptable behavior.
11. Men who lose their spouses generally need sexual activity more frequently than women who lose their spouses.
12. Women should not experience sexual intercourse with their mate prior to marriage.
13. I think people are too sexually active today.
14. Laws should be passed to ban pornography.
15. Too much information about sex and contraception is available to young people today.
16. Modern attitudes and morals about sex are responsible for the breakdown in the American family.

Senior Adult Sexuality Scales (SASS) (Part III)

Interest–Scale II

Part A

1. Having sex with someone I have recently met[b]
2. Stimulating my own genitals until climax (ejaculation, orgasm)
3. Having sex with someone other than my spouse or regular mate

4. Having sex with more than one partner at a time (group sex)
5. Having sex with partners considerably younger than myself
6. Watching sex movies
7. Reading sex books or magazines
8. Receiving oral sex to climax (ejaculation, orgasm)
9. Receiving oral sex until partner reaches climax
10. Extramarital sex activity

Part B

1. Kissing, cuddling, touching, petting
2. Having my breasts stroked or kissed
3. Body massage as sex play
4. Having sex in the shower
5. Extended foreplay that leads to intercourse
6. Sex only with someone of the opposite sex
7. Talking about sex with my partner

Senior Adult Sexuality Scales (SASS) (Part IV)

Activities–Scale III

1. How often do you engage in sexual intercourse?
   _____ times per day _____ times per week _____ times per month _____ times per year _____ never[c]
2. How often do you engage in touching, cuddling, petting as foreplay to sexual intercourse?
3. How often do you engage in oral sex as foreplay to sexual intercourse?
4. How often do you reach orgasm (climax)?
5. How often do you use a vibrator or other objects for sexual stimulation with a partner?
6. How often do you initiate (start) sexual activity with your partner?

Senior Adult Sexuality Scales (SASS) (Part V)

Biographical Information II

1. How would you rate your current participation in athletic activities?[d]
2. How would you rate your participation in athletic activities when you were 35-45 years old?
3. How would you rate your current participation in social functions?
4. How would you rate your participation in social functions when you were 35-45 years old?
5. How would you rate your current participation in sexual activities?
6. How would your rate your participation in sexual activities when you were 35-45 years old?
7. How would you rate your current interest in sexual activities, if it were available whenever you wanted it?[e]
8. How would you rate your interest in sexual activity when you were 35-45 years old?
9. How would you rate your current sexual attitudes?[f]
10. How would you rate your sexual attitudes when you were 35-45 years old?
11. (Circle the appropriate statement)
    Do you consider yourself a:
    Heterosexual person—(preference for sexual partner of opposite sex)
    Homosexual person—(preference for sexual partner of same sex)
    Bisexual person—(can prefer sexual partner of either sex)

In the space provided below please comment on any question you may have found difficult to understand, confusing, or offensive in any way. Be sure to include the number of the particular question.

Source. These scales are reprinted with permission of the author.
a. Each item in this section is followed by 7-point *strongly agree-strongly disagree* scales.
b. Each item in this section (both Parts A and B) is followed by 7-point *very interested-not interested* scales.
c. The remaining items in this section are followed by the same response options.
d. Items 1-6 are followed by 7-point *inactive-very active* scales.
e. Items 7 and 8 are followed by 7-point *not interested-very interested* scales.
f. Items 9 and 10 are followed by 7-point *very conservative-very liberal* scales.

Aging Sexual Knowledge and Attitudes Scale

Charles B. White,[1] *Trinity University*

The Aging Sexual Knowledge and Attitudes Scale (ASKAS) is designed to measure two realms of sexuality: (a) knowledge about changes (and nonchanges) in sexual response to advanced age in males and females and (b) general attitudes about sexual activity in older adults. The items are largely specific to elderly persons rather than a general sexual knowledge-attitudes scale. The ASKAS was developed for use in assessing the impact of group or individual interventions on behalf of sexual functioning in older adults using, for example, a pretest-posttest procedure. Furthermore, the measure may form the basis for group and individual discussion about sexual attitudes and sexual knowledge. The scale is also appropriate for use in educational programs for those working with older adults.

The actual numerical scores may be conveniently used for research purposes, but the individual items are also useful to assess the extent of an individual's knowledge on which to base clinical interventions, as well as identifying attitudinal obstacles to sexual intimacy in old age.

Description, Response Mode, and Timing

The ASKAS consists of 61 items, 35 true/false/don't know in format and 26 items responded to on a 7-point Likert-type scale as to degree of agreement or disagreement with the particular item. The 35 true/false questions assess knowledge about sexual changes and nonchanges that are or are not age related. The 26 agree/disagree items assess attitudes toward sexual behavior in older adults. The items are counterbalanced. The instrument takes 20-40 minutes to complete.

Scoring

The ASKAS may be given in an interview or paper-and-pencil format and may be group administered or individually administered. The nature of the scoring and items are readily adaptable to computer-scoring systems.

Scoring is such that a low knowledge score indicates high knowledge, and a low attitude score indicates a more permissive attitude. The rationale for the low knowledge score reflecting high knowledge is that we have given *don't know* a value of 3, indicating low knowledge. In the knowledge section, Questions 1 through 35, the following scoring applies: *true* = 1, *false* = 2, and *don't know* = 3. Items 1, 10, 14, 17, 20, 30, and 31 are reversed scored. In the exhibit, the correct answers are in parentheses for Items 1 through 35. The attitude questions, 36 through 61, are each scored according to the value selected by the respondent

---
[1]Address correspondence to Charles B. White, Department of Psychology, Trinity University, 715 Stadium Drive, San Antonio, TX 78212; email: cwhite@trinity.edu.

with the exception of Items 44, 47, 48, 50-56, and 59, in which the scoring is reversed.

Reliability

The reliability of the ASKAS has been examined in several different studies, and in varying ways, summarized in Table 1. As can be seen, reliabilities are very positive and at acceptable levels.

Table 1 Aging Sexual Knowledge and Attitudes Scale (ASKAS) Reliabilities

Type of reliability	Reliability coefficient	Sample size	Type of sample
		Knowledge	
Split-half[a]	.91	163	Nursing home staff
Split-half[a]	.90	279	Nursing home residents
Alpha	.93	163	Nursing home staff
Alpha	.91	279	Nursing home residents
Alpha	.92	30	Community older adults
Alpha	.90	30	Nursing home staff
Alpha	.90	30	Families of older adults
Test-retest	.97	15	Community older adults
Test-retest	.90	30	Staff of nursing home and families of older adults
		Attitudes	
Split-half[a]	.86	163	Nursing home staff
Split-half[a]	.83	279	Nursing home residents
Alpha	.85	163	Nursing home staff
Alpha	.76	279	Nursing home residents
Alpha	.87	30	Community older adults
Alpha	.87	30	Nursing home staff
Alpha	.86	30	Families of older adults
Test-retest	.96	15	Community older adults
Test-retest	.72	30	Staff of nursing home and families of older adults

a. These correlations have been corrected for test length.

Validity

Presented in Table 2 are the means and standard deviations of ASKAS scores from several studies. These means are not meant to be viewed as normative but rather are illustrative of group variation in ASKAS performance.

The validity of the ASKAS has been examined in a sexual education program for older persons, by individuals working with older persons, and by adult family members of aged persons in which each group received the psychological-educational intervention separately (White & Catania, 1981). Each experimental group had a comparable nonintervention control group. In all cases, the educational intervention resulted in significant increases in knowledge

Table 2 Aging Sexual Knowledge and Attitudes
Scale (ASKAS) Score Means and Standard
Deviations, by Group

Group	n	Mean	SD
Nursing home residents[a]	273		
Attitudes		84.56	23.32
Knowledge		65.62	15.09
Community older adults[b]	30		
Attitudes		86.40	17.28
Knowledge		73.73	12.52
Families of older adults[b]	30		
Attitudes		75.00	22.66
Knowledge		78.00	13.61
Persons who work with older adults[b]	30		
Attitudes		76.00	17.60
Knowledge		62.46	12.50
Nursing home staff[b]	163		
Attitudes		61.08	25.79
Knowledge		64.19	17.25

Note. The possible range of ASKAS scores are as follows: knowledge = 35-105;
attitudes = 26-182. All scores reported here are the pretest scores in cases where
both pretests and posttests were administered.
a. White (1981).
b. White and Catania (1981).

and significant changes in the direction of a more permissive
attitude, both relative to their own pretest scores and relative to the appropriate control group, whereas the control
group posttest scores were not significantly changed relative to their pretest scores. There was a 4- to 6-week period
between pre- and posttests.

Hammond (1979) used the ASKAS in a sexual education
program for professionals working with older adults. She
reported significant changes from pre- to posttest toward
increased knowledge and more permissive attitudes in the
interception group, as in the White and Catania (1981)
research, whereas the control group scores were unchanged
from pre- to posttest.

White (1982a), in a study of nursing home residents in
15 nursing homes, reported that both ASKAS attitude and
knowledge scores were associated with whether an individual was sexually active or not such that more activity was
associated with greater knowledge and with more permissive attitudes.

A factor analysis of the ASKAS results (White, 1982b)
from the studies in Table 2 resulted in a two-factor solution,
with each item loading most heavily on its hypothesized
membership in either the attitude or knowledge section of
the measure.

Other Information

It is requested that all findings using the ASKAS be shared
with the test author.

References

Hammond, D. (1979). *An exploratory study of a workshop on sex and
aging.* Unpublished doctoral dissertation, University of Georgia,
Athens.

White, C. B. (1982a). Interest, attitudes, knowledge, and sexual history
in relation to sexual behavior in the institutionalized aged. *Archives
of Sexual Behavior, 11,* 11-21.

White, C. B. (1982b). A scale for the assessment of attitude and
knowledge regarding sexuality in the aged. *Archives of Sexual Behavior, 11,* 491-502.

White, C. B., & Catania, J. (1981). Sexual education for aged people,
people who work with the aged, and families of aged people.
International Journal of Aging and Human Development, 15, 121-
138.

Exhibit

Aging Sexual Knowledge and Attitudes Scale

Knowledge Questions (Correct answer is shown in parentheses.)

  *1. Sexual activity in aged persons is often dangerous to their health. (F)
        True   False   Don't know[a]
   2. Males over the age of 65 typically take longer to attain an erection of their penis than do younger males. (T)
   3. Males over the age of 65 usually experience a reduction in intensity of orgasm relative to younger males. (T)
   4. The firmness of erection in aged males if often less than that of younger persons. (T)
   5. The older female (65+ years of age) has reduced vaginal lubrication secretion relative to younger females. (T)
   6. The aged female takes longer to achieve adequate vaginal lubrication relative to younger females. (T)
   7. The older female may experience painful intercourse due to reduced elasticity of the vagina and reduced vaginal
        lubrication. (T)
   8. Sexuality is typically a lifelong need. (T)
   9. Sexual behavior in older people (65+) increases the risk of heart attack. (F)
 *10. Most males over the age of 65 are unable to engage in sexual intercourse. (F)
  11. The relatively most sexually active younger people tend to become the relatively most sexually active older people. (T)
  12. There is evidence that sexual activity in older persons has beneficial physical effects on the participants. (T)
  13. Sexual activity may be psychologically beneficial to older person participants. (T)
 *14. Most older females are sexually unresponsive. (F)
  15. The sex urge typically increases with age in males over 65. (F)

16. Prescription drugs may alter a person's sex drive. (T)
*17. Females, after menopause, have a physiological-induced need for sexual activity. (F)
18. Basically, changes with advanced age (65+) in sexuality involve a slowing of response time rather than a reduction of interest in sex. (T)
19. Older males typically experience a reduced need to ejaculate and hence may maintain an erection of the penis for a longer time than younger males. (T)
*20. Older males and females cannot act as sex partners as both need younger partners for stimulation. (F)
21. The most common determinant of the frequency of sexual activity in older couples is the interest or lack of interest of the husband in a sexual relationship with his wife. (T)
22. Barbiturates, tranquilizers, and alcohol may lower the sexual arousal levels of aged persons and interfere with sexual responsiveness. (T)
23. Sexual disinterest in aged persons may be a reflection of a psychological state of depression. (T)
24. There is a decrease in frequency of sexual activity with older age in males. (T)
25. There is a greater decrease in male sexuality with age than there is in female sexuality. (T)
26. Heavy consumption of cigarettes may diminish sexual desire. (T)
27. An important factor in the maintenance of sexual responsiveness in the aging male is the consistency of sexual activity throughout his life. (T)
28. Fear of the inability to perform sexually may bring about an inability to perform sexually in older males. (T)
29. The ending of sexual activity in old age is most likely and primarily due to social and psychological causes rather than biological and physical causes. (T)
*30. Excessive masturbation may bring about an early onset of mental confusion and dementia in the aged. (F)
*31. There is an inevitable loss of sexual satisfaction in post-menopausal women. (F)
32. Secondary impotence (or non-physiologically caused) increases in males over the age of 60 relative to young males. (T)
33. Impotence in aged males may literally be effectively treated and cured in many instances. (T)
34. In the absence of severe physical disability males and females may maintain sexual interest and activity well into their 80s and 90s. (T)
35. Masturbation in older males and females has beneficial effects on the maintenance of sexual responsiveness. (T)

Attitude Questions (7-point Likert-type scale, where *disagree* = 1, *agree* = 7)

36. Aged people have little interest in sexuality. (Aged = 65+ years of age.)
37. An aged person who shows sexual interest brings disgrace to himself/herself.
38. Institutions, such as nursing homes, ought not to encourage or support sexual activity of any sort in their residents.
39. Male and female residents of nursing homes ought to live on separate floors or separate wings of the nursing home.
40. Nursing homes have no obligation to provide adequate privacy for residents who desire to be alone, either by themselves or as a couple.
41. As one becomes older (say, past 65) interest in sexuality inevitably disappears.

For Items 42, 43, and 44:

If a relative of mine, living in a nursing home, was to have a sexual relationship with another resident I would:
42. Complain to the management.
43. Move my relative from this institution.
†44. Stay out of it as it is not my concern.
45. If I knew that a particular nursing home permitted and supported sexual activity in residents who desired such, I would not place a relative in that nursing home.
46. It is immoral for older persons to engage in recreational sex.
†47. I would like to know more about the changes in sexual functioning in older years.
†48. I feel I know all I need to know about sexuality in the aged.
49. I would complain to the management if I knew of sexual activity between any residents of a nursing home.
†50. I would support sex education courses for aged residents of nursing homes.
†51. I would support sex education courses for the staff of nursing homes.
†52. Masturbation is an acceptable sexual activity for older males.
†53. Masturbation is an acceptable sexual activity for older females.
†54. Institutions, such as nursing homes, ought to provide large enough beds for couples who desire such to sleep together.
†55. Staff of nursing homes ought to be trained or educated with regard to sexuality in the aged and/or disabled.
56. Residents of nursing homes ought not to engage in sexual activity of any sort.
†57. Institutions, such as nursing homes, should provide opportunities for the social interaction of men and women.
58. Masturbation is harmful and ought to be avoided.

†59. Institutions, such as nursing homes, should provide privacy such as to allow residents to engage in sexual behavior without fear of intrusion or observation.

60. If family members object to a widowed relative engaging in sexual relations with another resident of a nursing home, it is the obligation of the management and staff to make certain that such sexual activity is prevented.

61. Sexual relations outside the context of marriage are always wrong.

a. These options are repeated for Items 2-35.

*Indicates that the scoring should be reversed such that 2 = 1, and 1 = 2 (i.e., a low score indicates high knowledge).

†Reverse scoring on these items. A low score indicates a permissive attitude.

The Sex Anxiety Inventory

Louis H. Janda,[1] *Old Dominion University*

The Sex Anxiety Inventory (SAI) measures anxiety regarding sexual matters, defined as a generalized expectancy for nonspecific external punishment for the violation of, or the anticipation of violating, perceived normative standards of acceptable sexual behavior. A major goal was to be able to distinguish sexual anxiety from sexual guilt, which Mosher (1965) defined as "a generalized expectancy for self-mediated punishment for violating, anticipating the violation of, or failure to attain internalized standards of proper behavior" (p. 162).

Description

The 25 items on the scale are in a forced-choice format with one alternative representing an anxiety response and the other a nonanxiety response. The form of the scale used by its developers includes 15 filler items. Items were included on the final version of the scale if they met the following criteria: (a) The correlation between the item and the total score of the SAI was significant at the .05 level (two-tailed); (b) the item-total correlation exceeded the correlation between that item and the score on the Sex Guilt subscale of the Mosher Forced-Choice Guilt Inventory; (c) the item-total correlation exceeded the correlation between that item and the score on the Crowne and Marlowe (1964) Social Desirability Scale; and (d) there was no significant difference between the item-total correlations for males and females. Of the 25 items that appear on the scale, only 4

were significantly correlated with social desirability, 2 in the positive direction and 2 in the negative direction. The scale was developed with a college student population.

Response Mode and Timing

The respondents circle the letter of the alternative that comes closest to describing their feelings. The scale rarely requires more than 15 minutes for completion.

Scoring

For Items 2, 3, 5, 6, 8, 11, 12, 13, 14, 15, 17, 22, 24, and 25, alternative "a" is the anxiety response. For the remaining items, alternative "b" is the anxiety response. Each anxiety response is scored as 1 point, resulting in a possible range of scores from 0 to 25.

Reliability

Janda and O'Grady (1980) reported that the internal consistency of the scale (using the Kuder-Richardson formula) was .86. Test-retest reliability, with a time interval of 10 to 14 days, was .85 for males and .84 for females.

Validity

Concurrent validity of the scale has been demonstrated by using it to predict self-reported sexual experiences of both men and women (Janda & O'Grady, 1980).

Other Information

A copy of the scale, complete with filler items, can be obtained at no cost from the author.

[1]Address correspondence to Louis H. Janda, Department of Psychology, Old Dominion University, Norfolk, VA 23508; email: lhj100f@viper.mgb.odu.edu.

References

Crowne, D. P., & Marlowe, D. (1964). *The approval motive: Studies in evaluative dependence.* New York: Wiley.

Janda, L. H., & O'Grady, K. E. (1980). Development of a sex anxiety inventory. *Journal of Consulting and Clinical Psychology, 48,* 169-175.

Mosher, D. L. (1965). Interaction of fear and guilt in inhibiting unacceptable behavior. *Journal of Consulting Psychology, 29,* 161-167.

Exhibit

The Sex Anxiety Inventory

1. Extramarital sex
   a. is OK if everyone agrees.
   b. can break up families.
2. Sex
   a. can cause as much anxiety as pleasure.
   b. on the whole is good and enjoyable.
3. Masturbation
   a. causes me to worry.
   b. can be a useful substitute.
4. After having sexual thoughts
   a. I feel aroused.
   b. I feel jittery.
5. When I engage in petting
   a. I feel scared at first.
   b. I thoroughly enjoy it.
6. Initiating sexual relationships
   a. is a very stressful experience.
   b. causes me no problem at all.
7. Oral sex
   a. would arouse me.
   b. would terrify me.
8. I feel nervous
   a. about initiating sexual relations.
   b. about nothing when it comes to members of the opposite sex.
9. When I meet someone I'm attracted to
   a. I get to know him or her.
   b. I feel nervous.
10. When I was younger
    a. I was looking forward to having sex.
    b. I felt nervous about the prospect of having sex.
11. When others flirt with me
    a. I don't know what to do.
    b. I flirt back.
12. Group sex
    a. would scare me to death.
    b. might be interesting.
13. If in the future I committed adultery
    a. I would probably get caught.
    b. I wouldn't feel bad about it.
14. I would
    a. feel too nervous to tell a dirty joke in mixed company.
    b. tell a dirty joke if it were funny.
15. Dirty jokes
    a. make me feel uncomfortable.
    b. often make me laugh.
16. When I awake from sexual dreams
    a. I feel pleasant and relaxed.
    b. I feel tense.
17. When I have sexual desires
    a. I worry about what I should do.
    b. I do something to satisfy them.
18. If in the future I committed adultery
    a. it would be nobody's business but my own.
    b. I would worry about my spouse's finding out.
19. Buying a pornographic book
    a. wouldn't bother me.
    b. would make me nervous.
20. Casual sex
    a. is better than no sex at all.
    b. can hurt many people.
21. Extramarital sex
    a. is sometimes necessary.
    b. can damage one's career.
22. Sexual advances
    a. leave me feeling tense.
    b. are welcomed.
23. When I have sexual relations
    a. I feel satisfied.
    b. I worry about being discovered.
24. When talking about sex in mixed company
    a. I feel nervous.
    b. I sometimes get excited.
25. If I were to flirt with someone
    a. I would worry about his or her reaction.
    b. I would enjoy it.

Source. This inventory is reprinted with permission of the author.

Sexual Arousability Inventory and Sexual Arousability Inventory–Expanded

Emily Franck Hoon,[1] *University of Florida*
Dianne Chambless, *Center for Psychotherapy Research*

The Sexual Arousability Inventory (SAI) and Sexual Arousability Inventory–Expanded (SAI-E) measure sexual arousability and anxiety. The SAI has clinical utility as it is capable of discriminating between a normal population and individuals seeking therapy for sexual dysfunction (Hoon, Hoon, & Wincze, 1976). The SAI-E can help determine if a client has an arousal dysfunction problem and/or sexual anxiety that may be inhibiting normal functioning. Furthermore, it can help pinpoint which erotic experiences may be problematic. The SAI is sensitive to therapeutic changes (e.g., Murphy, Coleman, Hoon, & Scott, 1980) and can, therefore, help to determine the efficacy of various therapy programs (or components thereof) for a given individual or group(s) of individuals.

The SAI-E is also a valuable research tool for determining the relationship of sexual arousability and anxiety to the characteristics, attitudes, and experiences of respondents (e.g., Burgess & Krop, 1978; Coleman, Hoon, & Hoon, 1983; Hoon & Hoon, 1982) and for investigating underlying dimensions of arousability (Chambless & Lifshitz, 1984; Hoon & Hoon, 1978).

Description

The SAI is a 28-item, self-report inventory measuring perceived arousability to a variety of sexual experiences. The SAI-E is the same inventory rated both on arousability and anxiety dimensions. The two dimensions are uncorrelated, providing independent information.

The SAI is suitable for either heterosexual women or lesbians. The SAI-E is suitable for administration to men or women regardless of sexual orientation or marital status. The items are descriptions of sexual experiences and situations, which are rated along a 7-point Likert-type scale on the basis of (a) how sexually aroused and (b) how anxious the respondent feels (or would feel) when engaged in the described activity. Response options on the arousability dimension range from −1, *adversely affects arousal; unthinkable, repulsive, distracting,* to 5, *always causes sexual arousal; extremely arousing.* Extremes of the anxiety scale are −1, *relaxing, calming,* to 5, *always causes anxiety; extremely anxiety producing.*

When frequent evaluations are desired, alternate forms of the arousability scale are available. Comprised of 14 items, each from the original scale, the shortened versions

of the SAI may be used interchangeably to assess sexual arousability throughout therapy for sexual dysfunction.

Response Mode and Timing

Using a paper-and-pencil format, respondents circle the number indicating their degree of arousal during each of the described activities. They then independently circle the numbers indicating their perceived anxiety during each of the same activities. A card sort format may also be used for individual assessment. The inventory takes an average of 10 minutes to complete by either method. It takes less than 5 minutes to complete the 14-item version.

Scoring

Arousability score is the sum of the arousability ratings (subtracting any −1s). Anxiety score is a sum of anxiety ratings (subtracting −1s). For ease of interpretation, available normative data are presented in Table 1.

Reliability

Arousability, female samples. Reliability information from the original research (Hoon et al., 1976) follows with additional information, as noted. Cronbach alpha coefficients for the original validation (N = 151) and cross-validation (N = 134) samples were .91 and .92, respectively. Spearman-Brown corrected split-half coefficients were .92 for each sample, indicating high internal consistency. A test-retest coefficient on a subsample (n = 48) with an 8-week interval was .69. Split-half reliability was later confirmed by Chambless and Lifshitz (1984), who obtained a Spearman-Brown corrected coefficient of .92 using a sample (N = 252) from another geographic location.

Cumulative percentile norms have remained remarkably consistent. The addition of a sample of women over the age of 25 to the original sample, and subsequent reanalysis of the data, did not appreciably alter the cumulative percentile distribution (M age = 28.4, revised N = 370). Similarly, the distributions obtained from independent samples (Chambless & Lifshitz, 1984) were remarkably similar with two minor differences. A slightly lower average arousability score was obtained from the younger sample (M age = 18.91, N = 252), and a slightly higher average score was obtained from the older sample (M age = 26.26, N = 90) (see Table 1).

Flax (1980) has provided reliability information on the 14-item shortened versions of the arousability scale for women. In a sample of 158 White married women, half

---
[1]Address correspondence to Emily Franck Hoon, 508 NW 35th Terrace, Gainesville, FL 32607; email: rmartin@vector.net

Table 1 Mean Arousability and Anxiety Score on the Sexual Arousability Inventory-Expanded (SAI-E)

| | | M SAI-E | | |
Group	N	score	SD	M age
Arousability				
Heterosexual females				
Validation group	370	82.00	23.30	25.80
Undergraduates	252	78.93	24.84	18.91
Community women	90	99.14	14.27	26.26
Lesbians	371	92.34	14.37	28.20
Heterosexual males	205	90.60	14.70	25.80
Anxiety				
Heterosexual females				
Undergraduates	252	34.34	33.14	18.91
Community women	90	6.36	16.11	26.26

with ileostomies, she obtained Cronbach alpha coefficients of .88 and .86 for Forms A and B, respectively. Test-retest coefficients after a 3-week interval were .97 and .98 ($N = 39$), respectively.

Anxiety, female samples. Split-half reliability was calculated on responses of 252 female undergraduates yielding an excellent corrected reliability coefficient of .94 (Chambless & Lifshitz, 1984). Test-retest data have yet to be collected.

Arousability and anxiety, male samples. Reliability information on the SAI-E and SAI for men is presently unavailable.

Validity

Arousability, female samples. Construct validity has been demonstrated by consistently high correlations with four criterion variables: awareness of physiological changes during sexual arousal, satisfaction with sexual responsiveness, frequency of intercourse, and total episodes of intercourse before marriage (Hoon et al., 1976). Separate factor analyses of the original SAI data and a subsequent independent heterosexual female sample both resulted in five highly interpretable solutions with similar factor loadings on the respective factors (Chambless & Lifshitz, 1984). Factor analysis of SAI data obtained on a sample of lesbians ($N = 407$) resulted in six underlying dimensions, three of which were analogous to factors found on the heterosexual samples. The other three factors were consistent with lesbian sexual practices, one differing in genitally oriented items, another representing oral sex, and the last representing nudity (Coleman et al., 1983).

Burgess and Krop (1978) found a significant correlation between SAI scores and satisfaction with intercourse frequency in heterosexual women ($N = 74$). They also found a significant positive relationship between sexual arousability and heterosexual attitude and significant negative relationships with sexual anxiety and trait anxiety. Trait anxiety was not significantly related to sexual anxiety, which implies that these two forms of anxiety are independent entities.

Discriminant validity has been demonstrated between normal and sexually dysfunctional women, the mean score of the latter falling at the 5th percentile of the former (Hoon et al., 1976). Significant and theoretically interpretable response differences to specific items have been found according to sex (Hoon & Hoon, 1977), experience with cohabitation (Hoon & Hoon, 1982), orientation (Coleman et al., 1983), and distinct styles of sexual expression (Hoon & Hoon, 1978).

Anxiety, female samples. Validation of the anxiety scale is in the initial stages, but available data are encouraging. Validity data were collected on two samples of women by Chambless and Lifshitz (1984), who predicted the anxiety scale should be negatively correlated with frequency of orgasm and with greater sexual experience. In the undergraduate sample ($N = 252$), the more sexually experienced were found to be significantly less anxious (tau = $-.14$), and in a sample of community women ($N = 90$), higher frequency of coital orgasm was significantly associated with lower anxiety (tau = $-.25$).

A principal components analysis with oblique rotation was conducted on the undergraduate responses. Three interpretable factors, accounting for 61% of the variance, were extracted. Factor 1 (45%) and Factor 3 (5%) were similar in being general factors defined more by their exclusion of pornography and masturbation than by items they included. Factor 1, however, seemed more related to intercourse and foreplay, whereas Factor 3 was weighted more heavily with items concerning noncoital genital stimulation. Factor 2 (12%) concerned pornography and masturbation. These factors are similar in content to three of those on the arousability scale, indicating these may be consistent dimensions of sexual stimuli. The two factors pertaining to partner sex were modestly negatively correlated with the masturbation factor.

Arousability and anxiety, male samples. Validity information on the SAI-E and SAI is presently unavailable.

Other Information

Samples of the measure, factor analytic information, item means, and standard deviation are available from the first author.

References

Burgess, D., & Krop, H. (1978, October). *The relationship between sexual arousability, heterosexual attitudes, sexual anxiety, and general anxiety in women.* Paper presented at the South East Regional American Association of Sex Educators, Counselors and Therapists, Asheville, NC.

Chambless, D. L., & Lifshitz, J. L. (1984). Self-reported sexual anxiety and arousal: The Expanded Sexual Arousability Inventory. *The Journal of Sex Research, 20,* 241-254.

Coleman, E., Hoon, P. W., & Hoon, E. F. (1983). Arousability and sexual satisfaction in lesbian and heterosexual women. *The Journal of Sex Research, 19,* 58-73.

Flax, C. C. (1980). *Comparison between married women with ileostomies and married women without ileostomies on sexual anxiety, control, arousability and fantasy.* Unpublished doctoral dissertation, New York University, New York.

Hoon, E. F., & Hoon, P. W. (1977, September). *Sexual differences between males and females on a self-report measure.* Paper presented at the Fifth Annual Canadian Sex Research Forum, Banff, Alberta.

Hoon, E. F., & Hoon, P. W. (1978). Styles of sexual expression in women: Clinical implications of multivariate analyses. *Archives of Sexual Behavior, 7,* 106-116.

Hoon, E. F., Hoon, P. W., & Wincze, J. P. (1976). The SAI: An inventory for the measurement of female sexual arousability. *Archives of Sexual Behavior, 5,* 291-300.

Hoon, P. W., & Hoon, E. F. (1982). Effects of experience in cohabitation on erotic arousability. *Psychological Reports, 50,* 255-258.

Murphy, W., Coleman, E., Hoon, E. F., & Scott, C. (1980). Sexual dysfunction and treatment in alcoholic women. *Sexuality and Disability, 3,* 240-255.

Exhibit

Sexual Arousability Inventory

Instructions: The experiences in this inventory may or may not be sexually arousing to you. There are no right or wrong answers. Read each item carefully, and then circle the number which indicates how sexually aroused you feel when you have the described experience, or how sexually aroused you think you would feel if you actually experienced it. *Be sure to answer every item.* If you aren't certain about an item, circle the number that seems about right. Rate feelings of arousal according to the scale below.

   −1 Adversely affects arousal; unthinkable, repulsive, distracting
    0 Doesn't affect sexual arousal
    1 Possibly causes sexual arousal
    2 Sometimes causes sexual arousal; slightly arousing
    3 Usually causes sexual arousal; moderately arousing
    4 Almost always sexually arousing; very arousing
    5 Always causes sexual arousal; extremely arousing

*   1. When a loved one stimulates your genitals with mouth and tongue[a]
*   2. When a loved one fondles your breasts with his/her hands
   3. When you see a loved one nude
   4. When a loved one caresses you with his/her eyes
*   5. When a loved one stimulates your genitals with his/her finger
*   6. When you are touched or kissed on the inner thighs by a loved one
   7. When you caress a loved one's genitals with your fingers
   8. When you read a pornographic or "dirty" story
*   9. When a loved one undresses you
*10. When you dance with a loved one
*11. When you have intercourse with a loved one
*12. When a loved one touches or kisses your nipples
 13. When you caress a loved one (other than genitals)
*14. When you see pornographic pictures or slides
*15. When you lie in bed with a loved one
*16. When a loved one kisses you passionately
 17. When you hear sounds of pleasure during sex
*18. When a loved one kisses you with an exploring tongue
*19. When you read suggestive or pornographic poetry
 20. When you see a strip show
 21. When you stimulate your partner's genitals with your mouth and tongue
 22. When a loved one caresses you (other than genitals)
 23. When you see a pornographic movie (stag film)
 24. When you undress a loved one
 25. When a loved one fondles your breasts with mouth and tongue
*26. When you make love in a new or unusual place
 27. When you masturbate
 28. When your partner has an orgasm

Note. Asterisks indicate those items comprising shortened Form A. Form B consists of items without asterisks.

a. The seven response options are repeated following each item.

Sexual Anxiety Inventory

Now rate each of the items according to how anxious you feel when you have the described experience. The meaning of anxiety is extreme uneasiness, distress. Rate feelings of anxiety according to the scale below.

- −1 Relaxing, calming
- 0 No anxiety
- 1 Possibly causes some anxiety
- 2 Sometimes causes anxiety; slightly anxiety producing
- 3 Usually causes anxiety; moderately anxiety producing
- 4 Almost always causes anxiety; very anxiety producing
- 5 Always causes anxiety; extremely anxiety producing

1. When a loved one stimulates your genitals with mouth and tongue[a]
2. When a loved one fondles your breasts with his/her hands
3. When you see a loved one nude
4. When a loved one caresses you with his/her eyes
5. When a loved one stimulates your genitals with his/her finger
6. When you are touched or kissed on the inner thighs by a loved one
7. When you caress a loved one's genitals with your fingers
8. When you read a pornographic or "dirty" story
9. When a loved one undresses you
10. When you dance with a loved one
11. When you have intercourse with a loved one
12. When a loved one touches or kisses your nipples
13. When you caress a loved one (other than genitals)
14. When you see pornographic pictures or slides
15. When you lie in bed with a loved one
16. When a loved one kisses you passionately
17. When you hear sounds of pleasure during sex
18. When a loved one kisses you with an exploring tongue
19. When you read suggestive or pornographic poetry
20. When you see a strip show
21. When you stimulate your partner's genitals with your mouth and tongue
22. When a loved one caresses you (other than genitals)
23. When you see a pornographic movie (stag film)
24. When you undress a loved one
25. When a loved one fondles your breasts with mouth and tongue
26. When you make love in a new or unusual place
27. When you masturbate
28. When your partner has an orgasm

---

a. The seven response options are repeated following each item.

Multiple Indicators of Subjective Sexual Arousal

Donald L. Mosher,[1] *University of Connecticut*

Three self-report measures of subjective sexual arousal were developed to serve as standard measures. Construction of the measures was designed to permit comparison of male and female subjective sexual arousal. To secure more uniform measurement across laboratories, item selection and analysis were guided by past research and theory, and careful attention was paid to the psychometric properties of the measures. From the perspective of involvement theory (Mosher, 1980), *subjective sexual arousal* is defined as a specific *affect-cognition* blend, in consciousness, of physiological sexual arousal with its accompanying sexual affects. The multiple indicators of self-reported sexual arousal were derived from past research that had variously used Likert-type rating scales (Jakobovits, 1965; Mosher & Abramson, 1977; Schmidt & Sigusch, 1970), adjective checklists (Mosher & Abramson, 1977; Mosher & Greenberg, 1969), and a checklist of genital sensations (Mosher & Abramson, 1977; Schmidt & Sigusch, 1970). Mosher, Barton-Henry, and Green (1988) developed the three measures of subjective sexual arousal presented here.

Descriptions and Scoring

Ratings of Sexual Arousal consist of the five items, selected from a pool of 11 items, yielding the highest alpha coefficients across self-reports to four types of erotic fantasies. The five items selected were sexual arousal, genital sensations, sexual warmth, nongenital physical sensations, and sexual absorption. Each item is further defined: for example, "Sexual Warmth—a subjective estimate of the amount of sexual warmth experienced in the genitals, breasts, and body as a function of increasing vasocongestion (i.e., engorgement with blood)." If a sixth item is desired, the next best item is "Sexual Tension—a subjective estimate of the sexual tension that presses toward release." A 7-point Likert-type format is used to rate the items with anchors of, for example, 1, *no sexual arousal at all*, to 7, *extremely sexually aroused*. This measure is appropriate for educated populations of men and women. The definitions of the concepts include technical vocabulary.

Respondents receive these instructions: "For each item, place a circle around the number that best describes how you felt during the experience." Average completion time is 2 minutes. Scores are summed, and a mean item score can be calculated. Higher scores indicate more subjective sexual arousal.

Affective Sexual Arousal consists of five adjective prompts selected from a pool of 10 items embedded in a 70-item adjective checklist patterned after the Differential Emotions Scale (Izard, Dougherty, Bloxom, & Kotsch, 1974; Mosher & White, 1981). The adjective prompts that were included, following the item analysis across the four erotic fantasies, were sexually aroused, sensuous, turned-on, sexually hot, and sexually excited. If a sixth item is needed, it should be "sexy." Each adjective prompt was rated on a 5-point Likert-type scale as follows: 1, *very slightly or not at all;* 2, *slightly;* 3, *moderately;* 4, *considerably;* and 5, *very strongly.* This measure of subjective sexual arousal contains standard and slang vocabulary understandable by both men and women, but it probably should be embedded within an affect adjective checklist.

Respondents answer by circling the number that best describes "how they felt during the experience." Completion time can be estimated at 10 items per minute if embedded in a larger affect checklist. Scores are summed across the five items, and a mean item score can be computed. Higher scores indicate more subjective sexual arousal.

Genital Sensations is an 11-item checklist modified from earlier versions of self-reports of genital sensations (Mosher & Abramson, 1977; Schmidt & Sigusch, 1970) by placing the items in an ordinal order and by writing brief descriptions of the genital sensations and bodily responses. The 11 items are as follows: no genital sensations, onset of genital sensations, mild genital sensations, moderate genital sensations, prolonged moderate genital sensations, intense genital sensations, prolonged intense genital sensations, mild orgasm, moderate orgasm, intense orgasm, and multiple orgasm. An example of the definitions given is "(4) Moderate genital sensations—vasocongestion sufficient to erect penis fully or to lubricate vagina fully." The vocabulary is appropriate for educated populations, but the arrangement into an ordered scale educates and helps a less educated group to respond.

Respondents check the peak or highest level of genital sensations experienced during the experience and, thus, achieve a score of 1 to 11. The measure requires 2 to 3 minutes to complete.

Reliability

Cronbach alpha coefficients for the two 5-item measures—Ratings of Sexual Arousal and Affective Sexual Arousal—in a sample of 120 male and 121 female college students, as measured across four fantasy conditions, ranged from .92 to .97 and were robust across erotic conditions (Mosher et al., 1988). Median Cronbach alpha coefficients for Ratings of Sexual Arousal were .97 and for Affective Sexual Arousal were .96.

Validity

Evidence of convergent validity between the measures when cast into an intercorrelation matrix was strong, with

[1]Address correspondence to Donald L. Mosher, 5051 North A1a, PH1-1, North Hutchinson Island, FL 34949; email: dlmosher@aol.com

a median validity coefficient—same scale across erotic conditions—of .52. Intercorrelations of the three measures of subjective sexual arousal within an erotic condition revealed median intercorrelations of approximately .81 for Ratings of Sexual Arousal with Affective Sexual Arousal, .74 for Ratings of Sexual Arousal with Sensations, and .69 for Affective Sexual Arousal with Genital Sensations (Mosher et al., 1988). Further evidence of construct validity is available in the body of literature cited above that used similar measures.

References

Izard, C. E., Dougherty, F. E., Bloxom, B. M., & Kotsch, W. E. (1974). *The Differential Emotions Scale: A method of measuring the subjective experience of discrete emotions.* Unpublished manuscript, Department of Psychology, Vanderbilt University.

Jakobovits, L. (1965). Evaluational reactions to erotic literature. *Psychological Reports, 16,* 985-994.

Mosher, D. L. (1980). Three dimensions of depth of involvement in human sexual response. *The Journal of Sex Research, 16,* 1-42.

Mosher, D. L. (1984). *Sexual desire in involvement theory: Sexual motivators.* Unpublished manuscript.

Mosher, D L., & Abramson, P. R. (1977). Subjective sexual arousal to films of masturbation. *Journal of Consulting and Clinical Psychology, 35,* 796-807.

Mosher, D. L., Barton-Henry, M., & Green, S. E. (1988). Subjective sexual arousal and involvement theory: Development of multiple indicators. *The Journal of Sex Research, 25,* 412-425.

Mosher, D. L., & Greenberg, I. (1969). Females affective responses to reading erotic literature. *Journal of Consulting and Clinical Psychology, 33,* 472-477.

Mosher, D. L., & White, B. B. (1981). On differentiating shame from shyness. *Motivation and Emotions, 5,* 61-74.

Schmidt, G., & Sigusch, V. (1970). Sex differences in responses to psychosexual stimulation by films and slides. *The Journal of Sex Research, 6,* 268-283.

Exhibit

Ratings of Sexual Arousal

Instructions: For each item, place a circle around one number that best described how you felt during the experience.

1. Sexual Arousal—a subjective estimate of your overall level of sexual arousal.

     1   2   3   4   5   6   7
   No sexual   Extremely
   arousal at all   sexually aroused

2. Genital Sensations—a subjective estimate of the amount and quality of sensation experienced in your genitals.

     1   2   3   4   5   6   7
   No sensation   Extreme
   at all   genital sensation

3. Sexual Warmth—a subjective estimate of the amount of sexual warmth experienced in the genitals, breasts, and body as a function of increasing vasocongestion, i.e., engorgement with blood.

     1   2   3   4   5   6   7
   No sexual   Extreme
   warmth at all   sexual warmth

4. Non-Genital Physical Sensations—a subjective estimate of the physical sensations such as tickling, floating, or fullness that accompany your experience of sexual arousal.

     1   2   3   4   5   6   7
   No sensation   Extreme non-genital
   at all   physical sensation

5. Sexual Absorption—a subjective estimate of your level of absorption in the sensory components of the experience.

     1   2   3   4   5   6   7
   No absorption   Extreme
   at all   absorption

Ratings of Affective Sexual Arousal

Instructions:[a] This scale consists of a number of words that describe different emotions or feelings. Please indicate the extent to which each word describes the way you felt during the preceding experiences. Record your answers by indicating the appropriate number on the five-point scale on the attached answer sheet. Presented below is the scale for indicating the degree to which each word describes the way you feel.

1	2	3	4	5
Very slightly	Slightly	Moderately	Considerably	Very strongly

In deciding on your answer to a given item or word, consider the feeling connoted or defined by that word. Then, if during the experience you felt that way *very slightly* or *not at all,* you would darken the blank under the number 1 on the scale; if you felt that way to a *moderate* degree, you would darken the blank under 3; if you felt that way *very strongly,* you would darken the circle under 5, and so forth.

Remember, you are requested to make your responses on the basis of the way you felt during the experience. Work at a good pace. It is not necessary to ponder; the first answer you decide on for a given word is probably the most valid. It should not take more than a few minutes to complete the scale.

Items:
1. Sexually aroused
2. Sensuous
3. Turned-on
4. Sexually hot
5. Sexually excited

Ratings of Genital Sensations

Instructions: Genital sensations refer to sensory sensations in the genital region that accompany any source of somatogenic or psychogenic sexual stimulation and that are a function of increasing vasocongestion in the genital area. Males experience these sensations as accompaniments of penile erections and females experience these sensations as a function of the engorgement of the labia and the orgasmic platform in the vagina with accompanying vaginal lubrication. Below, indicate the peak level of genital sensation that you felt during the experience. The items are:

_____ 1. No genital sensations.
_____ 2. Onset of genital sensations—onset of swelling of penis or vulva or nipple erection.
_____ 3. Mild genital sensations—vascongestion sufficient to begin penile erection or to begin vaginal lubrication.
_____ 4. Moderate genital sensations—vasocongestion sufficient to erect penis fully or to lubricate vagina fully.
_____ 5. Prolonged moderate genital sensations—maintain erection for several minutes or considerable vaginal lubrication for several minutes.
_____ 6. Intense genital sensations—hard or pulsing erection and elevation of testicles in the scrotum; or receptive, engorged vagina or sex flush, or breast swelling or retraction of clitoris or ballooning of vagina.
_____ 7. Prolonged intense genital sensations—near orgasmic levels of genital sensations; swelling of head of penis or high levels of muscular tension or heavy breathing or high heart rate; lasting several minutes and will produce orgasm if continued.
_____ 8. Mild orgasm—mild orgasmic release, slow reduction of vasocongestion, 3-5 contractions.
_____ 9. Moderate orgasm—moderate orgasmic release, average time to resolution of vasocongestion, 5-8 contractions.
_____ 10. Intense orgasm—intense orgasmic release with rapid resolution of vasocongestion, 8-12 contractions.
_____ 11. Multiple orgasm—repeated orgasmic release in a single sexual episode.

a. These instructions assume the five sexual prompts are embedded within a longer affect adjective checklist.

Hurlbert Index of Sexual Assertiveness

David F. Hurlbert,[1] *Adult and Adolescent Counseling Center*

The Hurlbert Index of Sexual Assertiveness (HISA) is described by Hurlbert (1991).

[1]Address correspondence to David F. Hurlbert, Adult and Adolescent Counseling Center, 619 North Main, Belton, TX 76513.

Reference

Hurlbert, D. F. (1991). The role of assertiveness in female sexuality: A comparative study between sexually assertive and sexually nonassertive women. *Journal of Sex & Marital Therapy, 17,* 183-190.

Exhibit

Hurlbert Index of Sexual Assertiveness

This inventory is designed to measure the degree of sexual assertiveness you have in the sexual relationship with your partner. This is not a test, so there are no right or wrong answers. Please answer each item as accurately as you can by placing a number by each question as follows:

> 0 = All of the time
> 1 = Most of the time
> 2 = Some of the time
> 3 = Rarely
> 4 = Never

1. I feel uncomfortable talking during sex.
2. I feel that I am shy when it comes to sex.
3. I approach my partner for sex when I desire it.
4. I think I am open with my partner about my sexual needs.
5. I enjoy sharing my sexual fantasies with my partner.
6. I feel uncomfortable talking to my friends about sex.
7. I communicate my sexual desires to my partner.
8. It is difficult for me to touch myself during sex.
9. It is hard for me to say no even when I do not want sex.
10. I am reluctant to describe myself as a sexual person.
11. I feel uncomfortable telling my partner what feels good.
12. I speak up for my sexual feelings.
13. I am reluctant to insist that my partner satisfy me.
14. I find myself having sex when I do not really want it.
15. When a technique does not feel good, I tell my partner.
16. I feel comfortable giving sexual praise to my partner.
17. It is easy for me to discuss sex with my partner.
18. I feel comfortable in initiating sex with my partner.
19. I find myself doing sexual things that I do not like.
20. Pleasing my partner is more important than my pleasure.
21. I feel comfortable telling my partner how to touch me.
22. I enjoy masturbating myself to orgasm.
23. If something feels good, I insist on doing it again.
24. It is hard for me to be honest about my sexual feelings.
25. I try to avoid discussing the subject of sex.

Source. This inventory was originally published in "The Role of Assertiveness in Female Sexuality: A Comparative Study Between Sexually Assertive and Sexually Nonassertive Women," by D. F. Hurlbert, 1991, *Journal of Sex & Marital Therapy, 17,* 183-190. Reprinted with permission.

Note. Reverse-score item numbers: 3, 4, 5, 7, 12, 15, 16, 17, 18, 21, 22, and 23.

Intimate Relationships Questionnaire

Georgia Yesmont,[1] *Hofstra University*

The Intimate Relationships Questionnaire (IRQ) was created to measure assertive, nonassertive, and aggressive tendencies specific to safer-sex behaviors in unmarried adolescents and young adults (Yesmont, 1992b). The AIDS epidemic has highlighted the serious health problems created by less fatal, yet more prevalent, sexually transmitted diseases (STDs). The rates of STDs are highest in the young adult population. The IRQ is a convenient and promising measure that is easily incorporated into assertiveness training to increase safer-sex behaviors and reduce the incidence of STDs. The IRQ offers a structured format that can be used in an individual or group setting, or with couples. It may be used in conjunction with role-play and rehearsal of precautionary behaviors and to identify those aspects of safer-sex behaviors that are especially difficult for respondents.

Description

The IRQ consists of 10 items, each with three response alternatives that measure assertive, nonassertive, and aggressive tendencies. The items describe intimate situations involving the precautionary behaviors of condom use, asking a date about his (her) STD history, asking about prior AIDS testing, and wanting to know a date better before engaging in sexual intercourse. The assertive, nonassertive, and aggressive responses are randomly sequenced throughout the items. There are an additional four items (1, 3, 5, and 8), pertaining to nonsexual intimate situations that are included as detractors. The IRQ items present the three types of responses in a 5-point Likert-type scale, from 1, *not at all like me,* to 5, *just like me.* Respondents are asked to rate each alternative according to their own probable cognitive or behavioral response in each scenario.

The precautionary sex situations were inspired by recent research in AIDS-prevention programs (Kelly, St. Lawrence, Hood, & Brasfield, 1989; Rotheram-Borus & Koopman, 1989). The assertive, nonassertive, and aggressive response alternatives were formulated from the most universally accepted definitions of these terms (Alberti & Emmons, 1986).

In a content validation procedure, a panel of clinicians rated the three response alternatives according to the given definitions of the three assertiveness dimensions. Further revisions resulted in the present content that had been unanimously rated by a second group of clinicians, according to the intended conceptualizations of assertiveness.

Although the IRQ was normed on predominantly heterosexual college students, its gender-nonspecific format renders it useful for individuals with other sexual orientations.

Response Mode and Timing

Respondents circle the number from 1 to 5 on each of the three alternatives to every test item, according to their self-perceived similarity to the proposed response. The IRQ requires approximately 10 minutes to complete.

Scoring

The numerical values of the Likert-type choices (1 to 5) are summed for each assertiveness dimension (assertiveness, nonassertiveness, and aggression) according to the response key. The answers to the detractor items (1, 3, 5 and 8) are not added into the score. The score range is from 10 to 50, with larger sums representing a stronger response tendency. Correlational analysis of the IRQ assertiveness dimensions revealed a significantly positive relationship between assertive and aggressive scores, $r = .15$, and a significantly negative relationship between assertiveness and nonassertiveness, $r = -.21$ (Yesmont, 1992a). Nonassertive and aggressive scores were unrelated.

Reliability

In a sample of 253 unmarried, predominantly White undergraduates (159 females, 94 males), the Cronbach alphas for the three assertiveness categories on the safer-sex questions were as follows: assertiveness, .77; aggressiveness, .67; and nonassertiveness, .71 (Yesmont, 1992b). Using a Spanish version of the IRQ, Batista (1995) reported similar alpha coefficients in a sample of 103 older high school students in Puerto Rico (assertiveness, .76; aggressiveness, .76; and nonassertiveness, .76).

Validity

In the Yesmont (1992b) study, the college students' IRQ assertiveness scores were significantly correlated with their degree of using Caution in a new, intimate relationship ($r = .35$) and Asking (inquiry about drug use, STD history, prior contact with high-risk partners, and AIDS testing; $r = .36$). Their aggressiveness scores also were significantly related to Caution, $r = .22$, and Asking, $r = .19$. As predicted, the students' nonassertiveness scores correlated negatively and significantly with their degree of Caution ($r = -.41$) and Asking ($r = -.34$).

IRQ assertiveness was significantly correlated to the percentage of time that condoms were used for coitus, $r = .24$. IRQ nonassertiveness had a significantly negative relationship to condom use, as expected, $r = -.25$.

The students who reported 100% condom use, as compared to nonusers, had higher assertiveness scores ($M = 35.01$ vs. $M = 33.74$), $t(87) = -2.17$, $p < .05$, and significantly lower nonassertiveness scores ($M = 14.65$ vs. $M = 19.53$), $t(85) = 4.95$, $p < .001$. The females were signifi-

---

[1] Address correspondence to Georgia Yesmont, Department of Psychology, Hofstra University, Hempstead, NY 11550.

cantly more assertive and aggressive on the IRQ than the males. Conversely, the males endorsed nonassertive responses to a significantly greater extent than the females.

References

Alberti, R. E., & Emmons, M. L. (1986). *Your perfect right: A guide to assertive living.* San Luis Obispo, CA: Impact.

Batista, N. (1995). *The design and evaluation of a counseling intervention program in sexual assertiveness in adolescents.* Unpublished doctoral dissertation. University of Puerto Rico, Rio Piedras.

Kelly, J. A., St. Lawrence, J. S., Hood, H. V., & Brasfield, T. L. (1989). Behavioral intervention to reduce AIDS risk activities. *Journal of Counseling and Clinical Psychology, 57,* 60-67.

Rotheram-Borus, M. J., & Koopman, C. (1989, January). *Research on AIDS prevention among runaways: The state of the art and recommendations for the future.* Paper presented at the National Institute of Child Health and Human Development Technical Review and Research Planning Meeting on Adolescents and HIV Infection, Bethesda, MD.

Yesmont, G. (1992a, April). *The development of the Intimate Relationships Questionnaire.* Paper presented at the annual meeting of the Eastern Psychological Association, Boston.

Yesmont, G. (1992b). The relationship of assertiveness to college students' safer sex behaviors. *Adolescence, 27,* 253-272.

Exhibit

Intimate Relationships Questionnaire

Each item below describes a situation and three responses that are thoughts or behaviors. These intimate situations involve a dating couple. Try to imagine a situation in your life that is as close to the one described as possible.

After reading each item, circle a number to the right of each response, indicating how similar it might be to the thought you might have or the behavior you might show, in the actual situation.

Please rate every response to each situation. Use the following scale for your ratings:

1	2	3	4	5
Not at all like me	Slightly like me	Somewhat like me	Mostly like me	Just like me

1. During the past few weeks your boyfriend (girlfriend) seems less enthusiastic and caring about your relationship.
   - (AG)[a] a. You'll decide to confront him (her) on your next date and let out your angry feelings. 1 2 3 4 5
   - (NON) b. You'll wait for him (her) to call you and you'll complain to your friends. 1 2 3 4 5
   - (AS) c. You'll decide to speak to him (her) frankly and suggest you try to work things out. 1 2 3 4 5
2. When your date says he (she) won't have sex with you if you insist on using a condom, you say . . .
   - (AS) a. O.K. Then how about trying some other things besides intercourse? 1 2 3 4 5
   - (AG) b. Your attitude doesn't make any sense! That's it for us. Let's go home. 1 2 3 4 5
   - (NON) c. O.K. You're more important to me, we don't need to use it. 1 2 3 4 5
3. You're at a party with your boyfriend (girlfriend) and notice that he (she) is very attentive to someone of the opposite sex that you've never seen before. You think . . .
   - (NON) a. I'll make the best of it—after all, he's (she's) going home with me tonight. 1 2 3 4 5
   - (AS) b. I really would like more of his (her) attention tonight and I'm going to tell him (her). 1 2 3 4 5
   - (AG c. How could he (she) ignore me like this—I'll find someone on my own I can talk to and make him (her) jealous. 1 2 3 4 5
4. You want to tell your date that you'd like to use a condom when making love tonight and you think . . .
   - (AS) a. If I can't convince him (her) to use a condom tonight, we can find other safe ways of enjoying ourselves for now. 1 2 3 4 5
   - (NON) b. Using a condom is a good idea but I don't think I have the nerve to ask him (her) to use one. 1 2 3 4 5
   - (AG) c. He (she) should do what I ask without any hesitation if he (she) loves me. 1 2 3 4 5
5. Your boyfriend (girlfriend) gets silent instead of saying what's on his (her) mind. You think . . .
   - (AG) a. Here it comes. The big silent treatment. I'm going to get mad and force him (her) to talk to me. 1 2 3 4 5
   - (NON) b. If I make a joke and distract him (her), maybe he'll (she'll) forget what's bothering him (her). 1 2 3 4 5

(AS)   c.   I'll tell him (her) it bothers me when he (she) gets silent because it leaves me confused about what he's (she's) thinking.   1 2 3 4 5

6. When you're asked by your date if you have any disease that you could give him (her) if you make love that night, you think . . .

   (AG)   a.   Who does he (she) think I am—some degenerate who runs around infecting people?   1 2 3 4 5

   (AS)   b.   I'm glad he (she) asked because it gives me a chance to ask the same question.   1 2 3 4 5

   (NON)   c.   I'd better answer or he (she) may get annoyed with me.   1 2 3 4 5

7. When your date asks you if you agree to using a condom when you both make love tonight, you think . . .

   (AG)   a.   This is a turn-off. I don't want anybody telling me what we should do when we make love.   1 2 3 4 5

   (NON)   b.   I'd better do what he (she) says or he'll (she'll) be frustrated tonight.   1 2 3 4 5

   (AS)   c.   I'm glad he (she) brought this up, now we're both protected.   1 2 3 4 5

8. Your boyfriend (girlfriend) has criticized your appearance in front of your friends. You say . . .

   (AS)   a.   It hurt my feelings when you criticized me. If you have something to say, please bring it up before we go out.   1 2 3 4 5

   (AG)   b.   How could you do such a rotten thing to me? If you do that again— we're through!   1 2 3 4 5

   (NON)   c.   I guess I don't look so great tonight since you criticized me in front of my friends.   1 2 3 4 5

9. When you suggest to your date that you both use a condom when you make love tonight, your date teases you about being such a worrier.

   (NON)   a.   You then become silent for a while, until he (she) comes around to agreeing with you.   1 2 3 4 5

   (AS)   b.   You then tell your date you'd love to make love with him (her), but you always use condoms.   1 2 3 4 5

   (AG)   c.   You then tell your date he's (she's) being really immature.   1 2 3 4 5

10. You want to ask if your date's been tested for AIDS and you say . . .

   (NON)   a.   I was wondering about . . . well, this is embarrassing to talk about . . . but . . . have you ever been tested for AIDS? You don't have to answer that if you don't want to.   1 2 3 4 5

   (AG)   b.   I want you to tell me right now if you've been tested for AIDS.   1 2 3 4 5

   (AS)   c.   I really like you a lot, but with all this talk about AIDS, I'd like to be a little careful. I've been tested for AIDS, have you?   1 2 3 4 5

11. If your date refuses to use a condom you think . . .

   (AS)   a.   I can find out what he (she) has against them and we can talk about it.   1 2 3 4 5

   (NON)   b.   I'm afraid he (she) won't want to see me again if I insist.   1 2 3 4 5

   (AG)   c.   If he (she) won't do what I say—that's it for us.   1 2 3 4 5

12. When neither you nor your date has any condoms one evening, you say . . .

   (NON)   a.   Oh . . . that's O.K. I suppose we can do it just once without one.   1 2 3 4 5

   (AG)   b.   That's irresponsible. If you like me you'd always have them when we're together.   1 2 3 4 5

   (AS)   c.   I don't have any either, but we can satisfy each other without intercourse tonight.   1 2 3 4 5

13. You tell your date that you'd like to wait until you know each other a little better before having sex. When he (she) gets annoyed you would . . .

   (AG)   a.   Tell your date that you couldn't go out with someone who argues with you about this.   1 2 3 4 5

   (AS)   b.   Re-state your feeling that you'd like to wait.   1 2 3 4 5

   (NON)   c.   Change your mind and have sex with him (her) sooner than you'd planned.   1 2 3 4 5

14. When you suggest to your date that you both use a condom when you make love tonight, he (she) says, "You don't trust me. I told you I've never been exposed to AIDS or herpes, or any other disease."

   (AS)   a.   You say, "I'm sorry, but we have no way of knowing that. I'd feel so much better if we used condoms."   1 2 3 4 5

   (AG)   b.   You say, "It's not a question of trust. You don't understand what I'm saying."   1 2 3 4 5

   (NON)   c.   You say, "I'm sorry. I do trust you. Let's drop the whole subject. I don't want to argue."   1 2 3 4 5

Source. This questionnaire was originally published in "The Relationship of Assertiveness to College Students' Safer Sex Behaviors," by G. Yesmont, 1992, *Adolescence, 27,* 253-272. Reprinted with permission.

a. Response classification: AG = aggressive; AS = assertive; NON = nonassertive.

Sexual Attitudes and Behavior

The Editors

This 100-item questionnaire, developed by Athanasiou and Sarkin (1974), covers a variety of sexuality-related attitude areas, including romance and liberal versus conservative sexual stances. It also includes a section on sexual behaviors and their frequency. The instrument appears in Athanasiou and Shaver (1969).

References

Athanasiou, R., & Sarkin, R. (1974). Premarital sexual behavior and postmarital adjustment. *Archives of Sexual Behavior, 3,* 207-225.

Athanasiou, R., & Shaver, P. (1969, July). A research questionnaire on sex. *Psychology Today,* pp. 64-69.

The Eysenck Inventory of Attitudes to Sex

The Editors

Eysenck's inventory was created to investigate the relationship between sexuality and personality and is specifically related to aspects of Eysenck's personality theory (Eysenck, 1967, 1981; Eysenck & Eysenck, 1985). He considers the inventory to be useful in the investigation of psychological factors as predictors of marital satisfaction (Eysenck & Wakefield, 1981), sexual abnormalities (Eysenck, 1977), masculinity-femininity issues (Eysenck, 1971b), and the special sexual adjustment of hysterical personality (Eysenck, 1971a).

There are both long and short versions. They are described in detail in Eysenck (1976). The long version consists of 158 questions. The short form contains 96 items. Factor analysis revealed 12 factors for both males and females: permissiveness, satisfaction, neurotic sex, impersonal sex, pornography, sexual shyness, prudishness, dominance-submission, sexual disgust, sexual excitement, physical sex, and aggressive sex. It takes from 20 minutes to an hour to complete the instrument.

Additional information and a copy of the instrument may be obtained from the first editor.

References

Eysenck, H. J. (1967). *The biological basis of personality.* Springfield, IL: Charles C Thomas.

Eysenck, H. J. (1970). Personality and attitudes to sex: A factorial study. *Personality, 1,* 355-376.

Eysenck, H. J. (1971a). Hysterical personality and sexual adjustment, attitudes and behavior. *The Journal of Sex Research, 7,* 274-281.

Eysenck, H. J. (1971b). Masculinity-femininity, personality and sexual and attitudes. *The Journal of Sex Research, 7,* 83-88.

Eysenck, H. J. (1971c). Personality and sexual adjustment. *British Journal of Psychiatry, 118,* 593-608.

Eysenck, H. J. (1972). Personality and sexual behavior. *Journal of Psychosomatic Research, 16,* 141-152.

Eysenck, H. J. (1973). Personality and attitudes to sex in criminals. *The Journal of Sex Research, 9,* 295-306.

Eysenck, H. J. (1976). *Sex and personality.* London: Open Books.

Eysenck, H. J. (1977). Personalidad y sex en grupo: Un estudio empirico. *Revista Latinoamericanan de Psiologia, 9,* 21-28.

Eysenck, H. J. (1981). *A model for personality.* New York: Springer.

Eysenck, H. J., & Eysenck, M. W. (1985). *Personality and individual differences.* New York: Plenum.

Eysenck, H. J., & Wakefield, H. A. (1981). Psychological factors are predictors of marital satisfaction. *Advances in Behaviour Research & Therapy, 3,* 151-192.

Eysenck, S. B. G., & Eysenck, H. J. (1971). Attitudes to sex, personality and lie scale scores. *Perceptual and Motor Skills, 33,* 216-218.

Sexual Attitude Scale

Walter W. Hudson,[1] *WALMYR Publishing Co.*
Gerald G. Murphy, *New Orleans, Louisiana*

The Sexual Attitude Scale (SAS) is a short-form scale designed to measure liberal versus conservative attitudes toward human sexual expression.

Description

The SAS contains 25 category-partition (Likert-type) items, 2 of which are worded negatively to partially offset the potential for response set bias. Each item is scored on a relative frequency scale as shown in the scoring key of the instrument. Obtained scores range from 0 to 100 where higher scores indicate greater degrees of conservatism and lower scores indicate more liberal attitudes. The SAS has a cutting score of 50, such that scores above that value indicate the presence of an increasingly conservative attitude toward human sexual expression and scores below that value indicate the presence of an increasingly liberal orientation. A score of 0 represents the most liberal position, and a score of 100 represents the most conservative position. The SAS can be used with all English-speaking populations aged 12 or older.

Readability statistics are as follows: Flesch Reading Ease: 63; Gunning's Fog Index: 10; and Flesch-Kincaid Grade Level: 7.

Response Mode and Timing

The SAS is a self-report scale that is normally completed in 5-7 minutes.

Scoring

Items noted below the copyright notation on the scale must first be reverse scored by subtracting the item response from $K + 1$, where K is the number of response categories in the scoring key. After making all appropriate item reversals, compute the total score as $S = (\Sigma X_i - N)(100) / [(K - 1)N]$, where X is an item response, i is item, K is the number of response categories, and N is the number of properly completed items. Total scores remain valid in the face of missing values (omitted items) provided the respondent completes at least 80% of the items. The effect of the scoring formula is to replace missing values with the mean item response value so that scores range from 0 to 100 regardless of the value of N.

Reliability

Cronbach's alpha = .94, and *SEM* = 4.20. Test-retest reliability is not available.

Validity

The known-groups validity coefficient is .73 as determined by the point-biserial correlation between group status (liberal vs. conservative criterion groups) and the SAS scores. Detailed information about content, factorial, and construct validity is reported in the *WALMYR Assessment Scale Scoring Manual*, which is available from the publisher.

Other Information

The SAS is a copyrighted commercial assessment scale and may not be copied, reproduced, altered, or translated into other languages. It may be obtained in tear-off pads of 50 copies per pad at $0.30 per copy ($15.00 per pad) by writing the WALMYR Publishing Co., P.O. Box 6229, Tallahassee, FL 32314-6229; phone and fax: (850) 656-2787; email: walmyr@syspak.com.

References

Hudson, W. W., Murphy, G. J., & Nurius, P. S. (1983). A short-form scale to measure liberal vs. conservative orientations toward human sexual expression. *The Journal of Sex Research, 19,* 258-272.

Nurius, P. S., & Hudson, W. W. (1993). *Human services practice, evaluation & computers.* Pacific Grove, CA: Brooks/Cole.

[1]Address correspondence to Walter W. Hudson, WALMYR Publishing Co., P.O. Box 6229, Tallahassee, FL 32314-6229; email: walmyr@syspac.com.

Exhibit

 SEXUAL ATTITUDE SCALE (SAS)

Name: _____ Today's Date: _____

This questionnaire is designed to measure the way you feel about sexual behavior. It is not a test, so there are no right or wrong answers. Answer each item as carefully and as accurately as you can by placing a number beside each one as follows.

1 = Strongly disagree
2 = Disagree
3 = Neither agree nor disagree
4 = Agree
5 = Strongly agree

1. ____ I think there is too much sexual freedom given to adults these days.
2. ____ I think that increased sexual freedom undermines the American family.
3. ____ I think that young people have been given too much information about sex.
4. ____ Sex education should be restricted to the home.
5. ____ Older people do not need to have sex.
6. ____ Sex education should be given only when people are ready for marriage.
7. ____ Pre-marital sex may be a sign of a decaying social order.
8. ____ Extra-marital sex is never excusable.
9. ____ I think there is too much sexual freedom given to teenagers these days.
10. ____ I think there is not enough sexual restraint among young people.
11. ____ I think people indulge in sex too much.
12. ____ I think the only proper way to have sex is through intercourse.
13. ____ I think sex should be reserved for marriage.
14. ____ Sex should be only for the young.
15. ____ Too much social approval has been given to homosexuals.
16. ____ Sex should be devoted to the business of procreation.
17. ____ People should not masturbate.
18. ____ Heavy sexual petting should be discouraged.
19. ____ People should not discuss their sexual affairs or business with others.
20. ____ Severely handicapped (physically and mentally) people should not have sex.
21. ____ There should be no laws prohibiting sexual acts between consenting adults.
22. ____ What two consenting adults do together sexually is their own business.
23. ____ There is too much sex on television.
24. ____ Movies today are too sexually explicit.
25. ____ Pornography should be totally banned from our bookstores.

Source. This scale is reprinted with permission of WALMYR Publishing Co.

Sexual Attitudes and Behaviors

The Editors

This questionnaire, developed by E. R. Mahoney, contains 96 items covering a wide range of sexual behaviors, including present and past behavior, frequency of behavior, sexual activity preferences, and several interpersonal and emotional-relationship dimensions of sexuality. Mahoney (1980) gives an extensive description.

Reference

Mahoney, E. R. (1980). Religiosity and sexual behavior among heterosexual college students. *The Journal of Sex Research, 16,* 97-113.

The Revised Attitudes Toward Sexuality Inventory

Wendy Patton[1] and Mary Mannison, *Queensland University of Technology*

In an attempt to develop a scale providing a focus for sexuality issues of the 1990s, we undertook the construction of this attitude scale, with a particular focus on sexual coercion.

Description

The 1980s and 1990s have seen a focus on attitudes toward sexual coercion, both in terms of their implications for female and male psychological development and their relationship to unintended pregnancy and sexually transmitted diseases (STDs). As such, a broad array of items focusing on attitudes toward sexual relationships, in addition to more specific issues, such as abortion, masturbation, homosexuality, contraception, sexuality in childhood and in elderly persons, and sexuality education, were seen as important for inclusion in the inventory.

The initial Attitudes Toward Sexuality Inventory (Patton & Mannison, 1993) was a 72-item questionnaire representing 10 attitudinal categories designed to evaluate a university course in human sexuality. There were 5 to 11 items in each category. The categories were selected to represent the main content areas of the course and included (a) contraception, (b) masturbation, (c) sexuality across the lifespan, (d) gender roles, (e) gay and lesbian relationships, (f) abortion, (g) STDs, (h) child sexual abuse, (i) rape, and (j) sexuality education.

Items in the initial inventory were derived from a number of different sources. These questionnaires included a number of the Burt (1980) scales, such as Sexual Conservatism, Rape Myth Acceptance, Interpersonal Violence, and Sex Role Stereotyping. Other measures used included those focusing on attitudes toward homosexuality (Herek, 1988), AIDS (Greiger & Ponterotto, 1988), rape (Deitz, Blackwell, Daley, & Bentley, 1982; Dull & Giacopassi, 1987; Feild, 1978), dating relationships (Giarusso, Johnson, Goodchild, & Zellman, 1979), and women (Spence, Helmreich, & Stapp, 1973).

As a result of preliminary research (Patton & Mannison, 1993, 1994), evaluations from independent experts in university sexuality education, and a review of item content and wording by a group of secondary school sexuality educators, changes were made. Several items were deleted, the focus of a number of items was changed, and other items were reworded to reflect subtle language shifts in the young adult population (Hall, Howard, & Boezio, 1986). Also, new items were added to capture various topical questions. In all, 35 items reflecting diverse issues in sexuality, including masturbation, sexuality in children and in

[1]Address correspondence to Wendy Patton, School of Learning and Development, Queensland University of Technology, Kelvin Grove Campus 4059, Brisbane, Australia; email: w.patton@qut.edu.au.

elderly persons, sexual coercion and assault in childhood and adulthood, homosexuality, abortion, and contraception were included in the revised inventory. Five items focusing on attitudes toward women (adapted from Spence et al., 1973) were also included, making a total of 40 items in the Revised Attitudes Toward Sexuality Inventory.

Three reliable and clear factors were found in a factor analysis, and two other factors were less clear (Patton & Mannison, 1995). The three factors were attitudes toward sexual coercion and assault (Items 2, 5, 6, 13, 17, 18, 25, 27, 29, 33, 37, 38), attitudes toward sexuality issues (Items 4, 7, 8, 15, 19, 20, 23, 35), and attitudes toward gender roles (Items 9, 28, 31, 32, 35).

Response Mode and Timing

The response format is a 6-point scale to which respondents reply from *strongly agree* to *strongly disagree*. The 6-point format was chosen to avoid a midpoint and invite a choice for one side or the other. The inventory typically requires 5-10 minutes to complete.

Scoring

Items were worded to counter any tendency to simply agree (or disagree) with all of them. This resulted in the reverse scoring of the following items: 4, 7, 13, 15, 19, 20, 23. On the attitudes toward sexual coercion and assault factor, higher scores reflect greater acceptance of rape myths and sexual coercion. Higher scores on the attitudes toward sexuality factor reflect less traditional attitudes toward sexuality. Higher scores on the attitudes toward gender roles factor reflect more traditional attitudes toward gender roles.

Reliability

The Cronbach alpha for the overall revised inventory was .85, and for the three clear factors, the alphas were .85, .79, and .68, respectively (Patton & Mannison, 1995).

Validity

The initial version of the Attitudes Toward Sexuality Inventory has been used to evaluate attitude change following a university course. Pre- and posttest data were received from 115 students (Patton & Mannison, 1993). Patton and Mannison (1994) also used the initial version of the inventory in a study designed to measure attitude and behavior change (measured by responses to problem situations) following a university human sexuality course. Patton and Mannison (1995) found significant differences. For Factor 1, there was a significant difference between men and women on all 12 items, with 10 of these at the $p < .001$ level. In every instance, men reported less disagreement with the item, indicating that women have a more negative response to sexual coercion. A similar pattern emerged with regard to the attitudes toward rape myths, as well as those items that reflected sexual coercion between people who knew each other. It must be noted that the difference was one of degree; all means were between 1.00 and 3.00, that is, between *strongly disagree* and *mildly disagree*.

On Factor 2 there were fewer items (four of eight) with a significant gender difference. The significant items showed women more accepting of the expression of sexuality in children and in elderly persons, and more rejecting of the notion that male and female homosexuality is a threat to society. Again, the difference was one of degree on most items.

In Factor 3, all five items showed significant differences between women and men. These differences reflected greater acceptance of traditional gender role attitudes by men—that women being whistled at in public is a compliment, intoxication in women is worse than in men, and homosexuality is a threat to societal institutions.

Analyses of variance were also performed on the summed factor scores for the reliable factors, Factors 1, 2, and 3. As expected, the consistent gender differences found on individual items generally remained for the total factor score, with Factors 1 and 3 showing significant gender differences. Overall means for Factor 2, the general attitudes toward sexuality factor, showed no significant difference between women and men. Although the items reflected specific area differences, the summed score results reflected a representative look at gender differences, illustrating differences on some dimensions of sexuality attitudes only.

Patton and Mannison (1995) indicated that additional redefinition of the measure is necessary. Although the first two factors may be used as independent measures, accepting the multidimensional complexity of attitudes toward sexuality suggests further refinement while continuing to include a wide range of content.

References

Burt, M. (1980). Cultural myths and supports for rape. *Journal of Personality and Social Psychology, 38,* 217-230.

Deitz, S. R., Blackwell, K. T., Daley, P. C., & Bentley, B. J. (1982). Measurement of empathy toward rape victims and rapists. *Journal of Personality and Social Psychology, 43,* 372-384.

Dull, R. T., & Giacopassi, D. (1987). Demographic correlates of sexual and dating attitudes: A study of date rape. *Criminal Justice and Behavior, 14,* 175-193.

Feild, H. S. (1978). Attitudes toward rape: A comparative analysis of police, rapists, crisis counselors, and citizens. *Journal of Personality and Social Psychology, 37,* 176-179.

Giarusso, R., Johnson, P., Goodchild, J., & Zellman, G. (1979, April). *Adolescent cues and signals: Sexual assault.* Paper presented at the annual meeting of the Western Psychological Association, San Diego, CA.

Greiger, I., & Ponterotto, J. G. (1988). Students' knowledge of AIDS and their attitudes toward gay men and lesbian women. *Journal of College Student Development, 29,* 415-422.

Hall, E., Howard, J., & Boezio, S. (1986). Tolerance of rape: A sexist or antisocial attitude? *Psychology of Women Quarterly, 10,* 101-118.

Herek, G. M. (1988). Heterosexuals' attitudes toward lesbians and gay men. *The Journal of Sex Research, 25,* 451-477.

Patton, W., & Mannison, M. (1993). Effects of a university subject on attitudes toward human sexuality. *Journal of Sex Education and Therapy, 19,* 93-107.

Patton, W., & Mannison, M. (1994). Investigating attitudes towards sexuality: Two methodologies. *Journal of Sex Education and Therapy, 20,* 185-197.

Patton, W., & Mannison, M. (1995). Sexuality attitudes: A review of the literature and refinement of a new measure. *Journal of Sex Education and Therapy, 21*, 268-295.

Spence, J. T., Helmreich, R., & Stapp, J. (1973). A short version of the Attitudes Toward Women Scale. *Bulletin of the Psychonomic Society, 2*, 219-220.

Exhibit

The Revised Attitudes Toward Sexuality Inventory

Your Attitudes

This page and the next asks you about your attitudes toward a number of sexual issues. Please offer your frank opinion by ticking one of the following options:

SA   Strongly agree
A   Agree
MA   Mildly agree
MD   Mildly disagree
D   Disagree
SD   Strongly disagree

	SA	A	MA	MD	D	SD
1. Some girls will only respond sexually if a little force is used.	☐	☐	☐	☐	☐	☐
2. Women falsely report rape in order to call attention to themselves.	☐	☐	☐	☐	☐	☐
3. Engaging in sex, e.g., for athletes, does not affect their energy and concentration.	☐	☐	☐	☐	☐	☐
4. A woman's decision to have an abortion is a good enough reason to have one.	☐	☐	☐	☐	☐	☐
5. A girl will often pretend she doesn't want intercourse because she doesn't want to seem loose, but she's really hoping the guy will force her.	☐	☐	☐	☐	☐	☐
6. In the majority of rapes, the woman already has a bad reputation.	☐	☐	☐	☐	☐	☐
7. Children should be encouraged to accept the practice of masturbation.	☐	☐	☐	☐	☐	☐
8. Easily accessible abortion will probably cause people to become unconcerned and careless.	☐	☐	☐	☐	☐	☐
9. There's nothing wrong with a little sweet talk to get what you want.	☐	☐	☐	☐	☐	☐
10. A woman cannot be forced to have intercourse against her will.	☐	☐	☐	☐	☐	☐
11. The primary goal of sexual intercourse should be to have children.	☐	☐	☐	☐	☐	☐
12. Sexual inaccessibility of a man's partner is a common cause of child sexual abuse in the home.	☐	☐	☐	☐	☐	☐
13. It's not okay for a guy to pressure for more sex even if he thinks the girl has led him on.	☐	☐	☐	☐	☐	☐
14. Normal males can commit rape.	☐	☐	☐	☐	☐	☐
15. Children should be ignored if found playing "doctors and nurses" or other games of sexual exploration.	☐	☐	☐	☐	☐	☐
16. It doesn't hurt children to have a little bit of sex play with their older relatives.	☐	☐	☐	☐	☐	☐
17. If the couple have dated a long time, it's only natural for the guy to pressure her for sex.	☐	☐	☐	☐	☐	☐
18. Women who are raped are usually a little to blame for the crime.	☐	☐	☐	☐	☐	☐
19. The elderly in nursing homes should have as much sexual access to each other as they want.	☐	☐	☐	☐	☐	☐
20. Contraceptives should be readily available to teenagers.	☐	☐	☐	☐	☐	☐
21. Even if the guy gets sexually excited, it's not okay for him to use force.	☐	☐	☐	☐	☐	☐
22. Rape is usually planned and premeditated.	☐	☐	☐	☐	☐	☐
23. Masturbation is a normal sexual activity throughout life.	☐	☐	☐	☐	☐	☐
24. Women should receive preferential treatment right now to make up for past discrimination.	☐	☐	☐	☐	☐	☐
25. If a guy spends a lot of money on a girl, he's got a right to expect a few sexual favors.	☐	☐	☐	☐	☐	☐
26. Forcing a woman to have sex when she doesn't want to is rape.	☐	☐	☐	☐	☐	☐
27. A woman who initiates a sexual encounter will probably have sex with anybody.	☐	☐	☐	☐	☐	☐
28. Being whistled at in public is like getting a compliment.	☐	☐	☐	☐	☐	☐
29. You can't blame a guy for not listening when the girl changes her mind at the last minute.	☐	☐	☐	☐	☐	☐

	SA	A	MA	MD	D	SD
30. No woman harbors a secret desire to be raped.	☐	☐	☐	☐	☐	☐
31. Sexuality education probably leads to experimentation and increased sexual activity.	☐	☐	☐	☐	☐	☐
32. Intoxication among women is worse than among men.	☐	☐	☐	☐	☐	☐
33. A girl should give in to a guy's advances so as not to hurt his feelings.	☐	☐	☐	☐	☐	☐
34. Rape has nothing to do with an uncontrollable desire for sex.	☐	☐	☐	☐	☐	☐
35. Male and female homosexuality is a threat to many of society's institutions.	☐	☐	☐	☐	☐	☐
36. *If there are rules about corporal punishment in schools, they should apply equally to boys and girls.*	☐	☐	☐	☐	☐	☐
37. If a girl engages in necking or petting and she lets things get out of hand, it is her own fault if her partner forces sex on her.	☐	☐	☐	☐	☐	☐
38. A woman who claims she was raped by a man she knows can be described as a "woman who changed her mind afterward."	☐	☐	☐	☐	☐	☐
39. Most adults who contract AIDS get pretty much what they deserve.	☐	☐	☐	☐	☐	☐
40. No clubs should be allowed to refuse membership, terms, or conditions of membership on the basis of gender.	☐	☐	☐	☐	☐	☐

Source. This scale was originally published in "Sexuality Attitudes: A Review of the Literature and Refinement of a New Measure," by W. Patton and M. Mannison, 1995, *Journal of Sex Education and Therapy, 21,* 268-295. Reprinted with permission.

Sexual Attitudes for Self and Others Questionnaire

Marilyn D. Story,[1] *University of Northern Iowa*

The Sexual Attitudes for Self and Others Questionnaire allows respondents to describe their emotional reactions to the idea of themselves or others participating in certain categories of sexual behaviors. Because it can be divided into a "self" and an "other" scale, it is a brief instrument to measure differences between sexual attitudes as applied to self and sexual attitudes as applied to others. Background information on the questionnaire enables demographic factors and attitude toward abortion to be related to attitudes on sexual behavior for self and for others.

Description

The Likert-type sexual attitude scale is constructed to allow university students (or other teenagers and adults) to indicate feelings about each of 12 categories of sexual behaviors for themselves and for others (24 items). The five

described points on the scale range from *I feel great about it* to *I feel repulsed by it* (see exhibit).

The questionnaire also includes an agree/disagree question related to abortion and demographic questions on classification, marital status, political affiliation, religious affiliation, sex, age, cumulative grade point average, and nudist/nonnudist affiliation.

Response Mode and Timing

Respondents mark the number indicating their answer on a machine-scorable answer sheet. If machine scoring is not desired, directions could be changed to have respondents mark their answers directly on the questionnaire. The attitude scale itself requires an average of 8 minutes for completion; the other background data on the questionnaire require another 4 minutes.

Scoring

Ratings on each of the items can range from 1 to 5 with lower number responses indicating more accepting atti-

[1]Address correspondence to Marilyn D. Story, 415 Broadwater Circle, Anderson, SC 29624-6537.

tudes. A "self" scale score may be obtained by summing the responses to the 12 categories of sexual behavior applied to self, and an "others" scale score may be obtained by summing the responses to the 12 categories of sexual behavior applied to others.

Reliability

Using 34 respondents, the test-retest reliability of the total attitude scale of 24 items over a 2-week period was .90. Based on 251 respondents, the self scale had a split-half internal consistency reliability coefficient of .55. Applying the Spearman-Brown formula, a reliability coefficient of .71 was obtained. Based on 251 respondents, the others scale had a split-half internal consistency reliability coefficient of .54 (Spearman-Brown formula = .70) (Story, 1979). Both the brevity of the scales and the comparatively narrow range of possible scores may have deflated the obtained reliability coefficients.

Validity

The questionnaire was reviewed by four university human sexuality instructors and pilot tested with a class of 34 university-level human sexuality students. Comments from instructor reviews and pilot testing indicated that the questionnaire was clearly written and had content (face) validity (Story, 1979).

Reference

Story, M. D. (1979). A longitudinal study of the effects of a university human sexuality course on sexual attitudes. *The Journal of Sex Research, 15*, 184-204.

Exhibit

Sexual Attitudes for Self and Others Questionnaire

Sexual Attitude Scale

Instructions: Please indicate your feelings about these specific activities, using the following alternative responses.

1 = I feel *great* about it
2 = I feel *comfortable* about it
3 = I feel *neutral* about it
4 = I feel *repulsed* by it

Mark the number of the response you prefer in each case on the answer sheet provided. Please also write your sex and the date on the answer sheet. Do not put your name on the answer sheet but write some identification code you will remember in the name space so you may later claim your paper.

I. Using masturbation as a form of sexual outlet:
   1)   1   2   3   4   5   for yourself[a]
   2)   1   2   3   4   5   for others
II. Mutual masturbation with someone of the opposite sex (An affectionate and tender relationship between the partners is assumed. It is also assumed that there is no danger of venereal disease.):
III. Mutual masturbation with someone of the same sex (An affectionate and tender relationship between the partners is assumed. It is also assumed that there is no danger of venereal disease.):
IV. Sexual intercourse with someone of the opposite sex (An affectionate and tender relationship between the partners is assumed. It is also assumed that there is no danger of venereal disease.):
V. Oral-genital stimulation with someone of the opposite sex (An affectionate and tender relationship between the partners is assumed. It is also assumed that there is no danger of venereal disease.):
VI. Oral-genital stimulation with someone of the same sex (An affectionate and tender relationship between the partners is assumed. It is also assumed that there is no danger of venereal disease.):
VII. Engaging in sex with your partner in the presence of others:
VIII. Three or more people engaging in intercourse and other sexual activity together:
IX. Maintaining more than one sexual relationship at a given time:
X. The woman in a heterosexual relationship being the more aggressive partner at times:
XI. Using erotica (erotic literature, pictures, films, live sex shows) to stimulate sexual arousal:
XII. Intercourse during the menstrual flow:

For the following question, mark number one on the answer sheet for *agree* or mark number two for *disagree*.

XIV. Abortion is an acceptable means of terminating an unwanted pregnancy.

Background Information Sheet

Instructions: Please complete the following information as it applies to you at the present time by marking the number of the correct response in each case on the answer sheet provided. Do not put your name on the answer sheet but write the same identification code in the name space that you wrote on the Sexual Attitude Scale answer sheet.

1. College Classification
   1. freshman
   2. sophomore
   3. junior
   4. senior
2. Marital Status
   1. single and never married
   2. married
   3. divorced
   4. widowed
3. Political Affiliation
   1. Democrat
   2. Republican
   3. Independent
   4. other
4. Religious Affiliation
   1. Catholic
   2. Protestant
   3. other
   4. none
5. Sex
   1. male
   2. female
6. Social Nudity Behavior
   1. Practice social nudity at nudist clubs and/or free beaches as well as at home
   2. Practice at-home nudity only, being generally nude with my family at home
   3. Practice neither social nor at-home nudity
7. Age _____
8. Cumulative Grade Point Average _____

a. These options are repeated for Items II-XII.

The Valois Sexual Attitude Scale

Robert F. Valois,[1] *University of South Carolina*
John C. Ory, *University of Illinois*

This scale was initially designed to evaluate the effects of a human sexuality program on the attitudes of university residence hall students (Valois, 1980).

[1] Address correspondence to Robert F. Valois, Department of Health Promotion & Education, 216 Health Sciences Building, University of South Carolina, Columbia, SC 29208; email: rvalois@sophe.sph.sc.edu.

Description

The instrument consists of two parts: 9 items concerning sociodemographic variables and 47, 5-point Likert-type items that reveal attitudes toward nine sexual topics. These subscale topics include (a) sexual stereotypes, (b) masturbation, (c) premarital intercourse, (d) homosexuality, (e) sexual communication, (f) college marriages, (g) abortion, (h) oral-genital sex, and (i) birth control. The five choices for each attitudinal item are *strongly agree, agree, uncertain, disagree,* and *strongly disagree.*

An extensive review of the sexuality literature on research findings facilitated instrument development. Questionnaire items written by Conley and O'Rourke (1973) and items from the instrument used by Bernard and Schwartz (1977) aided scale development.

Response Mode and Timing

Respondents answered each item by blackening the appropriate column of a standard computer-scored answer sheet. This scale requires an average of 20 minutes for completion.

Scoring

Scoring for each factor is keyed with a high score indicating acceptance, favorableness, or tolerance toward the respective sexual topic of each factor. A low score indicates unacceptance or a less tolerant standpoint toward the respective sexual topic.

Subscale scores were computed for each of the nine factor subscale topics. These mean subscale scores are average subscale scores computed by dividing the subscale total score, or the total item responses within a subscale factor, by the number of items contained in the subscale factor. Items 10, 11, 13, 16, 17, 19, 21, 23, 28, 30, 31, 33, 36, 37, 40, 41, 42, 44, 46, 48, 49, and 52 should be reverse scored.

The following is a breakdown of items belonging to the nine sexual subscale topics:

Subscale 1: Sexual Stereotypes—Questions 21, 17, 40, 43, 13, 36, 49, 41, and 21. These items refer to sexual items that tend to be stereotypic in nature and exist prior to formal sex education at the college or university level.

Subscale 2: Masturbation—Questions 34, 11, 24, and 34.

Subscale 3: Premarital Intercourse—Questions 15, 28, 38, and 51.

Subscale 4: Homosexuality—Questions 10, 23, 33, 46, and 56.

Subscale 5: Sexual Communication—Questions 32, 39, 44, and 45 deal with the process of sexual communication in a sexual situation and within a relationship.

Subscale 6: College Marriages—Questions 16, 29, and 52 refer to getting married while still in college.

Subscale 7: Abortion—Questions 19, 31, 42, and 54.

Subscale 8: Oral-Genital Sex—Questions 48, 25, 35, and 12.

Subscale 9: Birth Control—Questions 14, 26, 27, 37, and 50.

Reliability

Valois (1980) reported a 4-month stability coefficient of .85 for this scale. Internal consistency coefficients (Cronbach's alpha) for the subscales ranged from .66 to .92 (Valois & Ory, 1984).

Validity

Prior to use, a group of three university-level sex educator-researchers read and reviewed each scale item. The scale was judged to be content valid and representative of a postsecondary human sexuality curriculum.

Principal components analysis was used to examine the subscale structure of 56 items (Valois & Ory, 1984). The final components analysis with orthogonal rotation indicated nine viable dimensions accounting for 58% of the variance. Only those items having factor loadings of .30 or greater were considered as items belonging to a factor. Four items were eliminated because they were not evaluative items (18, 20, 22, and 53). The identification of these factors remained consistent with, and relevant to, the review of the sexual attitude literature. Each factor reflects an apparent dimension of the development of liberal sexual attitudes.

After viewing the nine factors identified, it becomes apparent that there is not one factor that could be identified as indicating a tolerant sexual attitude. Instead, the results (Valois & Ory, 1984) point to the conclusion that sexual attitude is not a unidimensional construct.

Other Information

Copyright to this scale belongs to both the Benjamin-Cummings Publishing Company (2424 Sand Hill Rd., Menlo Park, CA 94025) and the author. Permission for use may be obtained by contacting the publisher, who will in turn secure permission from the author. A nominal fee or no fee at all, depending on the use and reproduction or modification of the scale, would be determined by the author. Investigators using this scale for research purposes, who have given proper citation to the author, do not need written permission. In addition, the author would very much appreciate receiving a summary of any research study using this scale.

References

Bernard, H. W., & Schwartz, A. J. (1977). Impact of human sexuality program on sex related knowledge, attitudes, behavior and guilt of college undergraduates. *Journal of the American College Health Association, 25*(2), 182-185.

Conley, J. A., & O'Rourke, T. W. (1973). Attitudes of college students toward selected issues in human sexuality. *Journal of School Health, 43,* 286-292.

Valois, R. F. (1980). *The effects of a human sexuality program on the attitudes of university residence hall students.* Unpublished master's thesis, University of Illinois, Champaign-Urbana.

Valois, R. F. (1981). The Valois Sexual Attitude Questionnaire. In S. G. Cox, K. Doyle, S. K. Kammermann, & R. F. Valois (Eds.), *Wellness R.S.V.P.* (pp. 52-53). Menlo Park, CA: Benjamin-Cummings.

Valois, R. F. (1984). Assessment: What are your attitudes about sex? In M. R. Levy, M. Dignan, & J. H. Shirreffs (Eds.), *Life and health* (pp. 209-210). New York: Random House.

Valois, R. F., & Ory, J. C. (1984, May). An evaluation of the effects of a human sexuality program on the attitudes of university students. *Eta Sigma Gamma Monographs Series, 2*(2), 15-21.

Exhibit

Sexual Attitude Questionnaire

Please give us your cooperation by filling out the questionnaire. Completion is *not* mandatory. However, we do ask for your help, and we assure you this information will remain confidential. Please be as truthful as you can for it is important that we have valid answers to this questionnaire.

Directions: We ask that you place only your Social Security Number on the computer sheet, *no names*, please. The following questions (beginning with Question 10) deal with human sexuality in our culture. Each statement has a 5-point scale for answers. Indicate your reaction to each statement by blackening the appropriate column as follows:

     Column A = Strongly agree
     Column B = Agree
     Column C = Uncertain
     Column D = Disagree
     Column E = Strongly disagree

React as spontaneously as you can. Be sure to answer every question!

Thank you for your cooperation!

1. What is your sex?
   a. Male   b. Female
2. What is your age?
   a. 17-20   d. 27-29
   b. 21-23   e. 30-over
   c. 24-26
3. Marital status:
   a. Single   d. Divorced
   b. Married, living with spouse   e. Unmarried, living with partner
   c. Separated
4. In what year of college are you now?
   a. Freshman   d. Senior
   b. Sophomore   e. Graduate Student
   c. Junior
5. How much formal education did your father receive?
   a. Less than 12 years   d. College graduate
   b. High school graduate   e. Graduate or professional school
   c. Some college
6. How much formal education did your mother receive?
   a. Less than 12 years   d. College graduate
   b. High school graduate   e. Graduate or professional school
   c. Some college
7. What is your religious preference?
   a. None   d. Roman Catholic
   b. Jewish   e. Other
   c. Protestant
8. In the average month, how many times do you attend a church or synagogue?
   a. Never   d. Three times
   b. Once   e. Four or more times
   c. Twice
9. In which type of setting did you grow up in (grades 1-12)?
   a. Rural   b. Urban
10. Homosexuals should be put in a place where the rest of society does not have to put up with them.
11. Masturbation by a married person is a sign of poor marital adjustment.
12. Mouth-genital contact can provide a higher degree of effective erotic stimulation than can sexual intercourse.
13. Sex education should not be taught in the schools.
14. The practice of birth control is worthwhile.
15. Premarital intercourse between consenting adults is acceptable.

16. College marriages are usually doomed to failure.
17. Venereal disease is only contracted by lower socioeconomic people.
18. Rape is an easy crime to commit and never be convicted of this crime.
19. Abortion should be disapproved under all circumstances.
20. Pornography has a detrimental impact upon moral character and therefore is related to crimes of a sexual nature.
21. Living together is only practiced by white middle-class youth.
22. Sexual intercourse is a kind of communication.
23. Homosexuals should not be employed in occupations where they might serve as role models.
24. Masturbation is accepted when the objective is simply the attainment of sensory enjoyment.
25. Mouth-genital contact should be regarded as an acceptable form of erotic play.
26. Sex education should be as common a school subject as math or English.
27. Birth control is as much a man's responsibility as a woman's responsibility.
28. Sexual intercourse should occur only between married partners.
29. College marriages are no different than any other marriages.
30. Masturbation is generally unhealthy.
31. Preserving the physical health of the mother should be the only basis for abortion.
32. Communication barriers are the key factors causing sexual problems.
33. Homosexuality should be regarded as an illness.
34. Relieving tension by masturbation is a health practice.
35. Women should be as willing as men to participate in mouth-genital sex play.
36. Too much fuss is made over sex education.
37. The practice of birth control leads to increased sexual activity.
38. Women should experience sexual intercourse prior to marriage.
39. It takes a mature couple to make a college marriage work.
40. Venereal disease does not exist among upper- and middle-class people.
41. The ultimate goal of rape is sexual satisfaction.
42. Abortion is murder.
43. Pornography is not harmful to young children and there is no need to be concerned about their coming into contact with it.
44. Living together often indicates a strong sexual need for each partner.
45. The basis of sexual communication is touching.
46. Homosexuality repulses me.
47. Relieving tension by masturbation is a healthy practice.
48. Mouth-genital contact repulses me.
49. Sex education at the college-level serves no purpose.
50. Birth control pills should be available at a college health service.
51. Men should experience sexual intercourse prior to marriage.
52. College marriages add but one more problem to an already frustrating time of life.
53. A victim is usually raped within a mile of their home.
54. Abortion should be permitted whenever desired by the mother.
55. Masturbation should be encouraged under certain conditions.
56. Homosexuality is all right between two consenting adults.

Source. This scale is reprinted with permission of the authors.

Permissiveness of a Nurse's Sexual Attitudes

The Editors

This instrument is designed to assess nurses' attitudes toward sexual permissiveness. Sexual permissiveness was defined conceptually as the degree to which a woman feels free to act on her heterosexual impulses without acquiescence to social pressures and/or moralistic values that are in opposition to these impulses. The 20 items are statements advocating either conformity or nonconformity to social pressures and/or moralistic values limiting sexual behavior. A 5-point Likert-type response mode is used. The items of the scale are included in the Weinstein and Borok (1978) article.

Reference

Weinstein, S. A., & Borok, K. (1978). The permissiveness of nurses' sexual attitudes: Testing a stereotype. *The Journal of Sex Research, 14,* 54-58.

The Sexual Awareness Questionnaire

William E. Snell, Jr.,[1] *Southeast Missouri State University*
Terri D. Fisher, *Ohio State University at Mansfield*
Rowland S. Miller, *Houston State University*

The Sexual Awareness Questionnaire (SAQ; Snell, Fisher, & Miller, 1991) is an objective, self-report instrument designed to measure four personality tendencies associated with sexual awareness and sexual assertiveness: (a) *sexual consciousness*, defined as the tendency to think and reflect about the nature of one's sexuality; (b) *sexual preoccupation*, defined as the tendency to think about sex to an excessive degree; (c) *sexual monitoring*, defined as the tendency to be aware of the public impression that one's sexuality makes on others; and (d) *sexual assertiveness*, defined as the tendency to be assertive about the sexual aspects of one's life.

Description

The SAQ consists of 36 items arranged in a format whereby respondents indicate how characteristic of them

each statement is. A 5-point Likert-type scale is used, with each item being scored from 0 to 4: *not at all characteristic of me* (0), *slightly characteristic of me* (1), *somewhat characteristic of me* (2), *moderately characteristic of me* (3), and *very characteristic of me* (4). To create subscale scores (discussed below), the items on each subscale are summed. Higher scores thus correspond to greater amounts of the relevant tendency.

To confirm the conceptual dimensions assumed to underlie the SAQ, the questionnaire items were subjected to a principal axis factor analysis with varimax rotation. Four factors accounting for 42% of the variance were interpreted. The first factor contained items that pertained to sexual consciousness (Items 1, 4, 10, 13, 22, and 25). The items on the second factor (Items 2, 5, 14, 17, 23, 26, 28, 31, and 32) referred to sexual monitoring tendencies. The third factor was composed of items assessing sexual assertiveness (Items 3, 6, 9, 12, 15, 18, and 24), and the fourth factor was concerned with sex-appeal consciousness (Items 8, 11, and 29). A second cross-validation factor analysis reported by Snell et al. (1991) also showed that the SAQ subscales were factorially consistent with the anticipated

---

[1]Address correspondence to William E. Snell, Jr., Department of Psychology, Southeast Missouri State University, One University Plaza, Cape Girardeau, MO 63701; email: wesnell @semovm.semo.edu.

factor structure. The results of these statistical analyses provided strong preliminary evidence supporting the factor structure of the SAQ.

Response Mode and Timing

In most instances, people respond to the 36 items on the SAQ by marking their answers on separate machine-scorable answer sheets. The scale usually requires about 15-30 minutes to complete.

Scoring

All the SAQ items are coded so that A = 4, B = 3, C = 2, D = 1, and E = 0, except for six specific items that are reverse coded (Items 23, 31, 32, 30, 6, and 9); these items are designated with an R in the exhibit. The relevant items on each subscale are first coded so that A = 0, B = 1, C = 2, D = 3, and E = 4. Next, the items on each subscale are summed, so that higher scores correspond to greater amounts of each respective psychological tendency. Scores on the sexual-consciousness subscale can range from 0 to 24, sexual-monitoring scores can range from 0 to 32, sexual-assertiveness scores can range from 0 to 36, and scores on sex-appeal consciousness subscale can range from 0 to 12.

Reliability

The internal consistency of the four subscales on the SAQ was determined by calculating Cronbach alpha coefficients, using participants from two separate samples (Sample I consisted of 265 females, 117 males, and 4 gender unspecified; Sample II consisted of 265 females, 117 males, and 4 gender unspecified) drawn from lower division psychology courses at a small midwestern university (Snell et al., 1991). The average age of Sample I was 24.1, with a range of 17 to 60; the average age of Sample II was 24.07, SD = 6.87. Results indicated that all four subscales had clearly acceptable levels of reliability (Snell et al., 1991). In Sample I the alphas were: for sexual consciousness, alpha = .83 for males and .86 for females; for sexual monitoring, alpha = .80 for males and .82 for females; for sex-appeal

consciousness, alpha = .89 for males and .92 for females; and for sexual assertiveness, alpha = .83 for males and .81 for females. For Sample II, the internal consistency of the sexual-consciousness subscale was .85 for males and .88 for females; for sexual monitoring, .81 for males and .82 for females; for sex-appeal consciousness, .92 for males and .92 for females; and for sexual assertiveness, .80 for males and .85 for females.

Validity

Evidence for the validity of the SAQ comes from a variety of findings. Snell et al. (1991) provided evidence supporting the convergent and discriminant validity of the SAQ. All four SAQ subscales tended to be negatively related to measures of sex-anxiety and sex-guilt for both males and females, and sexual-consciousness was directly related to erotophilic feelings. Other findings indicated that women's and men's responses to the four SAQ subscales were related in a predictable fashion to their sexual attitudes, dispositions, and behaviors. Other findings indicated that men reported greater sexual assertiveness than did women, with no gender differences found for sexual consciousness, sexual monitoring, or sex-appeal consciousness. Snell (1994) revealed that sexual assertiveness in both males and females was predictive of greater contraceptive use, but only among males was sexual consciousness and sexual monitoring found to predict more favorable attitudes toward condom use. In addition, for both females and males, sexual consciousness, sexual monitoring, and sexual assertiveness were positively associated with a greater variety and a more extensive history of sexual experiences.

References

Snell, W. E., Jr. (1994, April). *Sexual awareness: Contraception, sexual behaviors and sexual attitudes.* Paper presented at the annual meeting of the Southwestern Psychological Association, Tulsa, OK.

Snell, W. E., Jr., Fisher, T. D., & Miller, R. S. (1991). Development of the Sexual Awareness Questionnaire: Components, reliability, and validity. *Annals of Sex Research, 4,* 65-92.

Exhibit

The Sexual Awareness Questionnaire

Instructions: The items listed below refer to the sexual aspects of people's lives. Please read each item carefully and decide to what extent it is characteristic of you. Give each item a rating of how much it applies to you by using the following scale:

A = *Not at all* characteristic of me.
B = *Slightly* characteristic of me.
C = *Somewhat* characteristic of me.
D = *Moderately* characteristic of me.
E = *Very* characteristic of me.

1. I am very aware of my sexual feelings.
2. I wonder whether others think I'm sexy.
3. I'm assertive about the sexual aspects of my life.
4. I'm very aware of my sexual motivations.

 5.   I'm concerned about the sexual appearance of my body.
 6.   I'm not very direct about voicing my sexual desires. (R)
 7.   I'm always trying to understand my sexual feelings.
 8.   I know immediately when others consider me sexy.
 9.   I am somewhat passive about expressing my sexual desires. (R)
10.   I'm very alert to changes in my sexual desires.
11.   I am quick to sense whether others think I'm sexy.
12.   I do not hesitate to ask for what I want in a sexual relationship.
13.   I am very aware of my sexual tendencies.
14.   I usually worry about making a good sexual impression on others.
15.   I'm the type of person who insists on having my sexual needs met.
16.   I think about my sexual motivations more than most people do.
17.   I'm concerned about what other people think of my sex appeal.
18.   When it comes to sex, I usually ask for what I want.
19.   I reflect about my sexual desires a lot.
20.   I never seem to know when I'm turning others on.
21.   If I were sexually interested in someone, I'd let that person know.
22.   I'm very aware of the way my mind works when I'm sexually aroused.
23.   I rarely think about my sex appeal. (R)
24.   If I were to have sex with someone, I'd tell my partner what I like.
25.   I know what turns me on sexually.
26.   I don't care what others think of my sexuality.
27.   I don't let others tell me how to run my sex life.
28.   I rarely think about the sexual aspects of my life.
29.   I know when others think I'm sexy.
30.   If I were to have sex with someone, I'd let my partner take the initiative. (R)
31.   I don't think about my sexuality very much. (R)
32.   Other people's opinions of my sexuality don't matter very much to me. (R)
33.   I would ask about sexually transmitted diseases before having sex with someone.
34.   I don't consider myself a very sexual person.
35.   When I'm with others, I want to look sexy.
36.   If I wanted to practice "safe sex" with someone, I would insist on doing so.

Source. This questionnaire is reprinted with permission of the authors.

Sexual Behavior

The Editors

These scales, developed by Bentler (1968a, 1968b), measure the extent to which a person has engaged in various heterosexual behaviors. The scales consist of 21 classes of heterosexual behavior, which form a cumulative, ordinal scale. Both graduate and undergraduate students were used in scale development. A 10-item form of each scale was also produced. Items for both scales are included in the Bentler (1968a, 1968b) articles.

References

Bentler, P. M. (1968a). Heterosexual behavior assessment—I, males. *Behavior Research & Therapy, 6,* 21-25.
Bentler, P. M. (1968b). Heterosexual behavior assessment—II, females. *Behavior Research & Therapy, 6,* 27-30.

Sexual Experience Inventory

The Editors

The questionnaire, developed by Brady and Levitt (1965), contains 16 items included in both heterosexual and homosexual behaviors, including kissing, breast and genital touching, oral-genital contact, and coitus. Respondents answer by checking whether they had experienced the activity sometime in life, during the last five years, or never. The questionnaire items are included in the Brady and Levitt article.

Reference

Brady, J. P., & Levitt, E. E. (1965). The relation of sexual preferences to sexual experiences. *The Psychological Record, 16,* 377-384.

Sexual Activity Questionnaire

E. Sandra Byers,[1] *University of New Brunswick*

Sexual activity occurs on a particular occasion as a result of individual and dyadic processes (see Byers & Heinlein, 1989, Figure 1). The Sexual Activity Questionnaire (SAQ) assesses the frequency of each step of the sequence of behaviors leading up to and during sexual interactions, as well as the specific behaviors used to initiate sexual activity and to respond to a sexual initiation. The SAQ has been used with married and cohabiting partners (Byers & Heinlein, 1989) and with dating partners (O'Sullivan & Byers, 1992). The term *sexual activity* includes all activities that are experienced as sexual, from holding hands to kissing to sexual intercourse. The SAQ could be easily adapted for use by same-sex couples.

Description

The SAQ is administered as a self-monitoring measure. At the end of each day, or as soon after a sexual interaction as possible, participants indicate (a) whether sexual activity had been initiated on that day, and, if so, by the man or by the woman; (b) if sexual activity was initiated, whether the noninitiator's first response was interest or disinterest in engaging in sexual activity at that time; and (c) if sexual activity was not initiated by either partner, whether the

respondent had considered initiating sexual activity. When used with dating, rather than cohabiting, partners, respondents first indicate on each day whether they had been on a "date" (defined as any social situation in which the person was with a member of the other sex).

Participants then provide detailed information about one or more of the sexual initiations that occurred that week. For example, participants can be asked to describe the first sexual initiation by the man and/or by the woman (O'Sullivan & Byers, 1992), the first sexual initiation to which the partner responded positively (if any), and/or the first sexual initiation to which the partner responded negatively (if any) (Byers & Heinlein, 1989). For the specified situation(s), respondents indicate the verbal and nonverbal behaviors used to initiate the sexual activity and to respond to the sexual initiation, as well as where the couple was and what they are doing when the initiation occurred. Respondents also indicate, from a list of 22 behaviors, those used by the initiator to demonstrate a desire for sexual activities. For the situation in which the partner initially was not interested in engaging in sexual activity, respondents indicate the reason(s) for the disinterest, how long the disagreement continued, and how the disagreement was resolved, and they rate how satisfied they were with their own and their partner's parts in resolving the disagreement. They also indicate whether they engaged in sexual activity at that time and, if so, why the initially disinterested person decided to engage in the activity. For the situation in which

---

[1]Address correspondence to E. Sandra Byers, Department of Psychology, University of New Brunswick, Fredericton, New Brunswick E3B 6E4, Canada; email: byers@unb.ca.

the partner was initially interested in engaging in the sexual activity, respondents indicate how satisfied they were with the way sex was initiated.

For those situations in which sexual activity resulted from the initiation, respondents indicate the types of sexual activities that resulted and their duration. They also rate how enjoyable the sexual interaction was for themselves and for their partner. Using an open-ended format, respondents are given the opportunity to provide additional information about the interaction they had described. Finally, they rate their confidence in the accuracy of their responses.

Dating partners are asked to provide information about their dating partner that is not included on the marital/cohabiting form. Questions assess their relationship with their dating partner (type of relationship, number of previous dates), their romantic interest in their date, and their perception of their date's romantic interest in them before they went on the date, and their own and their dates romantic interest at the end of the evening.

Response Mode and Timing

The SAQ takes approximately 10 minutes to complete. Most of the questions are objective. However, participants describe their activities and location at the time of the sexual initiation. Activities are coded for whether the partners are actively interacting. Location is coded as to whether the initiation occurred in a bedroom, other room in the house, or elsewhere. In addition, respondents describe the words and behaviors used to initiate sexual activity and to respond to a partner's initiation. The categories used to code descriptions of verbal initiations are no verbal initiation, indirect (ambiguous) statement, statement of feelings, and direct statement. Nonverbal initiations are coded as no nonverbal initiation, nonsexual touching or suggestive look, kissing, and sexual fondling. The checklist of 22 initiation behaviors is collapsed into five categories: direct verbal initiation, ambiguous verbal cues, physical contact, sexual cues, and suggestive movements and actions.

Different categories are used to code descriptions of negative and positive responses to initiations. For negative responses to initiations, the verbal responses are coded as no verbal response, verbal refusal without reason, refusal with physical reason, refusal indicating that there was not time, and refusal with a mood-related reason. The nonverbal responses are coded as no physical response, positive response to a lower level of sexual activity only, stopping or not responding to the partner's sexual advances, and moving away. For positive responses to initiations, the verbal responses are coded as no verbal response, agreement or invitation, and request for clarification. The nonverbal

responses are coded: no nonverbal response, initiated sexual activity, and continued sexual interaction. Alternately, ratings of positive and negative responses to initiations can be combined.

Reliability

The SAQ has good reliability. Byers and Heinlein (1989) found a mean interrater agreement for the open-ended questions of .86. In general, respondents were moderately or very sure that their responses were accurate ($M = 5.5$ on a 6-point scale). Eno (1994) found the average agreement between spouses from 36 couples to be .75 for initiations and .90 for responses to initiations. O'Sullivan and Byers (1992) found an average interrater agreement of .87 and an average confidence rating of 5.2, demonstrating good reliability with dating couples.

Validity

There is support for the validity of some aspects of the SAQ. Byers and Heinlein (1989) found that younger individuals, individuals newer to their relationships, and those who reported greater marital and sexual satisfaction reported more initiations. When number of initiations was controlled, more negative responses were associated with men and women who experienced less sexual pleasure, lower sexual satisfaction, and lower dyadic adjustment. Those individuals who had been in the relationship longer, and who reported less sexual pleasure for the woman and less sexual satisfaction, reported considering initiating sex despite not doing so more often. Eno (1994) found significant positive correlations between retrospective measures of the frequency of sexual initiations and positive responses in the week before self-monitoring and self-monitoring measures of these behaviors ($M = .71$). O'Sullivan and Byers (1992) found that respondents who had dated more frequently in the month before the study or who were in steady dating relationships reported more sexual initiations.

References

Byers, E. S., & Heinlein, L. (1989). Predicting initiations and refusals of sexual activity in married and cohabiting heterosexual couples. *The Journal of Sex Research, 26,* 210-231.

Eno, R. (1994). *Factors related to sexual initiations and responses to initiations within long-term heterosexual relationships.* Unpublished doctoral dissertation, University of New Brunswick, Fredericton.

O'Sullivan, L. F., & Byers, E. S. (1992). College students' incorporation of initiator and restrictor roles in sexual dating interactions. *The Journal of Sex Research, 29,* 435-446.

Exhibit

Sexual Activity Questionnaire (Married/Cohabiting Version)[a]

Instructions: We are interested in learning more about how couples initiate sexual activities, and how their partners respond to these initiations. By initiation of sexual activities, we mean any word and/or action that one person uses to indicate his or her interest in engaging in sexual activities, at a point in time when the couple is not engaging in any sexual activities. Notice that we are interested in initiations, whether or not any sexual activity results from the initiation. For example, one person may initiate sexual interactions by complimenting his or her partner on his or her looks or using a code phrase that the partner knows indicates sexual interest. Other examples of initiations would be if one person moved closer to their partner or if one person loosened or removed some of his or her own or the partner's clothing. We are interested in the initiation of all levels of sexual activity from kissing (if you consider it a sexual activity and not an expression of affection) to intercourse.

Please complete the attached questionnaire on a daily basis for one week. It is divided into 3 parts.

Part I. Part I of the questionnaire asks you to indicate, for each day of that particular week, whether either you or your partner initiated sexual activity. You are also asked to indicate for each "initiation" who initiated the sexual activity, and whether the noninitiator's *first response* was interest or disinterest in sex. By first response we mean the first thing he or she said or did in response to the initiation. In some cases, the noninitiator's first response might not be the same as his or her response a few seconds or minutes later. If sexual activity was not initiated by either partner on that day, please indicate whether you considered initiating and your reasons for not doing so. Further instructions for filling out this part of the questionnaire are on the questionnaire itself.

Part II. Fill in Part II of the questionnaire (the blue sheets) for the *first* occasion (if any) in that week on which sex was initiated, and the noninitiator's first response was that he or she was *not interested*. If no such initiation occurred in your relationship that week, leave this part of the questionnaire blank.

Part III. Fill in Part III of the questionnaire (the yellow sheets) for the *first* occasion (if any) in that week on which sex was initiated, and the noninitiator's first response was that he or she was *interested* in sex—that is, when both partners were interested from the outset. If no such initiation occurred that week, leave this part of the questionnaire blank.

Since it is easy to forget the specifics of any particular communication or interaction, it is important that you complete Parts II and III of the questionnaire as soon as possible after the initiation occurs. Try to be as accurate as possible in completing the questionnaire.

Definitions:

Sexual Activity: Any activity of a sexual (as opposed to purely affectionate) nature. Thus, this can include anything from kissing and touching to sexual intercourse. "SEX" is not necessarily intercourse.

Initiation: Any communication (verbal or nonverbal) of a "desire" to participate in sexual activity. Sexual activity may or may not follow.

Sexual Initiation Questionnaire

Part I. For each day of the week, please indicate the following (see Instruction Sheet for definitions):

(a) Whether sexual activity was initiated.
(b) If sexual activity was initiated, indicate whether it was initiated by you or by your partner (male or female). Then indicate what the first response was of the noninitiator. That is, if sex was initiated by you, indicate what your partner's first response was; if sex was initiated by your partner, indicate what your first response was.

(c) If neither you nor your partner initiated sex on that day, indicate if you considered initiating sex but did not do so. If you did change your mind, indicate the reasons for doing so.

Date and day of week	Was sex initiated?	If sex initiated		Did you consider initiating?	If sex not initiated
		By whom?	Noninitiator's first response		If yes, why didn't you initiate?
_____	_____ yes	_____ woman	_____ interested	_____ yes	_____
_____	_____ no	_____ man	_____ uninterested	_____ no	_____
_____	_____ yes	_____ woman	_____ interested	_____ yes	_____
_____	_____ no	_____ man	_____ uninterested	_____ no	_____
_____	_____ yes	_____ woman	_____ interested	_____ yes	_____
_____	_____ no	_____ man	_____ uninterested	_____ no	_____
_____	_____ yes	_____ woman	_____ interested	_____ yes	_____
_____	_____ no	_____ man	_____ uninterested	_____ no	_____
_____	_____ yes	_____ woman	_____ interested	_____ yes	_____
_____	_____ no	_____ man	_____ uninterested	_____ no	_____
_____	_____ yes	_____ woman	_____ interested	_____ yes	_____
_____	_____ no	_____ man	_____ uninterested	_____ no	_____
_____	_____ yes	_____ woman	_____ interested	_____ yes	_____
_____	_____ no	_____ man	_____ uninterested	_____ no	_____

The first of these days on which either you or your partner initiated sex and found that the noninitiator was *initially not interested* was _____ (write in day of the week). Please fill in Part II of the questionnaire on the *blue paper* for this occasion.

The first of these days on which either you or your partner initiated sex and found that the noninitiator was *initially interested* _____ (write in day of the week). Please fill in Part III of the questionnaire on the *yellow paper* for this occasion.

Part II. Complete Questions 1-14 (blue paper) if either you or your partner initiated sexual activity and the first response of the noninitiator was that he or she was *not interested.*

1. At the time of the initiation, where were you and your partner (e.g., in the kitchen of our home)? _____
2. Briefly describe the main thing(s) you and your partner were doing prior to the initiation (e.g., reading, talking). _____
3. The noninitiator indicated a desire for sexual activity by
   saying: _____
   doing: _____
4. The noninitiator responded to the initiator's initial advances by
   saying: _____
   doing: _____
5. The initiator then responded to this reaction by
   saying: _____
   doing: _____
6. How long did the disagreement continue? _____ minutes
7. How was the disagreement resolved? _____
8. (a) How satisfied are you with how sexual activity was initiated?
   _____ Very satisfied
   _____ Satisfied
   _____ Neutral
   _____ Dissatisfied
   _____ Very satisfied
   (b) Why? _____
9. (a) Overall, how satisfied are you with how the disagreement was resolved?
   _____ Very satisfied
   _____ Satisfied
   _____ Neutral

_____ Dissatisfied
_____ Very satisfied
(b) Why? _____

10. What behaviors did the initiator use to demonstrate a desire for sexual activities? (Check all that apply.)
_____ Asked directly
_____ Used some code words with which the man was familiar
_____ Used pet names
_____ Used more eye contact
_____ Touched her date
_____ Massaged or stroked
_____ Snuggled or cuddled
_____ Kissed date
_____ Shared a drink
_____ Moved closer
_____ Talked about the relationship
_____ Used "suggestive" body movements or postures
_____ Removed or loosened clothing
_____ Played with man's hair
_____ Lay down
_____ Changed tone of voice
_____ Made indirect talk of sex
_____ Set mood atmosphere (music, lighting, etc.)
_____ Played games or light "rough-housing"
_____ Made compliments
_____ Used some force
_____ Allowed hand to wander
_____ Looked at sexual material
_____ Others: _____

11. If you did engage in sexual activities at that time,
(a) Why did the person who was initially not interested decide to have sex? _____
(b) Which behaviors did you and your partner engage in at that time? (Check all that apply.)
_____ Hugging, cuddling
_____ Kissing
_____ Necking
_____ Fondling or kissing breast
_____ Fondling woman's genitals
_____ Fondling man's genitals
_____ Oral-genital stimulation
_____ Coitus
_____ Other (please specify)_____
(c) About how long did you and your partner spend in sexual activity at that time?
_____ Minutes
(d) How enjoyable was this occasion of lovemaking for you?
_____ Extremely unpleasant
_____ Moderately unpleasant
_____ Slightly unpleasant
_____ Slightly pleasant
_____ Moderately pleasant
_____ Extremely pleasant
(e) How enjoyable do you think this occasion of lovemaking was for your partner?
_____ Extremely unpleasant
_____ Moderately unpleasant
_____ Slightly unpleasant
_____ Slightly pleasant
_____ Moderately pleasant
_____ Extremely pleasant

12. If you did not engage in sexual activity at that time,
(a) Was sex initiated again later that day?
_____ Yes   _____ No
(b) If yes, by whom? _____ The man   _____ The woman   _____ Mutual consent

13. If there is any additional information that would help us to understand the situation that you described above, please provide it _____

14. How confident are you that your responses are accurate?

_____ Very unsure
_____ Moderately unsure
_____ Slightly unsure
_____ Slightly sure
_____ Moderately sure
_____ Very sure

Part III. Complete Questions 15-25 (yellow paper) if either you or your partner initiated sexual activity and the first response of the noninitiator was that he or she was *interested.*

15. At the time of the initiation, where were you and your partner (e.g., in the kitchen of our home)? _____ _____

16. Briefly describe the main thing(s) you and your partner were doing prior to the initiation (e.g., reading, talking). _____

17. The initiator indicated a desire for sexual activity by

saying: _____
doing: _____

18. The noninitiator responded to the initiator's initial advances by

saying: _____
doing: _____

19. (a) How satisfied are you with how sexual activity was initiated?

_____ Very satisfied
_____ Satisfied
_____ Neutral
_____ Dissatisfied
_____ Very satisfied

(b) Why? _____

20. What behaviors did the initiator use to demonstrate a desire for sexual activities? (Check all that apply.)

_____ Asked directly
_____ Used some code words with which the man was familiar
_____ Used pet names
_____ Used more eye contact
_____ Touched her date
_____ Massaged or stroked
_____ Snuggled or cuddled
_____ Kissed date
_____ Shared a drink
_____ Moved closer
_____ Talked about the relationship
_____ Used "suggestive" body movements or postures
_____ Removed or loosened clothing
_____ Played with man's hair
_____ Lay down
_____ Changed tone of voice
_____ Made indirect talk of sex
_____ Set mood atmosphere (music, lighting, etc.)
_____ Played games or light "rough-housing"
_____ Made compliments
_____ Used some force
_____ Allowed hand to wander
_____ Looked at sexual material
_____ Others: _____

21. Did you and your partner engage in sexual activity at that time?

_____ Yes _____ No

22. If you did have sex at that time,

(a) Which sexual behaviors did you and your partner engage in? (Check all that apply.)

_____ Hugging, cuddling

_____ Kissing
_____ Necking
_____ Fondling or kissing breast
_____ Fondling woman's genitals
_____ Fondling man's genitals
_____ Oral-genital stimulation
_____ Coitus
_____ Other (please specify) _____

(b) About how long did you and your partner spend in sexual activity at that time?
_____ Minutes

(c) How enjoyable was this occasion of lovemaking for you?
_____ Extremely unpleasant
_____ Moderately unpleasant
_____ Slightly unpleasant
_____ Slightly pleasant
_____ Moderately pleasant
_____ Extremely pleasant

(d) How enjoyable do you think this occasion of lovemaking was for your partner?
_____ Extremely unpleasant
_____ Moderately unpleasant
_____ Slightly unpleasant
_____ Slightly pleasant
_____ Moderately pleasant
_____ Extremely pleasant

23. If you did not engage in sexual activity at that time,
    (a) Was sex initiated again later that day?
    _____ Yes   _____ No
    (b) If yes, by whom? _____ The man   _____ The woman   _____ Mutual consent

24. If there is any additional information that would help us to understand the situation that you described above, please provide it _____

25. How confident are you that your responses are accurate?
    _____ Very unsure
    _____ Moderately unsure
    _____ Slightly unsure
    _____ Slightly sure
    _____ Moderately sure
    _____ Very sure

a. This version of the questionnaire is designed to be completed by cohabiting partners. The questionnaire can be modified for use by dating couples.

The Cowart-Pollack Scale of Sexual Experience

Debra Cowart-Steckler,[1] *Mary Washington College*
Robert H. Pollack, *University of Georgia*

The Cowart-Pollack Scale of Sexual Experience consists of two checklists of heterosexual activities: one for men and another for women. It was developed to assess the sexual experience of an individual or group of individuals in research, therapy, or the classroom.

Description

The checklists comprise a wide range of sexual activities for men and women, including oral contacts, masturbation, various intercourse positions, anal intercourse, and bondage. The female scale consists of 30 sexual activities. They range from "your nude breast felt by male" to "anal intercourse." The male scale consists of 31 sexual activities, ranging from "feeling female's nude breast" to "bondage."

Initially, the sexual experience scales consisted of 47 items drawn from previous studies (Bentler, 1968a, 1968b; Zuckerman, 1973). These 47-item scales were distributed to 153 men and 226 women during a group testing session. After completion, the items were ordered from most to least frequent according to the percentages of respondents who reported that they had engaged in such behavior. In accordance with the Cornell technique of Guttman scaling with two response categories, the top and bottom 10% of the items were discarded. This procedure yielded the present scales.

Investigations of the range of heterosexual experiences have shown a predictable sequence of experiences for men and women (Cowart & Pollack, 1979; Cowart-Steckler, 1984). These experiences can be described using the Cornell technique of Guttman scaling in which the behaviors are ordered from most frequent to least frequent (Guttman, 1947). Guttman scaling assumes that an individual who experiences a less frequent behavior previously has experienced the more common behavior (Edwards, 1957). Applying the Guttman scaling technique to sexual experiences suggests that heterosexual relationships progress through similar sequences of experiences. An individual who responds to this scale, then, can be compared to the normative sample and the level of sexual experience can be ascertained.

The Cowart-Pollack scale has been standardized using a college-aged sample (ages 18 to 21) and, therefore, is appropriate for people in that age group. Distributing the questionnaire to people of different ages may yield a different ordering in the sequence of behaviors.

Response Mode and Timing

When the scale is used in research, therapy, or to assess one's level of sexual experience the items are ordered randomly. Respondents indicate that they have or have not experienced each behavior by circling *yes* or *no* in answer to the question "Have you experienced the following?" The scale usually requires an average of 10 minutes for completion.

Scoring

No scoring per se is required. A comparison between the ordering of the respondent's experiences and the norms established by the Cowart-Pollack scale will give an accurate indication of the respondent's level of sexual experience.

Reliability and Validity

The Cowart-Pollack scale has been distributed twice to large groups of college-aged individuals. In 1979 (Cowart & Pollack, 1979), the 31-item scale for men and the 30-item scale for women were administered in a group testing situation to 199 men and 213 women. The coefficient of reproducibility for the male and female scales was .85 and .88, respectively. A coefficient of at least .85 indicates reliability in the ordering of behaviors (Edwards, 1957).

In 1983 the Cowart-Pollack scale was distributed to 197 men and 212 women (Cowart-Steckler, 1984). These respondents were demographically similar to the respondents in 1979. The coefficient of reproducibility was .88 for the male scale and .87 for the female scale.

The major difference in the results of the 1979 and 1983 distribution was not in the ordering of sexual experiences but in the numbers of men and women engaging in most types of sexual experiences. There were significantly more men and women from the 1983 sample engaging in sexual activities. This finding suggests that, at least for individuals aged 18 to 21, there has been an increase in sexual activity from 1979. As the coefficients of reproducibility indicate, the results of the 1983 distribution represent a reliable and stable sequence of events.

References

Bentler, P. M. (1968a). Heterosexual behavior assessment—I, males. *Behavior Research and Therapy, 6,* 21-25.

Bentler, P. M. (1968b). Heterosexual behavior assessment—II, females. *Behavior Research and Therapy, 6,* 27-30.

Cowart, D. A., & Pollack, R. H. (1979). A Guttman scale of sexual experience. *Journal of Sex Education and Therapy, 1,* 3-6.

Cowart-Steckler, D. (1984). A Guttman scale of sexual experience: An update. *Journal of Sex Education and Therapy, 10,* 49-52.

---

[1]Address correspondence to Debra Cowart-Steckler, Department of Psychology, Mary Washington College, Fredericksburg, VA 22401; email: dsteckle@s850.mwc.edu.

Edwards, A. L. (1957). *Techniques of attitude scale construction.* New York: Appleton-Century-Crofts.

Guttman, L. (1947). The Cornell technique of scale and intensity analysis. *Educational and Psychological Measurement, 7,* 247-280.

Zuckerman, M. (1973). Scales for sexual experience for males and females. *Journal of Consulting and Clinical Psychology, 11,* 27-29.

Exhibit

The Cowart-Pollack Scale of Sexual Experience

Men, N = 197   Women, N = 212

Activity	% Yes[a]	Activity	% Yes
Feeling female's nude breast	98	Your nude breast felt by male	91
Male mouth contact with female's nude breast	94	Male mouth contact with your breast	91
Exposure to erotic materials sold openly in newsstands	93	Penetration of vagina by male's finger	83
Male finger penetration of vagina	92	Male lying prone on female without penetration	83
Your observation of nude partner	91	Partner's observation of your nude body	80
Partner's observation of your nude body	91	Clitoral manipulation by male	79
Clitoral manipulation by male	90	Your observation of nude partner	78
Manipulation of penis by female	90	Male manipulation of vulva	77
Male lying prone on female without penetration	87	Manipulation of penis by female	76
Female mouth contact with penis	86	Sexual intercourse, male superior	67
Male manipulation of vulva	84	Female mouth contact with penis	67
Sexual intercourse, male superior	83	Male mouth contact with vulva	66
Masturbation	81	Male tongue manipulation of clitoris	66
Clitoral manipulation to orgasm by male	78	Male tongue penetration of vagina	66
Male mouth contact with vulva	77	Sexual intercourse, face to face, side	60
Sexual intercourse, partially clothed	77	Showering or bathing with partner	58
Male tongue penetration of vagina	76	Exposure to erotic materials sold openly in newsstands	58
Male tongue manipulation of clitoris	75	Sexual intercourse, partially clothed	56
Mutual oral stimulation of genitals to orgasm	74	Clitoral manipulation to orgasm by male	55
Sexual intercourse, face to face, side	73	Sexual intercourse, female superior	55
Exposure to hardcore erotic materials	72	Masturbation	54
Sexual intercourse, female superior	71	Sexual intercourse, vagina entered from rear	46
Showering or bathing with partner	68	Mutual oral stimulation if genitals to orgasm	45
Male tongue manipulation of female genitals to orgasm	66	Male tongue manipulation of your genitals to orgasm	45
Sexual intercourse, vagina entered from rear	63	Hand contact with partner's anal area	40
Hand contact with partner's anal area	61	Sexual intercourse, sitting position	37
Sexual intercourse, standing	48	Sexual intercourse, standing	28
Sexual intercourse, sitting	48	Exposure to hardcore erotic materials	24
Finger penetration of partner's anus	39	Finger penetration of partner's anus	19
Use of mild pain	16	Anal intercourse	13

a. From Cowart-Steckler (1984).

Sexual History Questionnaire

Caroline Cupitt,[1] *Warneford Hospital, Oxford, United Kingdom*

The Sexual History Questionnaire (SHQ) was devised to assess the degree to which an individual's sexual behavior is putting him or her at risk of infection by HIV, the virus that leads to AIDS. Respondents are asked to self-report such behavior and in addition are questioned regarding their beliefs about their risk of contracting HIV.

Description

The questionnaire first asks for information concerning basic demographic characteristics and is then divided into four sections. Section A begins by asking whether respondents have sex with men or women. This makes the important distinction between sexual identity and sexual behavior, which may be very different (Bancroft, 1989). Two questions follow asking whether the respondent had ever had protected or unprotected penetrative sex.

Section B asks for details of all sexual encounters over the past month. Because retrospective self-report of sexual behavior has been criticized for its unreliability, Section C then asks about the last occasion the respondent had sex. This also allows for more detailed questioning about interpersonal and situational variables involved in the last sexual encounter.

Finally, Section D includes a brief set of questions relating to contact with HIV counseling, sufferers, and risk assessment. There is substantial evidence that sexual behavior change is affected by knowing someone who has died of AIDS (e.g., Becker & Joseph, 1988) and some emerging evidence that it is affected by HIV antibody test counseling. Respondents are asked to make a general assessment of their perceived risk for HIV/AIDS using a standard scale.

Response Mode and Timing

A combination of multiple-choice, yes/no, 5-point scale, and numerical questions are used. The questionnaire takes between 5 and 10 minutes to complete, depending on the complexity of the respondent's sexual history.

Scoring

This questionnaire is not scored. However, the information in Section B gives an indication of a respondent's risk of HIV infection. If a respondent has had unprotected penetrative sex in the past month, he or she can be said to be at risk. This assumes that the risk from oral sex is not significant.

Reliability

By nature, the behavior this questionnaire seeks to measure is ever changing. In an endeavor to increase the reliability of the information gained, various means were used, such as asking about the last occasion a respondent had sex. In the original research (Cupitt, 1992) the final Section, D, was submitted to a test-retest reliability measurement. The questions in Section D were repeated over a 2-week interval with a group of 18 postgraduate students, and all were found to have an intraclass correlation of above 0.80 ($p <$ .001) indicating a high level of reliability.

Validity

Most of the questions are considered to have high face validity. To ensure that the respondent shared the same understanding of the different sexual practices mentioned, a summary of definitions was included at the beginning of the questionnaire. Critically, these definitions distinguish penetrative from nonpenetrative forms of sexual contact. The concept of *penetrative partner* has been advocated by Project SIGMA (Socio-sexual Investigations of Gay Men and AIDS; Hunt, Davies, Weatherburn, Coxon, & McManus, 1991). They argue that the notion of sexual partner per se is not valid to estimate risk behavior for HIV and that the concept of a penetrative sexual partner is considerably more accurate.

References

Bancroft, J. (1989). *Human sexuality and its problems* (2nd ed.). Edinburgh, Scotland: Churchill Livingstone.

Becker, M. H., & Joseph, J. G. (1988). AIDS and behavior change to reduce risk: A review. *American Journal of Public Health, 78,* 394-410.

Cupitt, C. (1992). *Cognitive factors in the decision to adopt safer sex practices.* Unpublished master's dissertation, University of London.

Hunt, A. J., Davies, P. M., Weatherburn, P., Coxon, A. P., & McManus, T. J. (1991). Sexual partners, penetrative sexual partners and HIV risk. *AIDS, 5,* 723-728.

---

[1]Address correspondence to Caroline Cupitt, Warneford Hospital, Headington Lane, Oxford OX3 7JX, United Kingdom.

Exhibit

Sexual History Questionnaire

Instructions: This questionnaire asks questions about your recent sexual history. Your answers are entirely confidential. Some words used in this questionnaire may not be familiar to you, or you may not be sure of their exact meaning. The following definitions may be helpful: *Vaginal sex* is sex in which the penis enters the vagina. *Oral sex* is sex in which the mouth or tongue is in contact with the genitals. *Anal sex* is sex in which the penis enters the anus, or back passage. *Penetrative sex* is sex in which the penis enters the vagina or anus. *Nonpenetrative sex* includes oral sex, and also many other forms of sex such as massage, touching, and mutual masturbation. *Protected sex* refers to penetrative sex with a condom or oral sex with a latex barrier or condom. *A regular partner,* for the purposes of this study, is someone with whom you have had sex more than once.

Please indicate your gender   male/female

your age   ____ years

your status   undergraduate/postgraduate

the religion which influences you most (please circle):
    1 Christianity,   2 Judaism,   3 Islam,   4 Hinduism,   5 Other

Section A

1. Who do you have sex with? (Please circle):
    1 only men,   2 mostly men,   3 equally men and women,   4 mostly women,   5 only women
2. Have you ever had penetrative sex (sex in which the penis penetrates the vagina or anus)?   yes/no
    If yes, at what age did you first have penetrative sex? _____
3. Have you ever had unprotected penetrative sex (penetrative sex without a condom)?   yes/no

Section B

The following questions relate to your sexual encounter(s) over the last month. This includes nonpenetrative sex such as oral sex and mutual masturbation. If you have not had sex in the last month please move on to Section C. If you have never had sex please move on to Section D.

4. In the last month how many sexual partners have you had? _____
5. How many of these were regular partners (people with whom you have had sex more than once)? _____
6. a) How many times have you had sex with a regular partner in the last month? _____
    b) On how many of these occasions did you have penetrative sex? _____
    c) On how many of these occasions did you use a condom? _____
7. a) How many times have you had sex with other partners in the last month? _____
    b) On how many of these occasions did you have penetrative sex? _____
    c) On how many of these occasions did you use a condom? _____

Section C

The following questions refer specifically to your last sexual encounter.

8. How long ago was your last sexual encounter? Please circle.
    1   less than a week ago
    2   between one week and one month ago
    3   between one month and three months ago
    4   between three months and six months ago
    5   between six months and one year ago
    6   more than one year ago

9. What kind(s) of sex did you have on this occasion? Please answer yes or no to the following activities:
   Unprotected vaginal sex: yes/no
   Vaginal sex with a condom: yes/no
   Unprotected anal sex: yes/no
   Anal sex with a condom: yes/no
   Oral sex: yes/no
   Other forms of nonpenetrative sex (such as massage and mutual masturbation): yes/no

10. What gender was your partner on this occasion? male/female

11. On this occasion did you or your partner mention using a condom?
    1   you
    2   your partner
    3   neither

12. On this occasion did you or your partner mention practicing nonpenetrative sex?
    1   you
    2   your partner
    3   neither

13. Was s/he a regular sexual partner (a partner with whom you have had sex more than once)? yes/no
    If yes, have you discussed practicing safer sex with this partner? (using condoms, latex barriers, or having nonpenetrative sex)?   yes/no

14. If you had heterosexual vaginal sex on this occasion, did you use a form of contraception? Please circle one or more:
    1   the condom
    2   the pill
    3   the diaphragm or cap
    4   IUD (the coil)
    5   spermicidal sponge, creams, or pessaries
    6   the rhythm (calendar) method
    7   the withdrawal method
    8   other (please specify) _____
    9   none

15. With this partner, have you discussed what kind of sex you like and don't like? yes/no

Using the scale below, write a number beside each statement to indicate how you felt.

        1   2   3   4   5
    not at all   a great deal

16. How much did you feel like having sex on this occasion? _____
17. How much did you feel like having unprotected sex on this occasion? _____
18. With this partner on this occasion, how able did you feel to express your wishes regarding sex? _____

Section D

Using the same scale answer the following, more general question.

        1   2   3   4   5
    not at all   a great deal

19. How much at risk do you consider yourself from HIV/AIDS? _____
20. Have you ever had an HIV antibody test? yes/no
21. Did you get the result of this test? yes/no/nonapplicable
22. To your knowledge, do you know or have you known anyone personally with HIV or AIDS? yes/no
23. Please feel free to add anything which you feel may give a clearer picture of your answers to this questionnaire.

_____

_____

Human Sexuality Questionnaire

Marvin Zuckerman,[1] *University of Delaware*

The experience scales are designed to measure cumulative heterosexual experience and homosexual experience in terms of the variety of sexual activities of each type and the frequency. Separate one-item scales assess the number of heterosexual partners and the number of homosexual partners. An orgasmic experience scale measures the variety of sexual activities leading to orgasm and their cumulative frequency. A one-item masturbation scale measures cumulative masturbatory experience.

The attitude scales are designed to measure (a) parental attitudes toward manifestations of sexual curiosity and behavior in children, (b) attitudes toward heterosexual activities as a function of the social relationship to the other person, (c) attitudes toward heterosexual activities as a function of the emotional relationship to the person, and (d) attitudes toward homosexuality in general.

EXPERIENCE SCALES

Description and Scoring of Subscales

1. The Heterosexual Experience scale is an extension of prior Guttman-type scales. It consists of 14 items, ranging from kissing to manual petting, oral stimulation of the breast, genital manipulation, oral-genital contact, and coitus in various positions. For each of the 14 items, the respondent rates his or her experience on a 5-point scale from 1 (*never*) to 5 (*10 times or more*). The score is the sum of the weighted item responses.

Reliability. Coefficients of reproducibility were .97 for males and females on a 12-item earlier version of the scale (Zuckerman, 1973) and .93 and .94 on the current 14-item version (Zuckerman, Tushup, & Finner, 1976). Coefficients of scalability in the latter study were .77 and .81 in males and females, respectively. Retest reliabilities after a 15-week interval were .80, .92, .94, and .95 in four groups (Zuckerman et al., 1976).

Validity. Respondents electing to take a course in human sexuality scored significantly higher than respondents in a personality course (Zuckerman et al., 1976). There were no initial sex differences. The males, but not the females, taking the sexuality course showed a greater increase than the control group. Heterosexual experience was positively correlated with all Sensation Seeking subscales in both males and females. Heterosexual college males scored higher than male members of a gay university group (Zuckerman & Myers, 1983). The scale correlated positively with levels of plasma testosterone and estradiol in college males (Daitzman & Zuckerman, 1980).

2. The Homosexual Experience scale consists of four items describing experiences of genital manipulation (active and passive) and oral-genital stimulation (active and passive) with members of one's own sex. The respondent answers on a 5-point scale for each item that ranges from 1 (*never*) to 5 (*10 times or more*). The score is the sum of the weighted item responses.

Reliability. Coefficients of reproducibility were .98 and 1.00 and coefficients of scalability were .76 and 1.00 for males and females, respectively (Zuckerman et al., 1976). Retest reliabilities after a 15-week interval were .84 and .49 for two groups of males (the lower one after taking a sexuality course), and .67 and .80 for two groups of females.

Validity. Males scored higher than females. Males, but not females, taking a course in human sexuality showed more increase than a control group (Zuckerman et al., 1976). Males in two gay groups scored higher than males in two heterosexual groups with practically no overlap in the two distributions (Zuckerman & Myers, 1983). The scales correlated positively with plasma estradiol levels in males, but not with testosterone (Daitzman & Zuckerman, 1980).

3. The Number of Heterosexual Partners scale consists of one item: "With how many different persons of the opposite sex have you had sexual relationships in your lifetime?" Respondents answer on a 5-point scale ranging from 1 (*none*) to 5 (*four or more*). The score is the weight (1 to 5) of the response choice.

Reliability. Retest reliabilities after a 15-week interval were .91 and .76 for two groups of males and .85 and .94 for two groups of females (Zuckerman et al., 1976).

Validity. Respondents taking a course in human sexuality scored higher than those taking a course in personality, and males scored higher than females (Zuckerman et al., 1976). The scale was unaffected by the course in human sexuality. It correlated positively with the Sensation Seeking subscales in both sexes. A heterosexual college male group scored higher than two gay male groups and a college church group (Zuckerman & Myers, 1983). The scale correlated positively with both plasma testosterone and estradiol levels in college males (Daitzman & Zuckerman, 1980).

4. The Number of Homosexual Partners scale consists of one item: "With how many different persons of your own sex have you had sexual relations in your lifetime?" Respondents answer on a 5-point scale from 1 (*none*) to 5 (*four or more*).

Reliability. Retest reliabilities were very low on this scale after a 15-week interval: .56 and .37 for males and .26 and .27 for females (Zuckerman et al., 1976). Instability may be due to changing interpretations of the term *sexual relations* in a homosexual context or more willingness to admit such relations on one occasion relative to another. Another reason is the highly restricted range; most persons respond

---

[1]Address correspondence to Marvin Zuckerman, Department of Psychology, 220 Wolf Hall, University of Delaware, Newark, DE 19711; email: zuckerma@brahms.udel.edu.

none, so the stability depends on the responses on the few individuals who respond *one or more.*

Validity. A group taking a sexuality course scored higher than a group taking a personality course. There were no sex differences (Zuckerman et al., 1976). Males taking the sexuality course increased on the scale relative to control males. Two groups of gay males scored higher than two groups of heterosexual males (Zuckerman & Myers, 1983). The scale did not correlate with either testosterone or estradiol levels in males (Daitzman & Zuckerman, 1980).

5. The Orgasmic Experience scale consists of eight items describing various ways in which orgasm can be achieved: masturbation, petting, genital manipulation, heterosexual and homosexual intercourse, oral stimulation from another, dreams, and fantasy alone. The scale is similar to Kinsey's (Kinsey, Pomeroy, & Martin, 1948) "total outlet" measure, which also includes all types of sexual activity. Respondents rate how many times they have reached orgasm by each of the specified methods on the scale ranging from 1 (*never*) to 5 (*10 times or more*). The score is the sum of weighted item responses.

Reliability. Retest reliabilities after a 15-week interval are .75 and .80 for males and .84 and .80 for females (Zuckerman et al., 1976).

Validity. Males scored significantly higher than females, but there was no difference between those taking sexuality and personality courses (Zuckerman et al., 1976). All Sensation Seeking subscales correlated with the scale in males, but only the Experience Seeking subscale correlated with Orgasmic Experience in females. Both gay groups (college and church affiliated) and the heterosexual college male group scored higher than the church-affiliated college male group on this scale (Zuckerman & Myers, 1983). Orgasmic experience correlated with plasma testosterone but not with estradiol levels in college males (Daitzman & Zuckerman, 1980).

6. The Masturbation scale is a one-item scale referring to "Manipulation of your own genitals." Respondents answer on a 5-point scale ranging from 1 (*once or twice*) to 5 (*10 times or more*). The score is the weighted item response.

Reliability. Retest reliabilities for a 15-week interval were .76 and .63 for males and .90 and .77 for females.

Validity. Males scored higher than females, but there were no differences between those taking sexuality and personality courses (Zuckerman et al., 1976). Males, but not females, increased more than a control group after taking a sexuality course. Gay groups had higher scores than the college church group but did not differ from the college heterosexual group (Zuckerman & Myers, 1983).

ATTITUDE SCALES

Description and Scoring of Subscales

1. The Parental Attitudes scale consisted of the five items in the Suppression of Sex scale from the Parental Attitude Research Instrument (PARI; Schaefer & Bell, 1958); the five corresponding reversed items from the reversed PARI (Zuckerman, 1959), constructed to control acquiescence

set in the PARI; and two additional items dealing with attitudes toward exposing children to pornography. The 12 items are in a four-response Likert-type format, *strongly disagree* to *strongly agree.* The score consists of the weighted sum of responses scored in the direction of permissiveness.

Reliability. Retest reliabilities after a 15-week interval were .63 and .64 for males and .44 and .56 for females (Zuckerman et al., 1976).

Validity. Students taking a sexuality course scored higher (more permissive) than those taking a personality course. There were no sex differences (Zuckerman et al., 1976). Females, but not males, taking a sexuality course showed significantly greater increases than a control group.

2. The Attitudes Toward Heterosexual Activities scales are modifications of the Reiss (1967) scale, which separates social relationships and emotional relationships as criteria for permissiveness.

a. The Social Relationship attitude scale consists of the 14 activities described in the Heterosexual Experience scale. For each item, respondents are asked to indicate the relationship of partners for which they would consider the particular activity *all right* or *not all right* for someone of their own sex. The response scale options are 1 = *never all right;* 2 = *all right with someone you are married to;* 3 = *all right with someone you are engaged to;* 4 = *all right with someone you know well;* and 5 = *all right with anyone, no matter how long you have known them.* The total score, in the direction of permissiveness, is the sum of the weighted responses to each of the items.

b. The Emotional Relationship attitude scale uses the same 14 sexual activities, but here respondents indicate whether the activity is all right under the following conditions: 1 = *never all right regardless of how much you love the person;* 2 = *all right if you are deeply in love with the person;* 3 = *all right if you feel strong affection toward the person;* 4 = *all right if you really like the person;* 5 = *all right, regardless of how you generally feel about the person.*

Reliabilities. For the Social Relationship scale, coefficients of reproducibility were .96 and 1.00, and coefficients of scalability were .89 and .96 for males and females, respectively. For the Emotional Relationship scale, coefficients of reproducibility were .96 and .98, and coefficients of scalability were .91 for both males and females. Retest reliabilities after a 15-week interval for the Social Relationship scale were .83 and .64 for males and .86 and .85 for females. For the Emotional Relationship scale retest reliabilities were .48 and .72 for males and .75 and .72 for females (Zuckerman et al., 1976).

Validity. Persons taking a sexuality course scored higher (more permissive) than those taking a personality course, and males scored higher than females on both attitude scales. The highly significant sex differences on the attitude scales were a marked contrast to the absence of difference on the Heterosexual Experience scale, which used the same activities in the items (Zuckerman et al., 1976). Attitude scales were more highly correlated with Experience scales for females than for males. Both males and females taking the sexuality course showed more change in the permissive attitude direction than did those in the control group. Permissive attitudes correlated positively with estradiol, but not testosterone, levels in males (Daitzman & Zuckerman, 1980).

3. The Attitudes Toward Homosexuality scale consists of four Likert-type items (*strongly disagree* to *strongly agree*) regarding the rights of homosexuals to marry or adopt children and whether homosexuals are regarded as normal or disturbed. The score is weighted based on the sum of the responses (1 to 4) for the items.

Reliability. No reliability data are available.

Validity. Unpublished data show no sex differences but do show a significant influence of a course in human sexuality in increasing permissiveness of attitudes toward homosexuality. Two gay groups had more permissive attitudes than two college heterosexual groups, and the heterosexual college group had more permissive attitudes than the heterosexual college church group (Zuckerman & Myers, 1983). Permissive attitudes correlated positively with estradiol, but not testosterone, levels in males (Daitzman & Zuckerman, 1980).

References

Daitzman, D., & Zuckerman, M. (1980). Disinhibitory sensation seeking and gonadal hormones. *Personality and Individual Differences, 1,* 103-110.

Kinsey, A. C., Pomeroy, W. B., & Martin, C. E. (1948). *Sexual behavior in the human male.* Philadelphia: Saunders.

Reiss, I. L. (1967). *The social context of premarital sexual permissiveness.* New York: Holt, Rinehart & Winston.

Schaefer, E. S., & Bell, R. Q. (1958). Development of the Parental Attitude Research Instrument. *Child Development, 29,* 339-361.

Zuckerman, M. (1959). Reversed scales to control acquiescence response set in the Parental Attitude Research Instrument. *Child Development, 30,* 523-532.

Zuckerman, M. (1973). Scales for sex experience for males and females. *Journal of Consulting and Clinical Psychology, 41,* 27-29.

Zuckerman, M., & Myers, P. L. (1983). Sensation seeking in homosexual and heterosexual males. *Archives of Sexual Behavior, 12,* 347-356.

Zuckerman, M., Tushup, R., & Finner, S. (1976). Sexual attitudes and experience: Attitude and personality correlates and changes produced by a course in sexuality. *Journal of Consulting and Clinical Psychology, 44,* 7-19.

Exhibit

Human Sexuality Questionnaire

Ordering of Scales: Generally, the Attitude scales are given before the Experience scales, beginning with the Parental Attitudes scale.

Parental Attitudes Scale

Response options for all items are:

A) Strongly agree
B) Mildly agree
C) Mildly disagree
D) Strongly disagree

1. A young child should be protected from hearing about sex.
2. Children should be taught about sex as soon as possible.
3. Children are normally curious about sex.
4. Young children should be prevented from contact with pornographic pictures.
5. There is usually something wrong with a child who asks a lot of questions about sex.
6. Sex play is a normal thing in children.
7. Sex is one of the greatest problems to be contended with in children.
8. Pornography is not harmful to young children and there is no need to be concerned about their coming into contact with it.
9. There is nothing wrong with bathing boys and girls in the same bathtub.
10. Sex is no great problem for child if the parent does not make it one.
11. It is very important that young boys and girls not be allowed to see each other completely undressed.
12. Children who take part in sex play become sex criminals when they grow up.

Scoring:

Items 2, 3, 6, 8, 9, and 10 are weighted: A = 1; B = 2; C = 3; D = 4
Items 1, 4, 5, 7, 11, and 12 are reversed weighted: A = 4; B = 3; C = 2; D = 1
Score is sum of weighted responses: range = 12-48.

Attitudes Toward Heterosexual Activities: I. Social Relationship

Instructions: Answer these based on what you feel is right for *most persons* of your own sex and age.

Response options for all items are:

      A)   Never
      B)   All right with someone you are married to
      C)   All right with someone you are engaged to, or intend to marry
      D)   All right with someone you have been going with for some time
      E)   All right with anyone, no matter how long you have known them

1. Kissing without tongue contact.
2. Kissing with tongue contact.
3. Male feeling covered female breasts.
4. Male feeling nude female breasts.
5. Male lying prone on the female, petting without penetration of her vagina.
6. Male mouth contact with female breast.
7. Female manipulation of male penis.
8. Male manipulation of female genitalia (vaginal and clitoral area).
9. Sexual intercourse in face-to-face position with the male on top.
10. Female mouth contact with male's penis.
11. Male mouth contact with female genitalia.
12. Sexual intercourse, face to face, with female on top.
13. Sexual intercourse, face to face, in side position.
14. Sexual intercourse, entering from the rear.

Scoring:
    Response options are weighted as follows for all items:
    A = 1; B = 2; C = 3; D = 4; E = 5
    Score is sum of weighted response: range = 14-70.

Attitudes Toward Heterosexual Activities: II. Emotional Relationship

Instructions: Answer these based on what you feel is right for *most persons* of your own sex and age.

Response options for all items are:

      A)   Never all right, regardless of how much you love the person
      B)   All right if you are deeply in love with the person
      C)   All right if you feel strong affection for the person
      D)   All right if you really like the person
      E)   All right, regardless of how you generally feel about the person

1. Kissing without tongue contact.
2. Kissing with tongue contact.
3. Male feeling covered female breasts.
4. Male feeling nude female breasts.
5. Male lying prone on the female, petting without penetration of her vagina.
6. Male mouth contact with female breast.
7. Female manipulation of male's penis.
8. Male manipulation of female genitalia (vaginal and clitoral area).
9. Sexual intercourse in face to face position with the male on top.
10. Female mouth contact with male's penis.
11. Male mouth contact with female genitalia.
12. Sexual intercourse, face to face, with female on top.
13. Sexual intercourse, face to face, in side position.
14. Sexual intercourse, entering vagina from the rear.

Scoring:
    Response options are weighted as follows for all items:
    A = 1; B = 2; C = 3; D = 4; E = 5
    Score is sum of weighted responses: range = 14-70.

Attitudes Toward Homosexuality

1. Do you think homosexuals (male or female) should have the right to legally marry?
   A) Definitely not
   B) No, I don't think so
   C) Yes, maybe
   D) Yes, definitely
2. Do you think homosexual couples (male or female) should have the right to adopt children?
   A) Definitely not
   B) No, I don't think so
   C) Yes, maybe
   D) Yes, definitely
3. Nearly all homosexuals are psychiatrically disturbed:
   A) Strongly agree
   B) Mildly agree
   C) Mildly disagree
   D) Strongly disagree
4. Except for differences in sexual preference, homosexuals are as normal as heterosexuals:
   A) Strongly agree
   B) Mildly agree
   C) Mildly disagree
   D) Strongly disagree

Scoring:

> Items 1, 2, and 4 are weighted: A = 1; B = 2; C = 3; D = 4
> Item 3 is reverse weighted: A = 4; B = 3; C = 2; D = 1
> Score is sum of weighted responses: range = 4-16.

Heterosexual Experience

Instructions: Heterosexual experience (with persons of the opposite sex). If you are male, substitute yourself for "male" in the item; if you are female, substitute yourself for "female" in the item (e.g., for a female, Item 4 is "having your nude breast felt by a male").

Response options for all items are:

> A) Never
> B) Once or twice
> C) Several times
> D) More than several times, less than ten times
> E) Ten times or more

How many times have you done the following?

1. Kissing without tongue contact.
2. Kissing with tongue contact.
3. Male feeling covered female breasts.
4. Male feeling nude female breasts.
5. Male lying prone on the female, petting without penetration of her vagina.
6. Male mouth contact with female breast.
7. Female manipulation of male's penis.
8. Male manipulation of female genitalia (vaginal and clitoral areas).
9. Sexual intercourse in face-to-face position with the male on top.
10. Female mouth contact with male's penis.
11. Male mouth contact with female genitalia.
12. Sexual intercourse, face to face, with female on top.
13. Sexual intercourse, face to face, in side position.
14. Sexual intercourse, entering vagina from the rear.

Scoring:

> Response options are weighted as follows:
> For all items A = 1; B = 2; C = 3; D = 4; E = 5
> Score is sum of weighted responses: range = 14-70.

Homosexual Experience

Instructions: Homosexual experience (with a person of your own sex).

Response options for all items are:

A)   Never
B)   Once or twice
C)   Several times
D)   More than several, less than ten times
E)   Ten times or more

How many times have you done the following?

1. Manipulating the genitals of a person of your own sex.
2. Having your genitals manipulated by a person of your own sex.
3. Performing mouth-genital contact on a person of your own sex.
4. Having mouth-genital contact performed on you by a person of your own sex.

Scoring:
Response options are weighted as follows:
A = 1; B = 2; C = 3; D = 4; E = 5
Score is sum of weighted responses: range = 4-20.

One-Item Scales

Masturbation Experience

How many times have you engaged in manipulation of your own genitals:
A)   Never
B)   Once or twice
C)   Several times
D)   More than several, less than ten times
E)   Ten times or more

Score is weighted response:
A = 1; B = 2; C = 3; D = 4; E = 5: range = 1-5

Number of Heterosexual Partners[a]

With how many different persons *of the opposite sex* have you had sexual intercourse in your lifetime?
A)   None
B)   One
C)   Two
D)   Three
E)   Four or more

Score is weighted response:
A = 1; B = 2; C = 3; D = 4; E = 5: range = 1-5

Number of Homosexual Partners

With how many different persons *of your own sex* have you had sexual relations in your lifetime?
A)   None
B)   One
C)   Two
D)   Three
E)   Four or more

Score is weighted response:
A = 1; B = 2; C = 3; D = 4; E = 5: range = 1-5

Orgasmic Experience[b]

Instructions: Orgasmic experience (orgasm = sudden spasmodic discharge of sexual tension usually accompanied by ejaculation in the male).

Response options for all items are:

    A)   Never
    B)   Once or twice
    C)   Several times
    D)   More than several, less than ten times
    E)   Ten times or more

How many times have you experienced orgasm through:

1. Masturbation
2. Petting, or body contact without manipulation of genitals
3. Manipulation of your genitals by someone else
4. Heterosexual intercourse
5. Homosexual relations
6. Oral stimulation by another
7. Dreams (nocturnal emissions)
8. Fantasy alone

Scoring:

    Response options are weighted as follows for all items:
    A = 1; B = 2; C = 3; D = 4; E = 5
    Score is sum of weighted responses: range = 8-40

a. Note that the Number of Partners scales may be used as a consistency check on the heterosexual sexual intercourse item and any of the homosexual experience items in regard to the report or denial of this type of experience.

b. Note that the Orgasmic Experience scale may be used for a consistency check on heterosexual and homosexual activities and partners scales.

Sexual Irrationality Questionnaire

The Editors

The Sexual Irrationality Questionnaire (SIQ) was developed to assess irrational beliefs in the realm of sexuality. It may be used with clients who have sexual problems (McCormick & Jordan, 1986) and by educators who wish to assess the extent to which sex education efforts succeed in diminishing students' erroneous and self-defeating beliefs about sexuality. The SIQ has 32 items and uses a 6-point Likert-type scale ranging from 0 = *strongly believing that a statement is false* to 5 = *strongly believing that a statement is true.* There is no neutral midpoint. It takes less than 10 minutes to complete the SIQ. The Cronbach alpha coefficient was .73 for the total scale. Concurrent validity was assessed by Jordan and McCormick (1986). A factor analysis revealed six factors.

The SIQ may be obtained from Naomi B. McCormick, 2717 Minnetonka Drive, Cedar Falls, IA 50613-1531; email: naomi.mccormick@uni.edu.

References

Jordan, T. J., & McCormick, N. B. (1986, November). *Development of a measure of irrational beliefs about sex.* Paper presented at the meeting of the Society for the Scientific Study of Sex, St. Louis, MO.

McCormick, N. B., & Jordan, T. J. (1986). Thoughts that destroy intimacy: Irrational beliefs about relationships and sexuality. In W. Dryden & P. Trower (Eds.), *Rational-emotive therapy: Recent developments in theory and practice* (pp. 47-62). Bristol, UK: Institute for RET.

Sexual Beliefs Scale

Charlene L. Muehlenhard,[1] *University of Kansas*
Albert S. Felts, *Houston, Texas*

We developed the Sexual Beliefs Scale (SBS) to measure five beliefs related to rape: the beliefs (a) that women often indicate an unwillingness to engage in sex when they are actually willing (the Token Refusal, or TR, subscale); (b) that if a woman "leads a man on," behaving as if she is willing to engage in sex when in fact she is not, then the man is justified in forcing her (the Leading On Justifies Force, or LOJF, subscale); (c) that women enjoy force in sexual situations (the Women Like Force, or WLF, subscale); (d) that men should dominate women in sexual situations (the Men Should Dominate, or MSD, subscale); and (e) that women have a right to refuse sex at any point, at which time men should stop their sexual advances (the No Means Stop, or NMS, subscale). There were existing scales that yielded one global score to measure a variety of beliefs related to rape (e.g., the Rape Myth Acceptance Scale; Burt, 1980) or that measured one particular belief related to rape (e.g., the Adversarial Sexual Beliefs Scale; Burt, 1980), but to our knowledge there were no scales that yielded separate scores for different beliefs related to rape.

Description

The short form of the SBS is a 20-item scale consisting of five 4-item subscales; the long form is a 40-item scale consisting of five 8-item subscales. Each item is rated on a 4-point scale, from *disagree strongly* (0) to *agree strongly* (3). Our experience suggests that respondents may find the long form repetitive, and correlations between the short and long forms are high, ranging from .955 to .981 for the five subscales ($N = 337$; all $ps < .0001$); thus, we recommend the short form for most purposes.

Response Mode and Timing

Respondents can write their answers directly on the questionnaire or mark their answers on machine-readable forms. The short form requires less than 5 minutes to complete; the long form requires less than 10 minutes.

Scoring

Items on each subscale are summed, yielding five subscale scores ranging from 0 to 12 (for the short form) or from 0 to 24 (for the long form). Higher subscale scores reflect greater agreement with the belief measured by that subscale.

---

[1]Address correspondence to Charlene L. Muehlenhard, Department of Psychology, University of Kansas, 426 Fraser Hall, Lawrence, KS 66045-2160; email: charlene @lark.cc.ukans.edu.

Reliability

For a sample of 337 university students, Cronbach's alphas for the short and long forms, respectively, were as follows: TR, .714 and .840; LOJF, .901 and .925; WLF, .921 and .952; MSD, .854 and .926; NMS, .944 and .959 ($n = 337$).

Validity

Jones and Muehlenhard (1990) investigated the effects of a 40-minute lecture aimed at changing students' attitudes related to rape. Four weeks after the lecture, students who had heard the lecture scored significantly lower than students who had not heard the lecture on the TR, LOJF, WLF, and MSD subscales (as well as on Burt's, 1980, Rape Myth Acceptance, Adversarial Sexual Beliefs, and Acceptance of Interpersonal Violence scales). The two groups did not differ significantly on the NMS subscale due to a ceiling effect; even the no-lecture control group had high NMS scores.

Muehlenhard and Hollabaugh (1988) found that sexually experienced women who reported having engaged in token refusal of sexual intercourse—indicating no when meaning yes—scored significantly higher on the TR subscale than sexually experienced women who had never engaged in such token refusals. Women who had engaged in this behavior were more likely than other women to view this behavior as common.

Muehlenhard and MacNaughton (1988) tested women whose LOJF scores fell at the lowest, middle, and highest 15% of the distribution. The high-belief group scored significantly higher than the low-belief group in how responsible they held a hypothetical rape victim for the rape, how justified they regarded the rape, and so forth. Furthermore, women in the medium- and high-belief groups were significantly more likely than women in the low-belief group to have engaged in unwanted intercourse because a man had become so aroused that they felt it was useless to stop him; perhaps they believed that they had "led him on" and thus were obligated to satisfy him.

Muehlenhard, Andrews, and Beal (1996) compared men with high LOJF scores (the Leading-On group), men with low LOJF scores but high TR scores (the Token-Refusal group), and men who scored low on both these scales (the Low-Myth group). The Leading-On group scored significantly higher than the Token-Refusal group, who in turn scored significantly higher than the Low-Myth group, in their ratings of how likely they would be to attempt sexual intercourse with a woman after she had said no. When asked to assume that the woman really meant no, however, the ratings of the TR group were no longer significantly different from the Low-Myth group, suggesting that men in the Token-Refusal group had not initially believed her refusal. Ratings of the Leading-On group remained higher than those of the Low-Myth group. The distinct pattern of results for each group illustrates the value of measuring each of these beliefs separately, which was our purpose for developing the SBS.

In summary, several studies have supported the validity of the SBS. The No Means Stop subscale, however, seems less useful than the others due to a ceiling effect. Some respondents endorse the items on the No Means Stop subscale, agreeing that a woman has a right to say no at any point, while also endorsing items on other subscales agreeing women who "lead men on" deserve to be forced or that women like to be forced. Similar patterns have been found by other researchers: For example, Goodchilds and Zellman (1984) found that 72% of the adolescents they questioned initially "with some righteous huffing and puffing" (p. 241) stated that forced intercourse was never justified, but when questioned about specific circumstances (e.g., what if a boy spends a lot of money on a girl), only 21% continued to maintain that forced intercourse was never justified. Some respondents seem to treat the NMS items

as virtuous sounding but empty statements that they endorse but also readily contradict.

References

Burt, M. R. (1980). Cultural myths and supports for rape. *Journal of Personality and Social Psychology, 38,* 217-230.

Goodchilds, J. D., & Zellman, G. L. (1984). Sexual signaling and sexual aggression in adolescent relationships. In N. M. Malamuth & E. Donnerstein (Eds.), *Pornography and sexual aggression* (pp. 234-243). Orlando, FL: Academic Press.

Jones, J., & Muehlenhard, C. (1990, November). *Using education to prevent rape on college campuses.* Paper presented at the annual meeting of the Society for the Scientific Study of Sex, Minneapolis, MN.

Muehlenhard, C. L., Andrews, S. L., & Beal, G. K. (1996). Beyond "just saying no": Dealing with men's unwanted sexual advances in heterosexual dating contexts. *Journal of Psychology and Human Sexuality, 8,* 141-168.

Muehlenhard, C. L., & Hollabaugh, L. C. (1988). Do women sometimes say no when they mean yes? The prevalence and correlates of women's token resistance to sex. *Journal of Personality and Social Psychology, 54,* 872-879.

Muehlenhard, C. L., & MacNaughton, J. S. (1988). Women's beliefs about women who "lead men on." *Journal of Social and Clinical Psychology, 7,* 65-79.

Exhibit

Sexual Beliefs Scale

Below is a list of statements regarding sexual attitudes. Using the scale below, indicate how much you agree or disagree with each statement. There are no right or wrong answers, only opinions.

(0)   Disagree strongly
(1)   Disagree mildly
(2)   Agree mildly
(3)   Agree strongly

*M	1.	Guys should dominate girls in bed.
N	2.	Even if a man really wants sex, he shouldn't do it if the girl doesn't want to.
L	3.	Girls who are teases deserve what they get.
*W	4.	By being dominated, girls get sexually aroused.
W	5.	A little force really turns a girl on.
N	6.	It's a girl's right to refuse sex at any time.
T	7.	Girls usually say "No" even when they mean "Yes."
L	8.	When a girl gets a guy obviously aroused and then says "No," he has the right to force sex on her.
W	9.	Girls really want to be manhandled.
*M	10.	Men should decide what should happen during sex.
*L	11.	A man is justified in forcing a woman to have sex if she leads him on.
M	12.	A man's masculinity should be proven in sexual situations.
*T	13.	Girls generally want to be talked into having sex.
*W	14.	Girls think it is exciting when guys use a little force on them.
*N	15.	A guy should respect a girl's wishes if she says "No."
M	16.	The man should be the one who dictates what happens during sex.
T	17.	Girls say "No" so that guys don't lose respect for them.
W	18.	Feeling dominated gets girls excited.
L	19.	A girl who leads a guy to believe she wants sex when she really doesn't deserves whatever happens.
*T	20.	Women often say "No" because they don't want men to think they're easy.
*N	21.	When girls say "No," guys should stop.
M	22.	During sex, guys should be in control.

*L   23. When a girl toys with a guy, she deserves whatever happens to her.
 T   24. Girls just say "No" so as not to look promiscuous.
*N   25. At any point, a woman always has the right to say "No."
*M   26. Guys should have the power in sexual situations.
*W   27. Women really get turned on by men who let them know who's boss.
*T   28. Girls just say "No" to make it seem like they're nice girls.
*L   29. Girls who tease guys should be taught a lesson.
*M   30. The man should be in control of the sexual situation.
 L   31. Girls who act like they want sex deserve it when the guy follows through.
*N   32. Even if a man is aroused, he doesn't have the right to force himself on a woman.
*L   33. Girls who lead guys on deserve what they get.
 N   34. If a woman says "No," a man has no right to continue.
 M   35. Men should exercise their authority over women in sexual situations.
*T   36. When girls say "No," they often mean "Yes."
 W   37. It really arouses girls when guys dominate them in bed.
 N   38. If a girl doesn't want sex, the guy has no right to do it.
 T   39. Girls who act seductively really want sex, even if they don't admit it.
*W   40. Girls like it when guys are a little rough with them.

Note. T = Token Refusal subscale; L = Leading On Justifies Force subscale; W = Women Like Force subscale; M = Men Should Dominate subscale; N = No Means Stop subscale.

*These items are on the short form.

Body Attitudes Questionnaire

Marilyn D. Story,[1] *University of Northern Iowa*

The Body Attitudes Questionnaire (BAQ) measures the respondent's degree of and reason(s) for satisfaction or dissatisfaction with 49 various parts or processes of the body and with "total body." Interpersonal and sexual relationship items, as well as sexual and elimination body parts not in previous instruments, are included in this instrument to make it more applicable to sex research. The BAQ is particularly useful for discriminant analyses on individual body-aspects items or for a principal components analysis to obtain factor structures accounting for the variance in body self-concept.

Description

The BAQ allows teenage and adult populations to rate each of 49 individual body parts or processes (see exhibit)

and one item labeled *total body* on a Likert-type scale. The five response options range from *have strong negative feelings and wish change could somehow be made* to *have strong positive feelings and desire no change to be made.* Respondents also mark a reason for each of their 50 ratings. In addition, the questionnaire contains two open-ended questions and demographic questions.

The questionnaire items are a combination of all those used in previous standard body-cathexis questionnaires (Mahoney & Finch, 1976a; Secord & Jourard, 1953) plus relationship items and sexual and elimination body parts not in previous instruments. A draft of the questionnaire was reviewed by midwestern university students ($N = 68$) for items difficult to understand, items difficult to rate, and items to add or delete. Three relationship items (ability to establish meaningful relationships, ability to keep meaningful relationships, and number of meaningful relationships) are included along with the sex activities item used by Secord and Jourard (1953) to cover a more complete range

[1]Address correspondence to Marilyn D. Story, 415 Broadwater Circle, Anderson, SC 29624-6537.

of relationships. Sexual and elimination parts were viewed as important aspects of body self-concept and included in spite of Secord and Jourard's (1953) fear that "their presence in the scale might give rise to an evasive attitude which would transfer to other items, resulting in avoidance of the two-answer categories representing negative feelings toward the body" (p. 344). Two forms of the questionnaire, one that included sexual and elimination parts and one that did not have those items, were each pilot tested on 100 midwestern university students. Because there were no differences between the groups' mean ratings of any item common to both forms or between the overall mean rating of the two groups, Secord and Jourard's fears were not supported. In contrast to Mahoney and Finch's (1976a) questionnaire, this questionnaire is the same for both sexes. Sex-differentiated parts are listed together as penis/vagina and chest/breasts so that differences between male and female body self-concept aspects can be more clearly tested.

The correlation matrices for responses to the 49 individual body parts or processes from 272 males and from 290 females were subjected to a principal components analysis (Story, 1984). Factors were extracted using Jöreskog's (1969) varimax procedure with orthogonal rotation. For males, seven factors were extracted accounting for 68% of the variance. The factors were labeled legs (16% of the variance), weight (12%), relationships (9%), face (9%), sex (9%), and height/torso (6%). For females, six factors were extracted accounting for 64% of the variance. The factors were labeled weight (24%), relationships (11%), legs (8%), face (8%), sex (7%), and health (5%). No other factor accounted for more than 5% of the variance for either males or females. Considering the additional items in the BAQ, compared to previous instruments, the extracted factors for both males and females are similar to those supported by previous literature (Mahoney & Finch, 1976a, 1976b). The relationships, sex, and health factors were formed from items not included by Mahoney and Finch.

When the components analysis was repeated using 150 social nudist males and 150 social nudist females (Story, 1984), no strong factors were found for either males or females. The strongest factor, relationships, accounted for 8% of the variance in nudist males' scores and 6% of the variance in nudist females' scores. No other factor accounted for more than 5% for either males or females. The failure to extract strong factors from the body self-concept ratings of social nudists should caution researchers that body self-concept factors may vary or even become nonexistent within different subcultures.

Response Mode and Timing

All questions are answered directly on the questionnaire and take an average of 20 minutes for completion. For each of the 49 individual body parts or processes and the total-body item, respondents first encircle the point on the 1-5 scale beneath the item that best indicates their degree of satisfaction or dissatisfaction according to the scale point descriptions given. Second, respondents encircle the letter beneath the item representing the factor that contributed more to their feelings of satisfaction or dissatisfaction on the item. If a respondent encircles the *other* factor as most important in determining his or her feelings, directions ask that the factor be named in the blank provided. Spaces are provided for answers directly after each of the two open-ended questions and each of the demographic questions.

Scoring

Ratings on each of the 49 individual body parts or processes and the total-body item range from 1-5 with higher-number responses indicating greater satisfaction. Factors contributing most to satisfaction/dissatisfaction are merely tabulated, but none of Story's (1984) 862 respondents used the *other* option. Answers to the questions "What part of your body do you like best?" and "What part of your body do you like least?" are categorized according to the following eight body self-concept factor groupings: no part, face, extremities, trunk, sexual parts, symbolic parts (soul, heart, brain, etc., as symbolic of qualities such as goodness, love, intelligence, etc.), overall build, and most or all parts.

Open-ended reasons given for liking a body part best or least are categorized into three possible reason groupings: attractiveness (looks good/bad), effectiveness (works well/poorly), both (attractiveness and effectiveness contribute equally).

Reliability

Sixty-five midwestern university students completed a test-retest over a 2-week period of satisfaction/dissatisfaction ratings on the 49 individual body parts and the total-body item. The test-retest reliability coefficient was .91 (Story, 1984).

Validity

The BAQ was pilot tested using 65 midwestern university students. Comments from pilot testing indicated that the questionnaire was clearly written and had content (face) validity. Concurrent validity was tested using 68 midwestern university students. A correlation coefficient of .88 was obtained between the mean satisfaction/dissatisfaction ratings from all items on Secord and Jourard's (1953) Body Cathexis Scale and from the 49 individual body parts or processes on the BAQ (Story, 1984).

References

Jöreskog, K. G. (1969). A general approach to confirmatory maximum likelihood factor analyses. *Psychometrika 34*(2), 183-202.

Mahoney, E. R., & Finch, M. D. (1976a). Body-cathexis and self-esteem: A reanalysis of the differential contribution of specific body parts. *Journal of Social Psychology, 99*, 251-258.

Mahoney, E. R., & Finch, M. D. (1976b). The dimensionality of body-cathexis. *Journal of Psychology, 92*, 277-279.

Secord, P. F., & Jourard, S. M. (1953). The appraisal of body-cathexis: Body-cathexis and the self. *Journal of Consulting Psychology, 17*, 343-347.

Story, M. D. (1984). Comparisons of body self-concept between social nudists and non-nudists. *Journal of Social Psychology, 118*, 99-112.

Exhibit

Body Attitudes Questionnaire

Please complete the following:

1. State of residence: _____
2. Age: _____
3. Sex: Male _____   Female _____
4. Nudity classification of your family:
    (1)   Nude both at camp and at home _____
    (2)   At home nudists only _____ (Please skip to number 6.)
    (3)   Normally clothed both socially and at home _____ (Please skip to number 9.)
5. Number of years you have been nude both at camp and at home: _____
6. Number of years you have been an at-home-only nudist: _____
7. Number of people living with you in your household on a regular basis: _____
8. Highest number of years of education completed by a family member: _____
9. Race or ethnic group:
    (1)   Black _____   (4)   Indian _____
    (2)   Caucasian _____   (5)   Oriental _____
    (3)   Chicano _____
10. Current marital status:
    (1)   Single (Never Married) _____   (3)   Divorced _____
    (2)   Married _____   (4)   Widowed _____

The following items are related to your body or your functioning.

For each item: *First,* encircle the number beneath it that best represents your feelings of satisfaction or dissatisfaction according to the following scale:

    1 = Have strong negative feelings and wish change could somehow be made.
    2 = Don't like, but can put up with.
    3 = Have no particular feelings one way or the other.
    4 = Am satisfied.
    5 = Have strong positive feelings and desire no change to be made.

Second, encircle the letter beneath the item that indicates what factor contributed most to your feelings of satisfaction or dissatisfaction according to the following scale:

    A = Attractiveness (looks good/bad)
    E = Effectiveness (works well/poorly)
    B = Both (attractiveness and effectiveness) contribute equally
    O = Other (when marking "other," please name the factor in the blank provided)

1. Hair 1 2 3 4 5   A   E   B   Oª _____
2. Facial complexion
3. Appetite
4. Hands
5. Distribution of hair over body
6. Nose
7. Fingers
8. Ability to establish meaningful relationships
9. Wrists
10. Waist
11. Energy level
12. Back
13. Ears
14. How others like my body
15. Chin
16. Ankles
17. Neck.
18. Shape of head

19. Body build
20. Profile
21. Height
22. Ability to keep meaningful relationships
23. Age
24. Shoulders
25. Arms
26. Breasts/chest
27. Eyes
28. Hips
29. Number of meaningful relationships I have
30. Skin texture
31. Lips
32. Legs
33. Teeth
34. Forehead
35. Feet
36. Health

37. Sex activities
38. Knees
39. Posture
40. Face
41. Weight
42. Sex (male or female)
43. Mouth
44. Skin color
45. Thighs

46. Stomach
47. Navel
48. Penis/Vagina
49. Buttocks
50. Total body
51. What part of your body do you like best? _____
    Why? _____
52. What part of your body do you like least? _____
    Why? _____

a. These options are repeated for Items 2-50.

Questionnaire on Young Children's Sexual Learning

Peggy Brick, *Center for Family Life Education*
Patricia Barthalow Koch,[1] *Pennsylvania State University*

Sexual development and sexual learning are ongoing processes from womb to tomb. Many adults, however, deny, misunderstand, or are uncomfortable with the sexual development and learning of young children. Yet this is an important time in life because it is the foundation for future development toward being a sexually healthy adult (Early Childhood Sexuality Education Task Force, 1995). Healthy Foundations is a nationwide initiative that includes a variety of resources designed to teach early childhood educators how to form a positive foundation for young children's growth toward healthy adult sexuality (Brick, Montfort, & Blume, 1993; Montfort, Brick, & Blume, 1993). The initiative includes a 1-day workshop designed for adults who deal with young children, including personnel in preschools, day care centers, and community agencies. The goals of the workshop include helping adults to become more knowledgeable about childhood sexual development and learning, to develop more positive attitudes and beliefs in these areas, and to become more comfortable and competent in dealing with these areas with young children and their families.

The Questionnaire on Young Children's Sexual Learning was developed to assess the knowledge, attitudes/beliefs, and comfort of adult caretakers regarding young children's

(infants to preschoolers) sexual development and learning. It has served as a useful tool in assessing the effectiveness of the Healthy Foundations professional development workshop. It also could be used in other educational, research, or clinical settings to determine the knowledge, attitudes/beliefs, or comfort levels of professionals, parents, students, or other groups of adults regarding young children's sexual development and learning. The terminology referring to the adult caretaker may be changed from "teacher" to "participant," for example, to make the items more appropriate for the group. Use with adults of differing backgrounds in various settings would help to further establish psychometric properties and norms for the scales.

Description

The Questionnaire on Young Children's Sexual Learning is composed of three separate scales. The Knowledge About Young Children's Sexual Learning Scale consists of 21 true-or-false statements designed to assess knowledge about young children's sexual development and learning. The Attitudes/Beliefs About Young Children's and Sexual Learning Scale contains 28 statements to which a respondent indicates on a 5-point Likert-type scale his or her attitudes and beliefs about sexual development and how young children should learn about various aspects of sexuality. The Comfort With Young Children's Sexual Learning Scale lists 10 topics with which adults typically need to discuss or deal when interacting with young children.

[1]Address correspondence to Patricia Barthalow Koch, Department of Biobehavioral Health, Pennsylvania State University, University Park, PA 16802; email: p3k@psu.edu.

Respondents indicate their comfort level with these topics on a 4-point Likert-type scale.

Response Mode and Timing

On the Knowledge About Young Children's Sexual Learning Scale, respondents choose the answer to each statement that best reflects their level of knowledge: 1 = *definitely true,* 2 = *probably true,* 3 = *probably false,* 4 = *definitely false,* and 5 = *don't know.* This scale requires no more than 10 minutes to complete.

Respondents choose the response that best reflects their attitudes/beliefs toward each statement on the Attitudes/ Beliefs About Young Children's Sexual Learning Scale: 1 = *strongly agree,* 2 = *agree,* 3 = *uncertain,* 4 = *disagree,* and 5 = *strongly disagree.* This scale requires no more than 15 minutes to complete.

On the Comfort With Young Children's Sexual Learning Scale, respondents indicate their comfort level in interacting with young children about each sexual topic: 1 = *very comfortable,* 2 = *somewhat comfortable,* 3 = *somewhat uncomfortable,* and 4 = *very uncomfortable.* Respondents can complete this scale in less than 5 minutes.

Scoring

One point is given for every correct answer on the Knowledge About Young Children's Sexual Learning Scale. Following are the correct answers for each item: definitely true, Items 1, 2, 3, 6, 8, 13, 16, 18; definitely false, Items 4, 5, 7, 9, 10, 11, 12, 14, 15, 17, 19, 20, 21. All other responses are counted as 0. Thus, the highest knowledge score would be 21. In a study of 183 participants attending eight different Healthy Foundations programs around the country, the average preworkshop knowledge score was 10 (Brick & Koch, 1996).

Scores on the Attitudes/Beliefs About Young Children's Sexual Learning Scale may range from 28, indicating the most negative or nonsupportive attitudes/beliefs, to 140, indicating the most positive and supportive attitudes toward young children's sexual learning. The following items need to be reverse scored: Items 3, 7, 10, 11, 12, 13, 15, 16, 19, 24, 25, 27, 28. The study of Healthy Foundations program participants found their preworkshop attitudes to be slightly negative to ambivalent (*M* = 78) (Brick & Koch, 1996).

On the Comfort With Young Children's Sexual Learning Scale, scores may range from 10, indicating the highest level of comfort, to 40, indicating the lowest level of comfort. Preworkshop comfort scores for a sample of Healthy Foundations program participants indicated that overall they felt somewhat comfortable in interacting with young children about various sexual topics (*M* = 17.6) (Brick & Koch,

1996). Respondents indicated most discomfort with masturbation.

Reliability

Internal reliability for each of the three scales, using Cronbach's alpha coefficient, was established with a nationwide sample of 183 Healthy Foundations participants (Brick & Koch, 1996). The alpha coefficients follow: for the Knowledge About Young Children's Sexual Learning Scale, .46; for the Attitudes/Beliefs About Young Children's Sexual Learning Scale, .92; for the Comfort With Young Children's Sexual Learning Scale, .93. Weak questions on the knowledge scale have been revised since that time.

Validity

The content validity for the three scales was determined through an extensive review of the literature on children's sexual development and learning. Initial items were constructed through collaboration of the researchers with the staff at the Center for Family Life Education. Items were then reviewed and content validity was established by a panel of experts that included practicing preschool teachers and professionals in the field of sexology.

Other Information

Information about the Healthy Foundations Program for Learning may be obtained from Peggy Brick, Center for Family Life Education, Planned Parenthood of Greater Northern New Jersey, Hackensack, NJ 07601.

References

Brick, P., Davis, N., Fischel, M., Lupo, T., MacVicar, A., & Marshall, J. (1993). *Bodies, birth, and babies: Developing healthy foundations for children's learning* [Video]. Hackensack, NJ: Planned Parenthood of Bergen Co.

Brick, P., Davis, N., Fischel, M., Supo, T., MacVicar, A., & Marshall, J. (1989). *Bodies, birth, babies: Sexuality education in early childhood programs.* Hackensack, NJ: Planned Parenthood of Bergen Co.

Brick, P., & Koch, P. B. (1996, November). *Healthy Foundations: An early childhood educators' sexuality program and it's effectiveness.* Paper presented at the annual meeting of the Society for the Scientific Study of Sexuality, Houston, TX.

Brick, P., Montfort, S., & Blume, N. (1993). *Healthy Foundations: The teacher's book—Responding to young children's questions and behaviors regarding sexuality.* Hackensack, NJ: Planned Parenthood of Greater Northern New Jersey.

Early Childhood Sexuality Education Task Force. (1995). *Right from the start: Guidelines for sexuality issues (birth to five years).* New York: Sexuality Information and Education Council of the United States.

Monfort, S., Brick, P., & Blume, N. (1993). *Healthy Foundations: Developing positive policies and programs regarding young children's learning about sexuality.* Hackensack, NJ: Planned Parenthood of Greater Northern New Jersey.

Exhibit

Questionnaire on Young Children's Sexual Learning

I. Knowledge About Young Children's Sexual Learning Scale

Please indicate if the following statements are "definitely true" (1), "possibly true" (2), "possibly false" (3), or "definitely false" (4) If you are unsure of the correct answer, circle "don't know" (5).

Scale[a]

1 = Definitely true; 2 = Possibly true; 3 = Possibly false; 4 = Definitely false; 5 = Don't know

1. Young children's sexual learning can affect how they feel about sexuality as adults.
2. Infants have sexual responses like clitoral/penile erections and orgasms.
3. Even if there is no formal program, children are learning about sexuality in their preschool.
4. It is unusual for young children to masturbate.
5. Most preschoolers are fearful of sexual topics.
6. By 3 years of age, most children can tell the difference between males and females.
7. It is O.K. for a child to be preoccupied with sex over a period of time.
8. Healthy and natural sex play usually occurs between friends and playmates of about the same age.
9. Children do not stimulate their own genitals until after they are 3 years old.
10. The vagina of female infants is not capable of lubrication.
11. Most 3- and 4-year-olds are really not curious about the differences in boys' and girls' bodies.
12. A person's body image does *not* begin to form until 4 years of age.
13. Children can be taught that it is O.K. to masturbate in private but not in public.
14. Young children understand human sexuality best when it is taught using plants and other animals as the examples rather than talking about people.
15. Adult responses to a child's sexual behavior have little affect upon how "good" or "bad" children think sex is.
16. Before answering a child's question about sexuality, you should try to find out what the child thinks.
17. When answering a child's questions about sexuality, you should only provide information and not deal with their feelings or attitudes.
18. Before responding to a child's sexuality-related behavior, you should try to find out what meaning this behavior has to the child.
19. The most effective method for dealing with sexuality-related behavior in children is to ignore the behavior.
20. It is too upsetting for preschoolers to tell them how babies are actually born.
21. Young children that have received age-appropriate sexuality education are more likely to be sexually exploited and abused.

II. Attitudes/Beliefs About Young Children's Sexual Learning Scale

Please circle the number that best represents your feelings or ideas toward the following statements.

Scale

1 = Strongly agree; 2 = Agree; 3 = Uncertain; 4 = Disagree; 5 = Strongly disagree

1. Preschool children can be sheltered from sexual messages in our society.
2. Biology is the main influence on a person's sexual attitudes and behaviors.
3. Masturbation is natural and healthy for children.
4. Sexual information is too complex for most preschool children to understand.
5. Adults/teachers must be careful not to allow little boys to act too much like girls.
6. Sexual learning for young children is primarily about where babies come from.
7. It is fine for young children to be curious about sexual topics.
8. Children receive positive messages about sexuality when adults use cute nicknames for genitals.
9. Most preschool children are too young to be able to use the correct names for their genitals (like "penis," "scrotum," "vulva," and "clitoris").
10. It is O.K. for preschool children to realize that their genitals feel good when they touch them.
11. It is better to use nonsexist language (i.e., "firefighter" instead of "fireman") with young children.
12. Children should feel positively about sexuality.

13. It is O.K. to allow children to touch their own genitals when their diapers or pants are being changed.
14. Teachers who have strong religious beliefs about sex should teach these to the children they care for.
15. It is important to begin discussing sexuality openly in early childhood.
16. Traditional gender role stereotypes discourage responsible sexual behaviors for both genders.
17. Anatomically detailed dolls or picture books promote unhealthy sexual curiosity in young children.
18. Talking about sexuality with young children encourages them to experiment.
19. Adults/teachers need to understand their own attitudes about sexual topics since these attitudes may influence their children.
20. Adults/teachers must be careful not to allow little girls to act too much like boys.
21. Seeing children of the other sex without clothes on encourages children to experiment with sexual behaviors.
22. Preschool programs should only deal with sexual information; dealing with sexual attitudes and values should be left up to parents.
23. Preschool teachers should refrain from affectionately touching their children.
24. Children have the right to choose who they want and do not want to touch their bodies.
25. A positive rather than a punitive approach is better when handling children's sexuality-related behaviors (like sex play and masturbation).
26. An early childhood sexuality program is adequate if it only deals with preventing sexual abuse.
27. Children should be encouraged to ask their teachers questions about sexuality.
28. A sexually healthy adult demonstrates tolerance for people with different sexual values, lifestyles, and orientations.

III. Comfort With Young Children's Sexual Learning Scale

Please circle the number that best represents how comfortable you currently feel in interacting with young children about the following sexuality topics.

Scale

   1 = Very comfortable; 2 = Somewhat comfortable; 3 = Somewhat uncomfortable; 4 = Very uncomfortable

1. Female and male roles and behavior.
2. Male and female body differences.
3. Names of genital or "sexual" body parts.
4. Being partially clothed (for example, changing diapers, going topless, nude swimming, etc.).
5. Masturbation.
6. Sex play (for example, "doctor," "mommies & daddies").
7. How babies are made ("get in").
8. How babies are born ("get out").
9. "Sexual" language use (for example, "poopy-head," "boobies").
10. The privacy of their bodies (for example, giving and receiving permission for touching, etc.).

---

a. The appropriate scale follows each item.

Survey of Unwanted Sexual Attention in University Residences

Kathleen V. Cairns[1] and Julie Wright, *University of Calgary*

The Survey of Unwanted Sexual Attention in University Residences is an amalgamation of several previous instruments (see below) with the addition of demographic descriptions and site-specific questions. It was used to identify the types of sexual harassment and coercion problems that occurred in undergraduate residence halls on campus and to determine how student attitudes and beliefs about sexual harassment and coercion were related to their occurrence. Specific outcomes of the study can be found in several published articles (Cairns, 1993a, 1993b, 1994a, 1994b). The narrative sections of the survey proved to be particularly valuable; qualitative analysis of the narratives confirmed and further developed the findings from the quantitative analyses.

Description

The final version of the survey contains 10 sections (only Sections D, G, H, and I appear in the exhibit), each of which addresses a different set of issues relevant to sexual harassment and coercion. Each of these sections is outlined below.

Section A. This section contains a series of general questions intended to provide a demographic picture of the sample population. The specific items selected for this section were chosen to reflect characteristics that the literature on harassment suggests may be useful in understanding variation in individual responses (i.e., age, gender) as well as information about issues unique to the residences, which might also be expected to systematically affect responses (i.e., type of residence, floor activity level, gender composition of the floor, length of time the participant had lived in residence). Additional questions elaborate on participants' backgrounds (i.e., length of time since leaving home, whether they had lived independently before moving into a university residence) and inquire about how content they were with their current living arrangements.

Section B. This section contains two standardized test instruments, the Sexual Harassment Attitude Scale (Lott, Reilly, & Howard, 1982) and the Attitudes Toward Sex, Dating and Rape Scale (Dull & Giacopassi, 1987). The items on these instruments include a range of beliefs about gender interaction and sex roles. Respondents indicate the extent of their agreement with each statement, using a 5-point Likert-type scale ranging from *strongly agree* to *strongly disagree.*

[1]Address correspondence to Kathleen V. Cairns, Department of Educational Psychology, University of Calgary, 2500 University Drive N.W., Calgary, Alberta T2N 1N4, Canada; email: kcairns@acs.ucalgary.ca.

Section C. This section was a modified version of Muehlenhard and Cook (1988), which provided a series of 16 possible reasons for engaging in unwanted sexual activity. Respondents were asked to indicate whether they had ever engaged in unwanted sexual activity for any of these reasons, and, if so, what type of sexual activity was involved.

Section D. Section D contains items that ask specifically about a series of 10 behaviors that the research literature indicates may be widely considered to constitute sexual harassment. The 10 behaviors are the use of sexually obscene language; display of sexually explicit, offensive, or pornographic materials; putting down women as a group; putting down men as a group; discussion or spreading rumors about the sexual activities of other residents; unwanted, sexually suggestive looks or gestures; unwanted sexual teasing, jokes, comments, or questions; unwanted pressure for social contact; unwanted deliberate touching or physical closeness; and unwanted attempts to kiss or fondle (Reilly, Lott, & Gallogly, 1986). An additional question, added by residents' focus groups prior to survey administration, asks about residents being exposed, against their wishes, to members of the opposite sex in states of undress.

For each problem behavior, residents are asked about whether and with what frequency the behavior had been observed, how offensive it was considered to be, and whether the respondent thought of it as sexual harassment. For Items 6 through 11, which were considered to be more problematic forms of harassment, an additional question was asked concerning frequency of occurrence; maximum number of times any one resident behaved in this manner; how upsetting the incidents were; how the person responded to the incidents; how the person thought he or she would have responded were the person precipitating the incident not another resident; whether responding person had ever engaged in the behavior him- or herself; and how often, why, and how upsetting the respondent thought the behavior was to the other person.

Section E. This section contains the Sexual Experiences Survey (Koss & Oros, 1982). Items on this instrument ask for information about eight types of unwanted sexual activity personally experienced by residents. These activities range from unwanted fondling, kissing, or petting to sexual intercourse. The questions consider possible sexual coercion, the involvement of alcohol and drugs, and the use of physical force. Because the literature indicates that offenders in these more serious types of offense are overwhelmingly likely to be men and that victims are almost exclusively women, the sections for each gender were written accordingly. Section E (Female) focuses on unwanted sexual activity as recipient, asking each woman whether she has had a particular experience, and, if so, how often, when, and where it occurred; to whom (if anyone) it was reported; and whether she considered it sexual assault. Section E (Male) asks about unwanted sexual activity from the perspective of the offender, using a comparable set of questions.

Section F. Section F requests further details about the most severe incident reported by the respondent in Section E, including the number of offenders involved, the relationship of the victim to the offender, where the offense had occurred, whether drugs or alcohol were involved, and various aspects of victim and offender perceptions of the incident. Again, this section is worded differently for female and male respondents reflecting the predominance of male offenders and female victims.

Qualitative Sections G, H, and I. Section G asks for written descriptions of incidents that the respondent felt had not been addressed in the previous sections. Section H provides descriptions of incidents of physical abuse of a nonsexual nature occurring between men and women in the residence complex. Section I requests narrative descriptions of a particular incident of sexually inappropriate behavior that the respondents felt had affected them most or that they remember best. The specific wording of the qualitative sections is contained in the exhibit.

Section J. The final section includes questions about the participants' perceptions of the level of their personal knowledge about sexual harassment and sexual assault, their judgments about current levels of education about these issues in the residences, and their impressions of their own personal safety in residences.

References

Cairns, K. V. (1993a). Sexual entitlement and sexual accommodation: Male and female responses to sexual coercion. *Canadian Journal of Human Sexuality, 2,* 203-214.

Cairns, K. V. (1993b). Sexual harassment in student residences: A response to Dekeseredy and Kelly. *Journal of Human Justice, 4,* 73-84.

Cairns, K. V. (1994a). A narrative study of qualitative data on sexual assault, coercion and harassment. *Canadian Journal of Counselling, 28,* 193-205.

Cairns, K. V. (1994b). Unwanted sexual attention in university residences. *Journal of College and University Student Housing, 24,* 30-36.

Dull, R. T., & Giacopassi, D. J. (1987). Demographic correlates of sexual and dating attitudes. *Criminal Justice and Behavior, 14,* 175-193.

Koss, M. P., & Oros, C. J. (1982). Sexual Experiences Survey: A research instrument investigating sexual aggression and victimization. *Journal of Consulting and Clinical Psychology, 50,* 455-457.

Lott, B., Reilly, M., & Howard, D. R. (1982). Sexual assault and harassment: A campus community case study. *Signs, 8,* 296-319.

Muehlenhard, C. L., & Cook, S. W. (1988). Men's self-reports of unwanted sexual activity. *The Journal of Sex Research, 24,* 58-72.

Reilly, M. E., Lott, B., & Gallogly, S. M. (1986). Sexual harassment of university students. *Sex Roles, 15,* 333-358.

Exhibit

Survey of Unwanted Sexual Attention in University Residences—Sections D, G, H, and I

Section D (adapted from Reilly, Lott, & Gallogly, 1986): In this section there are descriptions of several behaviors. Each description is followed by several questions regarding perceptions of and experience with the behavior.

Section G: Are there any other incidents that have occurred in the residence complex that you would classify as sexual harassment or sexually inappropriate that have not been addressed in the previous two sections? If so, please describe.

Section H: Have you ever experienced or been aware of physical abuse of a non-sexual nature occurring between men and women in the residence complex? If yes, please tell us about the incident or incidents.

Section I: Now we'd like you to think about the questions that have been asked and the types of behavior that have been addressed in this survey. We would like you to describe in your own words a particular incident of sexually inappropriate behavior that you feel has affected you the most or that you remember best. Please describe this incident as fully as possible (e.g., what occurred, why it occurred, how you felt, how you responded, the consequences of your response, how it affected your life and you personally, how it affected your relationships, etc.).

First Coital Affective Reaction Scale

Israel M. Schwartz,[1] *Hofstra University*

Research on premarital coital activity has generally focused on incidence, prevalence, and changing trends, with little attention given to the affective aspects of the experience. However, affective variables are an important component of human sexual behavior. The importance of assessing affect to facilitate a better understanding of the relationship between feelings (as predictors or consequences) and sexual behaviors, attitudes, and norms has been highlighted by the findings of several researchers (Byrne, Fisher, Lamberth, & Mitchell, 1974; Schwartz, 1993; Weis, 1983). Scales used by Byrne et al., and Weis (1983), in their assessment of affect, stimulated the development of the First Coital Affective Reaction Scale (FCARS). The scale was developed as part of a cross-cultural research project comparing first coital experiences of American and Swedish women from an affective, behavioral, and attitudinal perspective (Schwartz, 1993). This scale measures respondents' (male or female) reported affective reactions to their first coital experience.

Description

The FCARS consists of 13 bipolar items, using a 7-point Likert-type format for the measurement of each item. Respondents answering yes to the question "Have you ever had sexual intercourse (defined as penile-vaginal penetration)?" are asked to indicate the degree to which they had experienced the following feelings in reaction to their first coitus at the time that it occurred: confused, satisfied, anxious, guilty, romantic, pleasure, sorry, relieved, exploited, happy, embarrassed, excited, and fearful. The responses range from 1 (representing *not experiencing the feeling at all*) to 7 (representing *strongly experiencing the feeling*), with the numbers in between representing various gradations between these extremes. (To protect anonymity, two versions of the scale are provided to respondents. The respondents who have never engaged in sexual intercourse can complete a version asking about how they think they would feel during their first sexual intercourse. Thus far, only the version for coitally experienced participants has been used for analysis.)

In a cross-cultural study, the scale, included in a self-report anonymous questionnaire focusing on coital initiation and the circumstances surrounding the event, was administered to a sample of 217 female undergraduates drawn from institutions in the northeast, southeast, mideastern, and western regions of the United States (Schwartz, 1993). As part of the same study, the scale was administered to a sample of 186 female undergraduates from institutions in

the northern, middle, and southern regions of Sweden. The entire questionnaire, including the FCARS, was translated into Swedish. A complete description of the translation procedure is given in Schwartz's article.

Response Mode and Timing

Respondents are asked to circle the number (1 to 7) in each item that most closely represents the way they felt. The scale takes approximately 2 minutes to complete, making it easy to include in questionnaires in which time and length are important considerations.

Scoring

Each scale item uses a 7-point Likert-type response format yielding a possible score range of 1 to 7. Items 2 (satisfied), 5 (romantic), 6 (pleasure), 8 (relieved), 10 (happy), and 12 (excited) are reversed in scoring so that on all items 1 represents a positive response and 7 represents a negative response. Thus, greater positive FCARS affect would be represented by a lower total score and greater negative affect would be represented by a higher total score. Items may be scored and looked at separately to assess the degree to which a specific affective reaction was experienced (e.g., guilt, exploitation, pleasure, confusion).

Reliability

Internal consistency of the scale was estimated using Cronbach's alpha. The alpha coefficient with a sample of 217 female undergraduate students in the United States was .89 (Schwartz, 1993). With a sample of 186 female undergraduate students in Sweden (using the Swedish version of the scale), the alpha coefficient was .85. An unpublished pilot test of the research instrument used by Schwartz, with a sample of 37 female undergraduate students from a university in the New York metropolitan area, yielded an alpha coefficient of .87 for the FCARS.

Validity

For face validity the scale was reviewed by a panel of three sexuality experts. In addition, 10 of the participants in the pilot test were individually interviewed to get their opinions regarding format, readability, clarity, and possible bias. Recommendations were incorporated into the final version of the scale. The FCARS construct validity was supported by Schwartz's (1993) findings of expected differences between the American and Swedish samples (greater negative affect among the American group) based on Christensen's (1969) theoretical assertions. These findings were also consistent with Christensen's earlier findings comparing Danish and American cultures (Christensen & Carpenter, 1962a, 1962b; Christensen & Gregg, 1970).

[1]Address correspondence to Israel M. Schwartz, Department of Health, Physical Education and Recreation, Hofstra University, 1000 Fulton Avenue, Hempstead, NY 11550-1090; email: hprims@hofstra.edu.

Other Information

This scale is copyrighted by the author.

References

Byrne, D., Fisher, J. D., Lamberth, J., & Mitchell, H. E. (1974). Evaluations of erotica: Facts or feelings? *Journal of Personality and Social Psychology, 29,* 111-119.

Christensen, H. T. (1969). Normative theory derived from cross-cultural family research. *Journal of Marriage and the Family, 31,* 209-222.

Christensen, H. T., & Carpenter, G. R. (1962a). Timing patterns in the development of sexual intimacy: An attitudinal report on three modern Western societies. *Journal of Marriage and the Family, 24,* 30-35.

Christensen, H. T., & Carpenter, G. R. (1962b). Value-behavior discrepancies regarding premarital coitus in three Western cultures. *American Sociological Review, 27,* 66-74.

Christensen, H. T., & Gregg, C. F. (1970). Changing sex norms in America and Scandinavia. *Journal of Marriage and the Family, 32,* 616-627.

Schwartz, I. M. (1993). Affective reactions of American and Swedish women to their first premarital coitus: A cross-cultural comparison. *The Journal of Sex Research, 30,* 18-26.

Weis, D. L. (1983). Affective reactions of women to their initial experience of coitus. *The Journal of Sex Research, 19,* 209-237.

Exhibit

First Coital Affective Reaction Scale

1. Have you ever had sexual intercourse (defined as penile-vaginal penetration)?
   a. _____ Yes   b. _____ No

(If your answer to this question is "yes" then complete Question 2. If your answer to this question is "no" skip Question 2 and complete Question 3).

2. *Directions:* The following items deal with your feelings about your first sexual intercourse. Please try to answer as accurately and honestly as possible. Please answer *all items* "a" through "m" by using a 7-point scale, in which "1" represents not experiencing the feeling at all and "7" represents strongly experiencing the feeling with the numbers in between representing various gradations between these extremes. *Please circle the number in each item that most closely represents the way you felt.*

What were your reactions to your first sexual intercourse at the time that it occurred? I felt:

a.	Not at all confused	1	2	3	4	5	6	7	Very confused
b.	Not at all satisfied	1	2	3	4	5	6	7	Very satisfied
c.	Not at all anxious	1	2	3	4	5	6	7	Very anxious
d.	Not at all guilty	1	2	3	4	5	6	7	Very guilty
e.	Not at all romantic	1	2	3	4	5	6	7	Very romantic
f.	No pleasure at all	1	2	3	4	5	6	7	Much pleasure
g.	Not at all sorry	1	2	3	4	5	6	7	Very sorry
h.	Not at all relieved	1	2	3	4	5	6	7	Very relieved
i.	Not at all exploited	1	2	3	4	5	6	7	Very exploited
j.	Not at all happy	1	2	3	4	5	6	7	Very happy
k.	Not at all embarrassed	1	2	3	4	5	6	7	Very embarrassed
l.	Not at all excited	1	2	3	4	5	6	7	Very excited
m.	Not at all fearful	1	2	3	4	5	6	7	Very fearful

3. *Directions:* The following items deal with your anticipated reactions to your first sexual intercourse. Please answer *all items* "a" through "m" by using a 7-point scale, in which "1" represents not anticipating the feeling at all and "7" represents strongly anticipating the feeling with the numbers in between representing various gradations between these extremes. *Please circle the number in each item that most closely represents the way you anticipate feeling.*

How do you think you will react to your first sexual intercourse at the time that it occurs? I anticipate feeling:
(The 13 responses for Question 2 are repeated.)

Source. This scale is reprinted with permission of the author.

Dyadic Sexual Communication Scale

Joseph A. Catania,[1] *University of California, San Francisco*

The Dyadic Sexual Communication (DSC) scale is a Likert-type scale assessing respondents' perceptions of the communication process encompassing sexual relationships. The original 13-item scale discriminated people reporting sexual problems from those not reporting sexual problems (Catania, 1986). The shortened and modified versions of the DSC scales, which have been used in nationally sampled sexual-risk studies, discriminated significant differences in disclosure of extramarital sex (Choi, Catania, & Dolcini, 1994) and have also been correlated with incidence of multiple partners (Dolcini, Coates, Catania, Kegeles, & Hauck, 1995).

Description

The DSC scale is a 13-item scale that measures how respondents perceive the discussion of sexual matters with their partners. Items are rated on a 6-point Likert-type scale (1 = *disagree strongly*, 6 = *agree strongly*). When frequent evaluations are desired, shortened, modified versions of the DSC scale is available to assess respondents' quality of communication.

Response Mode and Timing

For each item respondents are instructed to choose the rating that most adequately describes their feelings. All forms of the DSC scale are interviewer administered. Scales are available in English and Spanish, and all versions of the DSC scale take 1-2 minutes to complete.

Scoring

Sum across items for a total score.

Reliability and Validity

The DSC scale has been administered to college and adolescent populations, as well as national urban probability samples constructed to adequately represent White, Black, and Hispanic ethnic groups, as well as high-HIV-risk factor groups (Choi et al., 1994; Dolcini et al., 1995). The DSC scale was assessed in a pilot study (N = 144 college students) that examined the internal consistency, test-retest reliability, and factor structure of the scale (Cronbach's alpha = .81 total sample, .83 cohabiting couples; test-retest = .89: a single factor was obtained) (Catania, Pollack, McDermott, Qualls, & Cole, 1990). In a larger study (N = 500), the scale was administered to respondents who had been recruited from pleasure parties in California's Bay Area (82%) and from church meetings and college classes in Colorado (18%). A slightly higher Cronbach's alpha was obtained (.87), and a factor analysis revealed that the DSC scale was composed of a single dimension. The communication measure discriminated people reporting sexual problems from those not reporting sexual problems, with the problem group (M = 53, SD = 13.0) reporting poorer sexual communication than the no-problem group (M = 63.7, SD = 10.2), t(416) = 9.32, p = .0001.

A shortened, four-item version of the DSC scale was examined in a study of the correlates of extramarital sex (Choi et al., 1994). The analysis was a part of the 1990-1991 National AIDS Behavior Survey (NABS) longitudinal study[2] (Catania, Coates, Kegeles, et al., 1992), which was composed of three interlaced samples designed to oversample African Americans and Hispanics for adequate representation. The interlaced samples included a national sample, an urban sample of 23 cities with high prevalences of AIDS cases, and a special Hispanic urban sample. To examine the correlates of extramarital sex, we restricted our analysis to married, 18- to 49-year-olds who reported having a primary sex partner. In Choi et al. (1994), the four-item version of the DSC scale was administered to those respondents (N = 5,900) who were married and between the ages of 18 and 49. Reliability was good (Cronbach's alpha = .62 for the total sample). Means, standard deviations, range, median, and reliabilities are given for White, Black, and Hispanic groups, males and females, and levels of education for both national and urban/high-risk city samples in Table 1. In the national sample, significant differences in test scores were found between education levels and gender. In the urban/high-risk city groups, differences were found between ethnic groups as well as levels of education and gender. A regression analysis revealed that Hispanics who scored poorly on the dyadic communication scale were more likely to report extramarital sex. A t test revealed gender differences (t = 2.02, p < .04) with women scoring higher than men.

A six-item version of the DSC scale was developed on 114 adolescent females who participated in a study that examined psychosocial correlates of condom use and multiple-partner sex (Catania, Coates, & Kegeles, 1989). Respondents, recruited from a family planning clinic in California, were White (92%), Hispanic (4%), and other (4%). The majority of respondents were heterosexual, unmarried, and sexually active. Reliability was good (Cronbach's alpha = .77).

[1]Address correspondence to Joseph A. Catania, Center for AIDS Prevention Studies, University of California, San Francisco, 74 New Montgomery, Suite 600, San Francisco, CA 94105.

[2] For further details on sample construction and weighting of the NABS cohort study, see Catania, Coates, Kegeles, et al. (1992).

Table 1 Normative Data for the Dyadic Sexual Communication Scale

	N	Mean	SD	Range	Median	Alpha
NABS[a] study						
National sample	1,217	13.35	2.21	11.0	14.0	.65
High-risk cities	4,683	13.14	2.26	12.0	13.0	.62
Ethnicity						
White						
National sample	843	13.48	2.14	11.0	14.0	.67
High-risk cities	1,816	13.20	2.22	12.0	13.0	.68
Black						
National sample	213	13.25	2.38	9.0	14.0	.64
High-risk cities	1,797	13.53	2.22	12.0	14.0	.58
Hispanic						
National sample	128	12.57	2.31	8.0	12.0	.53
High-risk cities	3,062	12.45	2.39	12.0	12.0	.59
Gender						
Male						
National sample	499	13.22	2.22	9.0	13.0	.65
High-risk cities	2,059	12.98	2.25	11.0	13.0	.62
Female						
National sample	723	13.48	2.17	11.0	14.0	.65
High-risk cities	2,617	13.32	2.24	12.0	14.0	.62
Education						
< 12 years						
National sample	125	13.46	2.37	9.0	14.0	.60
High-risk cities	694	12.39	2.31	11.0	12.0	.54
= 12 years						
National sample	330	13.09	2.23	11.0	13.0	.62
High-risk cities	1,163	13.20	2.30	12.0	13.0	.56
> 12 years						
National sample	765	13.46	2.13	11.0	14.0	.67
High-risk cities	2,286	13.32	2.18	12.0	14.0	.66
AMEN[b] study						
Total	558	20.73	2.97	14.0	21.0	.67
Ethnicity						
White	259	20.49	2.94	12.0	21.0	.73
Black	124	21.48	2.60	10.0	22.5	.53
Hispanic	124	20.59	3.35	14.0	21.5	.66
Gender						
Male	250	20.44	2.97	12.0	21.0	.67
Female	308	20.96	2.96	14.0	21.0	.66
Education						
< 12 years	58	20.45	3.44	14.0	21.0	.61
= 12 years	109	20.95	2.95	12.0	21.0	.66
> 12 years	390	20.71	2.91	14.0	15.0	.70

a. National AIDS Behavior Survey.
b. AIDS in Multi-Ethnic Neighborhoods.

The six-item DSC scale was also administered to 558 respondents who participated in a study (Dolcini et al., 1995) examining incidence of multiple partners and related psychosocial correlates, as part of the AIDS in Multi-Ethnic Neighborhoods (AMEN) study[3] (Catania, Coates, Stall,

[3]Respondents for the AMEN study were recruited from 16 census tracts of San Francisco that are characterized by high rates of STDs and drug use. For further information regarding sampling techniques, see Catania, Coates, Stall, et al. (1992) and Fullilove et al. (1992).

et al., 1992). The AMEN study is a longitudinal study (three waves) examining the distribution of HIV, sexually transmitted diseases (STDs), related risk behaviors, and their correlates across social strata. The multiple-partner study sample, which obtained data at Wave 2, was restricted to heterosexuals who reported having a primary sexual partner and being sexually active. Respondents ranged from 20 to 44 years of age. Reliability was good (Cronbach's alpha = .67). The mean, standard deviation, median, range, and reliabilities of ethnic groups, gender, and levels of education are provided in Table 1. The communication scale was relevant only to those with a primary partner. A multiple regression revealed the DSC scale to be associated with having two or more partners.

References

Catania, J. (1986). *Help-seeking: An avenue for adult sexual development.* Unpublished doctoral dissertation, University of California, San Francisco.

Catania J., Coates, T., Golden, E., Dolcini, M., Peterson, J., Kegeles, S., Siegel, D., & Fullilove, M. (1994). Correlates of condom use among Black, Hispanic, and White heterosexuals in San Francisco: The AMEN longitudinal survey. *AIDS Education and Prevention, 6,* 12-26.

Catania, J., Coates, T., & Kegeles, S. (1989). Predictors of condom use and multiple partnered sex among sexually active adolescent women: Implications for AIDS-related health interventions. *The Journal of Sex Research, 26,* 514-524.

Catania, J., Coates, T., Kegeles, S., Thompson-Fullilove, M., Peterson, J., Marin, B., Siegel, D., & Hulley, S. (1992). Condom use in multi-ethnic neighborhoods of San Francisco: The population-based AMEN (AIDS in Multi-Ethnic Neighborhoods) study. *American Journal of Public Health, 82,* 284-287.

Catania, J., Coates, T., Peterson, J., Dolcini, M., Kegeles, S., Siegel, D., Golden, E., & Fullilove, M. (1993). Changes in condom use among Black, Hispanic, and White heterosexuals in San Francisco: The AMEN longitudinal survey. *The Journal of Sex Research, 30,* 121-128.

Catania, J. A., Coates, T. J., Stall, R., Turner, H., Peterson, J., Hearst, N., Dolcini, M. M., Hudes, E., Gagnon, J., Wiley, J., & Groves, R. (1992). Prevalence of AIDS-related risk factors and condom use in the United States. *Science, 258,* 1101-1106.

Catania, J., Pollack, L., McDermott, L., Qualls, S., & Cole, L. (1990). Help-seeking behaviors of people with sexual problems. *Archives of Sexual Behavior, 19,* 235-250.

Choi, K. H., Catania, J. A., & Dolcini, M. M. (1994). Extramarital sex and HIV risk behavior among U.S. adults: Results from the National AIDS Behavior Survey. *American Journal of Public Health, 84,* 2003-2007.

Dolcini, M. M., Coates. T. J., Catania, J. A., Kegeles, S. M., & Hauck, W. W. (1995). Multiple sexual partners and their psychosocial correlates: The population-based AIDS in Multi-Ethnic Neighborhoods (AMEN) study. *Health Psychology, 14,* 1-10.

Fullilove, M., Wiley, J., Fullilove, R., Golden, E., Catania, J., Peterson, J., Garrett, K., Siegel, D., Marin, G., Kegeles, S., Coates, T., & Hulley, S. (1992). Risk for AIDS in multi-ethnic neighborhoods in San Francisco, California: The population-based AMEN study. *Western Journal of Medicine, 157,* 32-40.

Exhibit

Dyadic Sexual Communication Scale

Instructions: Now I am going to read a list of statements different people have made about discussing sex with their primary partner. As I read each one, please tell me how much you agree or disagree with it.

1. My partner rarely responds when I want to talk about our sex life.
2. Some sexual matters are too upsetting to discuss with my sexual partner.
3. There are sexual issues or problems in our sexual relationship that we have never discussed.
4. My partner and I never seem to resolve our disagreements about sexual matters.
5. Whenever my partner and I talk about sex, I feel like she or he is lecturing me.
6. My partner often complains that I am not very clear about what I want sexually.
7. My partner and I have never had a heart-to-heart talk about our sex life together.
8. My partner has no difficulty in talking to me about his or her sexual feelings and desires.
9. Even when angry with me, my partner is able to appreciate my views on sexuality.
10. Talking about sex is a satisfying experience for both of us.
11. My partner and I can usually talk calmly about our sex life.
12. I have little difficulty in telling my partner what I do or don't do sexually.
13. I seldom feel embarrassed when talking about the details of our sex life with my partner.

Note. The short, four-item questionnaire used in the NABS study includes Items 2, 8, 10, and 12. The six-item version used in the AMEN study and adolescent study includes Items 1, 2, 3, 8, 10, and 12. Questions in the original study have been modified for respondents who participated in subsequent studies.

The exact wording of the four-item version of the DSC scale is as follows: 1. Do you find some sexual matters too difficult to discuss with your spouse? 2. Does your spouse have difficulty in talking to you about what he/she likes during sex? 3. Is talking about sex with your spouse fun for the both of you? 4. Do you find that it is easy for you to tell your spouse what you do or do not like to do during sex?

The exact wording of the six-item version of the DSC scale is as follows: 1. I find some sexual matters are too upsetting to talk about with my primary partner. 2. I think it is difficult for my primary partner to tell me what (he/she) likes to do sexually. 3. It is easy for me to tell my primary partner what I do or don't like to do during sex. 4. My primary partner hardly ever talks to me when I want to talk about our sex life. 5. My primary partner really cares about what I think about sex. 6. Talking about sex with my primary partner is usually fun for the both of us.

Weighted Topics Measure of Family Sexual Communication

Terri D. Fisher,[1] *Ohio State University at Mansfield*

The Weighted Topics Measure of Family Sexual Communication was developed to enable researchers to assess quickly and objectively the amount of communication about sexuality that has occurred between parents and their adolescent children. This scale combines a relatively objective measure (number of topics discussed) with a more subjective one (extent of discussion).

[1]Address correspondence to Terri D. Fisher, Ohio State University at Mansfield, 1680 University Drive, Mansfield, OH 44906; email: fisher.16@osu.edu.

Description

This measure asks respondents to indicate the extent to which nine specific sexual topics have been discussed, using a scale of 0 to 4, with 0 corresponding to *none* and 4 corresponding to *a lot*. Possible scores range from 0 to 36 with higher scores indicating greater amounts of communication. Adolescents may be asked to give separate reports for communication with the mother and the father.

Response Mode and Timing

Respondents indicate the extent of communication about each topic by indicating which of the five possible ratings mentioned above best corresponds to the amount of communication experienced. This measure takes no more than 2 to 3 minutes to complete.

Scoring

To score the Weighted Topics Measure of Family Sexual Communication, simply add up the weights for each topic.

Reliability

In a study of 129 male and 234 female unmarried college students between the ages of 18 and 24, the Cronbach alpha reliability coefficient was found to be .89 for males reporting on communication with mothers, .91 for males reporting on communication with fathers, .90 for females reporting on communication with mothers, and .91 for females reporting on communication with fathers. Among the 336 mothers, the Cronbach alpha coefficient was .87, and for the 233 fathers it was .89.

Validity

In a validity study (Fisher, 1993) of nine measures of sexual communication using 129 male and 234 female college students between the ages of 18 and 24, the Weighted Topics measure was significantly correlated with general family communication as measured by the Openness in Family Communication subscale of Olson and Barnes's Parent-Adolescent Communication Scale (Olson et al., 1982), with correlation coefficients ranging from a low of .28 based on the fathers' reports of communication to a high of .53 based on the males' reports of communication with their mothers. This measure of family sexual communication was not significantly correlated with a measure of social desirability responding (Strahan & Gerbasi, 1972). The correlation between the various measures of sexual communication and the validity measures were generally nonsignificant, but this was largely due to the use of Bonferroni corrections to account for the very large number of correlation coefficients that were calculated. In general, for most analyses, the Weighted Topics Measure of Family Sexual Communication appeared to be the strongest of the measures.

Previous researchers have consistently found that when families are categorized as "high communication" and "low communication" families by means of a median split using this measure, adolescents and parents in the high-communication families have sexual attitudes that are much more strongly correlated than those in the low-communication families (Fisher, 1986, 1987, 1988).

References

Fisher, T. D. (1986). An exploratory study of parent-child communication about sex and the sexual attitudes of early, middle, and late adolescents. *Journal of Genetic Psychology, 147,* 543-557.

Fisher, T. D. (1987). Family communication and the sexual behavior and attitudes of college students. *Journal of Youth and Adolescence, 16,* 581-595.

Fisher, T. D. (1988). The relationship between parent-child communication about sexuality and the sexual behavior and attitudes of college students as a function of proximity to parents. *The Journal of Sex Research, 24,* 305-311.

Fisher, T. D. (1990). Characteristics of mothers and fathers who talk to their adolescent children about sexuality. *Journal of Psychology and Human Sexuality, 3,* 53-70.

Fisher, T. D. (1993). A comparison of various measures of family sexual communication: Psychometric properties, validity, and behavioral correlates. *The Journal of Sex Research, 30,* 229-238.

Olson, D. H., McCubbin, H. I., Barnes, H., Larsen, A., Muxen, M., & Wilson, M. (1982). *Family inventories.* St. Paul: University of Minnesota.

Strahan, R., & Gerbasi, K. C. (1972). Short, homogeneous versions of the Marlowe-Crowne Social Desirability Scale. *Journal of Clinical Psychology, 28,* 191-193.

Exhibit

Weighted Topics Measure

Using a scale from 1 to 4 with 0 = *none* and 4 = *a lot*, please indicate how much discussion you have had with your child about the following topics.

	None	0	1	2	3	4	A lot

_____ Pregnancy
_____ Fertilization
_____ Intercourse
_____ Menstruation
_____ Sexually transmitted (venereal) disease
_____ Birth control
_____ Abortion
_____ Prostitution
_____ Homosexuality

Hurlbert Index of Sexual Compatibility

David F. Hurlbert,[1] *Adult and Adolescent Counseling Center*

The Hurlbert Index of Sexual Compatibility (HISC) is described by Hurlbert, White, Powell, and Apt (1993).

[1]Address correspondence to David F. Hurlbert, Adult and Adolescent Counseling Center, 619 North Main, Belton, TX 76513.

Reference

Hurlbert, D. F., White, L. C., Powell, R. D., & Apt, C. (1993). Orgasm consistency training in the treatment of women reporting hypoactive sexual desire: An outcome comparison of women-only groups and couples-only groups. *Journal of Behaviour Therapy & Experimental Psychiatry, 24,* 3-13.

Exhibit

Hurlbert Index of Sexual Compatibility

1. My sexual beliefs are similar to those of my partner. (R)[a]
2. I think my partner understands me sexually. (R)
3. My partner and I share the same sexual likes and dislikes. (R)
4. I think my partner desires too much sex.
5. My partner is unwilling to do certain sexual things for me that I would like to experience.
6. I feel comfortable during sex with my partner. (R)
7. I am sexually attracted to my partner. (R)
8. My partner sexually pleases me. (R)
9. My partner and I argue about the sexual aspects of our relationship.
10. My partner and I share the same level of interest in sex. (R)
11. I feel uncomfortable engaging in some of the sexual activities that my partner desires.
12. When it comes to sex, my ideas and values are different from those of my partner.
13. I do not think I meet my partner's sexual needs.
14. My partner and I enjoy the same sexual activities. (R)
15. When it comes to sex, my partner and I get along well. (R)
16. I think my partner is sexually attracted to me. (R)
17. My partner enjoys doing certain sexual things that I dislike.
18. It is hard for me to accept my partner's views on sex.
19. In our relationship, my partner places too much importance on sex.
20. My partner and I disagree over the frequency in which we should have sex.
21. I have the same sexual values as my partner. (R)
22. My partner and I share similar sexual fantasies. (R)
23. When it comes to sex, my partner is unwilling to do certain things that I would like to experience.
24. I think I sexually satisfy my partner. (R)
25. My partner and I share about the same level of sexual desire. (R)

Note. This 25-item inventory is scored on the following 5-point Likert-type scale: *all of the time* (0); *most of the time* (+1); *some of the time* (+2); *rarely* (+3); *never* (+4).

a. R = reverse-scored items.

The Sexuality Scale

William E. Snell, Jr.,[1] *Southeast Missouri State University*

The Sexuality Scale (SS; Snell & Papini, 1989) is an objective, self-report instrument designed to measure three aspects of human sexuality: *sexual esteem,* defined as positive regard for and confidence in the capacity to experience one's sexuality in a satisfying and enjoyable way; *sexual depression,* defined as the experience of feelings of sadness, unhappiness, and depression regarding one's sex life; and *sexual preoccupation,* defined as the tendency to think about sex to an excessive degree.

Factor analysis confirmed that the items on the SS form three conceptual clusters corresponding to the three concepts (Snell & Papini, 1989). Other results indicated that all three subscales had clearly acceptable levels of reliability. Additional findings indicated that whereas there were no gender differences on the measures of sexual esteem and sexual depression, men reported higher levels of sexual preoccupation than did women. Other evidence showed that among both women and men, sexual esteem was negatively related to sexual depression, with the relationship being quite substantial among male respondents. Also, Snell and Papini (1989) found that women's sexual esteem was positively associated with sexual preoccupation, whereas among men sexual depression was directly related to their sexual preoccupation.

Description

The SS consists of 30 items arranged in a format allowing respondents to indicate how much they agree or disagree with that statement. A 5-point Likert-type scale is used, with responses being scored from +2 to –2: *agree* (+2), *slightly agree* (+1), *neither agree nor disagree* (0), *slightly disagree* (–1), and *disagree* (–2). To create subscale scores (discussed below), the items on each subscale are summed. Higher positive scores thus correspond to greater agreement with the statements, and more extreme negative scores indicate greater disagreement with the statements.

To confirm the three conceptual dimensions assumed to underlie the SS, the 30 items were subjected to a principal components factor analysis. A three-factor solution was specified and rotated to orthogonal simple structure with the varimax procedure. The first factor had an eigenvalue of 8.39 and accounted for 56% of the common variance; the first factor was characterized by the items on the sexual-esteem subscale. All 10 sexual-esteem items loaded on this factor with coefficients ranging from .52 to .82 (average coefficient, .69). The second factor had an eigenvalue of 4.75 and accounted for 32% of the common variance. All

10 of the sexual-preoccupation items loaded substantially on this factor (i.e., greater than .41), with an average loading of .65 (range = .41 to .86). The third factor, accounting for 13% of the common variance and having an eigenvalue of 1.88, dealt with the sexual-depression items; 8 of the 10 items on this sexual-depression subscale had loadings ranging from .48 to .84; average coefficient = .67. The other two items had loadings less than .20, and thus it was decided to consider them filler items.

Response Mode and Timing

In most instances, people respond to the 30 items by marking their answers on separate machine-scorable answer sheets. The scale usually requires about 15-20 minutes to complete.

Scoring

After several items are reverse coded (designated with an *R*), the relevant items on each subscale are then coded so that A = –2, B = –1, C = 2, D = +1, and E = +2. Next, the items on each subscale are summed, so that higher scores correspond to greater sexual esteem, sexual depression, and sexual preoccupation. Scores on the sexual-esteem and sexual-preoccupation scales can range from –20 to +20; scores on the sexual-depression scale range from –16 to +16. The items on the three SS subscales are as follows: sexual esteem (Items 1, 4, 7, 10R, 13R, 16, 19R, 22, 25R, 28R); sexual depression (Items 2, 5R, 8, 17, 20, 23R, 26, 29R); and sexual preoccupation (Items 3, 6, 9R, 12, 15, 18, 21R, 24R, 27R, 30R).

An abbreviated version of the three subscales was developed by Wiederman and Allgeier (1993). The 15-item SS short form includes the following items: sexual esteem (Items 1, 4, 16, 19R, 22); sexual depression (Items 2, 5R, 8, 17, 23R); and sexual preoccupation (Items 3, 6, 12, 15, 18).

Reliability

The internal consistency of the three subscales on the SS was determined by calculating Cronbach alpha coefficients, using a sample of 296 participants (209 females and 87 males) drawn from lower division psychology courses at a small midwestern university (Snell & Papini, 1989). The average age of the women in this study was 23.54 years (*SD* = 5.87), with a range of 19 to 53; the males averaged 23.71 years (*SD* = 4.44), with a range of 19 to 37. The alpha coefficients were computed for each of the three subscales for women and men separately and together. Each coefficient was based on 10-item scales, except for the measure of sexual depression, which consists of eight items. The alphas for the sexual-esteem scale were: .92 for women,

[1] Address correspondence to William E. Snell, Jr., Department of Psychology, Southeast Missouri State University, One University Plaza, Cape Girardeau, MO 63701; email: wesnell@semovm.semo.edu.

.93 for men, and .92 for all respondents. For the sexual-depression subscale, the alpha for women was .88 and the alpha for men was .94 (combined alpha = .90). The alphas for the sexual-preoccupation scale were: .88 for women, .79 for men, and .88 for all respondents.

Snell, Fisher, and Schuh (1992) also provided additional reliability evidence for the SS: sexual esteem (alpha range = .91 to .92), sexual depression (alpha range = .85 to .93), and sexual preoccupation (alpha range = .87 to .91). Test-retest reliability, as reported by Snell et al. (1992), was sexual esteem (range = .69 to .74), sexual depression (range = .67 to .76), and sexual preoccupation (range = .70 to .76). In brief, the three subscales had more than adequate internal consistency and test-retest reliability.

The 15-item short-form SS, five items per subscale, had Cronbach alphas for men and women, respectively, of .92 and .94 for sexual esteem, .89 and .89 for sexual depression, and .96 and .92 for sexual depression (Wiederman & Allgeier, 1993).

Validity

Evidence for the validity of the SS comes from a variety of sources. Snell and Papini (1989) found that among university students, women's and men's scores on sexual esteem and sexual depression were negatively correlated. However, for women, sexual preoccupation was positively correlated with sexual esteem. In contrast, for men, sexual preoccupation was positively correlated with sexual depression. Snell et al. (1992) provided evidence that the SS measures of sexual esteem, sexual depression, and sexual preoccupation were related in predictable ways to men's and women's sexual behaviors and attitudes; evidence for the discriminant validity of the SS was also documented by Snell et al. (1992). Wiederman and Allgeier (1993) indicated that men score higher than do women on both the sexual-esteem and sexual-preoccupation scales. Finally, other researchers have used the SS within a therapy treatment context (Hurlbert, White, Powell, & Apt, 1993).

References

Hurlbert, D. F., White, L. C., Powell, R. D., & Apt, C. (1993). Orgasm consistency training in the treatment of women reporting hypoactive sexual desire: An outcome comparison of women-only groups and couples-only groups. *Journal of Behavior Therapy and Experimental Psychiatry, 24,* 3-13.

Snell, W. E., Jr., Fisher, T. D., & Schuh, T. (1992). Reliability and validity of the Sexuality Scale: A measure of sexual-esteem, sexual-depression, and sexual-preoccupation. *The Journal of Sex Research, 29,* 261-273.

Snell, W. E., Jr., & Papini, D. R. (1989). The Sexuality Scale: An instrument to measure sexual-esteem, sexual-depression, and sexual-preoccupation. *The Journal of Sex Research, 26,* 256-263.

Wiederman, M. W., & Allgeier, E. R. (1993). The measurement of sexual-esteem: Investigation of Snell and Papini's (1989) Sexuality Scale. *Journal of Research in Personality, 27,* 88-102.

Exhibit

The Sexuality Scale

Instructions: The statements listed below describe certain attitudes toward human sexuality which different people may have. As such, *there are no right or wrong answers,* only personal responses. For each item you will be asked to indicate how much you agree or disagree with the statement listed in that item. Use the following scale to provide your responses:

(A)	(B)	(C)	(D)	(E)
Agree	Slightly agree	Neither agree nor disagree	Slightly disagree	Disagree

1. I am a good sexual partner.
2. I am depressed about the sexual aspects of my life.
3. I think about sex all the time.
4. I would rate my sexual skill quite highly.
5. I feel good about my sexuality. (R)
6. I think about sex more than anything else.
7. I am better at sex than most other people.
8. I am disappointed about the quality of my sex life.
9. I don't daydream about sexual situations. (R)
10. I sometimes have doubts about my sexual competence. (R)
11. Thinking about sex makes me happy.
12. I tend to be preoccupied with sex.
13. I am not very confident in sexual encounters. (R)
14. I derive pleasure and enjoyment from sex.
15. I'm constantly thinking about having sex.
16. I think of myself as a very good sexual partner.
17. I feel down about my sex life.
18. I think about sex a great deal of the time.

19. I would rate myself low as a sexual partner. (R)
20. I feel unhappy about my sexual relationships.
21. I seldom think about sex. (R)
22. I am confident about myself as a sexual partner.
23. I feel pleased with my sex life. (R)
24. I hardly ever fantasize about having sex. (R)
25. I am not very confident about my sexual skill. (R)
26. I feel sad when I think about my sexual experiences.
27. I probably think about sex less often than most people. (R)
28. I sometimes doubt my sexual competence. (R)
29. I am not discouraged about sex. (R)
30. I don't think about sex very often. (R)

Source. This scale is reprinted with permission of the author.

Attitude Toward Condoms Scale

The Editors

This scale, authored by Idalyn S. Brown, was published in Brown (1984).

Reference

Brown, I. S. (1984). Development of a scale to measure attitude toward the condom as a method on birth control. *The Journal of Sex Research, 20,* 255-263.

Exhibit

Attitude Toward Condoms Scale

The following items are intended to measure people's opinions about the use of condoms (rubbers) as contraceptive devices. There are no right or wrong responses to any of these statements. Please respond even if you are not sexually active or have never used (or had a partner who used) condoms. In such cases indicate how you think you would feel in such a situation.

Please read each of the following statements and indicate, on the answer sheet, the response that best fits your feeling about the statement. For example, if you agree with a certain statement, place an *A* in the blank. If you strongly disagree, put *SD,* and so forth.

    SD—Strongly disagree; *D*—Disagree; *U*—Undecided; *A*—Agree; *SA*—Strongly agree
1. In my opinion, condoms are too much trouble.
2. Condoms are unreliable.
3. Condoms are pleasant to use.
4. The neatness of condoms, for example, no wet spot on the bed, makes them attractive.
5. I see the use of a condom as adding to the excitement of foreplay if the female partner helps the male put it in place.
6. I would be willing to try a condom, even if I have never used one before.
7. There is no reason why a woman should be embarrassed to suggest a condom.
8. Women think men who use condoms show concern and caring.
9. I intend to try condoms.
10. I think proper use of a condom can enhance sexual pleasures.
11. Many people make use of the condom as an erotic part of foreplay.

12. All things considered, condoms seem safer to me than any other form of contraception except abstinence.
13. I just don't like the idea of using condoms.
14. I think condoms look ridiculous.
15. Condoms are inconvenient.
16. I see no reason to be embarrassed by the use of condoms.
17. Putting a condom on an erect penis can be a real sexual turn-on.
18. Condoms are uncomfortable.
19. Using a condom makes sex unenjoyable.
20. I would avoid using condoms if at all possible.
21. I would be comfortable suggesting that my partner and I use a condom.
22. Condoms ruin the sex act.
23. Condoms are uncomfortable for both partners.
24. Women think men who use condoms are jerks.
25. The idea of using a condom doesn't appeal to me.
26. Use of the condom is an interruption of foreplay.
27. What to do with a condom after use is a real problem.
28. The thought of using a condom is disgusting.
29. Having to stop to put on a condom takes all the romance out of sex.
30. Most women don't like for their partner to use condoms.
31. I don't think condoms interfere with the enjoyment of sex.
32. There is no way that using a condom can be pleasant.
33. Using a condom requires taking time out of foreplay, which interrupts the pleasure of sex.
34. I think condoms are an excellent means of contraception.
35. Condoms seem unreliable.
36. There is no reason why a man should be embarrassed to suggest using a condom.
37. To most women, a man who uses a condom is sexier than one who leaves protection up to the woman.
38. The condom is a highly satisfactory form of contraception.
39. I would have no objection if my partner suggested that we use a condom.
40. The skillful woman can make placing a condom a highly erotic experience.

Source. This scale is reproduced here by permission of the author and *The Journal of Sex Research.*

Note. Items 1, 2, 13, 14, 15, 18, 19, 20, 22, 23, 24, 25, 26, 27, 28, 29, 30, 32, 33, and 35 are scored negatively. Items 3, 4, 5, 6, 7, 8, 9, 10, 11, 12, 16, 17, 21, 31, 34, 36, 37, 38, 39, and 40 are scored positively.

Condom Embarrassment Scale

Karen Vail-Smith[1] and Thomas W. Durham, *East Carolina University*
H. Ann Howard, *University of North Carolina–Chapel Hill*

Embarrassment as a construct inhibiting effective contraceptive use has been supported in the literature (Baffi, Schroeder, Redican, & McCluskey, 1989; Herold, 1981; Hingson, Strunin, Berlin, & Heeren, 1990; Hughes & Torre, 1987; Kallen & Stephensen, 1980; Valdiserri,

[1]Address correspondence to Karen Vail-Smith, Department of Health Education, East Carolina University, Greenville, NC 27858-4353; email: vail-smithk@mail.ecu.edu.

Arena, Proctor, & Bonati, 1989) The Condom Embarrassment Scale (CES) was developed to measure the level of embarrassment in college men and women regarding condom use (Vail-Smith, Durham, & Howard, 1992). Condom embarrassment is here defined as the psychological discomfort, self-consciousness, and feeling of being ill-at-ease associated with condom use. We hypothesized that this psychological discomfort would be experienced when an individual makes acquisition of condoms, negotiates with a partner to use condoms, and actually uses a condom as a part of a sexual encounter.

Description

The 18-item CES employs a Likert-type scale (5 point) with response options labeled from *strongly disagree* to *strongly agree*. From the responses of a sample of 256 college students, a principal components factor analysis with varimax rotation revealed three major components of condom embarrassment, which accounted for 59% of the total variance. Items 1, 2, 3, 4, 5, 6, 7, and 12 loaded on the first factor. This factor accounted for 45% of the shared variance explained by the three factors and appears to be characterized by embarrassment associated with acquiring, purchasing, obtaining, or possessing condoms. Items 14, 15, 16, 17, and 18 loaded on the second factor, which accounted for 30% of the common variance and appears to be associated with actually using condoms. Items 8, 9, 10, 11, and 13 loaded on the third factor. The third factor appears to be associated with negotiating the use of condoms and accounts for 25% of the explainable variance.

Response Mode and Timing

Respondents indicate their level of agreement with each item by circling the number (1-5) corresponding with their answer choice. The CES requires approximately 10 minutes to complete.

Scoring

Each item on the CES is scored from 1 to 5 with 1 corresponding to *strongly disagree* (low embarrassment) and 5 corresponding to *strongly agree* (high embarrassment). Point values for all answers were summed to provide the CES score. The possible range of CES scores is from 18 to 90 with 90 indicating the highest embarrassment and 18 indicating the lowest. Among the 256 college students who participated in the original study, the mean score on the CES was 44.88 (SD = 14.85). Women (M = 46.54, SD = 14.65) scored significantly higher than men (M = 41.81, SD = 14.74), $t(254) = 2.48$, $p = .0138$.

Reliability

To assess the stability of the test over time, a Pearson product-moment correlation coefficient was computed using the scores from the 256 college students who completed two administrations of the CES over a 3-week period. The obtained correlation was .78, ($p < .001$). The Cronbach alpha for the summed scores from the 18 items was .92.

Validity

As expected, Vail-Smith et al. (1992) found that the summed score of the CES was significantly correlated with the Sex Anxiety Inventory (Janda & O'Grady, 1980), $r = .39$. It was also predicted that those persons with greater knowledge about condom use and sexually transmitted diseases (STDs) would feel less embarrassed about buying, discussing, and using condoms. When comparing the scores on an STD/condom knowledge test (Solomon & DeJong, 1989) and the CES across both men and women, the Pearson product-moment correlation for these two variables was .34 ($p < .01$) also indicating a significant correlation in the predicted direction. The relationship of CES scores with the STD/condom knowledge test scores differs by gender, however. For the 163 women, the correlation between the two variables was −.35 ($p < .001$), indicating that women who scored higher on the knowledge test felt less embarrassment about condom acquisition and use. For the 93 men, this correlation was −.13 ($p > .20$), revealing no significant relationship between the variables.

In addition to the attitude measures described above, variation on CES scores as a function of various behaviors was also examined. As expected, those who have actually purchased a condom do feel less condom embarrassment than those who have not made such a purchase and consequently scored significantly lower on the CES. Another factor supporting construct validity is that sexually active respondents have a lower embarrassment score than those who are not sexually active.

Other Information

The use of the CES for educational or research purposes is encouraged. The authors would appreciate receiving information about the results.

References

Baffi, C. R., Schroeder, K. K., Redican, K. J., & McCluskey, L. (1989). Factors influencing selected heterosexual male college students' condom use. *Journal of American College Health, 38*, 137-141.

Herold, E. S. (1981). Contraceptive embarrassment and contraceptive behavior among young single women. *Journal of Youth and Adolescence, 10*, 233-242.

Hingson, R. W., Strunin, L., Berlin, M., & Heeren, T. (1990). Beliefs about AIDS, use of alcohol and drugs, and unprotected sex among Massachusetts adolescents. *American Journal of Public Health, 80*, 295-299.

Hughes, C. B., & Torre, C. (1987). Predicting effective contraceptive behavior in college females. *Nurse Practitioner, 12*, 44-54.

Janda, L. H., & O'Grady, K. E. (1980). Development of a sex anxiety inventory. *Journal of Consulting and Clinical Psychology, 48*, 169-175.

Kallen, J. D., & Stephensen J. (1980). The purchase of contraceptives by college students. *Family Relations, 29*, 358-364.

Solomon, M. Z., & DeJong, W. (1989). Preventing AIDS and other STDs through condom promotion: A patient education intervention. *American Journal of Public Health, 79*, 453-458.

Vail-Smith, K., Durham, T. W., & Howard, H. A. (1992). A scale to measure embarrassment associated with condom use. *Journal of Health Education, 29*, 209-214.

Valdiserri, R. O., Arena, V. C., Proctor, D., & Bonati, F. A. (1989). The relationship between women's attitudes about condoms and their use: Implications for condom promotion programs. *American Journal of Public Health, 79*, 499-501.

Exhibit

Condom Embarrassment Scale

1. I am embarrassed or would be embarrassed about buying a condom from a drug store near campus.
2. I am embarrassed or would be embarrassed about buying a condom from a drug store close to where my parents live.
3. I am embarrassed or would be embarrassed about buying a condom from a place where I could be certain no one I know would see me.
4. I am embarrassed or would be embarrassed about obtaining condoms from Student Health Services (Infirmary).
5. I am embarrassed or would be embarrassed about obtaining condoms from a local health department.
6. I am embarrassed or would be embarrassed about asking a pharmacist or drug store clerk where condoms are located in the store.
7. I am embarrassed or would be embarrassed about asking a doctor or other health care professional questions about condom use.
8. I am embarrassed or would be embarrassed about stopping during foreplay and asking my partner to use a condom.
9. I would be embarrassed if a new partner insisted that we use a condom.
10. I am embarrassed or would be embarrassed to tell my partner during foreplay that I am not willing to have sexual intercourse unless we use a condom.
11. I am embarrassed or would be embarrassed about being prepared and providing a condom during lovemaking if my partner didn't have one.
12. I am embarrassed or would be embarrassed about carrying a condom around in my wallet/purse.
13. I am embarrassed or would be embarrassed about talking to my partner about my thoughts and feelings about condom use.
14. I am embarrassed or would be embarrassed if my partner watched me dispose of a condom after we had used it.
15. (FEMALE:) I am embarrassed or would be embarrassed about watching my partner put on a condom.
    (MALE:)   I am embarrassed or would be embarrassed if my partner watched me put on a condom.
16. (FEMALE:) I am embarrassed or would be embarrassed about helping my partner put on a condom.
    (MALE:)   I am embarrassed or would be embarrassed if my partner helped me put on a condom.
17. (FEMALE:) I am embarrassed or would be embarrassed about watching my partner remove a condom.
    (MALE:)   I am embarrassed or would be embarrassed if my partner watched me remove a condom.
18. (FEMALE:) I am embarrassed or would be embarrassed about helping my partner remove a condom.
    (MALE:)   I am embarrassed or would be embarrassed if my partner helped me remove a condom.

Source. This scale is reprinted with permission of the authors.

Sexual Situation Questionnaire

E. Sandra Byers,[1] *University of New Brunswick*
Lucia F. O'Sullivan, *Toledo, Ohio*

The Sexual Situation Questionnaire (SSQ) measures behavior during interactions in which heterosexual dating partners disagree about the level of sexual intimacy in which they desire to engage (Byers & Lewis, 1988; O'Sullivan & Byers, 1993, 1996). It also assesses coercive and noncoercive behaviors individuals use to influence a reluctant partner to engage in the disputed sexual activity. Parallel forms measure disagreement situations in which the male or the female is the reluctant partner and differ only in the pronouns used to designate the initiating and the reluctant partner. The term *sexual activity* is defined to include all activities that the participants experience as sexual, ranging from holding hands and kissing to sexual intercourse. *Dating* is defined broadly as any social situation in which the respondent was with a member of the other sex, even if it was not part of what they would consider to be a true date. The SSQ could easily be adapted to assess same-sex sexual interactions.

Description

The SSQ can be administered retrospectively (O'Sullivan & Byers, 1993, 1996) or as a self-monitoring device (Byers & Lewis, 1988). The self-monitoring version requires participants to keep a daily record of whether they had been on a date, whether the date involved sexual activity, and whether they and their partner differed about the desired level of sexual activity. The retrospective version requires participants to indicate whether they have ever experienced the designated type of disagreement situation (i.e., a disagreement situation in which the woman desired the higher level of sexual activity or a disagreement situation in which the man desired the higher level of sexual activity). There are male and female versions of each questionnaire.

Respondents who report having experienced such an interaction then complete a 19-item questionnaire assessing characteristics of the first (self-monitoring) or most recent (retrospective) incident. Questions assess their relationship with their dating partner (i.e., type of relationship, number of previous dates, romantic interest in their partner), where they were at the time of the disagreement, the disputed level of sexual activity, whether they had engaged in the disputed sexual activity with that partner on a previous occasion, and the consensual sexual activities preceding the disagreement (if any). Respondents also provide the reasons why the reluctant partner did not want to engage in the initiated sexual activity. Respondents provide detailed information

regarding the communication about the disputed sexual activity by reporting the verbal and/or nonverbal behaviors used by (a) the man or woman to indicate his or her desire to engage in the sexual activity (i.e., initiation behaviors), (b) the reluctant partner to indicate unwillingness to engage in the initiated sexual activity (i.e., response behaviors), and (c) the initiator in response to the noninitiating partner's reluctance (i.e., influence behaviors). Respondents rate how clearly the initiator had indicated a desire for the sexual activity and how clearly the partner had indicated reluctance. Respondents also indicate, from a list of 34 possible influence strategies, those strategies (if any) used to influence the reluctant partner to engage in the unwanted sexual activity. For each strategy endorsed, respondents indicate whether the impact on the reluctant partner was positive (i.e., pleasing), negative (i.e., displeasing), or neutral (i.e., neither pleasing nor displeasing). Respondents indicate whether they had engaged in the disputed level of sexual activity following the disagreement, and they rate the pleasantness associated with the disagreement interaction both at the time of the disagreement and at the time the questionnaire is completed. They also rate the amount of romantic interest felt toward their dating partner both before and after the disagreement.

Using an open-ended format, respondents are given the opportunity to provide additional information about the interaction they had described. Finally, they rate their confidence in the accuracy of their responses.

Response Mode and Timing

The SSQ takes approximately 10 minutes to complete. The format is primarily multiple choice. Five items are open ended: location of incident, reasons for reluctance to engage in the disputed level of sexual activity, and the verbal and nonverbal components of the disagreement. Location was rated as occurring in a bedroom or not in a bedroom. The following categories are used to rate reasons for reluctance to engage in the sexual activity: unknown, timing in relationship, inappropriate relationship, situational (wrong time or location), moral beliefs, physical reasons, and mood. Verbal initiation behavior is categorized as no verbal initiation, indirect verbal initiation, or direct verbal initiation. Nonverbal initiation is categorized as no nonverbal initiation, suggestive look or action, kissing or sexual fondling, or coercion using physical tactics. Responses can be rated categorically (O'Sullivan & Byers, 1993, 1996) or on two definiteness scales (Byers & Lewis, 1988). Categories for verbal responses are no verbal response, refusal without reason, refusal with situation reason, and refusal with personal reason. Categories for nonverbal responses are no

---

[1]Address correspondence to E. Sandra Byers, Department of Psychology, University of New Brunswick, Fredericton, New Brunswick E3B 6E4, Canada; email: byers@unb.ca.

nonverbal response, no resistance, passive acceptance, physical counteraction, or nonsexual touch. The verbal definiteness scale consists of the following 4-point scale: no verbal refusal, refusal implying advances might be accepted at some other time or place, unqualified refusal, and refusal with anger or threat that date should leave. Nonverbal definiteness is scored on the following 4-point scale: no physical refusal, blocked or did not perform sexual activity, moved away or pushed partner away, and got up or slapped. Similarly, influence behaviors can be rated categorically (O'Sullivan & Byers, 1993, 1996) or on a compliance scale (Byers & Lewis, 1988). The categories for influence behaviors are compliance using no influence behaviors, compliance using influence behaviors, or noncompliance. Alternately, compliance is scored on a 5-point scale consisting of stopped without questioning, stopped and asked for clarification, stopped and attempted to persuade partner, stopped and expressed displeasure or anger, and continued unwanted advances.

Reliability and Validity

The SSQ has good reliability. The mean interrater agreement for open-ended questions was .87 (range .83 to 1.0) (O'Sullivan & Byers, 1993, 1996) and .85 (range .71 to 1.00) (Byers & Lewis, 1988).

Respondents' mean confidence ratings of 5.1 (O'Sullivan & Byers, 1993) and 5.2 (Byers & Lewis, 1988; O'Sullivan & Byers, 1996) on a 6-point scale provide evidence for the validity of the responses. Men have been found to rate themselves as less likely to comply with women's refusal of their sexual advances in response to less definite than to more definite verbal responses, providing evidence for the validity of the definiteness scale. More traditional men have been found to be less compliant in their responses to a woman's refusal of their sexual advances, providing evidence for the validity of the compliance scale.

References

Byers, E. S., & Lewis, K. (1988). Dating couples' disagreements over the desired level of sexual intimacy. *The Journal of Sex Research, 24,* 15-29.

O'Sullivan, L. F., & Byers, E. S. (1993). Eroding stereotypes: College women's attempts to influence reluctant male sexual partners. *The Journal of Sex Research, 30,* 270-282.

O'Sullivan, L. F., & Byers, E. S. (1996). Gender differences in responses to discrepancies in desired level of sexual intimacy. *Journal of Psychology & Human Sexuality, 8*(1/2), 49-67.

Exhibit

Sexual Situation Questionnaire for Men (Reluctant Woman Version)[a]

Instructions: We are interested in learning more about communication in dating situations in which you, a man, wished to engage in a higher level of sexual activity than your date, a woman, wanted to engage in at that time. For example, you may have wanted to kiss a woman when she did not wish to kiss you. Another example would be if you wanted to have intercourse and your date only wanted to go as far as sexual fondling. Notice that we are interested in communication about *all* levels of sexual activity from holding hands and kissing to intercourse. And, while we use the term "date," we are interested in any sexual situation that you are in with a member of the other sex, even if it is not part of what you may consider to be a true "date." Also, when we use the term "disagreement," we are referring to those situations in which you indicate a desire to engage in a higher level of sexual activity than a woman wanted—even if she later changed her mind and engaged in the sexual activity anyway or she was convinced to engage in the sexual activity some other way. In other words, the term "disagreement" means that you and your date differed in the level of sexual activity desired. It does not imply that you argued or fought about this issue.

1. Have you ever been on a date where you wanted to engage in a higher level of sexual activity than your date, a woman, did? _____ Yes _____ No
   If *No,* then you do not need to complete the rest of the questionnaire.
   If *Yes,* please complete the rest of the questionnaire for the *most recent* time that this occurred.
2. How long ago was the *most recent* time that you wanted to engage in a higher level of sexual activity than your date did?
   _____ (specify number and whether it was days, weeks, or months).
3. Prior to the disagreement, how many previous dates had you and this woman had together? _____
4. What type of relationship did you have with your date prior to the disagreement?
   _____ First date
   _____ Casual date
   _____ Steady date
5. Where were you and your date at the time of the disagreement?

6. The sexual activity that you wished to engage in but your date did not wish to engage in was: (check all that apply)
   _____ Hugging
   _____ A kiss

_____ Necking
_____ You fondling or kissing your date's breasts
_____ You fondling your date's genitals
_____ Your date fondling your genitals
_____ Oral sex (male to female)
_____ Oral sex (female to male)
_____ Intercourse
_____ Anal sex
_____ Other (please specify) _____

7. Why did your date *not* wish to engage in this sexual activity?

_____ _____

8. Had you ever engaged in this sexual activity before with this woman?
_____ Yes _____ No

9. The sexual activity (or activities) that you and your date were engaging in *immediately prior* to the disagreement
   was (were): (check as many as apply)
   _____ No sexual activity
   _____ Hugging
   _____ A kiss
   _____ Necking
   _____ Your date fondling or kissing your breasts
   _____ Your date fondling your genitals
   _____ You fondling her genitals
   _____ Oral sex (male to female)
   _____ Oral sex (female to male)
   _____ Intercourse
   _____ Anal sex
   _____ Other (please specify) _____

10. How clearly did you indicate to your date that you wanted to engage in the higher level of sexual activity that you
    specified in Question 6?
    _____ Extremely clearly
    _____ Moderately clearly
    _____ Somewhat clearly
    _____ Somewhat unclearly
    _____ Moderately unclearly
    _____ Extremely unclearly

11. What did you say and/or do to indicate that you wanted to engage in the higher level of sexual activity that you
    specified in Question 6? (Please write the exact words you used [if any] and/or describe the actions that you used
    [if any] to indicate that you wanted to engage in the sexual activity.)
    I said: _____
    I did: _____

12. How clearly did your date indicate that she did not want to engage in this sexual activity?
    _____ Extremely clearly
    _____ Moderately clearly
    _____ Somewhat clearly
    _____ Somewhat unclearly
    _____ Moderately unclearly
    _____ Extremely unclearly

13. What did she say and/or do to indicate that she did not want to engage in this sexual activity? (Please write the exact
    words she used [if any] and/or describe the actions that she used [if any] to indicate that she did not want to engage
    in the sexual activity.)
    She said: _____
    She did: _____

14. How did you respond after she had indicated that she did *not* want to engage in this sexual activity? (Please write the
    exact words you used [if any] and/or describe the actions that you used [if any] after she had indicated that she did
    not want to engage in the sexual activity.)
    I said: _____
    I did: _____

15. Did you and your date end up engaging in the sexual activity that you had disagreed upon?
    Yes, then _____
    Yes, later on that date _____
    No, not on that date _____

16. Please indicate which of the following behaviors you used (if any) in attempting to influence your date to engage in the higher level of sexual activity once she had indicated that she did not want to by placing a check mark in the lefthand column below.

Then, for each behavior you used, indicate the impact of the behavior on your date *at that time.* Use a "P" if the impact of the behavior was positive or pleasing to your date, a "D" if the impact of the behavior was negative or displeasing, or an "N" if the impact of the behavior was neutral. (Check as many behaviors as occurred.)

Did you use this?	Impact on woman (P, D, or N)	
_____	_____	Asked her if she found you sexually attractive
_____	_____	Pouted, sulked, or refused to talk
_____	_____	Told her that you were too sexually aroused to stop
_____	_____	Said things to her that you did not really mean (e.g., told her that you loved her and you do not)
_____	_____	Talked about your real feelings toward her (e.g., told her that you loved her and you do)
_____	_____	Threats (e.g., to end the date, end the relationship, or tell others)
_____	_____	Discontinued all sexual activity
_____	_____	Complimented her on her body or sexuality
_____	_____	Made negative comments (e.g., about her sexuality, her personality, her appearance, or the relationship)
_____	_____	Pinched, poked her
_____	_____	Tickled her
_____	_____	Pleaded
_____	_____	Tried to reason with her
_____	_____	Bargained, negotiated, or suggested a compromise
_____	_____	Took off or loosened clothing
_____	_____	Flirted
_____	_____	Pretended to become disinterested in the sexual activity that you had wanted to engage in previously
_____	_____	Cried
_____	_____	Grabbed her or used some other form of physical pressure
_____	_____	Touched, stroked her
_____	_____	Tried to get her drunk, stoned
_____	_____	Started an argument
_____	_____	Made positive comments about her appearance
_____	_____	Made positive comments about her personality
_____	_____	Made positive comments about the relationship
_____	_____	Told her how enjoyable it would be
_____	_____	Made her feel guilty
_____	_____	Used humor
_____	_____	Moved away from her
_____	_____	Made her jealous (e.g., flirted with someone else)
_____	_____	Ignored refusal and engaged in the higher level of sexual activity anyway
_____	_____	Asked her why she didn't want to do it
_____	_____	Put on clothing, music that you hoped she would find arousing
_____	_____	Danced, moved seductively
_____	_____	Other (please specify) _____

17. *At the time* when you wanted to engage in the higher level of sexual activity than your date did, how pleasurable was it being with your date?
    _____Extremely unpleasant
    _____Moderately unpleasant
    _____Slightly unpleasant
    _____Slightly pleasant
    _____Moderately pleasant
    _____Extremely pleasant

18. How do you *now* evaluate this time with your date (when you wanted to engage in a higher level of sexual activity)?
    _____Extremely unpleasant
    _____Moderately unpleasant

_____ Slightly unpleasant
_____ Slightly pleasant
_____ Moderately pleasant
_____ Extremely pleasant

19. Before this incident, how romantically interested did you feel toward your date?
_____ No romantic interest
_____ Slightly romantically interested
_____ Moderately romantically interested
_____ Very romantically interested
_____ Extremely romantically interested

20. After this incident, how romantically interested did you feel toward your date?
_____ No romantic interest
_____ Slightly romantically interested
_____ Moderately romantically interested
_____ Very romantically interested
_____ Extremely romantically interested

21. If there is any additional information that would help us to understand the incident that you described above, please provide it. _____

22. How confident are you that your responses are accurate?
_____ Very unsure
_____ Moderately unsure
_____ Slightly unsure
_____ Slightly sure
_____ Moderately sure
_____ Very sure

a. This version of the questionnaire is designed for men to report on incidents in which they desired a higher level of sexual activity than did their female partner. Men can also be asked to report on situations in which their female partner desired to engage in a higher level of sexual activity than they did, and women can be asked to report on either of these disagreement situations by altering the pronouns and use of the terms *man* and *woman*.

Styles of Conflict Inventory for Personal Relationships

Michael E. Metz,[1] *University of Minnesota*

General theories of sexual dysfunction and dissatisfaction have emphasized the role of relationship conflict in the etiology, maintenance, and therapeutic treatment of sexual problems. The Styles of Conflict Inventory (SCI) is a brief self-report measure designed to aid in the assessment of couples' conflict. It gives a broad, initial overview of the

[1] Address correspondence to Michael E. Metz, Department of Family Practice & Community Health, University of Minnesota Medical School, 1300 South 2nd Street, Suite 180-3, Minneapolis, MN 55454; email: MMetzMPLS@aol.com

basic types of cognitive and behavioral responses between partners, and it provides a general screen of a couple's interactions when discord or disagreement occurs in the relationship. As such, the SCI may be helpful to sex and relationship therapists to determine the possible role that conflict may play in a sexual problem, or the severity of effect a sexual problem may have on the relationship. In research situations, it may also be used with specialized directions such as "When you experience disagreement or conflict in your *sexual* relationship, how often do you have the following . . . [responses]?"

Description

The SCI organizes conflict resolution styles according to two basic dimensions: (a) the classic engaging versus avoiding conflict styles composed of three engaging styles (assertion, aggression, adaptation) and three avoiding styles (withdrawal, submission, denial); and (b) constructive versus destructive styles, which may promote (assertion, adaptation, submission) or contaminate (verbal aggression, physical aggression, withdrawal, denial) beneficial conflict resolution, and subsequently, overall relationship satisfaction. These two dimensions define the styles according to their function or role in conflict resolution; for example, assertion is classified as a constructive, engaging style, whereas withdrawal is categorized as a destructive, avoiding style.

Part 1 of the inventory consists of the 12-item Appraisal of Conflict form that assesses the context of relationship conflict. Part 2 of the inventory consists of 126 items measuring the Styles of Conflict. The Appraisal of Conflict items are 7-point Likert-type items that measure the climate or context of conflict (such as relationship satisfaction, conflict frequency, intensity, estimates of power, level of distress, effort to resolve differences), and the SCI Styles of Conflict scales, composed of 5-point Likert-type items (*never* to *very often*), measure four cognition styles, and seven behavior and seven corresponding perception (i.e., perception of partner's behavior) styles. By design, scales were intended to be efficient measures of the construct and were composed of three to seven items per scale. A lower score indicates a lower amount and a higher score indicates a higher amount of an item or style. Cognition scales measure the respondent's self-reported styles of thinking or "self-statements" in reaction to relationship conflict; behavior scales assess the self-reported styles of action or physical enactment when conflict occurs; and perception scales measure the impressions one forms about the other person's actions in response to the conflict. Sample behavior items include the following: "Calmly ask your partner to talk," "Push or slap your partner," "Withdraw or stay away from your partner," and "Verbally blame your partner." Because the items in the behavior and perception sections directly correspond, Partner X's self-reported behavior scales (B_x) can be compared to Partner Y's perception scales (P_y) and produce discrepancy (D) or "difference scores" ($B_x - P_y = D_x$) for each partner's behavior scales. The SCI test booklet/answer sheet is eight pages in length (four pages front and back). It comes in color-coded duplicate forms so that the test administrator can tear the booklet in half, giving each partner a four-page questionnaire in a different color. The complete cost of the SCI test ($8 per couple) includes the test booklet and the mail-in computer scoring report, which yields a 12-page summary with graphs presenting partner profiles and couple comparisons.

Response Mode and Timing

The partners complete the computer-scored test booklet/answer sheet by indicating the frequency of using a particular response to relationship conflict. The SCI takes approximately 15-20 minutes to complete, and its reading level is approximately fifth grade.

Scoring

Because of the complexity of computing interpartner discrepancy scores, only mail-in computer scoring is available. The SCI is scored by mailing the test booklet/answer sheet to the publisher to obtain the SCI Computer Report, which concisely conveys the couple's results. The 12-page computer report includes a cover page explaining the scores in language suitable for the couple to understand and six sections of results that present graphs of the partner's scores from a variety of perspectives: (a) The appraisal of conflict items report partner's side-by-side results of relationship satisfaction, conflict frequency, intensity, estimates of power, level of distress, and efforts to resolve differences; (b) individual graphs profile each partner's self-thoughts, behaviors, and perceptions of the partner's actions; (c) side-by-side graphs compare partner's styles of conflict; (d) graphic profiles compare the differences between each partner's self-reported behaviors and the other's perceptions of those behaviors; (e) a listing of "critical items," which are items that received extreme scores; and (f) raw scores.

Two types of scores are reported throughout the report. The average frequency score indicates how often the partner indicated experiencing a particular style of response. It is derived by averaging all the items on a scale. The T score is a standard score that relates partner scores to a larger norm group.

The computer report has separate scoring report norms for heterosexual, gay, and lesbian couples.

Reliability

Internal consistency reliability (Cronbach's alpha) for the SCI scales ranged from .85 (Verbal Aggression, Perception of Partner) to .61 (Submission Behavior), with the majority of scales within the .73 to .80 range. The mean alpha for the SCI scales was .78, and alpha coefficients were comparable for women and men, with no scale difference greater than .08., indicating good internal consistency for most subscales, particularly for scales consisting of small numbers of items (3-7). The test-retest reliability coefficients with a 4-week test interval with a community sample averaged .74, with individual scales ranging from .90 to .59. Test-retest reliability coefficients with a 2-week test interval with clinical couples averaged .75, with individual scales ranging from .93 to .53. These results indicate that most SCI scales possess good temporal stability—especially for brief scales.

Validity

SCI scales were constructed by item-to-scale assignments by seven expert raters who assigned 95% of items to scales (e.g., assertion, aggression) with total agreement, whereas the remaining 5% received agreement ratings from six of seven raters. The construct validity of these SCI scales was subsequently examined using confirmatory factor analyses (LISREL 7). For both women and men, factor loadings for each item in the cognition, behavior, and perception analyses confirmed the expert rater item-to-scale assignments for all SCI scales. All items had significant t values at $p < .05$. The goodness-of-fit indexes for the cognition, behavior, and perception scales were very good: for items comprising the cognition scales, the goodness-of-fit index was .92 for both women and men, and for the behavior scales, .89 for women and .88 for men. For items comprising the perception scales, the goodness-of-fit index was .83 for women and .88 for men. These results of confirmatory factor analyses support the SCI scale structure and indicate that the scale structure is valid for each gender.

Data regarding concurrent validity studies (e.g., Straus's Conflict Tactics Scale, Spanier's Dyadic Adjustment Scale, Locke and Wallace's Marital Adjustment Test, Olson's EN-RICH scales), clinical populations discriminant analyses, and regression analyses are reported in the SCI manual.

Other Information

The SCI is published by Consulting Psychologists Press, 3803 East Bayshore Road, Palo Alto, CA 94303. Complimentary sample copies are available from the publisher at 1-800-624-1765 by ordering SCI Sampler #0980N.

References

Metz, M. E. (1993). *The Styles of Conflict Inventory (SCI) for personal relationships*. Palo Alto, CA: Consulting Psychologists Press.

Metz, M. E. (1995, June). Results from empirical studies of couples conflict resolution. *Minnesota Association for Marital & Family Therapy Newsletter, 13*(1), 4-5.

Metz, M. E., & Dwyer, S. M. (1993). Relationship conflict management patterns among sex dysfunction, sex offender, and satisfied couples. *Journal of Sex & Marital Therapy, 19*(2), 104-122.

Metz, M. E., & Epstein, N. (1998). *The Styles of Conflict Inventory (SCI): New evidence of its validity*. Manuscript submitted for publication.

Metz, M. E., Rosser, B. R. S., & Strapko, N. (1994). Differences in conflict resolution styles between heterosexual, gay, and lesbian couples. *The Journal of Sex Research, 31*, 293-308.

Contraceptive Attributes Questionnaire

The Editors

The Contraceptive Attributes Questionnaire was developed by Beckman, Harvey, and Murray (1992) "to assess the subjective importance of specific contraceptive attributes and the perceived characteristics of specific contraceptives" (p. 243). Eighteen attributes of three birth control methods (sponge, pill, and diaphragm) are judged by respondents. The scales are multidimensional, and the factors identifying the subscales have moderate internal consistency. Respondents' judgments were related to use of each method.

Reference

Beckman, L. J., Harvey, S. M., & Murray, J. (1992). Dimensions of the Contraceptive Attributes Questionnaire. *Psychology of Women's Quarterly, 16*, 243-259.

The Contraceptive Utilities, Intention, and Knowledge Scale

Larry Condelli,[1] *University of California, Santa Cruz*

The Contraceptive Utilities, Intention, and Knowledge Scale (CUIKS) was developed to test a social psychological model of contraceptive behavior developed by Condelli (1984). This model combined elements of the health belief model (Rosenstock, 1974), Luker's (1975) model of contraceptive risk taking, and Fishbein and Ajzen's (1975) behavioral intention model. Consequently, it is appropriate for use when examining any of these models or the unified model. It can also be used to study women's knowledge and perceptions about contraceptive methods and their attitudes about pregnancy and to measure intention to use contraception.

Description

The scale is designed to be used with women and is divided into three parts. Part one has nine items (Questions 1-6 in the exhibit) and measures perceived likelihood of becoming pregnant, both when the respondent is using her chosen method of contraception and with unprotected intercourse. It also asks the likelihood she will use her method at each act of intercourse over the next year. This item is designed to measure intention to use contraception. One item measures attitude about becoming pregnant at the present time. This part of the scale also has the respondent rate the degree of subjective social support she expects from "people who are most important" to her for using each of four methods of contraception (diaphragm, IUD, the pill, and condoms). Part one also includes an item asking the respondent to state her current method of contraception.

Part two of the scale (Questions 7 and 8 in the exhibit) has 16 items and measures respondent attitudes about four methods of contraception. The respondent indicates her perceptions of the effectiveness of each method. Her concerns about effects from using each method are also measured. The third part of the scale is a multiple-choice knowledge test. This test is divided into two parts. The first part is an eight-item test of general knowledge of conception and contraception. The second part is a four-item test that measures the respondent's knowledge of the primary birth control method she is currently using. Although the test contains four items for each of the four methods of contraception, the respondent answers *only* the four questions dealing with her method. (In the original instrument, there were four items for the IUD. Because of the infrequent use of the IUD by women in the United States today, these items

have been removed from this edition of the exhibit, to save space.)

The CUIKS was developed to be used in a family planning clinic. It was tested at the clinic on over 600 women of highly diverse age and educational backgrounds. Consequently, it can be used on any population of women.

Response Mode and Timing

The scale is designed to be self-administered either individually or in a group setting. Respondents indicate their answers by circling the number that best represents their feelings. For the knowledge scale portion, respondents circle the letter that indicates what they believe to be the correct answer. The scale requires an average of 15 minutes to complete.

Scoring

For parts one and two of the scale, the number circled on the scale is used as the respondent's score on the item. Items 1 and 4 represent the respondent's perceived susceptibility to becoming pregnant, with higher scores indicating a greater likelihood. Item 3 measures intention to use the chosen contraceptive method; Item 6 measures the degree of subjective normative support expected by the respondent for using each method. Both items are positively scaled. Item 5 measures the perceived severity of pregnancy for the respondent and is scored by assigning a value of 7 to the first, most negative statement (*It would be the worst thing that could happen to me*) and a value of 1 to the last, most positive statement (*It would be the best thing that could happen to me*). The intermediate statements decrease in value consecutively according to their order listed in the item (e.g., the third statement down, *It would be sort of bad but not terrible*, is assigned a value of 5, the following statement a 4, etc.).

For part two of the scale, the value circled by the respondent is the score for that item. The scores for Item 7 on effectiveness and convenience of the methods are reverse scored.

For the knowledge portion of the scale, items are scored as correct or incorrect. Two scores are then derived by summing the number of correct answers. Items 1 through 8 comprise the general knowledge subscale; the four items relating to the respondent's chosen contraceptive method make up the specific knowledge subscale. A total score is computed by adding general and subscale scores. The correct answers are indicated by an asterisk in the exhibit. No response on an item is scored as incorrect.

[1]Address correspondence to Larry Condelli, CRS Incorporated, Suite 600, 1400 Eye Street N.W., Washington, DC 20005.

Reliability and Validity

The reliability of the knowledge scale was computed using responses from 632 women visiting a suburban family planning clinic. For the total knowledge scale, Condelli (1986) reported the Kuder-Richardson 20 was .62. The reliability is somewhat low due to the varied nature of the topics covered in the scale.

The validity of the scale has been demonstrated through its ability to predict contraceptive behavior and contraceptive choice. Condelli (1984) obtained four measures of contraceptive behavior from women who had completed the scale an average of 6 months previously. Using multiple regression, a significant proportion of variance of each behavioral measure was accounted for using Items 1, 5, 6, 7, and 8 as predictor variables. For Items 7 and 8, only the respondent's rating of the effectiveness, convenience, concern about minor side effects, and concern about major side effects of her own chosen contraceptive method were used in the analysis.

The behavioral measures examined included whether the respondent had unprotected intercourse at any time since completing the scale (coded 0 or 1; $R = .21$); frequency of use of her chosen contraceptive method on a 4-point scale (1 = *every time*, 4 = *less than half the time*; $R = .36$); period of time in weeks the respondent had been sexually active without using contraception ($R = .42$); and ranked actual use of effectiveness of the chosen contraceptive method ($R = .38$). All multiple Rs were significant at the .05 level or less.

Condelli (1986) also used the scale to predict choice of contraceptive. Women who chose to use the pill were compared with diaphragm users in a discriminant function analysis, with the scale items and total knowledge test score as predictors. The scale significantly distinguished pill users from diaphragm users on their reported belief the diaphragm was more inconvenient to use and the pill more convenient, expressing less concern about the pill's side effects, believing they were more protected from pregnancy when using the pill and more susceptible when not using it, and having less knowledge about contraception. More than 60% of the variance between the groups was explained by the discriminant function.

References

Condelli, L. (1984). *A unified social psychological model of contraceptive behavior.* Unpublished doctoral dissertation, University of California, Santa Cruz.

Condelli, L. (1986). Social and attitudinal determinants of contraceptive choice: Using the health belief model. *The Journal of Sex Research, 22*, 478-491.

Fishbein, M., & Ajzen, I. (1975). *Belief attitude intention and behavior: An introduction to theory and research.* Reading, MA: Addison-Wesley.

Kirby, D. (1979). *An analysis of U.S. sex education programs and evaluation methods.* Washington, DC: U.S. Department of Health, Education, and Welfare.

Luker, K. (1975). *Taking changes: Abortion and the decision not to contracept.* Berkeley: University of California Press.

Rosenstock, I. (1974). The health belief model and preventive health behavior. *Health Education Monographs, 2*, 354-386.

Exhibit

The Contraceptive Utilities, Intention, and Knowledge Scale

Attitude Survey

1. If you were *not* to use birth control, how likely do you think it is that you would become pregnant during the next year? (Circle one category)

1	2	3	4	5
Very unlikely	Somewhat unlikely	Neutral, neither likely nor unlikely	Somewhat likely	Very likely

2. What form of birth control have you chosen to use? _____

3. How likely do you think it is that you will use the above method every time you have intercourse over the next year?

1	2	3	4	5
Very unlikely	Somewhat unlikely	Neutral, neither likely nor unlikely	Somewhat likely	Very likely

4. If you were to continue using this form of birth control, how likely do you think it is that you would become pregnant during the next year? (Circle one category)

1	2	3	4	5
Very unlikely	Somewhat unlikely	Neutral, neither likely nor unlikely	Somewhat likely	Very likely

5. Below are a number of statements about how you might feel about becoming pregnant within the next year. Please place a check in front of the one that best represents how you feel. (Check one only)

   If I were to get pregnant within the next year:

   _____ It would be the worst thing that could happen to me.

   _____ It would be very bad.

   _____ It would be sort of bad but not terrible.

_____ It would be O.K.
_____ It would be sort of good but not terrific.
_____ It would be very good.
_____ It would be the best thing that could happen to me.

6. People who are important to you may have feelings about the type of birth control you might use. For each birth control method below, please indicate how the people who are most important to you would feel about your using that form of contraception. (Circle the number from 1 to 5 that best represents *their* feelings.)
   They would be:

   1 = Very much opposed (would discourage use)
   2 = Somewhat opposed
   3 = Neither opposed nor in favor (neutral)
   4 = Somewhat in favor
   5 = Very much in favor (would encourage use)

Foam/condoms	1	2	3	4	5
Diaphragm	1	2	3	4	5
IUD	1	2	3	4	5
Birth control pills	1	2	3	4	5

7. Different birth control methods vary in how *effective* or ineffective they are in preventing pregnancy. They also vary in how *convenient* they are to use. For each birth control method listed below, please rate how *effective* you think they would be in *preventing you* from becoming pregnant, and how *convenient or inconvenient* they would be for you to use. (Circle the number from 1 to 5 that best represents your feelings.)

1 = Very effective (definitely prevents pregnancy)	1 = Very convenient (no trouble at all)
2 = Pretty effective	2 = Pretty convenient
3 = Unsure	3 = Unsure
4 = Pretty ineffective	4 = Pretty inconvenient
5 = Ineffective (would not prevent pregnancy)	5 = Very inconvenient (too much trouble to use)

	Effectiveness					*Convenience*				
Foams/condoms	1	2	3	4	5	1	2	3	4	5
Diaphragm	1	2	3	4	5	1	2	3	4	5
IUD	1	2	3	4	5	1	2	3	4	5
Birth control pills	1	2	3	4	5	1	2	3	4	5

8. Different forms of birth control vary in terms of how likely they are to have side effects. Some side effects may be *minor*, such as irritation of or skin problems, while others may be *major*, such as increasing risk of serious illness. For each method of birth control below, please rate how concerned you would be about the occurrence of both *minor* and *major* side effects. (Circle the number from 1 to 5 that best represents your feelings.)

   1 = Not at all concerned
   2 = Slightly unconcerned
   3 = Unsure
   4 = Pretty concerned
   5 = Very concerned

	Minor side effects					*Major side effects*				
Foams/condoms	1	2	3	4	5	1	2	3	4	5
Diaphragm	1	2	3	4	5	1	2	3	4	5
IUD	1	2	3	4	5	1	2	3	4	5
Birth control pills	1	2	3	4	5	1	2	3	4	5

Knowledge Survey

Circle the correct response.

1. The pill:
   *a.   prevents ovulation
   b.   keeps cervical mucus very thin
   c.   changes the lining of the uterus to make implantation unlikely
   d.   both a and c
   e.   all of the above
2. According to the most accepted current thought, the IUD's effectiveness is due to:
   a.   changing levels of hormones
   b.   changed functioning of the fallopian tubes

*c.   preventing implantation of the fertilized egg
   d.   preventing ovulation
   e.   all of the above
3. A diaphragm should be used:
   a.   without any cream or jelly
   b.   with any type of lubricant
*c.   with spermicidal jelly or cream inside it
   d.   either with or without spermicidal jelly
4. Contraceptive foam is most effective in preventing pregnancy when inserted inside the vagina:
*a.   right before intercourse
   b.   2-4 hours before intercourse
   c.   right after intercourse
   d.   all of the above
5. The use of a condom when having sexual intercourse is recommended because:
   a.   if used right, it usually prevents getting or giving gonorrhea
   b.   it can be bought in a drug store by both men and women
   c.   it does not have dangerous side effects
*d.   all of the above
6. A woman can get pregnant:
   a.   a few minutes after sexual intercourse
   b.   a few hours after sexual intercourse
   c.   a few days after sexual intercourse
*d.   all of the above
   e.   a and b
7. Over a one-year period, what is the likelihood that a sexually active woman who uses no birth control will become pregnant?
   a.   1 in 10
   b.   5 in 10
   c.   7 in 10
*d.   9 in 10
8. A woman is most likely to become pregnant (no matter how long or short her menstrual cycle) if she has sexual intercourse about:
   a.   1 week before menstruation begins
   b.   2 weeks after menstruation begins
*c.   2 weeks before menstruation begins
   d.   1 week after menstruation begins

If you decided on the *pill* as your primary method of birth control, answer the questions on page 3 only.

If you decided on the *IUD* as your primary method of birth control, answer the questions on page 4 only.

If you decided on the *diaphragm* as your primary method of birth control, answer the questions on page 5 only.

If you decided on *foam* and/or *condoms* as your primary method of birth control, answer the questions on page 6 only.

Answer these questions *only* if you decided on the *pill* as your primary method of birth control.

1. Some warning signs that may signal the onset of pill-related problems are:
   a.   chest pain
   b.   yellowing of the skin
   c.   pain in the calf of the leg
*d.   all of the above
   e.   none of the above
2. Medical conditions that make it dangerous for a woman to use the pill are:
   a.   high blood pressure
   b.   heavy smoking
   c.   diabetes
   d.   both a and b
*e.   all of the above

3. Present evidence indicates that the most serious side effect of the pill is:
   a. cancer
   *b. blood clotting problems
   c. chloasma
   d. nausea
   e. creating permanent sterility
4. Which of the following group of women has the highest risk of side effects if they use the pill?
   a. women who have never had children
   *b. women over 40 who smoke
   c. women who have severe menstrual cramps and are 10-20 lbs. overweight
   d. women who have been on the pill for more than 5 years.

This completes the survey. Thank You!

Answer these questions *only* if you have decided on the *IUD* as your primary method of birth control:

1. Serious side effect(s) of the IUD include:
   a. perforation of the uterus
   b. uterine infection
   c. tubal infection
   d. both a and b
   *e. all of the above
2. The IUD is not recommended for:
   a. women with severe menstrual cramping
   b. teenagers
   c. women who have had pelvic infections
   *d. all of the above
   e. none of the above
3. Once an IUD is inserted, it is important to check periodically for the string because:
   a. if it *can* be felt, it indicates the IUD is out of place
   *b. if it *cannot* be felt, it indicates the IUD may be out of place
   c. if it *can* be felt, it indicates it should be removed immediately
   d. if it *can* be felt, it will interfere with sexual intercourse
   e. none of the above
4. A drawback of using an IUD is:
   *a. it may be expelled by the body without the woman's knowledge
   b. it may interfere with orgasm by making uterus contractions painful
   c. its effectiveness is dependent on the age and pregnancy history of the user
   d. none of the above

This completes the survey. Thank You!

Answer these questions *only* if you have decided on the *diaphragm* as your primary method of birth control.

1. After intercourse, a diaphragm:
   a. should be removed immediately to prevent infection
   b. can be taken out after 2 hours
   *c. must be left in place for at least 8 hours
   d. must be left in place for at least 12 hours
2. A problem that may result from using a diaphragm is:
   a. increased pelvic infection
   b. increased cervical infection
   *c. increased urinary tract infection
   d. all of the above
   e. none of the above
3. When a diaphragm is properly in place:
   *a. the woman *will not* be able to feel it
   b. the woman *will* be able to feel it
   c. both partners will be able to feel it
   d. both b and c

4. A diaphragm must be fitted by a health professional because:
    a.   the risk of complication is high
    *b.   it must fit properly over the cervix
    c.   it is a difficult and risky medical procedure
    d.   all of the above
    e.   both a and b

This completes the survey. Thank You!

Answer these questions *only* if you have decided on *foam* and/or *condoms* as your primary method of birth control.

1. The actual user effectiveness rate of foam and condoms is equal to or better than the actual user rates of:
    a.   an IUD
    b.   a diaphragm
    c.   the pill
    *d.   all of the above
    e.   none of the above
2. To use a condom correctly, a person must:
    a.   leave some space at the tip for the sperm
    b.   use one every time sexual intercourse occurs
    c.   hold it on the penis while withdrawing from the vagina
    *d.   all of the above
3. When having sexual intercourse, the use of both contraceptive foam and condoms is recommended because:
    a.   the man and the woman are sharing the responsibility for avoiding pregnancy
    b.   the woman is less likely to become pregnant than if only one of these is used
    c.   they can both be purchased at the drug store without prescriptions
    *d.   all of the above
    e.   a and c
4. Contraceptive (birth control) foam is most effective for the repeated acts of sexual intercourse:
    a.   if a single application is used
    *b.   if an additional application is used before each act of sexual intercourse
    c.   if a woman douches after each act of intercourse
    d.   all of the above
    e.   b and c

This completes the survey. Thank you!

Contraceptive Knowledge Inventory

Robert L. DelCampo,[1] *Eastern Michigan University*
Diana S. DelCampo, *Madonna College*

The purpose of this inventory is to measure an individual's knowledge of selected natural, mechanical, and chemical contraceptive techniques.

Description

The scale is a 25-item multiple-choice test. Each question has five response choices, the fifth being *do not know*. The *do not know* choice for each question is particularly useful when the instrument is used in research.

The following areas are tested using this scale: calendar and basal body temperature techniques of the rhythm method, viability of sperm and ova, motility of sperm, physician-prescribed versus over-the-counter methods of contraception, use and types of spermicidal agents, oral contraception, mechanical and hormonal methods of contraception, effectiveness of various contraceptive techniques, and contraceptive methods that prevent sperm and egg from uniting.

The instrument (DelCampo, Sporakowski, & DelCampo, 1976) was originally developed and used with a college student sample of freshmen through seniors. However, it would be appropriate for groups of high school students through adults. Questions are worded in a straightforward manner and the use of jargon is minimized. Some familiarity with basic human sexuality vocabulary, such as menstrual cycle, sperm, ejaculation, and coitus, is essential.

Response Mode and Timing

The updated, 25-item instrument requires approximately 25 minutes to complete. Respondents can circle their choice of answer for each question, or they can be given a separate scoring sheet to accompany the questionnaire so as to facilitate machine scoring.

Scoring

The test has five response choices per question; each response choice is mutually exclusive of the others. There is only one correct answer per item. Higher scores indicate greater knowledge of contraceptive devices and techniques than do lower ones. The scoring key is shown with the exhibit.

Reliability

The reliability of the instrument was determined in two ways. For the original 26-item scale, a sample of college students ($N = 21$) was administered the test once and then given the same test 17 days later. Using Spearman's rho, the coefficient of reliability for this group was .89. For the modified, revised 25-item scale, an internal reliability measure, the Kuder-Richardson 20 technique, was used with another group of college students ($N = 176$), and the reliability coefficient was .86.

Validity

Because the original and revised instruments are concerned exclusively and directly with questions regarding knowledge of contraceptive devices and techniques, face validity is assumed.

The original 26-item scale has successfully predicted differences in knowledge of contraceptive devices and techniques between men and women, Blacks and Whites, and college students of various ages and income levels (DelCampo, 1973; DelCampo et al., 1976).

Other Information

A keyed copy of the instrument can be secured by writing to the first author. Please include $3.00 to cover postage, handling, and printing charges.

References

DelCampo, R. L. (1973). *The relationship between college students' knowledge of contraceptive devices and techniques and their attitudes toward premarital sexual permissiveness.* Unpublished master's thesis, Virginia Polytechnic Institute and State University.

DelCampo, R. L., Sporakowski, M. J., & DelCampo, D. S. (1976). Premarital sexual permissiveness and contraceptive knowledge: A biracial comparison of college students. *The Journal of Sex Research, 12,* 180-192.

[1]Address correspondence to Robert L. DelCampo, Department of Human, Environmental and Consumer Resources, Eastern Michigan University, Ypsilanti, MI 48917.

Exhibit

Contraceptive Knowledge Inventory

Directions: Answer each of the following questions by circling the letter that corresponds to the correct answer.

1. Of the following, the most important factor in successfully implementing the calendar method of rhythm is:
   - *a) the punctuality of the woman's menstrual cycle
   - b) the number of days per cycle the woman menstruates
   - c) the length of the safe period
   - d) the number of days between the safe period and the first day of menstruation
   - e) do not know

2. After ejaculation, sperm cells live, on the average, approximately _____ within the vagina.
   - a) less than 1 day
   - *b) 1-2 days
   - c) 3-5 days
   - d) 1 week to 10 days
   - e) do not know

3. It takes about _____ from the time of ejaculation for sperm to get through the cervix and into the uterus.
   - a) 30-45 minutes
   - b) 15-20 minutes
   - c) 5-10 minutes
   - *d) 1-3 minutes
   - e) do not know

4. Which of the following contraceptive devices is fitted by a physician?
   - a) Lippes loop
   - b) Cu-7
   - c) diaphragm
   - *d) all of the above
   - e) do not know

5. All of the following ingredients may be found in birth control pills except:
   - a) estrogen
   - b) iron
   - c) progesterone
   - *d) testosterone
   - e) do not know

6. Which of the following, when used as a douche, can kill sperm cells?
   - a) Coca-Cola
   - b) vinegar
   - c) soapy water
   - *d) all of the above
   - e) do not know

7. The temperature method of rhythm refers to a change in basal body temperature of the female:
   - a) before menstruation
   - *b) before ovulation
   - c) after menstruation
   - d) after ovulation
   - e) do not know

8. This method of contraception may cause irritation to the mucous lining of the vagina.
   - a) intrauterine device
   - b) withdrawal
   - *c) postcoital douching
   - d) diaphragm
   - e) do not know

9. Some researchers hypothesize that which of the following birth control methods prevents a fertilized egg from implanting in the uterus, thus acting as an abortifacient?
   - a) oral contraceptive (the pill)
   - *b) IUD
   - c) contraceptive foam
   - d) diaphragm
   - e) do not know

10. The IUD, when properly positioned, would be found in the:
    - a) cervix
    - b) vagina
    - *c) uterus
    - d) urethra
    - e) do not know

11. The diaphragm covers this:
    - a) fallopian tubes
    - *b) cervix
    - c) vagina
    - d) ovaries
    - e) do not know

12. If a woman using this form of contraception is experiencing pain in her lower back, cramps, and spotting, she is probably using:
    - *a) IUD
    - b) diaphragm
    - c) cervical cap
    - d) oral contraceptive (pill)
    - e) do not know

13. Which of the following is rated the most effective method of contraception?
    - a) IUD
    - b) oral contraceptive (pill)
    - *c) salpingectomy (tubal ligation)
    - d) abortion
    - e) do not know

14. The diaphragm should be left in place at least _____ after sexual intercourse to obtain maximum contraceptive effectiveness.
  a) 1-3 hours
  *b) 7-9 hours
  c) 12-15 hours
  d) 2-3 days
  e) do not know
15. Which of the following contraceptive preparations kill sperm?
  a) creams
  b) jellies
  c) suppositories
  *d) all of the above
  e) do not know
16. When using a condom (rubber), to insure maximum contraceptive effectiveness one should:
  a) lubricate it thoroughly with petroleum jelly if it is not of the prelubricated variety
  b) leave a space between the end of the penis and the end of the condom
  c) hold onto the open end when withdrawing after ejaculation
  *d) both b and c
  e) do not know
17. Which of the following contraceptives is sold in a drug store without a doctor's prescription?
  a) IUDs
  b) latex diaphragms
  *c) vaginal suppositories
  d) "morning after" pills
  e) do not know
18. The action of the condom is most similar to:
  a) intrauterine device
  *b) diaphragm
  c) contraceptive jelly
  d) contraceptive foam
  e) do not know
19. The IUD should be:
  a) inserted before intercourse and removed several hours later
  *b) checked regularly to see if it is in place
  c) cleaned on a regular basis
  d) removed when a woman menstruates
  e) do not know
20. In general, a woman's "safe" period (when she cannot become pregnant even though she has sexual intercourse) is:
  a) the first 15 days after menstruation ceases
  b) the first 15 days before menstruation begins
  *c) the first 5 days before and after menstruation
  d) the first 5 days before and after ovulation
  e) do not know
21. A female ovum (egg) is viable (capable of being fertilized) for approximately _____ after it is released.
  a) 6-7 days
  b) 4-5 days
  c) 2-3 days
  *d) 12 hours-1 day
  e) do not know
22. The main function of the oral contraceptive (pill) is to:
  a) kill sperm
  *b) suppress ovulation
  c) inhibit the implantation of the egg
  d) regulate ovulation
  e) do not know
23. The contraceptive method of withdrawal can be an ineffective method of birth control because:
  *a) there can be a small amount of sperm released prior to ejaculation
  b) it places great demands on the self-control of the female
  c) it can lead to premature ejaculation
  d) it can lead to postmature ejaculation
  e) do not know
24. A contraceptive, as well as a protectant against venereal disease (VD), is:
  a) IUD (intrauterine device)
  *b) condom (rubber)
  c) vaginal douche
  d) contraceptive foam
  e) do not know
25. Used as a method of birth control, surgical sterilization (vasectomy in the male, tubal ligation in the female) usually affects the person's sex drive:
  a) as a reduced desire for intercourse
  b) as a reduced desire for intercourse in a sterilized male but not in a sterilized female
  c) as a reduced desire for intercourse in a sterilized female but not in a sterilized male
  *d) by increasing it
  e) do not know

Note. The asterisked (*) choices are the correct answers to the questions.

A Scale to Assess University Women's Attitudes About Contraceptive Acquisition and Use

William A. Fisher,[1] *University of Western Ontario*

In the course of research on affective and cognitive determinants of contraceptive behavior, a scale was developed to assess university women's attitudes regarding contraceptive acquisition and use (Fisher et al., 1979; see also Fisher, Byrne, & White, 1983).

Description

Scale development was guided by the assumption that attitudes toward specific *behaviors* (as opposed to attitudes toward objects, values, etc.) will be most strongly predictive of these behaviors (Fishbein, 1972; Fishbein & Ajzen, 1975). Consequently, a pool of 17 items that assessed university women's beliefs and evaluations about contraceptive acquisition and use was assembled by Fisher et al. (1979). Each item presents a belief or evaluation about using or acquiring contraception, and respondents answer using 7-point Likert-type scales to indicate the degree of their belief or evaluation. Ten of the items were adapted from research (Jaccard & Davidson, 1972) that elicited salient beliefs about oral contraceptive use in a sample of undergraduate women. The remaining seven items were created to assess additional beliefs and evaluations about contraceptive use in general and acquisition of contraception at a university health service, which was the major provider of contraception at the university where the research took place.

This scale was created specifically to assess university women's attitudes about contraceptive use and contraceptive acquisition at a university health service. Nonetheless, applications of this technique of assessing beliefs and evaluations about contraceptive acquisition and use may be adapted to a variety of populations and behaviors. For example, Fisher (1984) elicited salient beliefs about condom use in a group of university men, and measurement of beliefs and evaluations about condom use predicted this behavior in an independent sample of men (for additional discussion of the technique, based on Fishbein and Ajzen's theory of reasoned action, see Ajzen & Fishbein, 1980; Davidson & Jaccard, 1975, 1979).

Response Mode and Timing

In the scale development research (Fisher et al., 1979), items were presented with a number of other questions regarding respondents' sexual and contraceptive history, normative beliefs, dating relationships, and so on and the Sexual Opinion Survey (see Fisher's chapter in this volume).

[1]Address correspondence to William A. Fisher, Department of Psychology, University of Western Ontario, London, Ontario N6A 5C2, Canada; email: fisher@sscl.uwo.ca.

For future research use, the items may be presented by themselves in the format indicated; instructions for the use of Likert-type scales may be appended for respondents who are not familiar with this response format. The 17-item scale should take less than 10 minutes to complete.

Scoring

The attitude scale is to be scored as follows. For Items 2, 3, 4, 5, 6, 8, 9, 10, 11, 13, 15, 16, and 17, score from 1 = left-most response to 7 = right-most response on the 7-point Likert-type scale. For Items 1, 7, 12, and 14, reverse score (i.e., 1 = right-most response to 7 = left-most response). The total score is simply the sum of these individual item scores, minus 17. To avoid possible confusion, it should be noted that in the original scale development research (Fisher et al., 1979) the value 17 was not subtracted from total scale scores. This procedure has been introduced merely to simplify use of this scale. Missing data may be dealt with by calculating the respondent's mean response to the attitude items and substituting this value for the missing data, provided that only a small number of data points are missing. Scores range from 0 (most negative attitude toward contraceptive acquisition and use) to 102 (most positive attitude toward contraceptive acquisition and use) with a numerical midpoint of 51. It should be noted that the numerical midpoint of the attitude scale (51) may not be particularly meaningful in interpreting scores; comparisons with sample means, and relative differences within samples, may be more meaningful in interpreting scale scores. For example, in Fisher et al.'s (1979) research, both users ($M = 86.16$) and nonusers ($M = 74.99$) of a contraception clinic scored on the positive side of the numerical scale midpoint but differed significantly relative to one another and fell on the appropriate sides of the sample mean (79.41). In scale development research with a sample of 230 university women, Fisher et al. (1979) reported a mean response of 79.41 on the attitude ($SD = 14.87$).

Reliability

A Cronbach's alpha coefficient of .83 has been reported, and each of the item-total score correlations (with item deletion) is significant (Fisher et al., 1979), indicating that the attitude scale is highly internally consistent. Test-retest reliability data are not available for this scale.

Validity

Concurrent validity data are based on scale development research (Fisher et al., 1979) that involved administering the measure of contraceptive attitudes, as well as various criterion measures, to a sample of 230 university women. Attitude scale scores were correlated with contraceptive behavior such that women with more negative attitudes toward contraceptive acquisition and use were less likely to acquire contraception at the campus clinic, $r(228) = .37$, $p < .001$; less likely to be aware that the campus clinic provided contraceptive services, $r(227) = .37$, $p < .001$; and (for those who were sexually active) less likely to report the consistent use of contraception, $r(145) = .31, p < .001$. Additional findings showed that the measure of attitudes toward contraceptive acquisition and use correlated with conceptually related variables such as erotophobia-erotophilia, $r(228) = .36, p < .001$ (those with negative attitudes to contraception were more erotophobic) and normative beliefs about whether respondents perceived significant others as approving their use of contraception, $r(228) = .44, p < .001$ (those with negative attitudes toward contraception perceived less normative approval for contraceptive use). Attitude scale scores were also correlated with background variables such that those who had more negative attitudes toward contraceptive acquisition and use were younger, $r(228) = .28, p < .001$; had less frequent sexual intercourse, $r(225) = .26, p < .001$; were more likely to regret having had intercourse, if they had done so, $r(139) = .53, p < .001$; and did not expect their frequency of intercourse to increase, $r(192) = .25, p < .001$. Persons with more negative attitudes toward contraception also intended to have more children, $r(199) = .14, p < .03$; were less likely to have had an abortion in the past, $r(221) = .16, p < .007$; and were more likely to use sanitary napkins (vs. tampons) during menstruation, $r(202) = .30$, $p < .001$.

References

Ajzen, I., & Fishbein, M. (1980). *Understanding attitudes and predicting social behavior.* Englewood Cliffs, NJ: Prentice Hall.

Davidson, A. R., & Jaccard, J. J. (1975). Population psychology: A new look at an old problem. *Journal of Personality and Social Psychology, 31,* 1073-1082.

Davidson, A. R., & Jaccard, J. J. (1979). Variables that moderate the attitude-behavior relation: Results of a longitudinal study. *Journal of Personality and Social Psychology, 37,* 1364-1376.

Fishbein, M. (1972). Toward an understanding of family planning behaviors. *Journal of Applied Social Psychology, 2,* 214-227.

Fishbein, M., & Ajzen, I. (1975). *Belief, attitude, intention, and behavior: An introduction to theory and research.* Reading, MA: Addison-Wesley.

Fisher, W. A. (1984). Predicting contraceptive behavior among university men: The role of emotions and behavioral intentions. *Journal of Applied Social Psychology, 14,* 104-123.

Fisher, W. A., Byrne, D., Edmunds, M., Miller, C. T., Kelley, K., & White, L. A. (1979). Psychological and situation-specific correlates of contraceptive behavior among university women. *The Journal of Sex Research, 15,* 38-55.

Fisher, W. A., Byrne, D., & White, L. A. (1983). Emotional barriers to contraception. In D. Byrne & W. A. Fisher (Eds.), *Adolescents, sex and contraception* (pp. 207-239). Hillsdale, NJ: Lawrence Erlbaum.

Jaccard, J. J., & Davidson, A. R. (1972). Toward an understanding of family planning behaviors: An initial investigation. *Journal of Applied Social Psychology, 2,* 288-235.

Exhibit

A Scale to Assess Attitudes About Contraceptive Acquisition and Use Among University Women

1. Using a method of birth control is:
   Good _____ | _____ | _____ | _____ | _____ | _____ | _____ Bad
2. Using a method of birth control is:
   Wrong _____ | _____ | _____ | _____ | _____ | _____ | _____ Right
3. Using birth control leads to major negative side effects.
   Probable _____ | _____ | _____ | _____ | _____ | _____ | _____ Improbable
4. Using birth control would have a negative effect on my sexual morals.
   Probable _____ | _____ | _____ | _____ | _____ | _____ | _____ Improbable
5. Using birth control is immoral.
   Probable _____ | _____ | _____ | _____ | _____ | _____ | _____ Improbable
6. Using birth control methods is unnatural.
   True _____ | _____ | _____ | _____ | _____ | _____ | _____ Untrue
7. Using birth control would enable me to regulate the size of my family.
   Probable _____ | _____ | _____ | _____ | _____ | _____ | _____ Improbable
8. Birth control methods are unreliable.
   Probable _____ | _____ | _____ | _____ | _____ | _____ | _____ Improbable
9. Using birth control would give me guilty feelings.
   Probable _____ | _____ | _____ | _____ | _____ | _____ | _____ Improbable
10. Using birth control will produce children who are born with something wrong with them.
    Probable _____ | _____ | _____ | _____ | _____ | _____ | _____ Improbable
11. Using birth control would decrease my sexual pleasure.
    Probable _____ | _____ | _____ | _____ | _____ | _____ | _____ Improbable

12. Using birth control would remove the worry of becoming pregnant.
    Probable _____ |_____| _____ | _____ | _____ | _____ | _____ Improbable
13. Using birth control would make sex less romantic.
    Probable _____ |_____| _____ | _____ | _____ | _____ | _____ Improbable
14. Going to the Student Health Service to obtain a method of birth control is:
    Good _____ |_____| _____ | _____ | _____ | _____ | _____ Bad
15. Being required to attend an educational information session in order to obtain birth control is inconvenient.
    Probable _____ |_____| _____ | _____ | _____ | _____ | _____ Improbable
16. Going to the Student Health Service in order to obtain birth control will let others know that I am engaging in sexual intercourse.
    Probable _____ |_____| _____ | _____ | _____ | _____ | _____ Improbable
17. Going to the Student Health Service in order to obtain birth control would be embarrassing.
    Probable _____ |_____| _____ | _____ | _____ | _____ | _____ Improbable

Attitudes Toward Contraceptive Methods

The Editors

The Attitudes Toward Contraceptive Methods questionnaire is designed to assess attitudes toward and preferences among 10 contraceptive methods: condom, abstention, diaphragm, rhythm, foam or jelly, withdrawal, vasectomy, IUD, tubal ligation, pill.

Respondents rate each for its personal acceptability, using a 5-point scale. Four types of method were identified by factor analysis: coitus-dependent, surgical, coitus-inhibition, and coitus-independent. The instrument can be completed in less than 5 minutes.

Additional information and the scale may be obtained from the first editor.

References

Gough, H. G. (1973). A factor analysis of contraceptive preferences. *Journal of Psychology, 84,* 199-210.

Gough, H. G. (1979). Some factors related to men's stated willingness to use a male contraceptive pill. *The Journal of Sex Research, 15,* 27-37.

Lazzari, R., & Gough, H. G. (1974). Studio sulle preferenze per differenti metodi contraccettivi. *Sessuologia, 15*(3), 26-34.

Westoff, C. F. (1972). The modernization of U.S. contraceptive practice. *Family Planning Perspectives, 4*(3), 9-12.

Attitude Toward Using Birth Control Pills Scale

Edward S. Herold[1] and Marilyn Shirley Goodwin, *University of Guelph*

The birth control pill is one of the most commonly used methods of contraception, especially among young single females. Attitudes toward the pill, mainly with respect to safety and effectiveness, are important considerations in the decision to use the pill as well as in the decision to continue or discontinue its use. The purpose of this scale is to measure attitudes toward using birth control pills, including the components of effectiveness, safety, and anxiety about pill usage.

A problem in attitude-behavior research is that researchers have assumed they could predict behavior by measuring general attitudes. Measures of general attitudes, however, are poor predictors of specific behavior. For example, Fishbein and Jaccard (1973) found that the correlation between attitude toward contraception and intention to use a specific contraceptive method was not significant. The attitude toward each specific contraceptive method, however, was significantly correlated with the intention to use that method.

Description and Response Mode

Herold and Goodwin (1980) developed the Attitude Toward Using Birth Control Pills Scale with a sample of 486 females, ages 13 to 20, who were attending birth control centers in Ontario, Canada. The scale uses the semantic differential format. The concept "I think that using birth control pills is:" was rated on 14 pairs of bipolar adjectives by means of 7-point scales. The choice of adjectives was based on their relevance to the concept and for their representativeness of the three factors of evaluation, potency, and activity.

The 14 items were subjected to a principal components analysis in which all factors achieving an eigenvalue of greater than 1.0 were retained. The resulting three orthogonal factors, accounting for 62% of the common variance, were subjected to a varimax rotation. Only items with factor loadings of .50 or higher were included in the interpretation of the three factors.

Factor 1 accounted for 45% of the common variance and was defined by loadings on the potency items of reliable-unreliable, effective-ineffective, efficient-inefficient, and adequate-inadequate. This factor is labeled *effectiveness*.

Factor 2 contained the evaluation items of good-bad, healthy-sick, beneficial-harmful, positive-negative, safe-dangerous, and useful-useless, and it accounted for 10% of the common variance. This factor is labeled *safety*.

Factor 3 accounted for 7% of the common variance. It included the items of calm-anxious, restful-nervous, pleasant-unpleasant, and strong-weak. This factor is labeled *anxiety* because it appears to measure subjective feelings of anxiety about using birth control pills.

Timing

The scale takes 5-10 minutes to complete.

Scoring

Factor scores and a total score may be computed by summing items on each factor or the total 14 items. Weighted factor scores could also be computed.

Reliability and Validity

Factor scores were used to construct three composite indexes representing the theoretical dimensions associated with the factors. Internal consistencies of the dimensions were determined by using Cronbach's alpha. The reliability coefficient for the separate dimensions were as follows: effectiveness, .88; safety, .85; and anxiety, .84.

The three dimensions had high intercorrelations, suggesting that they tap a common dimension. The 14-item Attitude Toward Using Birth Control Pills Scale was constructed by adding each of the items from the effectiveness, safety, and anxiety dimensions. The reliability coefficient of the total scale was .91.

Using the known-groups approach to concurrent validation, two separate validity tests were made by selecting criterion groups. In the first validity test, the attitude scores of 68 continuing pill users were contrasted with those of 17 discounting pill users. The continuing pill users were using the birth control pill and were renewing their pill prescription. The discontinuing pill user had used the pill but now intended to use the IUD instead. The mean scores of the Pills Scale and its subscales were significantly different for the two groups, with the continuers having more favorable attitudes.

In the second validity test, the attitude scores of 48 virgin pill users were contrasted with those of 12 sexually active pill nonusers. The virgin pill users were using the birth control pill before they began having sexual intercourse. The pill nonusers consisted of women who were at the clinic for pregnancy testing and who had never used the pill and did not intend to use the pill. The mean scores of the Pills Scale and its subscales were significantly different for the two groups with the virgin pill users having more favorable attitudes.

[1]Address correspondence to Edward S. Herold, Department of Family Studies, University of Guelph, Guelph, Ontario N1G 2W1, Canada; email: eherold@facs.uoguelph.ca.

References

Fishbein, M., & Jaccard, J. (1973). Theoretical and methodological considerations in the prediction of family planning intentions and behavior. *Representative Research in Social Psychology, 4,* 37-51.

Herold, E. S., & Goodwin, M. S. (1980). Development of a scale to measure attitudes toward using birth control pills. *Journal of Social Psychology, 110,* 115-122.

Exhibit

Attitude Toward Using Birth Control Pills

Please indicate your feelings toward using birth control pills by placing a ✓ in the interval along the scale. Example: I think that school is:

			U					
		1	2	3	4	5	6	7	
1)	good	✓	___	___	___	___	___	___	bad
2)	good	___	___	___	___	✓	___	___	bad

The first answer indicates that one feels very strongly that school is good. The second answer indicates that one feels mildly that school is bad. If you find that a pair of adjectives does not apply to your feelings toward using birth control pills, or if you are undecided, place a ✓ in the center space (4).

I think that using birth control pills is:

					U				
		1	2	3	4	5	6	7	
a)	good	___	___	___	___	___	___	___	bad
b)	useful	___	___	___	___	___	___	___	useless
c)	healthy	___	___	___	___	___	___	___	sick
d)	reliable	___	___	___	___	___	___	___	unreliable
e)	beneficial	___	___	___	___	___	___	___	harmful
f)	positive	___	___	___	___	___	___	___	negative
g)	effective	___	___	___	___	___	___	___	ineffective
h)	safe	___	___	___	___	___	___	___	dangerous
i)	adequate	___	___	___	___	___	___	___	inadequate
j)	pleasant	___	___	___	___	___	___	___	unpleasant
k)	strong	___	___	___	___	___	___	___	weak
l)	calm	___	___	___	___	___	___	___	anxious
m)	efficient	___	___	___	___	___	___	___	inefficient
n)	restful	___	___	___	___	___	___	___	nervous

Contraceptive Embarrassment Scale

Edward S. Herold,[1] *University of Guelph*

Embarrassment about going to a physician or pharmacist for contraception can be a significant barrier to contraceptive use. The purpose of this scale is to measure the level of contraceptive embarrassment among single young people. Contraceptive embarrassment is defined as embarrassment over having to visit a physician or pharmacy to obtain contraceptive devices. Because many young people fear situations where parents might find out about their contraceptive use, it is important to differentiate situations in which parents would be likely to discover contraceptive use from those in which parents would be unlikely to find out.

Description and Response Mode

The scale is an eight-item Likert-type scale (9-point) with response options labeled from *strongly agree* to *strongly disagree*. There is a neutral category. The items are preceded by the following statement: "I am embarrassed or would be embarrassed about the following." Respondents circle the number indicating their agreement or disagreement with each statement.

The scale can be divided into two subscales of four items each. One subscale consists of items measuring embarrassment over obtaining contraception close to the parental home (close embarrassment). The other subscale measures embarrassment over obtaining contraception distant from home (distant embarrassment).

---

[1]Address correspondence to Edward S. Herold, Department of Family Studies, University of Guelph, Guelph, Ontario N1G 2W1, Canada; email: eherold@facs.uoguelph.ca.

Timing

The scale requires an average of 2-3 minutes for completion.

Scoring

The possible range of scores is from 8 to 72 with 8 indicating low embarrassment.

Reliability and Validity

Herold (1981) found with a sample of 265 high school and college females who were sexually experienced that the Cronbach alpha coefficient of reliability was 0.88 for the total scale and 0.87 and 0.79 for the close and distance subscales, respectively. The mean scale scores were 31.7 for the total scale and 19.5 and 12.2 for the close and distant subscales, respectively. The scale and the two subscales predicted significant differences in contraceptive behavior. Higher correlations with contraceptive use were found for the close embarrassment subscale than for the distant embarrassment subscale.

Herold (1981) found that for each situation there was greater embarrassment about obtaining contraceptive devices near to the parental home. In particular, three times as many respondents indicated they would be embarrassed to obtain the pill from a pharmacy close to home than from one distant from home. Of the specific methods, greatest embarrassment was for obtaining condoms and least embarrassment was for obtaining birth control pills.

Reference

Herold, E. S. (1981). Contraceptive embarrassment and contraceptive behaviour among young single women. *Journal of Youth and Adolescence, 10,* 233-242.

Exhibit

Contraceptive Embarrassment Scale

I am embarrassed or would be embarrassed about the following:

1. Obtaining condoms from a pharmacy close to where my parents live.
2. Obtaining contraceptive foam from a pharmacy close to where my parents live.
3. Obtaining birth control pills from a pharmacy close to where my parents live.
4. Obtaining a prescription for the birth control pill from my family doctor.
5. Obtaining condoms from a pharmacy distant from where my parents live.
6. Obtaining contraceptive foam from a pharmacy distant from where my parents live.
7. Obtaining birth control pills from a pharmacy distant from where my parents live.
8. Obtaining a prescription for the birth control pill from a clinic doctor.

Affective Responses Toward Contraceptive Topics and Behavior Scale

Kathryn Kelley,[1] *University at Albany, State University of New York*

The scale of Affective Responses Toward Contraceptive Topics and Behavior was designed to assess affective responses toward a variety of contraceptive topics and behaviors. To accomplish this, respondents were presented with concepts and activities involved in contraceptive use and expressed their affective responses toward them on semantic differential scales. A distinctive feature of the stimuli used in developing the scale was their theoretical relevance to genital versus nongenital manipulative behavior that occurs in contraceptive use (Kelley, 1979). Regarded as an individual-difference variable (Balassone, 1991), these affective responses toward contraception also interrelate as attitudinal domains (Severy, 1979) and provide an avenue for testing a model of their convergence and predictiveness (Morrison, 1985).

Description

The scale consists of a series of statements about contraception, each of which is followed by the two 7-point, semantic differential scales, *negative-positive* and *disgusted-not at all disgusted*. Kelley (1985) determined that these two affective scales corresponded to positive and negative components of feelings, respectively. The different forms for males and females, designed for the college student sample, include 12 statements about performing genitally manipulative techniques and 4 for genitally nonmanipulative acts. Examples of the former are females' diaphragm insertion and males' condom placement, and of the latter, taking a contraceptive pill.

Response Mode and Timing

Respondents indicate their affective response to each item on the paper-and-pencil scale by indicating how accurately an endpoint on the rating format describes their feelings. They place an X in the appropriate space on the semantic differential scale. Response times average about 8 to 10 minutes.

Scoring

Responses are scored by coding the endpoints *disgusted* or *negative* as 1 and *positive* or *not at all disgusted* as 7.

Intervening responses are coded as 2-6. Scores on the two scales are summed as responses to each statement. Higher scores indicate a more favorable affective response.

Reliability

Test-retest reliability of the scale responses over a 1-month period was .83 among 14 females and .78 among 18 males, in unpublished data that I collected. From the same source, the Cronbach alpha coefficient for all scale responses was .72 among females and .67 among males at the first administration of the scale.

Validity

The scale's construct validity is supported by the finding that the degree of genital manipulation involved in contraceptive use related to responses toward explicit heterosexual (Items 1, 2, 3, and 5A) or masturbatory stimuli (Items 4A through 4E and 5B through 5H; Kelley, 1979). Mosher and Vonderheide (1985) expanded the rating scale to include more negative emotions, such as fear, and demonstrated that scale responses correlated with sex and masturbation guilt.

References

Balassone, M. L. (1991). A social learning model of adolescent contraceptive behavior. *Journal of Youth and Adolescence, 20,* 593-616.

Bancroft, J., & Sartorius, N. (1990). The effects of oral contraceptives on being and sexuality. *Oxford Review of Reproductive Biology, 12,* 57-92.

Gold, D., & Berger, C. (1983). The influence of psychological and situational factors on the contraceptive behavior of single men: A review of the literature. *Population and Environment, 6,* 113-129.

Kelley, K. (1979). Socialization factors in contraceptive attitudes: Roles of affective responses, parental attitudes, and sexual experience. *The Journal of Sex Research, 15,* 6-20.

Kelley, K. (1985). Sex, sex guilt, and authoritarianism: Differences in responses to explicit heterosexual and masturbatory slides. *The Journal of Sex Research, 21,* 68-85.

Morrison, D. M. (1985). Adolescent contraceptive behavior: A review. *Psychological Bulletin, 98,* 538-568.

Morrison, D. M. (1989). Predicting contraceptive efficacy: A discriminant analysis of three groups of adolescent women. *Journal of Applied Social Psychology, 19,* 1431-1452.

Mosher, D. L., & Vonderheide, S. (1985). Contributions of sex guilt and masturbation guilt to women's contraceptive attitudes and use. *The Journal of Sex Research, 21,* 24-39.

Severy, L. J. (1979). Sex, contraception, and fertility attitudes and behavior: An overview. *The Journal of Sex Research, 15,* 76-83.

[1]Address correspondence to Kathryn Kelley, Department of Psychology, State University of New York at Albany, Social Science 112, Albany, NY 12222; email: kelley@cnsibm.albany.edu.

Exhibit

Affective Responses Toward Contraceptive Topics and Behavior

Instructions for Scales

These are directions for filling out the 7-point scales used in this study. Important: A 7-point scale is one with adjectives at both ends, and 7 points between them. See the examples below, and read them carefully. If your feelings seem very closely described by the adjective at one end of the scale or the other, you should place your check mark as follows:

positive |___X___|_____|_____|_____|_____|_____|_____| negative

or

positive |_____|_____|_____|_____|_____|_____|___X___| negative

If your feelings seem quite closely described by one or the other end of the scale (but not extremely), you should place your check mark as follows:

positive |_____|___X___|_____|_____|_____|_____|_____| negative

or

positive |_____|_____|_____|_____|_____|___X___|_____| negative

If your feelings seem only slightly described by one side as opposed to the other (but not really neutral), then you should check as follows:

positive |_____|_____|___X___|_____|_____|_____|_____| negative

or

positive |_____|_____|_____|_____|___X___|_____|_____| negative

The direction toward which you check, of course, depends on which of the two ends of the scale seem most characteristic of your feelings.

If you consider your feelings neutral on the scale, both sides of the scale equally associated with your feelings, or if the scale if completely irrelevant, unrelated in any way to your feelings, then you should place your check mark in the middle space, as shown here:

positive |_____|_____|_____|___X___|_____|_____|_____| negative

Survey of Attitudes About Contraception

(Items 1, 2, and 3 apply to both female and male respondents.)

1. How would you feel about doing the following thing?
   Asking a doctor for a contraceptive
   positive |_____|_____|_____|_____|_____|_____|_____| negative*
   disgusted |_____|_____|_____|_____|_____|_____|_____| not at all disgusted*
2. How do you feel about the use of birth control techniques in general?
3. How do you feel about the use of contraception in your own experience?

(Items 4, A through E, apply to male respondents.)

4. How would you feel about doing the following things?
   A. Asking for a condom
   B. Buying a condom
   C. Putting a condom on
   D. Using withdrawal
   E. Having a vasectomy

(Items 5, A through G, apply to female respondents.)

5. How would you feel about doing the following things?
   A. Taking a contraceptive pill
   B. Having an IUD (intrauterine device) inserted into your uterus
   C. Wearing an IUD (intrauterine device) in your uterus
   D. Inserting contraceptive foam into your vagina
   E. Inserting a diaphragm into your vagina
   F. Having an abortion
   G. Asking for contraceptive foam
   H. Buying contraceptive foam

a. The two scales are repeated after each item.

Contraceptive Attitude Scale

Kelly Black Kyes,[1] *University of Washington*

The Contraceptive Attitude Scale (CAS) is a measure of attitudes toward the use of contraceptives in general as opposed to attitudes toward a specific type of contraceptive (Brown, 1984), or toward the premarital use of contraceptives (Parcel, 1975). Potentially, the scale could help distinguish between an attitude toward using a particular method of contraception (e.g., the condom) and an attitude toward using any contraceptive.

Description

The CAS consists of 17 positively and 15 negatively worded items to which respondents indicate their agreement or disagreement. The final set of statements was selected based on the responses of 75 male and 60 female college students to a larger set of 80 statements.

Response Mode and Timing

Participants respond to each item by indicating their level of agreement with each statement. Possible responses range from 1 (*strongly disagree*) to 5 (*strongly agree*). The scale requires about 10 minutes to complete.

Scoring

All statements are scored using a 5-point scale. For positively worded statements, *strongly disagree* receives a score of 1 and *strongly agree* receives a score of 5. Negatively worded statements are reverse scored so that *strongly disagree* receives a score of 5 and *strongly agree* receives a score of 1. The total score is the sum of the responses to each item. Lower scores indicate more negative attitudes toward contraception.

Reliability

Test-retest reliability of the 32-item scale is very good, $r(166) = .88, p < .001$. Internal reliability, as measured by corrected item-total correlations, is also good (rs range from .26 to .68; Black & Pollack, 1987).

Validity

Scores from the CAS correlated significantly with scores from the Premarital Contraceptive Attitude Evaluation Instrument (Parcel, 1975), $r = .72$. It also correlated with reported frequency of contraceptive use among nonvirgin male and female college students, $r = .60$.

References

Black, K. J., & Pollack, R. H. (1987, April). *The development of a contraceptive attitude scale.* Paper presented at the annual meeting of the Southern Society for Philosophy and Psychology.

[1]Address correspondence to Kelly Black Kyes, Department of Health Services, XD-47, School of Public Health and Community Medicine, 1914 N. 34th Street, Suite 402, University of Washington, Seattle, WA 98103; email: kkyes@u.washington.edu.

Brown, I. S. (1984). Development of a scale to measure attitudes toward the condom as a method of birth control. *The Journal of Sex Research, 20,* 255-263.

Parcel, G. S. (1975). Development of an instrument to measure attitudes toward the personal use of premarital contraception. *Journal of School Health, 45,* 157-160.

Exhibit

Contraceptive Attitude Scale

Below are several statements about the use of contraceptives (birth control). We are interested in knowing your opinion about each statement. Using the scale below, please indicate your level of agreement or disagreement with each statement. Keep in mind that there are no right or wrong answers. Also remember that we are interested in your personal opinion. Therefore, we want to know how you feel about these statements and not how you think your family or friends might feel about these statements.

SA = Strongly agree; A = Agree; U = Undecided; D = Disagree; SD = Strongly disagree

_____ 1. I believe that it is wrong to use contraceptives.
_____ 2. Contraceptives reduce the sex drive.
_____ 3. Using contraceptives is much more desirable than having an abortion.
_____ 4. Males who use contraceptives seem less masculine than males who do not.
_____ 5. I encourage my friends to use contraceptives.
_____ 6. I would not become sexually involved with a person who did not accept contraceptive responsibility.
_____ 7. Teenagers should not need permission from their parents to get contraceptives.
_____ 8. Contraceptives are not really necessary unless a couple has engaged in intercourse more than once.
_____ 9. Contraceptives makes sex seem less romantic.
_____ 10. Females who use contraceptives are promiscuous.
_____ 11. I would not have intercourse if no contraceptive method was available.
_____ 12. I do not believe that contraceptives actually prevent pregnancy.
_____ 13. Using contraceptives is a way of showing that you care about your partner.
_____ 14. I do not talk about contraception with my friends.
_____ 15. I would feel embarrassed discussing contraception with my friends.
_____ 16. One should use contraceptives regardless of how long one has known his/her sexual partner.
_____ 17. Contraceptives are difficult to obtain.
_____ 18. Contraceptives can actually make intercourse seem more pleasurable.
_____ 19. I feel that contraception is solely my partner's responsibility.
_____ 20. I feel more relaxed during intercourse if a contraceptive method is used.
_____ 21. I prefer to use contraceptives during intercourse.
_____ 22. In the future, I plan to use contraceptives any time I have intercourse.
_____ 23. I would practice contraception even if my partner did not want me to.
_____ 24. It is no trouble to use contraceptives.
_____ 25. Using contraceptives makes a relationship seem too permanent.
_____ 26. Sex is not fun if a contraceptive is used.
_____ 27. Contraceptives are worth using, even if the monetary cost is high.
_____ 28. Contraceptives encourage promiscuity.
_____ 29. Couples should talk about contraception before having intercourse.
_____ 30. If I or my partner experienced negative side effects from a contraceptive method, we would use a different method.
_____ 31. Contraceptives make intercourse seem too planned.
_____ 32. I feel better about myself when I use contraceptives.

Contraceptive Self-Efficacy Scale

Ruth Andrea Levinson,[1] *Skidmore College*

The Contraceptive Self-Efficacy (CSE) scale assesses motivational barriers to contraceptive use among sexually active teenage women. The self-efficacy construct has been used by Bandura and his associates to understand motivations for apparently dysfunctional or avoidance behavior (Bandura, 1990; Bandura, Adams, Hardy, & Howells, 1980; Kazdin, 1974; McAlister, Perry, & Maccoby, 1979; Rosenthal & Bandura, 1978; Strecher, DeVellis, Becker, & Rosenstock, 1986). The nonuse of contraceptives by sexually active teenage women who say that they do not desire a pregnancy is similar to other types of phobic behaviors. Thus, teenage women's contraceptive behavior was treated as a special behavioral domain for application of the construct.

According to the self-efficacy construct, a person's expectations about whether she should and can execute a component behavior will determine initiation and persistence in achieving a desired goal (Bandura, 1977; Fishbein & Ajzen, 1975). The CSE scale measures the strength of a sexually active teenage woman's conviction that she should and can control sexual and contraceptive situations to achieve a contraceptively protected priority. Stressors are embedded within items to ascertain individual differences among young women who may have different issues that inhibit feelings of self-efficacy. The scale was designed to be used both diagnostically by educators and clinicians as a tool for designing and assessing interventions and as a research instrument.

Description

CSE statements evaluate the respondent's perceptions of her ability to take responsibility for sexual and contraceptive behaviors across a variety of situations. CSE is assessed using 18 items, which respondents rate on a 5-point Likert-type scale ranging from (1) *not at all true of me* to (5) *completely true of me*. The scale has been significantly and independently correlated with contraceptive use among diverse samples of young girls and women ranging in age from 13 to 22 years, including inner-city African American youth, White French Canadian youth, and suburban European American and Latina American youth in settings such as family planning clinics, high school classrooms, and college campuses. The results, spanning more than a 10-year period, indicate that a variety of methods for assessing CSE (e.g., either the sum or the average of the 18-item CSE scale, or a four-factor scoring solution) have been predictive of contraceptive behavior among all groups of young women (Bilodeau, Forget, & Tétreault, 1994;

Heinrich, 1993; Levinson 1986, 1995; Levinson, Beamer, & Wan, 1996; Wright, 1992).

To determine the best measure of the CSE scale, we explored the scale's relationship to contraceptive behavior with four diverse samples (see Levinson et al., 1996). A series of correlational analyses was conducted with each sample to examine scale properties. A pattern of low correlations among CSE items emerged (averaging near 0.15 with a small standard deviation), indicating that use of the total item set separately as the basis for CSE was warranted. Zero-order and partial correlations revealed which CSE items were correlated with contraceptive behavior, as well as which items explained unique variance in contraceptive behavior for each sample. This analytic strategy was used because the dependent measure assessing contraceptive behavior was on a different metric in each sample.

These results with the CSE scale suggest that diverse groups of women and girls have different issues that inhibit their ability to use contraceptives effectively or to postpone unprotected sexual activity. It is recommended that the CSE scale be used prior to interventions to adjust interventions appropriately to meet the particular needs of the participants. Another finding was that Item 8 was consistently predictive of contraceptive behavior across three of the four samples. The predictive power of this one item suggests that the "discourse of desire" (Fine, 1988) is a very important aspect to be explored in sexuality education for the development of healthy sexual behaviors and skills (Levinson et al., 1996). Other items uniquely related to contraceptive behavior were those items that assessed confidence in the ability to confront oneself or significant others (e.g., parents, partner, pharmacist) about issues related to sexual needs (e.g., Items 2, 3, 6, 10, 11, 12, 13c, and 14). These findings are congruent with earlier research outcomes, thereby highlighting persistent issues that seem to affect young women's contraceptive behavior.

Response Mode and Timing

Respondents circle the number indicating how true or not true that statement is for them. The CSE scale requires approximately 10 minutes to complete.

Scoring

The scale is scored such that higher scores represent higher CSE. The scoring direction requires that Items 2, 5, 6, 8, 9, 11, 12, 14, and 15 be reverse scored.

Reliability

Reliability was estimated using Cronbach's alpha. It has equaled .73 or higher across investigations.

[1]Address correspondence to Ruth Andrea Levinson, Education Department, Skidmore College, Skidmore, NY 12866; email: rlevinso@skidmore.edu.

Validity

In the initial phases of instrument construction, CSE items were scrutinized for face and content validity. The validity of the instrument was inspected according to two major criteria: (a) Did the items simulate the events that were both common and critical to teenage women's successful use of contraceptives, and (b) were the content and response formats of each item conducive to collecting information on expected behavior in a manner that corresponds to self-efficacy assessments of that behavior? The appearance and content of the original CSE instrument were changed several times based on information derived from pretesting the instrument among different populations and from personal communication with Bandura and associates.

In current research with the CSE scale, items pertaining to obsolete methods of birth control (e.g., the sponge) are being deleted from the content of the scale items as presented here. We are exploring adding items that pertain to more accessible methods of birth control (e.g., the condom, Norplant, Depo Provera, and emergency contraception). The impact of drug use on CSE and contraceptive behavior is also under investigation.

Other Information

The instrument is copyrighted. It can be used for research, clinical, or educational purposes by obtaining permission from the author.

References

Bandura, A. (1977). Self-efficacy: Toward a unifying theory of behavioral change. *Psychological Review, 84,* 191-215.

Bandura, A. (1990). Perceived self-efficacy in the exercise of control over AIDS infection. *Evaluation and Program Planning, 13,* 9-17.

Bandura, A., Adams, N. E., Hardy, A. B., & Howells, G. N. (1980). Tests of the generality of self-efficacy theory. *Cognitive Therapy and Research, 4,* 39-66.

Bilodeau, A., Forget, G., & Tétreault, J. (1994). L'auto-efficacité relative à la contraception chez les adolescentes et les adolescents: La validation d'une échelle de mesure. *Canadian Journal of Public Health, 85*(2), 115-120.

Fine, M. (1988). Sexuality, schooling, and adolescent females: The missing discourse of desire. *Harvard Educational Review, 58*(1), 29-53.

Fishbein, M., & Ajzen, I. (1975). *Belief, attitude, intention, and behavior.* Reading, MA: Addison-Wesley.

Heinrich, L. B. (1993). Contraceptive self-efficacy in college women. *Journal of Adolescent Health, 14,* 269-276.

Kazdin, A. E. (1974). Effects of covert modeling and reinforcement on assertive behavior. *Journal of Abnormal Psychology, 83,* 240-252.

Levinson, R. A. (1984). Contraceptive self-efficacy: A primary prevention strategy. *Journal of Social Work and Human Sexuality, 3,* 1-15.

Levinson, R. A. (1986). Contraceptive self-efficacy: A perspective on teenage girls' contraceptive behavior. *The Journal of Sex Research, 22,* 347-369.

Levinson, R. A. (1995). Reproductive and contraceptive knowledge, contraceptive self-efficacy, and contraceptive behavior among teenage women. *Adolescence, 30,* 65-85.

Levinson, R. A., Beamer, L. A., & Wan, C. K. (1996, June). *The contraceptive self-efficacy scale in four samples.* Paper presented at the 17th annual conference of the National Women's Studies Association, Saratoga Springs, NY.

McAlister, A., Perry, C. L., & Maccoby, N. (1979). Adolescent smoking: Onset and prevention. *Pediatrics, 67,* 650-688.

Rosenthal, T. L., & Bandura, A. (1978). Psychological modeling: Theory and practice. In S. L. Garfield & A. E. Bergin (Eds.), *Handbook of psychotherapy and behavior change: An empirical analysis* (pp. 621-658). New York: Wiley.

Strecher, V. J., DeVellis, B. M., Becker, M. H., & Rosenstock, I. M. (1986). The role of self-efficacy in achieving health behavior change. *Health Education Quarterly, 13*(1), 73-91.

Wright, C. (1992). *Factors associated with contraceptive behavior among Black college students.* Unpublished doctoral dissertation, University of Oregon.

Exhibit

Contraceptive Self-Efficacy Scale

The items on the following page are a list of statements. Please rate each item on a 1 to 5 scale according to how true the statement is of you. Using the scale, circle one number for each question:

1 = Not at all true of me
2 = Slightly true of me
3 = Somewhat true of me
4 = Mostly true of me
5 = Completely true of me

1.	1	2	3	4	5	When I am with a boyfriend, I feel that I can always be responsible for what happens sexually with him.
2.	1	2	3	4	5	Even if a boyfriend can talk about sex, I can't tell a man how I really feel about sexual things.
3.	1	2	3	4	5	When I have sex, I can enjoy it as something that I really wanted to do.
4.	1	2	3	4	5	If my boyfriend and I are getting "turned-on" sexually and I don't really want to have sexual intercourse (go-all-the-way, get-down), I can easily tell him "no" and mean it.
5.	1	2	3	4	5	If my boyfriend didn't talk about the sex that was happening between us, I couldn't either.

6.	1	2	3	4	5	When I think about what having sex means, I can't have sex so easily.
7.	1	2	3	4	5	If my boyfriend and I are getting "turned-on" sexually and I don't really want to have sexual intercourse (go-all-the-way, get-down), I can easily stop things so that we don't have intercourse.
8.	1	2	3	4	5	There are times when I'd be so involved sexually or emotionally, that I could have sexual intercourse even if I weren't protected (using a form of birth control).
9.	1	2	3	4	5	Sometimes I just go along with what my date wants to do sexually because I don't think I can take the hassle of trying to say what I want.
10.	1	2	3	4	5	If there were a man (boyfriend) to whom I was very attracted physically and emotionally, I could feel comfortable telling him that I wanted to have sex with him.
11.	1	2	3	4	5	I couldn't continue to use a birth control method, if I thought my parents might find out.
12.	1	2	3	4	5	It would be hard for me to go to the drugstore and ask for foam (Encare Ovals, a diaphragm, a pill prescription, etc.) without feeling embarrassed.
13.						If my boyfriend and I were getting really heavy into sex and moving towards intercourse and I wasn't protected . . .
a.	1	2	3	4	5	I could easily ask him if he had protection (or tell him that I didn't).
b.	1	2	3	4	5	I could excuse myself to put in a diaphragm or foam (if I used them for birth control).
c.	1	2	3	4	5	I could tell him that I was on the pill or had an IUD (if I used them for birth control).
d.	1	2	3	4	5	I could stop things before intercourse, if I couldn't bring up the subject of protection.
14.	1	2	3	4	5	There are times when I should talk to my boyfriend about using contraceptives; but, I can't seem to do it in the situation.
15.	1	2	3	4	5	Sometimes I end up having sex with a boyfriend because I can't find a way to stop it.

(Thank you very much for your time and thought. The answers you gave will help us prepare better services for others.)

Source. This scale was originally published in "Contraceptive Self-Efficacy: A Perspective on Teenage Girls' Contraceptive Behavior," by R. A. Levinson, 1986, *The Journal of Sex Research, 22,* 347-369; and "Reproductive and Contraceptive Knowledge, Contraceptive Self-Efficacy, and Contraceptive Behavior Among Teenage Women," by R. A. Levinson, 1995, *Adolescence, 30,* 65-85. Reprinted with permission.

Male Birth Control Practice and Sex Role Stereotypes Regarding Female Contraceptive Responsibility

The Editors

Two scales were developed. The first scale measures attitudes toward male birth control practice (ABC), and the second scale measures attitudes toward sex role stereotypes regarding female contraceptive responsibility (SRS). The ABC, having 12 items, is defined as the degree to which the respondents agree with statements of commonly expressed objections to use of the condoms, withdrawal, vasectomy, and rhythm methods of birth control. The SRS, having eight items, is defined as the degree to which the respondents agree with statements placing responsibility for birth control on the female. A five-choice scoring system is used to measure the degree of agreement or disagreement with each statement.

Reference

Weinstein, S. A., & Goebel, G. (1979). The relationship between contraceptive sex role stereotyping and attitudes toward male contraception among males. *The Journal of Sex Research, 15,* 235-242.

The Juhasz-Schneider Sexual Decision-Making Questionnaire

Anne McCreary Juhasz,[1] *Loyola University of Chicago*
Mary Sonnenshein-Schneider, *National Teachers College*

The Juhasz-Schneider Sexual Decision-Making Questionnaire (JSSDMQ) is a self-administered paper-and-pencil questionnaire on factors influencing sexual decisions of high school students.

Description

The JSSDMQ was developed from the original Juhasz Sexual Decision-Making Questionnaire (Juhasz & Kavanagh, 1978) based on a chain of sexual decision making (Juhasz, 1975). This chain includes six major sexual decisions: (a) having intercourse, (b) having children, (c) using contraception, (d) delivering a child or having an abortion, (e) keeping or giving a child up for adoption, and (f) marrying. The questionnaire deals with practical, emotional, and psychological aspects of influences on the six decisions and attempts to determine the strength of each influence (i.e., how important it is on the final decision).

The original questionnaire used college students. Minor revisions were needed for use with adolescents. Vocabulary, sentence structure, and content were revised making the questionnaire appropriate for use with all grade levels in high school.

The adolescent sample (*N* = 484) consisted of 220 male and 264 female, primarily White, respondents attending Catholic high schools in a large midwestern city. Age ranged from 13 to 19 years, with a mean of 15.4. In terms of the Warner Reviewed Scale for Rating Occupation (Warner, Mecker, & Ellis, 1957), respondents were middle and lower-middle class. Few respondents claimed to be nonreligious or very religious; the majority displayed a moderate degree of religiosity.

The resulting questionnaire consists of 135 items arranged on a 5-point Likert-type scale ranging from an indication of *strong influence* on the decision to *no influence* on the decision.

Response Mode and Timing

Respondents indicate how important each factor would be by circling the number (1-5) reflecting their reaction to the item. The instrument requires approximately 45 minutes for completion.

Scoring

Scores on each factor may be computed by summing the item scores for those items loading on the factor or by using factor scores. A profile chart is also available from Juhasz for use in interpreting the data and providing counseling on the individual level.

Reliability and Validity

Construct validity was established through a principal components analysis. The eigenvalues resulting from the analysis were examined and the scree test (Gorsuch, 1974) indicated that a six-factor solution was appropriate. The first six principal components were submitted to a varimax rotation. Four experts in the field discussed the nature of each factor arriving at a consensus of opinion regarding the name to be allocated to each. Factors were named on the basis of their item content and on the relationship between each factor and personality as measured by the High School Personality Questionnaire dimensions (Cattell & Cattell, 1969).

The following six factors emerging on the JSSDMQ accounted for 35% of the variance (see the exhibit for item loadings):

1. Family establishment competence
2. External morality
3. Consequences of childbearing
4. Self-enhancement through sexual intercourse
5. Intimacy considerations regarding intercourse
6. Consequences of marriage

Reliability for each factor was determined using Cronbach's alpha. Variables loading .30 and above were employed. Reliability coefficients of the JSSDMQ factors are .91, .89, .92, .86, .81, and .90 for the six factors, respectively.

References

Cattell, R. B., & Cattell, M. D. L. (1969). *Handbook for the Jr.-Sr. high school personality questionnaire.* Champaign, IL: Institute for Personality and Testing.

Gorsuch, R. L. (1974). *Factor analysis.* Philadelphia: Saunders.

Juhasz, A. M. (1975). A chain of sexual decision-making. *The Family Coordinator, 24,* 43-49.

Juhasz, A. M., & Kavanagh, J. A. (1978). Factors which influence sexual decisions. *Journal of Sex Education and Therapy, 4,* 35-35.

Warner, W. L., Mecker, M., & Ellis, K. (1957). *Social class in America.* Boston: Peter Smith.

---

[1]Address correspondence to Anne McCreary Juhasz, 4300 Marine Drive, #706, Chicago, IL 60613.

Exhibit

The Juhasz-Schneider Sexual Decision-Making Questionnaire

Using the code below, circle the number that indicates how important the factors would be in influencing your decision.

1—of no importance   4—quite important
2—of little importance   5—extremely important
3—of some importance

How important would each of the following be in influencing your decision?

Decision 1: To have or not to have sexual intercourse

1.	My partner's personality.	4—.39[a]
2.	My partner's sex appeal.	5—.40
3.	My partner is single or married.	2—.48
4.	My partner's religion.	
5.	My partner's age.	
6.	My desire to be a virgin when I marry.	2—.49
7.	My desire to marry a virgin.	2—.46
8.	My religious beliefs regarding premarital sexual intercourse.	5—.58
9.	My feeling that I should be in love to have sexual intercourse.	5—.49
10.	My worry that my partner is only interested in me for sexual reasons.	5—.49
11.	My desire for sexual intercourse.	4—.32
12.	My partner's desire for sexual intercourse.	4—.43
13.	My partner's physical appearance.	4—.35
14.	I (or my partner) am having my period.	5—.38
15.	The possibility of getting V.D.	
16.	The fear that I might lose my partner if we don't have sex.	4—.48

How important would these be in influencing your decision?

17.	This is our first date.	5—.47
18.	We are going steady.	5—.46
19.	We are living together.	5—.44
20.	We are engaged.	5—.47
21.	We feel that we are committed to one another.	5—.48
22.	My partner is dating other people.	5—.53
23.	My partner is having sex with other people.	5—.45
24.	My fear that my partner might gain control over me.	2—.38
25.	My desire to get sexual experience.	4—.50
26.	It will boost my ego.	4—.61
27.	I can compare my experiences with friends.	4—.54
28.	It will keep me from masturbating (touching myself to get sexual pleasure).	4—.48
29.	It will help me avoid homosexual relationships.	4—.42
30.	It will give me the feeling of being close and belonging to someone.	4—.48
31.	It will help me know myself better.	4—.52
32.	It will be fun and pleasurable.	4—.64
33.	It will get rid of my sexual tensions.	4—.65
34.	It will make me want more intercourse.	4—.54
35.	My partner will expect us to get married.	
36.	My partner will expect us to date only each other.	5—.42
37.	It will reduce my chances of getting married later on.	2—.37
38.	My partner's feelings about me afterwards.	5—.39
39.	My friends' feelings about me afterwards.	2—.45
40.	My parents' feelings about me afterwards.	2—.57

How important would these be in influencing your decision?

41.	My feeling that love can cause you to lose control of yourself.	4—.38

42.	My feeling that love is a mysterious force that I must follow no matter where it takes me.	4—.45
43.	My feeling that love is very hard to find, and when you do you must do everything possible to keep it.	4—.45

How important would each of the following be in influencing this decision?

Decision 2: To have or not to have children

44.	I have the characteristics of a good parent.	1—.46
45.	My partner has the characteristics of a good parent.	1—.46
46.	There might be negative physical effects on the mother.	
47.	It would interfere with my social life.	
48.	My friends' feelings about this.	2—.52
49.	My parents' feelings about this.	2—.57
50.	My partner's feelings about this.	1—.37
51.	I feel that every woman should have a child because it is a woman's destiny.	4—.44

How important would each of the following be in influencing this decision?

Decision 3: To use or not to use birth control

52.	The risks involved in using birth control.	1—.40
53.	Birth control would prevent an unwanted pregnancy.	
54.	It would reduce my fear of pregnancy and make sex more enjoyable.	4—.42
55.	My parents' feelings about me using birth control.	2—.64
56.	My friends' feelings about me using birth control.	2—.56
57.	My partner's feelings about me using birth control.	
58.	My church's teachings about the use of birth control.	2—.59

How important would each of the following be in influencing this decision?

Decision 4: If pregnant, to deliver the child or have an abortion

59.	There might be negative physical effects of delivery on the mother.	3—.43
60.	The psychological effects of delivery on the mother.	3—.48
61.	The psychological effects of delivery on the father.	3—.42
62.	Having a child will limit the female's independence.	3—.62
63.	Having a child will limit the female's personal development.	3—.65
64.	Having a child will limit the female's social life.	3—.61
65.	Having a child will limit the female's education.	3—.71
66.	Having a child will limit the female's career.	3—.69
67.	Having a child will limit the male's independence.	3—.58
68.	Having a child will limit the male's personal development.	3—.62
69.	Having a child will limit the male's social life.	3—.59
70.	Having a child will limit the male's education.	3—.63
71.	Having a child will limit the male's career.	3—.62
72.	There will be financial problems for the male.	3—.62
73.	There will be financial problems for the female.	3—.62
74.	The female has the ability to be a good parent.	1—.52
75.	The female wants to be a parent.	1—.50
76.	The male has the ability to be a good parent.	1—.57
77.	The male wants to be a parent.	1—.50
78.	People's opinions of an unwed mother.	2—.43
79.	The father and mother will marry now or later.	
80.	No other man will want to marry an unwed mother.	3—.37
81.	The male will stick by the pregnant female.	1—.44
82.	The male feels that the female became pregnant to trap him to marriage.	
83.	I am afraid of having an abnormal child.	3—.45
84.	The child will have problems whether we marry or not.	3—.45
85.	The cost of delivery.	3—.42
86.	The nine months' time involved in carrying a pregnancy.	3—.52

Regarding the decision to have an abortion:

87.	Abortion is a quick solution to pregnancy.	3—.45
88.	The cost of the abortion.	3—.40
89.	My partner doesn't want to have a child.	3—.43
90.	My religious beliefs against abortion.	2—.56
91.	My friends' feelings about my abortion.	2—.46
92.	My parents' feelings about my abortion.	2—.62
93.	The abortion might have negative psychological effects on the female.	1—.54
94.	The abortion might have negative physical effects on the female.	1—.53
95.	The abortion might have negative psychological effects on the male.	1—.48
96.	The effect of the abortion on my relationship with my partner.	1—.49

How important would each of the following be in influencing this decision?

Decision 5: If you (or your partner) delivered a child . . . to keep the baby or give it up for adoption

97.	Our decision to stay together.	1—.53
98.	Our decision not to marry.	
99.	The emotional stability of the female.	1—.50
100.	The emotional stability of the male.	1—.47
101.	The female's desire to raise a child.	1—.65
102.	The female's ability to raise a child	1—.64
103.	The male's desire to raise a child.	1—.68
104.	The male's ability to raise a child.	1—.64
105.	The fear that the child may change our relationship for the worse.	3—.35
106.	My feeling that the child may improve our relationship.	1—.40
107.	The psychological effects on the female if she gives up the child.	1—.65
108.	The psychological effects on the male if he gives up the child.	1—.60
109.	I would have guilt feelings.	1—.45
110.	My parents' reaction and feelings would influence me.	2—.64
111.	My friends' reaction and feelings would influence me.	2—.53
112.	My partner's race.	2—.30
113.	My partner's religion.	2—.57
114.	My partner is a virgin.	2—.49
115.	My partner is divorced.	2—.55
116.	My partner has children from a former relationship.	
117.	Our compatibility.	1—.37
118.	Our respect for one another.	1—.53
119.	Our mutual desire for marriage.	1—.47
120.	Our commitment to one another.	1—.53
121.	My parents' opinions about the marriage.	2—.58
122.	My friends' opinions about the marriage.	2—.54
123.	My feeling that marriage may change our relationship.	6—.38
124.	My feeling that marriage would limit the female's educational plans.	6—.50
125.	My feeling that marriage would mean less freedom for the female.	6—.54
126.	My feeling that marriage would limit the female's chances for personal growth.	6—.68
127.	My feeling that marriage would limit the female's social contacts.	6—.60
128.	My feeling that marriage would limit the male's educational plans.	6—.69
129.	My feeling that marriage would limit the male's career chances.	6—.66
130.	My feeling that marriage would limit the male's chances for personal growth.	6—.76
131.	My feeling that marriage would mean less freedom for the male.	6—.66
132.	My feeling that marriage would change the man's lifestyle.	6—.56
133.	My feeling that there is an ideal mate for most people and when you find him/her you must marry.	
134.	My feeling that two people should be friends before they marry.	
135.	My feeling that you should be in love to marry.	1—.32

a. Identifies factor number and loading. Where there is no indicator, the item did not load ≥ .30 on any factor.

Hurlbert Index of Sexual Desire

David F. Hurlbert,[1] *Adult and Adolescent Counseling Center*

The Hurlbert Index of Sexual Desire (HISD) is described by Apt and Hurlbert (1992).

[1]Address correspondence to David F. Hurlbert, Adult and Adolescent Counseling Center, 619 North Main, Belton, TX 76513.

Reference

Apt, C., & Hurlbert, D. F. (1992). Motherhood and female sexuality beyond one year postpartum: A study of military wives. *Journal of Sex Education and Therapy, 18,* 104-114.

Exhibit

Hurlbert Index of Sexual Desire

1. Just thinking about having sex with my partner excites me. (R)
2. I try to avoid situations that will encourage my partner to want sex.
3. I daydream about sex. (R)
4. It is difficult for me to get in a sexual mood.
5. I desire more sex than my partner does. (R)
6. It is hard for me to fantasize about sexual things.
7. I look forward to having sex with my partner. (R)
8. I have a huge appetite for sex. (R)
9. I enjoy using sexual fantasy during sex with my partner. (R)
10. It is easy for me to get in the mood for sex. (R)
11. My desire for sex should be stronger.
12. I enjoy thinking about sex. (R)
13. I desire sex. (R)
14. It is easy for me to go weeks without having sex with my partner.
15. My motivation to engage in sex with my partner is low.
16. I feel I want sex less than most people.
17. It is easy for me to create sexual fantasies in my mind. (R)
18. I have a strong sex drive. (R)
19. I enjoy thinking about having sex with my partner. (R)
20. My desire for sex with my partner is strong. (R)
21. I feel that sex is not an important aspect of the relationship I share with my partner.
22. I think my energy level for sex with my partner is too low.
23. It is hard for me to get in the mood for sex.
24. I lack the desire necessary to pursue sex with my partner.
25. I try to avoid having sex with my partner.

Source. This inventory was originally published in "Motherhood and Female Sexuality Beyond One Year Postpartum: A Study of Military Wives," by C. Apt and D. F. Hurlbert, 1992, *Journal of Sex Education and Therapy, 18,* 104-114. Reprinted with permission.

Note. (R) = reverse scored. Scoring system responses: 0 points = *all of the time,* +1 point = *most of the time,* +2 points = *some of the time,* +3 points = *rarely,* +4 points = *never.*

Sexual Desire Inventory

Ilana P. Spector,[1] *Douglas Hospital and McGill University*
Michael P. Carey, *Syracuse University*
Lynne Steinberg, *Oklahoma State University*

The Sexual Desire Inventory (SDI) is a self-administered questionnaire developed to measure sexual desire. To date, sexologists have had difficulty measuring this construct. Previous measurement of sexual desire involved either indirect measurement through examining frequency of sexual behavior or broad self-report of cognitions such as "rate your level of sexual desire." Both these methods are less accurate measures of sexual desire because first, sexual desire is theoretically a multidimensional construct, and second, no empirical data are available to suggest that sexual desire and behavior are perfectly correlated. For the purposes of this questionnaire, sexual desire was defined as interest in sexual activity, and it was measured as primarily a cognitive variable through amount and strength of thought directed toward approaching or being receptive to sexual stimuli.

Description

The items of the SDI were selected by considering theoretical models of desire and clinical experience in assessing sexual desire disorders. They were presented initially to sexologists and then to a small pilot sample ($N = 20$ students), who rated the clarity and content validity of the items. Next, a sample of 300 students completed the SDI. Based on factor analytic data, items were eliminated or reworded to measure two dimensions of sexual desire: dyadic sexual desire (interest in behaving sexually with a partner) and solitary sexual desire (interest in behaving sexually by oneself).

To date, the 11-item SDI has been administered to three samples for the purpose of collecting psychometric data. These samples include 380 students (Spector, Carey, & Steinberg, 1996), 40 respondents living in geriatric long-term care facilities (Spector & Fremeth, 1996), and 40 couples (Spector & Davies, 1995). The SDI can be used to measure sexual desire both in the general population and in clinical samples. It has been used to measure sexual desire with both younger (M age = 20.8) and older (M age = 82.5) samples, and individuals and couples.

Response Mode and Timing

For each item, respondents are asked to circle the number that best reflects their thoughts and feelings about their

---
[1]Address correspondence to Ilana P. Spector, Community Psychiatric Center, Douglas Hospital, 6875 LaSalle Boulevard, Verdun, Quebec H4H 1R3, Canada; email: mdis@musica. mcgill.ca.

interest in or wish for sexual activity. They are asked to used the last month as a referent. For the three frequency items (Items 1, 2, and 10), respondents circle one of seven options. For the remaining eight strength items, respondents rate their level of sexual desire on an 8-point Likert-type scale. Most respondents complete the scale within 5 minutes.

Scoring

Items 1-8 are summed to obtain a dyadic sexual desire score. Items 9-11 are summed to obtain a solitary sexual desire score. Within a couple, female dyadic scores can be subtracted from male dyadic scores to obtain a desire discrepancy score.

Reliability

Internal consistency estimates (using Cronbach's alpha coefficients) were calculated for the Dyadic scale ($r = .86$) and the Solitary scale ($r = .96$), indicated strong evidence of reliability (Spector et al., 1996). Test-retest reliability was calculated at $r = .76$ over a 1-month period (Carey, 1995).

Validity

Evidence for factor validity has been examined. Factor analyses revealed that Items 1-8 loaded high (i.e., > .45) on the dyadic factor, whereas Items 9-11 loaded high on the solitary factor. Both factors had eigenvalues > 1 (Spector et al., 1996).

Concurrent validity evidence, collected from 380 students, revealed that solitary sexual desire is correlated with the frequency of solitary sexual behavior ($r = .80$, $p < .0001$), and with erotophilia ($r = -.28, p < .0001$) (Spector, 1992). Dyadic desire is correlated with the frequency of dyadic sexual behavior ($r = .34$, $p < .0001$). Note that neither dyadic nor solitary desire is perfectly correlated with sexual behavior, indicating that measuring desire indirectly through behavior would be inaccurate. Discriminant validity evidence reveals that neither subscale of the SDI is correlated with social desirability (Spector, 1992).

A second study conducted on 40 couples revealed that for females, dyadic desire is positively correlated with relationship adjustment as measured by the Dyadic Adjustment Scale (Spanier, 1976) ($r = .54, p < .001$), with sexual satisfaction as measured by the Index of Sexual Satisfaction (Hudson, Harrison, & Crosscup, 1981) ($r = .63, p < .001$), with sexual daydreams as measured by the Sexual Daydreams Scale (Giambra, 1980) ($r = .53, p < .001$), and with sexual arousal as measured by the Sexual Arousal Inventory

(Hoon, Hoon, & Wincze, 1976) ($r = .71, p < .001$). With males, dyadic sexual desire is only correlated with sexual satisfaction ($r = .36, p < .01$) (Spector & Davies, 1995).

Gender differences have been noted on the SDI. Males have significantly higher levels of dyadic, $F(1, 374) = 5.79$, $p < .05$, and solitary, $F(1, 376) = 55.15, p < .0001$, desire than do females. This difference is also found in geriatric samples (Spector & Fremeth, 1996).

References

Carey, M. P. (1995). [Test-retest reliability of the Sexual Desire Inventory]. Unpublished raw data.

Giambra, L. M. (1980). A factor analysis of the items of the Imaginal Processes Inventory. *Journal of Clinical Psychology, 36*, 383-409.

Hoon, E. F., Hoon, P. W., & Wincze, J. P. (1976). The SAI: An inventory for the measurement of female sexual arousability. *Archives of Sexual Behavior, 5*, 291-300.

Hudson, W. W., Harrison, D. F., & Crosscup, P. C. (1981). A short-form scale to measure sexual discord in dyadic relationships. *The Journal of Sex Research, 17*, 157-174.

Spanier, G. B. (1976). Measuring dyadic adjustment: New scales for assessing the quality of marriage and similar dyads. *Journal of Marriage and the Family, 38*, 15-28.

Spector, I. P. (1992). *Development and psychometric evaluation of a measure of sexual desire*. Unpublished doctoral dissertation, Syracuse University, New York.

Spector, I. P., Carey, M. P., & Steinberg, L. (1996). The Sexual Desire Inventory: Development, factor structure, and evidence of reliability. *Journal of Sex & Marital Therapy, 22*, 175-190.

Spector, I. P., & Davies, S. (1995). *The experience of sexual desire in couples*. Manuscript in preparation.

Spector, I. P., & Fremeth, S. M. (1996). Sexual behaviors and attitudes of geriatric residents in long-term care facilities. *Journal of Sex & Marital Therapy, 22*, 235-246.

Exhibit

Sexual Desire Inventory

This questionnaire asks about your level of sexual desire. By desire, we mean *interest in* or *wish for sexual activity*. For each item, please circle the number that best shows your thoughts and feelings. Your answers will be private and anonymous.

1. During the last month, *how often* would you *have liked* to engage in sexual activity with a partner (for example, touching each other's genitals, giving or receiving oral stimulation, intercourse, etc.)?

   0) Not at all
   1) Once a month
   2) Once every two weeks
   3) Once a week
   4) Twice a week
   5) 3 to 4 times a week
   6) Once a day
   7) More than once a day

2. During the last month, *how often* have you had sexual thoughts involving a partner?

   0) Not at all
   1) Once or twice a month
   2) Once a week
   3) Twice a week
   4) 3 to 4 times a week
   5) Once a day
   6) A couple of times a day
   7) Many times a day

3. When you have sexual thoughts, *how strong* is your desire to engage in sexual behavior with a partner?

   0 1 2 3 4 5 6 7 8
   No desire   Strong desire

4. When you first see an attractive person, *how strong* is your sexual desire?

   0 1 2 3 4 5 6 7 8
   No desire   Strong desire

5. When you spend time with an attractive person (for example, at work or school), *how strong* is your sexual desire?

   0 1 2 3 4 5 6 7 8
   No desire   Strong desire

6. When you are in romantic situations (such as a candle-lit dinner, a walk on the beach, etc.), *how strong* is your sexual desire?

   0 1 2 3 4 5 6 7 8
   No desire   Strong desire

7. *How strong* is your desire to engage in sexual activity with a partner?

   0 1 2 3 4 5 6 7 8
   No desire   Strong desire

8. *How important* is it for you to fulfill your sexual desire through activity with a partner?

   0 1 2 3 4 5 6 7 8
   Not at all   Extremely
   important   important

9. Compared to other people of your age and sex, how would you rate your desire to behave sexually with a partner?

   0 1 2 3 4 5 6 7 8
   Much less desire   Much more desire

10. During the last month, *how often* would you *have liked* to behave sexually by yourself (for example, masturbating, touching your genitals, etc.)?

    0) Not at all   4) Twice a week
    1) Once a month   5) 3 to 4 times a week
    2) Once every two weeks   6) Once a day
    3) Once a week   7) More than once a day

11. *How strong* is your desire to engage in sexual behavior by yourself?

         0   1   2   3   4   5   6   7   8
      No desire   Strong desire

12. *How important* is it for you to fulfill your desires to behave sexually by yourself?

         0   1   2   3   4   5   6   7   8
    Not at all   Extremely
    important   important

13. Compared to other people of your age and sex, how would you rate your desire to behave sexually by yourself?

         0   1   2   3   4   5   6   7   8
    Much less desire   Much more desire

14. *How long* could you go comfortably without having sexual activity of some kind?

    0) Forever   5) A week
    1) A year or two   6) A few days
    2) Several months   7) One day
    3) A month   8) Less than one day
    4) A few weeks

Source. This inventory was originally published in "The Sexual Desire Inventory: Development, Factor Structure, and Evidence of Reliability," by I. P. Spector, M. P. Carey, and L. Steinberg, 1996, *Journal of Sex & Marital Therapy, 22,* 175–190. Reprinted with permission.

Perception of Diabetes Mellitus Questionnaire

Barbara A. Pieper,[1] *Wayne State University*

The purpose of the Perception of Diabetes Mellitus questionnaire (PDM) is to measure the perceived impact of diabetes on life and sexuality. For the person with diabetes, an understanding of the perceived effect of diabetes on sexuality, along with assessment of physical sexual functioning, may enhance understanding of the diabetic experience and thus aid teaching and counseling.

Description

The PDM consists of 35 statements about the effect of diabetes; this represents the refinement of a 43-item questionnaire (Pieper, 1980) by means of factor analysis. The PDM is a modification of Hanson's (1982) questionnaire exploring the effect of chronic lung disease on sexuality and life.

The PDM has a modified Porter (1962) format. Each of the 35 stem statements explores the effect of diabetes, its treatment, and symptoms on life and sexuality. Stem statements represent three factors: Psychosocial, 18 items; Relationship-Sexual Function, 9 items; and Blood Sugar-Diet, 8 items. For each stem, four questions are asked concerning the effect (see below).

Responses for each question are quantified on 7-point Likert-type scales with response options ranging from *great effect* (score of 7) to *minimal effect* (score of 1) for Questions 1 and 3; *very positive effect* (score of 7) to *very negative effect* (score of l) for Question 2; *very important* (score of 7) to *not important* (score of 1) for Question 4.

[1]Address correspondence to Barbara A. Pieper, College of Nursing, 5557 Cass Avenue, Wayne State University, Detroit, MI 48202; email: piepwin@mail.ic.net.

The PDM is designed to be used with adults who have diabetes. It has been successfully administered to men and women who ranged in age from 18 to 83 years. Participants have primarily (85%) had a high school education or greater (Pieper, 1980, 1982; Pieper et al., 1983).

Because the items are worded in terms of marriage, sexual partner, or sexual activity, only persons who are married or sexually active within the previous year can respond to the Relationship-Sexual Function items. Diabetes, especially in the male, has a high association with impotence. These items allow examination of potential change in the marriage and/or sexual function for the person as a result of diabetes.

Persons who were diagnosed as diabetic for 5 years or longer prior to testing often have difficulty remembering what it was like not to have diabetes, thus affecting the validity of the response to "What effect did you expect?"

The PDM may be self-completed or used in an interview format. Individuals are told that the questionnaire explores how diabetes affects a person's life and sexuality and that there are no right or wrong answers.

Response Mode and Timing

Respondents circle the number on the scale best representing the perceived impact of diabetes on the questions for the stem item. The PDM requires an average of 30 to 45 minutes to complete.

Scoring

Four scores are possible for each factor. These are obtained by summing responses across stem items for each question. The following scores may be obtained:

1. Effect score—the sum total of the responses to "What effect does it have?" The higher the effect score, the greater the effect/interference of diabetes on that factor. The effect score quantifies the effect of diabetes.

2. Rating score—the sum total of the responses to "How would you rate the effect?" The higher the rating score, the more positive was the perceived effect of diabetes in terms of that factor.

3. Expected effect score—the sum total of the responses to "What effect did you expect?" The higher the expected effect score, the greater the expected interference of diabetes in terms of that factor.

4. Importance score—the sum total of the responses to "How important is this effect on your life to you?" The higher the importance score, the greater the importance of the effect on diabetes in terms of that factor for the individual.

Possible ranges for the above scores are 18 to 126 for the Psychosocial factor, 9 to 63 for the Relationship-Sexual Function factor, and 8 to 56 for the Blood Sugar-Diet factor. The PDM may be used to obtain a total life-sexuality score by summing across all three factor items for specific questions. The total scores for each question may range from 35 to 245.

Reliability

Coefficient alpha values for internal consistency for 177 respondents range, for the Psychosocial factor, from .92 to .96; for the Blood Sugar-Diet factor, from .81 to .89; and for the Relationship-Sexual Function factor, from .84 to .93.

Split-half (odd-even) reliabilities for a total sexuality-life score are .88 for the effect score, .96 for the rating score, .91 for the expected effect score, and .95 for the importance score. Each half correlated highest with its respective half.

Validity

Content (face) validity was established by experts in sexual counseling and diabetes. Factor analysis was used to assess the structure of the ratings. The effect scores were chosen in preference to the other scores because the former is specific to the effect of diabetes on life and sexuality, whereas the latter were qualifiers on the effect. Nine factors were extracted during the principal components analyses. After examination of item intercorrelations and factor loadings, it was decided to rotate three factors. A varimax orthogonal rotation was performed. The factor on which the item loaded highest and a loading greater than .40 were the criteria used to associate items with factors. The structure revealed by factor analysis lends support to content validity of the PDM.

The Psychosocial factor contains the following 18 items: life, employment, home, income, children, social life, self-worth, interest in life, energy, care for self, personal business, rely on others, moods, get along with others, woman/man, urine testing on life, insulin on life, and all treatments on life. Urine testing on life (.31) and insulin on life (.36) loaded less than .40, however. They were retained because they are common care practices in diabetes management. The effect of diabetes on energy level conceptually overlaps with blood sugar and diet; as expected, this item loaded in the Psychosocial (.54) and Blood Sugar-Diet (.37) factors.

The Relationship-Sexual Function factor[2] contains the following nine items: closeness to spouse, care for spouse, insulin on relationship, diet on relationship, all treatments on relationship, interest in sex, satisfaction with sex, and all treatments on sex. Because of their psychosocial nature, closeness to spouse and care for spouse loaded on the Psychosocial factor (.31 and .34, respectively) as well as the Relationship-Sexual Function factor (.72 and .70, respectively).

The Blood Sugar-Diet factor contains the following eight items: meal schedule; diet; high blood sugar on life, relationship, and sex; low blood sugar on life, relationship, and sex. High blood sugar on relationship, high blood sugar on sexual function, and low blood sugar on sexual function loaded on the second factor (.39 to .50) because of their sexual nature. Meal schedule (.34) and diabetic diet (.36) loaded less than .40, but were retained because of their crucial role in diabetes care.

---

[2]In previous reports of the PDM, the Relationship-Sexual Function factor was separated in two. This was determined by content wording of the items and a preliminary factor analysis.

Construct validity is tentative but has been examined in comparison to other research. The effect score for the Psychosocial items correlated in a low moderate manner with the Profile of Mood States (McNair, Lorr, & Droppleman, 1971): Tension Anxiety ($r = .43$, $p < .001$) and Depression-Dejection ($r = .36$, $p < .001$) scores. This may reflect the effect of moods on perception. Men ($M = 16.16$) scored significantly higher on the effect score for Relationship-Sexual Function items than women ($M = 11.70$), $t(119) = 2.30$, $p < .05$. This may document the effect of altered sexual functioning (e.g., diabetic impotence) in the male.

Other Information

Although the PDM is specific to diabetes, it is easily modified for use with other conditions. Kehle (1985) modified it for use with perception of chronic back pain, and Clarke (1983) modified it for body weight. Pieper and Mikols (1996) modified the PDM to examine the perceived effect of having a fecal stoma. The Perceived Effect of an Ostomy questionnaire has 46 items. Items explore the effect of an ostomy on self-care, body image, and participation in work, home, leisure, and sexual activity. Prior to the hospital discharge, persons responded to each item with the question "What effect do you think your ostomy will have?" The postdischarge response was to the question "What effect does your ostomy have?" Response options ranged from *minimal/no effect/not a concern* (score of 1) to *very great effect/very great concern* (score of 7). Coefficient alpha values were .97 for both. Prior to discharge, five sexual items occurred in the top 15 concerns; after discharge, one item. Eight items were of high concern both

pre- and postdischarge. This questionnaire format may help to identify patient concerns for teaching and counseling in both inpatient and outpatient settings.

The PDM is copyrighted.

_____

References

Clarke, P. (1983). *Body weight: Perceived effect on life, conversational distance, and self-actualization.* Unpublished doctoral dissertation, Wayne State University, Detroit, MI.

Hanson, E. I. (1982). Effects of chronic lung disease on life in general and on sexuality: Perceptions of adult patients. *Heart and Lung, 11*, 435-441.

Kehle, M. (1985). *Perception of chronic back pain.* Unpublished doctoral dissertation, Arizona State University.

McNair, D., Lorr, M., & Droppleman, L. (1971). *EITS manual profile of mood states.* San Diego, CA: Educational and Industrial Testing Service.

Pieper, B. A. (1980). *The relationship between health status and perceived sexuality among females with diabetes mellitus.* Unpublished doctoral dissertation, Wayne State University, Detroit, MI.

Pieper, B. A. (1982). Women's perceived effect of diabetes mellitus on sexual function and relationship to spouse. *Journal of Sex Education and Therapy, 8*, 18-21.

Pieper, B. A., Clarke, P. N., Caldwell, M. H., Bryan, J. B., Vincent, M. K., & Miner, M. (1983). Perceived effect of diabetes on relationship to spouse and sexual function. *Journal of Sex Education and Therapy, 9*, 46-50.

Pieper, B., & Mikols, C. (1996). Predischarge and postdischarge concerns of persons with an ostomy. *Journal of Wound, Ostomy, and Continence Nursing, 23*(2), 105-109.

Porter, L. W. (1962). Job attitude in management: Perceived deficiencies in need fulfillment as a function of job level. *Journal of Applied Psychology, 46*, 375-384.

Exhibit

Perceptions of Diabetes Mellitus Questionnaire

This questionnaire contains 35 items about the effect of diabetes mellitus on life, marriage, and sexual function. Please circle the number on the scale which represents how you feel about the question. Please answer each item as best as you can. There are no right or wrong answers.

1. The effect of diabetes on your life in general.[a]

What effect does it have?	Minimal effect	1	2	3	4	5	6	7	Great effect
How would you rate the effect?	Very negative	1	2	3	4	5	6	7	Very positive
What effect did you expect diabetes to have?	Minimal effect	1	2	3	4	5	6	7	Great effect
How important is this effect to you?	Not important	1	2	3	4	5	6	7	Very important

2. The effect of diabetes on your ability to be employed outside the home now or prior to your retirement.
3. The effect of diabetes on your ability to carry out your home responsibilities.
4. The effect of diabetes on your income/budget.
5. The effect of diabetes on your ability to care for children/grandchildren.
6. The effect of diabetes on your social life.
7. The effect of diabetes on your feelings of self-worth.
8. The effect of diabetes on your interest in life.
9. The effect of diabetes on your energy level.
10. The effect of diabetes on your ability to care for yourself such as bathing, dressing, and grooming.
11. The effect of diabetes on your ability to take care of personal business such as attending school, banking, or shopping.
12. The effect of diabetes on your need to rely on others.
13. The effect of diabetes on your moods.

14. The effect of diabetes on your ability to get along with people.
15. The effect of diabetes on your feelings about yourself as a man/woman.
16. Your diabetic meal schedule on your life in general.
17. Your diabetic food selection on your life in general.
18. Urine testing on your life in general.
19. Injecting insulin or taking oral hypoglycemic agents on your life in general.
20. All treatments related to your diabetes on your life in general.
21. Symptoms you associate with high blood sugar on your life in general.
22. Symptoms you associate with low blood sugar on your life in general.

The following questions relate to the effect of diabetes on your marriage, relationship to sexual partner, and sexual activity. Please answer if you are married and/or sexually active.

23. The effect of diabetes on your marriage.
24. The effect of diabetes on your feelings of closeness and tenderness for your spouse/partner.
25. The effect of your diabetes on your ability to care for your spouse/partner.
26. The effect of injecting insulin or taking oral hypoglycemic agents on your relationship with your spouse/partner.
27. Your diabetic diet on your relationship with your spouse/partner.
28. All treatments related to your diabetes on your relationship with spouse/partner.
29. Symptoms you associate with high blood sugar on your relationship with your spouse/partner.
30. Symptoms you associate with low blood sugar on your relationship with your spouse/partner.
31. The effect of diabetes on your interest in sex.
32. The effect of diabetes on your feelings of satisfaction after sexual intercourse.
33. All treatments related to your diabetes on your sexual love play/intercourse.
34. Symptoms you associate with high blood sugar on your sexual love play/intercourse.
35. Symptoms you associate with low blood sugar on your sexual love play/intercourse.

a. This scale is repeated after each question.

Sexuality After Spinal Cord Injury Questionnaire

Paul A. Kettl,[1] *Pennsylvania State University and Milton S. Hershey Medical Center*

Few injuries are as personally devastating as a spinal cord injury. From the moment of injury, the patient's life and body are changed, often forever, as the patient loses sensation and motor control over the lost portions of his or her body, which are now strangely distant. Sexual changes after spinal cord injury accompany the physical and psychological sequelae that occur. It is, in fact, in these sexual changes where the physical and psychological disabilities of the spinal cord injury merge and present the patient with a great challenge in rehabilitation.

In rehabilitation from a spinal cord injury, the goal of therapy is to return the patient as fully as possible to his or her premorbid level of functioning. The same goal is present in assessing and restoring sexual functioning as well. To do this effectively, however, the treatment team must have information about the patient's sexual past as well as how that person views his or her sexual present.

The Sexuality After Spinal Cord Injury Questionnaire is designed to obtain information about how the patient viewed his or her sexual life before the injury compared to

[1]Address correspondence to Paul A. Kettl, Pennsylvania State University College of Medicine, Milton S. Hershey Medical Center, P.O. Box 850, Hershey, PA 17033.

how he or she views sexual life in rehabilitation after the injury. Using that information, the therapist has knowledge about how sexually disabled the patient views himself or herself. With this information, rehabilitation in sexuality after spinal cord injury can further progress.

Description

The Sexuality After Spinal Cord Injury Questionnaire is designed to obtain a broad array of information about sexuality in those persons disabled by spinal cord injury. Beginning with demographic information, questions seek information on the quality of one's social life, sexual frequency and sexual difficulties, sexual satisfaction, and information about body image and physical health. Information is obtained comparing current views of one's sexual life to sexual life before spinal cord injury. The questionnaire was developed in a university hospital rehabilitation center by all members of the treatment team (i.e., nurses, occupational therapists, physical therapists, and a psychiatrist) to assess and assist sexual rehabilitation after spinal cord injury.

Response Mode and Timing

The instrument is spread out over several pages and designed to be answered by simple pencil marks to make it easiest to answer for those whose arm movements may be partially or completely paralyzed. Respondents answer items on a 5-point scale or by circling the response that is most appropriate. In most cases, the questionnaire can be answered by the respondent without assistance, and it takes about 15 minutes to complete. If the respondent is not physically able to answer on his or her own, it can be administered orally with responses marked by the interviewer.

Scoring

The questionnaire seeks to measure the perceived difference in sexuality before and after spinal cord injury. Questions are therefore linked to behavior before, and then after, spinal cord injury. Measures are obtained to reveal respondents' perceived decline in different aspects of sexuality after injury compared with perceptions of their preinjury sexuality. For example, a change from a 3 before injury to a 1 after injury would represent a 50% decline in that area of functioning.

Reliability

No data are available on either the internal consistency or test-retest reliability of the instrument.

Validity

The questionnaire was developed by administering it to 390 spinal cord-injured patients being followed by the Milton S. Hershey Medical Center. Information from the questionnaire has been useful in assessing sexuality in women after spinal cord injury (Kettl et al., 1990; Kettl, Zarefoss, Jacoby, et al., 1991) as well as men (Kettl, Zarefoss, Garman, et al., 1991). Women and men show similar response rates to the questionnaire (Kettl, Zarefoss, Garman, et al., 1991).

The instrument's greatest strength is its face validity in being able to assess the perceived disability from the patient's viewpoint. However, we acknowledge that the patient's perception of his or her sexual life before injury may be presented in an overly favorable light and likewise that their view of body image and sexuality after injury may be presented in a darker context. This information, although perhaps not objectively unassailable, presents important data on how the patient views his or her life so further therapeutic work can be done in rehabilitation.

References

Kettl, P. A., Zarefoss, S., Garman, C., Jacoby, K., Hulse, C., Rowley, R., Sredy, M., & Bixler, E. O. (1990). Female sexuality after spinal cord injury. In *Abstracts Digest*. Orlando, FL: American Spinal Injury Association.

Kettl, P. A., Zarefoss, S., Garman, C., Jacoby, K., Hulse, C., Rowley, R., Sredy, M., Bixler, E. O. (1991). Differences between male and female sexuality after SCI [Abstract]. *Journal of the American Paraplegic Society, 14,* 74.

Kettl, P. A., Zarefoss, S., Jacoby, K., Garman, C., Hulse, C., Rowley, R., Corey, R., Sredy, M., & Bixler, E. O. (1991). Female asexuality after spinal cord injury. *Journal of Sexuality and Disability, 9,* 287-295.

Exhibit

Sexuality After Spinal Cord Injury Questionnaire

Sex: Male   Female
Date of birth: _____
Level of injury: Para Quad   //   Complete   Incomplete
Marital status: Single _____   Married _____   Divorced _____   (0-5)   (6-10)   (11-15)   (16-20) Years
                              Widowed _____   Number of children _____
Present living situation: Who lives with you?—Circle those that apply
     (girlfriend, boyfriend, spouse, parents, brothers, sisters, live alone) .
     other _____
Level of schooling completed: Grade school _____   High school _____   College _____   Postgraduate _____
Are you presently: In school (full time) (part time) _____
Employed (full time) (part time) _____
Unemployed _____

(Mark the most appropriate response)

				Very often— a great deal
Not at all 0	1	2	3	4

How often do you go out socially?
    –before your injury   (0   1   2   3   4)
    –after your injury   (0   1   2   3   4)
How enjoyable was your social life?
    –before your injury   (0   1   2   3   4)
    –after your injury   (0   1   2   3   4)
How close were your relationships with your friends?
    –before your injury   same sex   (0   1   2   3   4)
                                                       opposite sex   (0   1   2   3   4)
    –after your injury   same sex   (0   1   2   3   4)
                                                       opposite sex   (0   1   2   3   4)
How important was sexual activity?
    –before your injury   (0   1   2   3   4)
    –after your injury   (0   1   2   3   4)
How often did you engage in sexual activity?
    –before your injury   (0   1   2   3   4)
    –after your injury   (0   1   2   3   4)
If female, during sexual activity, have you experienced any physical
difficulties that hinder intercourse? (i.e., inadequate lubrication, painful
intercourse, bleeding, etc.)
    –before your injury   (0   1   2   3   4)
    –after your injury   (0   1   2   3   4)
If male, have you experienced any difficulty getting an erection during
sexual activity?
    –before your injury   (0   1   2   3   4)
    –after your injury   (0   1   2   3   4)
If male, have you experienced any difficulty maintaining an erection during
sexual activity?
    –before your injury   (0   1   2   3   4)
    –after your injury   (0   1   2   3   4)
How satisfying was sexual activity?
    –before your injury   (0   1   2   3   4)
    –after your injury   (0   1   2   3   4)
How well do you feel you satisfied your partner?
    –before your injury   (0   1   2   3   4)
    –after your injury   (0   1   2   3   4)

How satisfied were you with the frequency of your sexual activity?
  –before your injury   (0   1   2   3   4)
  –after your injury   (0   1   2   3   4)
Compared to before your injury, have you: (Circle most appropriate)
  –been sexually active   never   less than   the same   more often
  –had intercourse   never   less than   the same   more often
  –engaged in oral sex   never   less than   the same   more often
  –engaged in anal sex   never   less than   the same   more often
  –engaged in masturbation   never   less than   the same   more often
What was your most pleasurable sexual activity before your injury? (Please circle)
    kissing and caressing   intercourse   oral sex   anal sex   masturbation
Since your injury, have you been able to have an orgasm? (Circle one)
          Yes   No
If yes, was it (Circle one)?
      the same   similar   different
Are you presently using any form of birth control? (Please circle)
          Yes   No
If yes, which type? _____
In your estimation how attractive do you feel your body was?
  –before your injury   (0   1   2   3   4)
  –after your injury   (0   1   2   3   4)
How healthy were you?
  –before your injury   (0   1   2   3   4)
  –after your injury   (0   1   2   3   4)
How well were your sexual concerns addressed during rehabilitation?   (0   1   2   3   4)
During rehab, how comfortable were you in discussing sex with the staff?   (0   1   2   3   4)
Has your spinal cord injury contributed to the break-up of relationships with a significant other?
          Yes   No
If yes, was it with: _____ a spouse_____ a friend?
If yes, how much do you feel sexual difficulties contributed to the break-up?   (0   1   2   3   4)
Based on your experience, what is important for us to be teaching newly injured spinal cord injury patients?_____

Double Standard Scale

Sandra L. Caron,[1] *University of Maine*
Clive M. Davis, *Syracuse University*
William A. Halteman, *University of Maine*
Marla Stickle, *University of Maine*

The purpose of the Double Standard Scale is to measure acceptance of the traditional sexual double standard.

[1]Address correspondence to Sandra L. Caron, Department of Human Development, University of Maine, 15 Merrill Hall, Orono, ME 05469; email: scaron@maine.edu.

Description

The Double Standard Scale consists of 10 items arranged in a 5-point Likert-type format with response options labeled from (1) *strongly agree* to (5) *strongly disagree.*

Response Mode and Timing

Respondents circle the number from 1 to 5 corresponding to their answer. The scale requires an average of 5 minutes for completion.

Scoring

A total score for the instrument is obtained by summing each of the item scores, including reversing the negative item (Item 8). Scores can range from 10 to 50 points. A lower score indicates greater adherence to the traditional double standard.

Reliability

In a sample of 330 college men and women (Caron, Davis, Halteman, & Stickle, 1993), the Cronbach alpha for the summed scores from the 10 items was .72.

Validity

In addition to the face validity of the questions, Caron et al. (1993) obtained results consistent with expectations about how those men and women who held a double standard would behave regarding some aspects of condom use.

Reference

Caron, S. L., Davis, C. M., Halteman, W. A., & Stickle, M. (1993). Predictors of condom-related behaviors among first-year college students. *The Journal of Sex Research, 30,* 252-259.

Exhibit

Double Standard Scale

Instructions: Please circle your response to the following questions about your attitudes about the sex roles of men and women. Please keep in mind that there are no right or wrong answers. Please answer honestly.

1 = Strongly agree
2 = Agree
3 = Undecided
4 = Disagree
5 = Strongly disagree

1	2	3	4	5	1.	It is expected that a woman be less sexually experienced than her partner.
1	2	3	4	5	2.	A woman who is sexually active is less likely to be considered a desirable partner.
1	2	3	4	5	3.	A woman should never appear to be prepared for a sexual encounter.
1	2	3	4	5	4.	It is important that the men be sexually experienced so as to teach the woman.
1	2	3	4	5	5.	A "good" woman would never have a one-night stand, but it is expected of a man.
1	2	3	4	5	6.	It's important for a man to have multiple sexual experiences in order to gain experience.
1	2	3	4	5	7.	In sex the man should take the dominant role and the woman should assume the passive role.
1	2	3	4	5	8.	It is acceptable for a woman to carry condoms.
1	2	3	4	5	9.	It is worse for a woman to sleep around than it is for a man.
1	2	3	4	5	10.	It is up to the man to initiate sex.

Indicators of a Double Standard and Generational Difference in Sexual Attitudes

Ilsa L. Lottes,[1] *University of Maryland, Baltimore County*
Martin S. Weinberg, *Indiana University*

Description

The Indicators of a Double Standard and Generational Difference in Sexual Attitudes were developed by Weinberg as part of a 1992 comparative study of sexual attitudes and behaviors of university students in the United States and Sweden. Compared with the United States, Sweden is considered a much more homogeneous society, and the double standard of sexuality is also thought to be less evident in Sweden (see Reiss, 1980; Weinberg, Lottes, & Shaver, 1995). Thus, the indicators were used to test these expectations. In general, the indicators can be used to assess the perceived heterogeneity of sexual attitudes of a population by generation and gender or to compare two or more populations with respect to such generational and gender differences.

The indicators of sexual attitudes consist of six, 5-point Likert-type items. For each item, respondents compare their sexual attitudes with those of their mother, father, close female friends, close male friends, female students their own age, and male students their own age. The response options for each item are that the specified individual(s) is (are) *much more liberal* (1), *slightly more liberal* (2), *the same* (3), *slightly more conservative* (4), or *much more conservative* (5). Because the evaluation of parent and peer sexual attitudes is provided by respondents, not respondents' parents and peers, this instrument should be regarded as providing indirect measures of a lack of homogeneity—a perception of a double standard and/or a generational difference in sexual attitudes. When evaluating a double standard of sexual behavior, researchers often ask the same respondents identical questions about acceptable sexual behavior for women and men. These types of questions make it obvious to respondents that female-male comparisons may be made, and respondents influenced by "social desirability" and "political correctness" pressures may be careful to put the same response to corresponding pairs of female-male questions. We believe that the wording of items of the indicators make such a social desirability bias less likely because it is less obvious that comparisons to assess a double standard will be made.

The indicators of sexual attitudes would be appropriate to administer to high school or university students.

[1]Address correspondence to Ilsa L. Lottes, Department of Sociology and Anthropology, University of Maryland, Baltimore County, 5401 Wilkens Avenue, Baltimore, MD 21228; email: lottes@umbc2.umbc.edu.

Response Mode and Timing

Respondents circle the number from 1 to 5 corresponding to their rating of the similarity of their sexual attitudes to those of their parent or peer group. This takes less than 5 minutes to complete.

Scoring

In a society characterized by the traditional double standard of sexual behavior, men are subjected to more permissive or liberal sexual norms than women. In such a society we would expect the sexual attitudes of men to be more liberal than the sexual attitudes of women. In operationalizing the double standard, we assume that if sexual attitudes of women and men are judged to be similar with respect to a liberal-conservative dimension, then this will indicate lack of support for a double standard. If the sexual attitudes of men are judged to be more liberal than women, then this will indicate a male-permissive double standard; similarly, if the attitudes of women are judged to be more liberal than men, then this will indicate a female-permissive double standard.

For ease of interpretation and also to identify the extent of more substantial or "real" generational and gender differences in sexual attitudes, responses to the six items were recoded as follows: 1 to -1, 2 to 0, 3 to 0, 4 to 0, and 5 to 1. With this coding, a minus one indicates that a respondent rated a parent or peer groups to have sexual attitudes *much more liberal* than his or her own attitudes, and a plus one indicates that a respondent rated a parent or peer group to have sexual attitudes *much more conservative* than his or her own attitudes. A zero indicates that a respondent rated a parent or peer group to have sexual attitudes similar to his or her own, where "similar" includes the *slightly more liberal, slightly more conservative,* and *the same* responses.

To assess the extent of a double standard of sexual behavior for women and men, three new variables—Dparent, Dfriend, and Dstudent—are created by taking the difference of corresponding female and male items. Using the variable names, Dparent = Mother − Father, Dfriend = Ffriend − Mfriend, and Dstudent = Fstudent − Mstudent. Shown in Table 1 are the possible numerical values of these three double standard difference variables. A value of 0 for a double standard difference variable indicates a similar rating of sexual attitudes for a pair of female-male variables and is interpreted as an indicator of egalitarian sexual attitudes and no double standard. A negative difference (of −1 or −2) indicates that women's sexual attitudes were rated more

Table 1 Variable Values and Difference Variable Interpretation

Female variable Mother Ffriend Fstudent Values	Male variable Father Mfriend Mstudent Values	Difference variable[a] Dparent Dfriend Dstudent Values	*Interpretation of difference variables*
−1	1	−2	Female more liberal, female-permissive double standard
−1	0	−1	Female more liberal, female-permissive double standard
0	1	−1	Female more liberal, female-permissive double standard
−1	−1	0	Egalitarian, no double standard
0	0	0	Egalitarian, no double standard
1	1	0	Egalitarian, no double standard
0	−1	1	Male more liberal, male-permissive double standard
1	0	1	Male more liberal, male-permissive double standard
1	−1	2	Male more liberal, male-permissive double standard

a. The difference variable equals the female variable minus the male variable.

liberal than those of men—a female-permissive double standard. A positive difference (of 1 or 2) indicates that men's sexual attitudes were rated more liberal than those of women—an indicator of a male-permissive double standard.

Reliability

Principal components factor analyses were performed on the six items using all five of the original responses with samples of male and female university students in the United States and Sweden. Factor analyses for each of the four country/gender groups revealed two factors—a parental factor composed of the mother and father items and a peer factor composed of the four friend and student items. For samples of male university students in the United States and Sweden, Cronbach alphas for the parental factor were .60 and .80, respectively; for these samples, Cronbach alphas for the peer factor were .85 and .84, respectively. For samples of female university students in the United States and Sweden, Cronbach alphas for the parental factor were .64 and .77, respectively; for these samples, Cronbach alphas for the peer factor were both .78.

Validity

Construct validity of the Indicators of a Double Standard and Generational Difference in Sexual Attitudes was supported by significant differences in the predicted direction for groups of Swedish and American university students. Greater proportions of Swedish than American students responded in the similar category. Between 77% and 89% of Swedish students rated their parents' sexual attitudes as similar to their own compared with between 54% and 65% for American students. Thus, these findings support the view that with respect to sexual attitudes, Sweden is a more homogeneous society, characterized by less of a generational difference in such attitudes than the United States. With respect to parents' sexual attitudes, the proportion rated *much more conservative* was higher than the proportion rated *much more liberal* (especially for Americans).

Between 80% and 94% of Swedish students rated their male peers as having sexual attitudes similar to their own compared to between 55% and 79% for American students. For comparison with male peers, there were higher homogeneity ratings for Sweden than for the United States, as expected. For ratings of male peer sexual attitudes, nonsimilar responses for each country and gender tended to occur in the *much more liberal* rather than *much more conservative* category. For comparisons with female peer sexual attitudes, similar responses were high for all four country/gender groups. Thus, with respect to comparisons with female peers, the expectation regarding greater homogeneity in Sweden was only partially supported. A greater proportion of Swedish women (88%) compared to American women (78%) rated female students their own age as having sexual attitudes similar to their own. But no greater homogeneity was found in ratings of close female friends. More than 90% of all country/gender groups rated the sexual attitudes of their close female friends as similar to their own.

For the mother-father comparison, a higher proportion of American males rated their mother as having much more conservative sexual attitudes than their father than rated their mother as having much more liberal attitudes than their father (27% vs. 10%). For the double standard variables involving gender differences for friends and students, all four country/gender groups reported a higher proportion of much more conservative female peers than much more liberal female peers. However, the ratings of *much more conservative* female peers and the difference between the *much more conservative* and *much more liberal* ratings were larger for the American students than for the Swedish students. These findings support the expectation that a male-permissive double standard of sexual behavior is more prevalent in the United States. Nevertheless, about three fourths of American students and more than 90% of Swedish students gave similar evaluations of the sexual attitudes of male and female peers. Thus, only a minority of respondents in both countries (less than 10% in Sweden and about

25% in the United States) indicated perception of a male-permissive double standard of sexual attitudes.

References

Reiss, I. R. (1980). Sexual customs and gender roles in Sweden and America: An analysis and interpretation. In H. Lopata (Ed.), *Research on the interweave of social roles: Women and men* (pp. 191-220). Greenwich, CT: JAI.

Weinberg, M. S., Lottes, I. L., & Shaver, F. M. (1995). Swedish or American heterosexual college youth: Who is more permissive? *Archives of Sexual Behavior, 24,* 409-437.

Exhibit

Indicators of a Double Standard and Generational Difference in Sexual Attitudes

Directions: Circle the number that corresponds to your answer. Do you think the sexual attitudes of the following people are more liberal or conservative than your own?

Theirs are:	Much more liberal	Slightly more liberal	The same	Slightly more conservative	Much more conservative
1. Mother	1	2	3	4	5
2. Father	1	2	3	4	5
3. Close female friends	1	2	3	4	5
4. Close male friends	1	2	3	4	5
5. Female students your own age	1	2	3	4	5
6. Male students your own age	1	2	3	4	5

Sexual Double Standard Scale

Charlene L. Muehlenhard,[1] *University of Kansas*
Debra M. Quackenbush, *University of Utah*

We developed the Sexual Double Standard Scale (SDS; Muehlenhard & Quackenbush, 1996) to measure the extent to which respondents adhere to the traditional sexual double standard. This double standard allows men more sexual freedom than women regarding premarital sex, multiple partners, and sex at a young age or in a new or uncommitted relationship (DiIorio, 1989; Komarovsky, 1976; Reiss, 1960; Sprecher, McKinney, & Orbuch, 1987).

[1]Address correspondence to Charlene L. Muehlenhard, Department of Psychology, University of Kansas, 426 Fraser Hall, Lawrence, KS 66045-2160; email: charlene@lark.cc.ukans.edu.

Description

The SDS consists of 26 items, each rated on a 4-point scale ranging from *disagree strongly* (0) to *agree strongly* (3). There are six individual items that compare attitudes toward women's and men's sexual behavior within the same item (e.g., "A man should be more sexually experienced than his wife," keyed positively, or "A woman's having casual sex is just as acceptable to me as a man's having casual sex," keyed negatively). There are 20 items that occur in pairs, with parallel items about women's and men's sexual behavior (e.g., "A girl who has sex on the first date is 'easy.'" and "A guy who has sex on the first date is 'easy.' ").

Response Mode and Timing

Researchers can select a response mode to meet their needs. For example, respondents can write their responses on the questionnaire, or they can use machine-readable answer sheets. Completing the scale requires about 5 minutes.

Scoring

For the individual items, responses to negatively keyed items are reversed. For the items that occur in pairs, responses to items critical of sexually active men are subtracted from responses to items critical of sexually active women, and responses to items affirmative toward sexually active women are subtracted from responses to items affirmative toward sexually active men; difference scores reflect discrepancies in the amount of sexual freedom respondents regard as appropriate for women and men. Total scores are then calculated by summing the responses to the six individual items and the difference scores from the 10 pairs of items (see exhibit). Scores can range from 48 (indicating acceptance of the traditional sexual double standard allowing men more sexual freedom than women) to 0 (indicating identical standards for women and men, whether restrictive or permissive) to –30 (indicating acceptance of greater sexual freedom for women than for men). For one sample of university students, women's mean score was 11.99 ($n = 461$); men's mean score was 13.15 ($n = 255$).

Reliability

In a sample of university students (Muehlenhard & Quackenbush, 1996), coefficient alpha was .733 for women's reports of their own acceptance of the double standard ($n = 463$), .817 for women's predictions about how their male partners would have responded ($n = 461$), .764 for men's reports of their own acceptance of the double standard ($n = 255$), and .620 for men's predictions about how their female partners would have responded ($n = 255$). (These alphas were calculated using 16 values for each respondent: their responses to the 6 individual items after the responses to the negatively keyed items were reversed and the 10 difference scores from paired items; they were not calculated using the 26 original responses.)

Validity

We initially developed the SDS to investigate the relationship between the sexual double standard and condom use (Muehlenhard & Quackenbush, 1996). We hypothesized that "if a woman believes that her partner accepts the sexual double standard, she might be reluctant to provide or suggest using a condom, lest she appear too eager or experienced" (p. 2). Men, we predicted, would not be faced with a similar dilemma. We asked respondents about condom use during their first sexual encounter with their most recent sexual partner. We also asked them to complete the SDS twice, first as they—and then as their partner—would have completed it at the time. As expected, women who had engaged in intercourse without suggesting, providing, or using a condom believed that their partners were more accepting of the sexual double standard (i.e., they predicted that their partners would have had higher SDS scores) than did women who had provided or suggested using condoms. Also as expected, this relationship did not hold for men's condom use or their predictions about their partners' SDS scores.

Muehlenhard and McCoy (1991) used the SDS to investigate the relationship between the sexual double standard and what has been called "token resistance" (TR) to sex—indicating unwillingness to engage in sex when one is, in fact, willing. Muehlenhard and McCoy predicted that women interested in sexual intercourse would be most likely to engage in TR when they believed that their partner accepted the sexual double standard: "A woman who wants to have sexual intercourse with a man but believes that he accepts the double standard faces a double bind: She can either openly acknowledge her desire for sex and face negative sanctions (e.g., being labeled 'easy'), or else she can refuse and be labeled 'respectable' " (p. 449). In contrast, women would be most likely to openly acknowledge (OA) their interest in sexual intercourse when they believed that their partner had more egalitarian attitudes toward sex. In a study of 403 university women, Muehlenhard and McCoy asked women who had ever been in TR and/or OA situations to complete the SDS twice for each situation, first as they—and then as their partner—would have completed it at the time. As expected, women rated their partners as more accepting of the sexual double standard (i.e., as having higher SDS scores) in TR situations than in OA situations. Women's own SDS scores did not differ significantly between the two situations.

Muehlenhard and McCoy (1991) also found that the SDS correlated significantly (—.36, $p < .001$) with the Attitudes Toward Women Scale-Short Form (AWS; Spence, Helmreich, & Stapp, 1973). The AWS measures acceptance of traditional gender roles, with higher scores reflecting more nontraditional gender role attitudes. Thus, greater acceptance of the sexual double standard, as measured by the SDS, was associated with greater acceptance of traditional gender roles, as measured by the AWS.

In the studies discussed above, the scale's title was not printed on the questionnaire. Because many people claim to reject the sexual double standard (even those who endorse it when asked specific questions; Komarovsky, 1976), it seems likely that using the title on the questionnaire would bias respondents' answers and thus lower the scale's validity.

References

DiIorio, J. A. (1989). Being and becoming coupled: The emergence of female subordination in heterosexual relationships. In B. J. Risman & P. Schwartz (Eds.), *Gender in intimate relationships: A microstructural approach* (pp. 94-107). Belmont, CA: Wadsworth.

Komarovsky, M. (1976). *Dilemmas of masculinity: A study of college youth.* New York: Norton.

Muehlenhard, C. L., & McCoy, M. L. (1991). Double standard/double bind: The sexual double standard and women's communication about sex. *Psychology of Women Quarterly, 15,* 447-461.

Muehlenhard, C. L., & Quackenbush, D. M. (1996). *The social meaning of women's condom use: The sexual double standard and*

women's beliefs about the meaning ascribed to condom use. Unpublished manuscript.

Reiss, I. L. (1960). *Premarital sexual standards in America.* New York:
Free Press.

Spence, J. T., Helmreich, R., & Stapp, J. (1973). A short version of
the Attitudes Toward Women Scale (AWS). *Bulletin of the Psychonomic Society, 2,* 219-220.

Sprecher, S., McKinney, K., & Orbuch, T. L. (1987). Has the double
standard disappeared? An experimental test. *Social Psychology
Quarterly, 50,* 24-31.

Exhibit

Sexual Double Standard Scale[a]

0) Disagree strongly,   1) Disagree mildly,   2) Agree mildly,   3) Agree strongly

1. It's worse for a woman to sleep around that it is for a man.
2. It's best for a guy to lose his virginity before he's out of his teens.
3. It's okay for a woman to have more than one sexual relationship at the same time.
4. It is just as important for a man to be a virgin when he marries as it is for a woman.
5. I approve of a 16-year-old girl's having sex just as much as a 16-year-old boy's having sex.
6. I kind of admire a girl who has had sex with a lot of guys.
7. I kind of feel sorry for a 21-year-old woman who is still a virgin.
8. A woman's having casual sex is just as acceptable to me as a man's having casual sex.
9. It's okay for a man to have sex with a woman with whom he is not in love.
10. I kind of admire a guy who has had sex with a lot of girls.
11. A woman who initiates sex is too aggressive.
12. It's okay for a man to have more than one sexual relationship at the same time.
13. I question the character of a woman who has had a lot of sexual partners.
14. I admire a man who is a virgin when he gets married.
15. A man should be more sexually experienced than his wife.
16. A girl who has sex on the first date is "easy."
17. I kind of feel sorry for a 21-year-old man who is still a virgin.
18. I question the character of a guy who has had a lot of sexual partners.
19. Women are naturally more monogamous (inclined to stick with one partner) than are men.
20. A man should be sexually experienced when he gets married.
21. A guy who has sex on the first date is "easy."
22. It's okay for a woman to have sex with a man she is not in love with.
23. A woman should be sexually experienced when she gets married.
24. It's best for a girl to lose her virginity before she's out of her teens.
25. I admire a woman who is a virgin when she gets married.
26. A man who initiates sex is too aggressive.

Source. This scale is used with permission of the author.

Note. Scoring: Total = #1 + #15 + #19 + (3 − #4) + (3 − #5) + (3 − #8) + (#2 − #24) + (#12 − #3) + (#10 − #6) + (#17 − #7) + (#9 − #22) + (#11 − #26) + (#13 − #18) + (#25 − #14) + (#16 − #21) + (#20 − #23).

a. Do not use the title of the scale on the form completed by the respondents; this might bias their responses.

Attitudes Related to Sexual Concerns Scale

Patricia Barthalow Koch,[1] *Pennsylvania State University*

The Attitudes Related to Sexual Concerns Scale (ASCS) was developed to measure those attitudes that have been conceptually, empirically, or clinically associated with specific sexual concerns/dysfunctions of men and women. Although a number of scales have previously been developed to measure overall sexual attitudes or some particular attitudes, none targeted those attitudes that were specifically associated with sexual concerns/dysfunctions. The ASCS can be used as a research tool in examining the attitudes of various subsamples of differing gender, sexual orientation, age, relationship status, ethnicity, and so forth (Cowden & Koch, 1995). It could also serve as a clinical tool for counselors and therapists in assessing the attitudes related to the sexual concerns/dysfunctions their clients are experiencing.

Description

The ASCS consists of 30 items with responses on a 5-point Likert-type format ranging from 1 (*strongly agree*) to 5 (*strongly disagree*). Each statement is written in a personalized manner to measure the most proximal attitude, rather than a generalized one, because proximal attitudes are more closely related to one's own personal behavior (Ajzen & Fishbein, 1980). Through pilot testing with approximately 400 college students, principal components factor analysis with promax rotation extracted eight factors that were identified as attitudes toward (a) sexual self-understanding (14% explained variance), (b) body image (8%), (c) gender roles (4%), (d) commitment (6%), (e) communication with a sexual partner (10%), (f) masturbation (42%), (g) sexual guilt (11%), and (h) sexual performance (5%) (Koch; 1983, Koch & Cowden, 1990).

Response Mode and Timing

The respondent is instructed to indicate the choice (*strongly agree* = 1, *agree* = 2, *uncertain* = 3, *disagree* = 4, *strongly disagree* = 5) that best represents his or her attitudes toward each statement. The statements represent attitudes that might be expressed in a variety of situations. The respondents are instructed that if they have never personally been in such a situation, they are to imagine themselves in it and think of how they might react. The term *partner* refers to whomever the respondent might share his or her sexuality. The scale takes approximately 15 minutes to complete.

Scoring

Scores on the ASCS range from 30, indicating the least negative attitudes, to 150, indicating the most negative

attitudes. Thus, the higher a person's score, the more she or he exhibits attitudes associated with experiencing high levels of various relationship and sexual functioning concerns. The subscales consist of the following items (those with an asterisk must be reversed scored): Body Image (1, 9, *17); Self-Understanding (*2, 10, *18, 25), Gender Roles (*3, *11, 19), Communication (*4, 12, *20, *26), Guilt (*5, *13, 21, 27), Commitment (6, *14, *22, *28), Masturbation (7, 15, *23), and Sexual Performance (*8, *16, *24, *29/*30—29 is for females only; 30 is for males only). In administering the scale to homosexually oriented respondents, the Gender Roles subscale is deleted because some items refer to other-gender pairings.

Reliability

Internal reliability during pilot testing with male and female college students, using Cronbach's alpha coefficient, has been established at .70 for the entire scale (Koch & Cowden, 1990). Subscale reliability coefficients are as follows: Body Image, .74; Self-Understanding, .84; Gender Roles, .64; Communication, .73; Guilt, .75; Commitment, .80, Masturbation, .91; and Sexual Performance, .66.

Validity

Content validity was ensured by performing a content analysis of over 40 major sexuality education, counseling, and therapy textbooks and over 250 scientific articles written about sexual concerns/dysfunctions. Repeated pilot testing was used to determine the most reliable and valid subscales and items. Construct validity was established through factor analysis (described above). Concurrent validity for the ASCS was determined through its significant positive correlations with other established questionnaires measuring various sexual attitudes, including the Mosher Sex Guilt Inventory (Mosher, 1966), the Derogatis Sexual Attitudes Scale (Derogatis & Melisaratos, 1979), and the Sex Anxiety Inventory (Janda & O'Grady, 1980). The ASCS has also been shown to discriminate persons experiencing high levels of relationship concerns from those with low levels of such concerns, $t(402.87) = 6.58$, $p < .001$, and persons experiencing high levels of sexual functioning concerns/dysfunctions from those with little concern with their sexual functioning, $t(400.98) = 3.50$, $p < .001$ (Koch, 1988; Koch & Cowden, 1990).

References

Ajzen, I., & Fishbein, M. (1980). *Understanding attitudes and predicting social behaviors.* Englewood Cliffs, NJ: Prentice Hall.

Cowden, C. R., & Koch, P. B. (1995). Attitudes related to sexual concerns: Gender and orientation comparisons. *Journal of Sex Education and Therapy, 21*(2), 78-87.

[1]Address correspondence to Patricia Barthalow Koch, Department of Biobehavioral Health, Pennsylvania State University, University Park, PA 16802; email: p3k@psu.edu.

Derogatis, L. R., & Melisaratos, N. (1979). The DSFI: A multidimensional measure of sexual functioning. *Journal of Sex & Marital Therapy, 5,* 244-281.

Janda, L. H., & O'Grady, K. E. (1980). Development of a Sex Anxiety Inventory. *Journal of Consulting and Clinical Psychology, 48,* 169-175.

Koch, P. B. (1983). The relationship between sex-related attitudes and beliefs and sexual concerns of college students. *Dissertation Abstracts International, 44.* (University Microfilms No. DA83-20895)

Koch, P. B. (1988). The relationship of first intercourse to later sexual functioning concerns of adolescents. *Journal of Adolescent Research, 3,* 345-362.

Koch, P. B., & Cowden, C. R. (1990). *Development of a measurement of attitudes related to sexual concerns.* Unpublished manuscript.

Mosher, D. L. (1966). The development and multitrait-multimethod matrix analysis of three measures of three aspects of guilt. *Journal of Consulting Psychology, 30,* 25-29.

Exhibit

Attitude Related to Sexual Concerns Scale

Respond to the following statements by circling the choice which best represents your attitudes. These statements represent feelings that might be experienced in a variety of situations. If you have not been in such a situation, imagine yourself in it and think of how you might feel. The term "partner" refers to whomever you might choose to share your sexuality with.

1 = Strongly agree	4 = Disagree
2 = Agree	5 = Strongly disagree
3 = Uncertain	

1. Overall, I feel that my body is sexually attractive.[a]
2. It is difficult for me to explain my sexual thoughts, attitudes, and feelings to someone else because I really don't understand them myself.
3. When a male and female are having a sexual relationship, I feel it is the female's responsibility to set the sexual limits since the male will try to get as much as possible.
4. I would feel very uncomfortable expressing my negative feelings about our sexual relations to a partner.
5. I would feel guilty if I did *not* follow religious pronouncements about sexual behavior.
6. I would *not* be afraid of becoming involved in a committed relationship at this point in time.
7. I would *not* feel ashamed to use masturbation as a sexual release.
8. I would worry that my partner would leave me if I did not do what she or he wanted me to do in bed.
9. I feel a partner would be sexually attracted to my nude body.
10. I am *not* confused about my sexual feelings.
11. It is more acceptable to me for a male to have a one-night stand than for a female to have a one-night stand.
12. It would *not* be difficult for me to make suggestions to a partner on ways to improve his or her sexual techniques.
13. I would feel guilty if I did *not* follow my family's teachings about sexual behavior.
14. I would feel trapped if I was in a committed relationship at this time.
15. I would feel good about exploring and learning about my own body through masturbation.
16. If my partner did not reach orgasm, I would feel like a failure.
17. Because of the way my body looks, I would feel uncomfortable in the nude with a sexual partner.
18. It bothers me that I really do not understand why I behave sexually as I do.
19. I do *not* believe that males usually use love to get sex and females usually use sex to get love.
20. I would feel hurt if a sexual partner told me that something I do during lovemaking turns her or him off.
21. I would *not* feel guilty if I had genital sexual relations (such as intercourse) with a partner.
22. I am afraid to trust anyone in a sexual relationship at this time in my life.
23. I would feel guilty about masturbating.
24. I would worry that if I did not perform well sexually, my partner would look for someone else.
25. It is *not* difficult for me to sort out my sexual feelings, values, and behaviors.
26. There probably would be some aspects of our sexual relationship that I just could *not* talk about with my partner.
27. I would *not* feel guilty fantasizing about sexual experiences.
28. I would feel like a failure if I found out that my sexual partner also engaged in solitary masturbation.

    Females Only
29. I would feel inadequate if I could not reach orgasm during vaginal penetration (such as vaginal intercourse) and needed other kinds of stimulation in order to reach an orgasm.

    Males Only
30. I would feel humiliated if I was unable to get an erection during a sexual encounter.

a. A scale from 1 to 5 follows each item.

Sexual Dysfunction Scale

Marita P. McCabe,[1] *Deakin University*

The Sexual Dysfunction Scale (SDS) is designed to evaluate the factors associated with each of the sexual dysfunctions among males and females. Respondents are asked a general question about which sexual dysfunctions they are experiencing, and then they complete a set of more specific questions on their particular sexual dysfunction(s).

Description

The SDS consists of the following eight sections (see Table 1 for additional detail): (a) nature of the problem, (b) premature ejaculation, (c) erectile problems, (d) retarded ejaculation, (e) orgasmic dysfunction, (f) female unresponsiveness, (g) vaginismus, and (h) lack of sexual interest.

Table 1 Areas Included in the Sexual Dysfunction Scale and the Reliability of These Scales

	No. of respondents in reliability study	Coefficient alpha
1. Nature of the sexual problem (30 items)	120	.63
2. Premature ejaculation (33 items)	26	.71
3. Erectile problems (33 items)	38	.72
4. Retarded ejaculation (31 items)	11	.69
5. Orgasmic dysfunction (48 items)	26	.63
6. Female unresponsiveness (51 items)	18	.73
7. Vaginismus (31 items)	14	.72
8. Lack of sexual interest (91 items)	24	.61

For each dysfunction, respondents answer questions about medical and lifestyle factors, quality of the respondent's relationship (if the person is in a relationship), length of time the dysfunction has been in place, the frequency and severity of the dysfunction, attitudes to sexual activities and responses to these activities, response to the dysfunction, and impact of the dysfunction on the respondent's relationship (if relevant).

The SDS has been in the process of development for the past 10 years. The items were initially drawn from the factors that were claimed in the literature to be associated

with each particular sexual dysfunction. This resulted in the construction of a guided-interview measure that elicited responses to open-ended questions. Respondents were also asked about whether the questions were relevant to their particular sexual dysfunction. This instrument was tested on 55 people with sexual dysfunction (with at least 6 respondents within any particular dysfunctional category). The measure was then converted into a forced-choice format and administered to a sexually dysfunctional population (both clinical and nonclinical respondents) (McCabe, 1994a, 1994b). The scale was further modified as a result of these studies and administered to an additional 120 clinically dysfunctional respondents.

Response Mode and Timing

The scale is completed as a questionnaire measure and, depending on the number of sexual dysfunctions experienced by the respondent, takes from 10 minutes to 50 minutes to complete. All items are objectively scored and consist of either yes/no responses or 5-point Likert-scale responses.

Scoring

Responses on items may be summed to provide an index of severity (nature of problem × length of time problem has been in place × frequency of problem). There are also separate questions on the medical, lifestyle, and relationship factors surrounding the problem and questions on the impact of the problem on the relationship.

Reliability and Validity

Coefficient alpha for each of the subscales was calculated for 120 respondents who presented to the Sexual Behaviour Clinic for treatment of their sexual problem and is shown in Table 1. The number of respondents with each dysfunction is also listed in the table. Because some respondents experienced more than one sexual dysfunction, the number of dysfunctions is greater than 120. Respondents with a partner ($n = 89$) were asked to report on the nature of their partner's problem. The concordance rate between their report and their partner's report was 82%, thus demonstrating the validity of the scale. Further validity is ensured by the process of the scale construction.

Other Information

The scale, along with the scoring code, can be purchased from the author for a cost of U.S.$10.

[1]Address correspondence to Marita P. McCabe, School of Psychology, Deakin University, 221 Burwood Highway, Burwood, Victoria 3125, Australia; email: maritam@deakin.edu.au.

References

McCabe, M. P. (1994a). Childhood, adolescent and current psychological factors associated with sexual dysfunction. *Sexual and Marital Therapy, 9,* 267-276.

McCabe, M. P. (1994b). The influence of the quality of relationship on sexual dysfunction. *Australian Journal of Marriage and the Family, 15,* 2-8.

The GRISS: A Psychometric Scale and Profile of Sexual Dysfunction

John Rust,[1] *Goldsmiths College*
Susan Golombok, *City University, London*

The Golombok Rust Inventory of Sexual Satisfaction (GRISS) is a short measure of sexual dysfunction that may be administered to heterosexual couples or individuals who have a current heterosexual relationship. It provides overall scores, for men and women separately, of the quality of sexual functioning within a relationship. In addition, subscale scores of impotence, premature ejaculation, anorgasmia, vaginismus, infrequency, noncommunication, male dissatisfaction, female dissatisfaction, male nonsensuality, female nonsensuality, male avoidance, and female avoidance can be obtained and represented as a profile. The GRISS can be used to assess improvement as a result of sexual or marital therapy and for comparing the efficacy of different treatment methods. It can also be used to investigate the relationship between sexual dysfunction and extraneous variables. The subscales are particularly helpful in providing a profile for diagnosis of the pattern of sexual functioning within the couple, which can be of great benefit in designing a treatment program. The GRISS has a companion scale, the Golombok Rust Inventory of Marital State (GRIMS), which provides a single scale of marital discord.

Description

The GRISS, in separate forms for men and women, appears on a single sheet and has standard format, thus making it easy for the respondent to complete. The male version is blue and the female version is green. There are 28 items in each, and the items are all Likert type (5-point) with response options labeled *never, hardly ever, occasionally, usually,* and *always.* GRISS forms are carbon backed with an adhered scoring sheet to be detached by the user and contains a scoring and standardization format and a profile blank.

The test specification for the GRISS draws on the accumulated expertise and understanding of practicing sex therapists and, therefore, tends toward a functional rather than a theoretical base. Clinical experience enables the sex therapist to identify the areas in a couple's sexual relationship that could be improved. This test specification was designed by a "think tank" of sex therapists at the Sexual Dysfunction Clinic of the Maudsley Hospital, London. It specified seven major areas of interest: frequency, satisfaction, interest, dysfunction, anxiety, communication, and touching. An initial 96-item version was piloted on 51 client couples at the Maudsley Sexual Dysfunction Clinic and 36 nonclinical couples. After item analysis to eliminate items with extreme scores or with a large amount of response refusal, promax oblique factor analysis was used to identify subscales. The identified subscale items were then factor analyzed separately for each subscale, using orthogonal rotations. The final subscales had four items each, selected using the following criteria: (a) stability of the factor structure, with a common factor accounting for more than 50% of the variance; (b) an equal number of items (four), two with positive and two with negative loadings; (c) content continuity along the full length of the indicated dimension; (d) factorial consistency between the clinical and student samples; and (e) face validity. Four of the subscales generated in this manner concerned the specific problems of anorgasmia, vaginismus, impotence, and premature ejacu-

[1] Address correspondence to John Rust, Department of Psychology, Goldsmiths College, Lewisham Way, New Cross, London SE16 6NW, England.

lation. All of these diagnostic categories proved to be continuous with minor degrees of disturbance in the normal population. Six other subscales gave separate male and female scores for avoidance, dissatisfaction, and nonsensuality. The remaining two subscales measured infrequency and noncommunication about sex within the couple.

Orthogonal factor analysis of the scored subscales, together with the remaining items from the pilot inventory, yielded an orthogonal two-factor solution. On the basis of this, single overall scales for men and women separately were constructed. Some of the items retained in the questionnaire, generally those dealing with level of interest in sex, contribute toward these two main scales but are not included in the subscales.

The GRISS was standardized on a sample of 88 sex therapy clients from clinics throughout the United Kingdom. The factor structure was stable across both the pilot and standardization samples. A combination of norm referencing and criterion referencing yielded transformed scales giving a good indication of the existence and severity of any problems. Transformations are to a pseudo-stanine scale (from 1 to 9) with a score of 5 being borderline and a score of above 5 indicating a problem. Distributions of these transformed scales are approximately normal for the clinical sample, but skewed toward the lower end of the scale to facilitate measurement in nonclinical populations.

Response Mode and Timing

Respondents circle the number indicating the frequency with which each statement applies. The GRISS normally takes between 4 and 10 minutes to complete.

Scoring

The GRISS is provided by the publishers in self-scoring carbon-backed form with a detachable confidential sheet for scoring and drawing the profile. For the two main scales and the 12 subscales, there are equal numbers of positive and negative items. When these have been reversed, as appropriate, and scored, each scale and subscale must be standardized. This rather complex operation is made simple by the structured procedure of the scoring sheet and should take about 3 minutes per GRISS. For larger studies, the procedure can be computerized, using the scoring instructions in the handbook (Rust & Golombok, 1986a).

Reliability

For the main scales, the split-half reliabilities were found to be extremely high, .94 and .87 for the female and the male scales, respectively. For the subscales, split-half reliabilities average .74; they range between .61 for noncommunication and .83 for anorgasmia. Test-retest reliabilities were calculated for the pre- and posttherapy data on 41 clinical couples, 20 of whom had marital therapy (Bennun, Rust, & Golombok, 1985), and 21 sex therapy. Both these groups showed significant improvement with therapy, so that the figures obtained are underestimates. The values obtained were .76 for the male scale and .65 for the female scale. Subscale test-retest reliabilities ranged from .47 for

female dissatisfaction to .84 for premature ejaculation (M = .65).

Validity

For 68 men and 63 women from sexual dysfunction clinics, of whom 62 were couples, therapists completed validation questionnaires in which they were asked to define the severity and nature of any sexual problems for men and women separately. Those respondents (n = 42 for women, n = 57 for men) who had been diagnosed as having a problem were compared with a control group of 59 respondents (29 men and 30 women) taken from a random sample of people attending their family doctor for the usual variety of medical and social problems (Golombok, Rust, & Pickard, 1984). Both the overall female scale (point biserial r = .63, p < .001) and the overall male scale (point biserial r = .37, p < .005) were found to discriminate between the clinical and nonclinical groups. The specific dysfunctional groups as diagnosed by the therapists (impotence, premature ejaculation, vaginismus, and anorgasmia) were also compared with the control group. All clinical groups differed from the control group on their target subscale.

A further measure of validity was obtained by correlating the therapists' ratings of severity of problems (0 = *no problem*, 1 = *slight problem*, 2 = *moderate problem*, and 3 = *severe problem*) with the overall male and female scales. These correlations were r = .56 (n = 63, p < .001) for women and r = .53 (n = 63, p < .001) for men, good for an instrument of this type.

Follow-up validation of the main scales against therapists' estimates of improvement during the therapy was conducted on 30 clinical couples after their fifth sex therapy session. The therapists, blind to the GRISS results, rated both the man and the woman separately on a 5-point scale, where 0 = *improved a great deal*, 1 = *improved moderately*, 2 = *slightly improved*, 3 = *not improved at all*, and 4 = *got worse*. For the men, the correlation between the therapists' ratings of improvement and the change in the main male score was .54 (p < .005). For the women, the equivalent correlation was .43 (p < .01). Both male and female scales are, therefore, clearly valid as measures of outcome of therapy.

Other Information

The copyright of the GRISS is held by the publisher, NFER-Nelson (Darville House, 2 Oxford Road East, Windsor, Berkshire SL4 1DF, England) from whom it may be purchased. There is a separate handbook, which includes full details of construction and use. The authors would welcome any information from users of the GRISS, particular details or publications.

References

Bennun, I. (1985). Behavioural marital therapy: An outcome evaluation of conjoint group and one spouse treatment. *Scandinavian Journal of Behavior Therapy, 14,* 157-168.

Bennun, I., Rust, J., & Golombok, S. (1985). The effects of marital therapy on sexual satisfaction. *Scandinavian Journal of Behaviour Therapy, 14,* 65-72.

Golombok, S., Rust, J., & Pickard, C. (1984). Sexual problems encountered in general practice. *British Journal of Sexual Medicine, 11,* 65-72.

Rust, J., Bennun, I., Crowe, M., & Golombok, S. (1986). The Golombok Rust Inventory of Marital State. *Sexual and Marital Therapy, 1,* 55-60.

Rust, J., & Golombok, S. (1985). The Golombok Rust Inventory of Sexual Satisfaction (GRISS). *British Journal of Clinical Psychology, 24,* 63-64.

Rust, J., & Golombok, S. (1986a). *The Golombok Rust Inventory of Sexual Satisfaction.* Windsor, UK: NFER-Nelson.

Rust, J., & Golombok, S. (1986b). The GRISS: A psychometric instrument for the assessment of sexual dysfunction. *Archives of Sexual Behavior, 15,* 153-165.

Exhibit

Golombok Rust Inventory of Sexual Satisfaction (GRISS)

Copyright forbids the reproduction of the GRISS in full. However, sample items are "Do you have sexual intercourse as often as you would like?" "Do you feel uninterested in sex?" "Are there weeks in which you don't have sex at all?" "Do you become tense and anxious when your partner wants to have sex?" "Do you lose your erection during intercourse?" "Do you fail to reach orgasm during intercourse?" "Does your vagina become moist during lovemaking?" "Do you ejaculate by accident just before your penis is about to enter your partner's vagina?" Instructions on the GRISS run as follows:

Each question is followed by a series of possible answers: N = *never,* H = *hardly ever,* O = *occasionally,* U = *usually,* A = *always.* Read each question carefully and decide which answer best describes the way things have been for you recently, then circle the corresponding letter. Please answer every question. If you are not completely sure which answer is most accurate, circle the answer which you feel is most appropriate. Do not spend too long on each question. Please answer the questionnaire without discussing any of the questions with your partner. In order for us to obtain valid information it is important for you to answer each question as honestly and as accurately as possible. All the information will be treated in the strictest confidence.

Segraves Sexual Symptomatology Interview

Kathleen A. Segraves,[1] *MetroHealth Medical Center*

The Segraves Sexual Symptomatology Interview (SSSI; Segraves, Segraves, & Schoenberg, 1987) is a brief structured interview to help differentiate psychogenic from organogenic erectile dysfunction. The self-report questions concern the presence of adequate early morning erections, adequate masturbatory erections, and adequate noncoital erections.

In the original study (Segraves et al., 1987), we used questions derived from prior sexual symptomatology research (Abel, Becker, Cunningham-Rathner, Mittelman, & Primack, 1982; Kockott, Feil, Revenstorf, Aldenhoff, & Besinger, 1980) and combined these with the University of Chicago interview to identify the most predictive subset of questions. Three out of the initial 18 sexual history questions differentiated reliably between organic and psychogenic erectile problems. The single best predictor was the question regarding morning erections. The presence or absence of early morning erections correctly assigned 100%

[1] Address correspondence to Kathleen A. Segraves, Department of Psychiatry, MetroHealth Medical Center, 2500 Metro-Health Drive, Cleveland, OH 44109; email: kathy123@aol.com.

of the men with biogenic erectile problems and 86% of the men with psychogenic difficulties.

Simply stated, the ability to experience an erection under any circumstance supports the assumption of a psychogenic etiology to the erectile complaint. Under this assumption, a full medical exam might best be postponed until an adequate trial of cognitive behavioral treatment is given in an effort to ameliorate the problem.

Description

The SSSI is a brief structured interview containing five forced-choice questions. An affirmative answer to any of the first four questions suggests a psychogenic component to the erectile disorder. Although the last question is not predictive of psychogenic erectile disorder, it is included to serve as a prompt for the investigator to evaluate the patient for male sexual desire disorder if the patient responds with a *no* to Question 5.

Response Mode and Timing

All five questions require a positive or negative response. The interview requires approximately 3 to 7 minutes to complete. The interviewer's task is to help the patient understand the questions and elicit the most truthful responses.

Scoring

Except for the last question, any positive response is associated with a psychogenic component to the erectile dysfunction. The most predictive question is Question 1.

Reliability

Thirty-two patients entered the original study. Self-report reliability was checked by comparing responses given during the investigational interview with information in the medical chart gathered earlier during a psychiatric interview with an independent interviewer. The patient's self-report and medical record agreed except for one patient, producing a phi coefficient of .92 for morning erections. (The one exception was a patient reporting episodic firm morning erections, not quite meeting the criteria of firm erections twice weekly.) Agreement was 100% for alternative partners; reliability concerning masturbatory erections resulted in a phi of .61 showing discrepancies in four patients.

The sleep technician's rating of penile turgidity was checked in two ways. A correlation between the rating and nocturnal penile tumescence (NPT) circumference was computed, resulting in a correlation of .9. Second, both centimeter change and technician ratings were compared for their correlation with an independent dimension, the patient's self-report of turgidity of early morning erections. Both the centimeter change and the technician's ratings were highly correlated: cm change, $r = .56$, $p < .01$; rating, $r = .65$, $p < .01$.

Validity

All patients were independently classified based on NPT recording, a sleep lab technician's rating of penile turgidity of erections, and Doppler determination of penile blood flow, serum prolactin, and testosterone levels. Using stringent criteria, patients were assigned to either a psychogenic or organic group. All patients with psychogenic impotence had nocturnal erections rated by the technician as 100% fully capable of vaginal penetration. The average circumference change was 2.4 cm ($SD = 0.4$), and the range was from 2 to 3 cm.

Every question from the SSSI was evaluated by computing its specificity, sensitivity, and efficiency. The questions with the best efficiencies and acceptable sensitivities were Questions 1, 2, and 4. The sexual history question permitting maximal discrimination between the groups is the question concerning adequacy of morning erections. Use of this question alone correctly assigned all of the men with organic impotence (100%) and 86% of the men with psychogenic impotence. The inclusion of the other questions did not increase the discriminatory power. One reason why the addition of other questions did not increase the discriminatory power of the sexual interview is that none of the men with psychogenic impotence who denied early morning erections reported erections under any condition.

A partial replication study is being conducted in Canada by Blanchette and colleagues. The research team has collected data on 375 patients for the complete analysis. The research team plans on collecting data on 500 patients. Preliminary results of the first 250 patients using the SSSI were reported by Blanchette, Alarie, and Dominique (1989). This group divided the sample into three groups: organogenic erectile dysfunction, psychogenic erectile dysfunction, and both psychogenic and organogenic erectile dysfunction, thus adding a third group. Although this group did not find a single question that could correctly assign 100% of the patients in any one of the three groups, Blanchette et al. reported the most discriminating variables concerned the presence of self-reported full early morning erection and full nocturnal erections. These results support the premise that an affirmative response to the question of morning erections suggests a psychogenic component to the erectile etiology.

References

Abel, G. G., Becker, J. U., Cunningham-Rathner, J., Mittelman, M., & Primack, M. (1982). Differential diagnosis of impotence in diabetics. *Neurological Urodynamics, 1*, 57-69.

Blanchette, F., Alarie, P., & Dominique, A. (1989, Winter). Differential diagnosis of erectile dysfunction using sexual symptomatology: Preliminary results of 250 patients studied. *SIECCAN Journal, 4*(4), 35-46.

Kockott, G., Feil, W., Revenstorf, D., Aldenhoff, J., & Besinger, U. (1980). Symptomatology and psychological aspects of male sexual inadequacy: Results of an experimental study. *Archives of Sexual Behavior, 9*, 457-475.

Segraves, K. A., Segraves, R. T., & Schoenberg, R. T. (1987). Use of sexual history to differentiate organic from psychogenic impotence. *Archives of Sexual Behavior, 16*, 125-137.

Exhibit

Segraves Sexual Symptomatology Interview

Instructions: I will be asking you questions to document your penile capacity and specific sexual history questions. You will need to answer with either a yes or no. If you do not understand the question or how to respond, I will try to reword the question to help you determine your specific answer.

1. During the last month, did you experience erections upon wakening greater than or equal to 2/wk? yes/no
1b. If you experienced 2/wk erections upon wakening was the erection sufficient for vaginal penetration? yes/no
2. During masturbation, are your erections sufficient for vaginal penetration? yes/no
3. With someone other than your regular partner, are your erections sufficient for vaginal penetration? yes/no
4. Do you have frequent and lasting erections during noncoital activity or fantasy (for example, during foreplay; during the night)? yes/no
5. Do you still have the same interest or desire for sex (in your mind) (decreased sexual desire, drive, or libido)? yes/no

Source. This questionnaire was originally published in "Use of Sexual History to Differentiate Organic From Psychogenic Impotence," by K. A. Segraves, R. T. Segraves, and R. T. Schoenberg, 1987, *Archives of Sexual Behavior, 16,* 125-137. Used with permission of Plenum Press.

Sex Education Inventory: Preferred and Actual Sources

Susan M. Bennett,[1] *California State Department of Education*
Winifred B. Dickinson, *University of Steubenville*

The Sex Education Inventory (SEI) measures preferred and actual sources of sex education, family environment for sexual learning, and recent sexual experiences.

Description

The SEI is a 1983 revision of the Student Sex Education Survey (SSES) developed by Bennett and Dickinson (1980). Fifty-seven items assess college students' preferred and actual sources of sex education, satisfaction with actual sex education, aspects of family environment for sexual learning (e.g., rapport with parents, family affection, permissiveness for expression of sexuality, and discussion of sex-related topics), and heterosexual activities in the past 2 years. Tests of general knowledge about sex, birth control, and

venereal disease developed for the SSES are not included in the SEI.

The SSES and several revised instruments preceding the SEI were developed by the authors for research use in populations of 18- to 23-year-old college students. Items measuring rapport were inspired by similar items in Sorensen's (1973) questionnaire, and the items measuring sexual experiences were suggested by Spanier's (1977) analyses of similar measures reflecting recognized subdimensions of attitude toward premarital sexual permissiveness (Reiss, 1967). The SEI includes standard precoded and open-ended questionnaire items as well as checklists, Likert-type scales, and true-false questions.

Response Mode, Scoring, and Timing

Selecting from lists of possible sources, respondents indicate preferred and actual sources for each of five aspects of sex education (Items 1-10). Responses to each item are coded as nominal data, and two scores, 0 to 5, indicate the

[1]Address correspondence to Susan M. Bennett, Administrator, Adult Education Field Assistance Unit, California Department of Education, 560 J Street, Suite 290, Sacramento, CA 95814; email: sbennett@cde.ca.gov.

total number of aspects of sex education for which a given source (e.g., parents, teachers, male friends) was preferred and the total number of aspects for which it was the actual source.

More detailed information on sex-related topics discussed with each parent and/or studied in high school or college is assessed by a checklist of 16 sex-related topics (Item 11). Separate scores are given for the total number of topics (of the 16), the total number of birth control and venereal disease topics (of 3 each) discussed with parents, and the total number of topics studied in high school and in college.

Rapport and discussion of sexuality with each parent and parents' expression of affection are measured by 5-point Likert-type items (Items 12-22 concern father; 26-36 concern mother). Scores are given for each item with response values reversed for Items 13, 15, 17, 20, 27, 29, 31, and 34. Higher scores indicate more positive rapport, more open discussion of sexuality, and more affectionate family relationships.

Two index scores for rapport with each parent have been developed. The first, General Rapport, is the sum of the responses to four items for each parent (Items 12-15 for father; 26-29 for mother) minus 3. The second index score, Sex-Related Rapport, is the sum of the General Rapport score and scores for three additional items (Items 16-18 for father; 30-32 for mother) minus 2. Scores range from 1 to 29.

A third index score, Family Affection, is computed by summing scores for Items 22, 23, 24, and 36 and subtracting 3. Scores range from 1-17.

Items 37-44 provide additional information concerning the discussion of sex-related topics with each parent. All responses, except the respondent's age (Items 39 and 42), are coded as nominal data. Items 40 and 43 are also scored to indicate the total number of factors discouraging the discussion of sexual topics with each parent (range = 0-12).

Satisfaction with mode of sex education and with current knowledge of things pertaining to sex is measured by two 7-point Likert-type items (Items 45 and 46). Respondents also indicate attitudes toward their own children's sex education compared to their sex education (Item 47). Written comments can be coded following content analysis procedures.

Parental permissiveness for expression of sexuality is measured by Item 25 concerning parental caution and instruction regarding appropriate behavior. The response options of *true*, *false*, and *can't say* are scored 3, 1, 2, respectively. An index score, Parental Caution, is derived separately for male and female respondents by summing the scores for four items (Items 48, 49, 50, and 51 for males; 48, 49, 52, and 53 for females) and subtracting 3 (range = 1-9). Higher scores indicate a greater amount of parental caution and instruction.

Heterosexual involvement in the past 2 years is measured by Items 54-57, the Sexual Experiences Inventory (SEXI; Bennett, Dickinson, Price, & Karwoski, 1980). Responses indicate the frequency of each of four types of sexual activity on a 4-point scale. Scores for individual items, as well as a Guttman-scaled score for all four items, are used in data analysis.

The average time to complete the SEI is 25 minutes.

Reliability

Test-retest reliability of individual items and index scores has been assessed in four samples of students from Pennsylvania State University and the University of Steubenville. Bennett and Dickinson (1980) reported a median coefficient of stability of .87 (r = .58-.95, N = 55, interval = 2 weeks) for ordinal scales including the five discussion scores (Item 11) and the four rapport indexes (Items 12-18 and 26-32). Coefficients for the rapport indexes are higher (r = .90-.95) for the original *true/false/can't say* SSES response format (Bennett & Dickinson, 1980) than for the 5-point Likert-type SEI response format (r = .76-.73, N = 55, interval = 4 weeks).

Median coefficients of stability for the single-item measures of rapport, discussion, affection, and permissiveness in the SEI (Items 12-18, 23, 25, and 26-32) are .73 (r = .79-.89, N = 27) and .78 (r = .60-.86, N = 55) for 1-week and 4-week intervals, respectively.

Additional coefficients of stability for specific SEI scales administered with a 4-week interval (N = 55) are .80 and .89 for Items 1-10 (aspects of sex education for which parents were the preferred or actual scores), .85 for Items 40 and 43 (factors discouraging discussion of sexuality), and .62 and .64 for the Parental Caution and Family Affection scales derived from Items 48-53 and 22-24 and 36, respectively. Coefficients for other scales administered with a 1 ½-week interval (N = 72) are .75 for Items 29 and 42 (age when a parent was last asked a question about sex) and .85-.91 for Items 54-57 (sexual activity scales). Coefficient for scales administered with a 1-week interval (N = 27) are .88 and .90 for Items 45 and 46 (satisfaction with sex education), respectively.

The Guttman-scaled score for Items 54-57 has a coefficient of reproducibility of .99 (Bennett et al., 1980).

Test-retest reliability, indicated by the median percentage of agreement for the nominal scales for Items 1-10 (preferred and actual sources of sex education) and Items 37, 38, 41, and 44 (parents' roles in sex education and discussion), is 74% (range 56%-89%, N = 27, interval = 1 week).

Validity

Construct validity of the SEI measures has been demonstrated by intercorrelations among SEI scores and by correlations between SEI scores and measures of sexual knowledge, attitudes to sex, and patterns of parental responsibility. For example, Bennett et al. (1980) reported that the number of aspects of sex education for which parents should be responsible correlates with the number of aspects for which they were responsible (r = .32-.47 for males and females), with number of sex-related topics discussed with each parent (r = .15-.40 for four student-parent combinations), with the Allgeier Sexual Knowledge Scale (Allgeier, 1978) (r = .44), and with attitudes measured by Eysenck's (1970) Inventory of Attitudes to Sex (r = .23-.31 for males; −.45-.38 for females). Indexes of rapport with parents correlate with sex-related topics discussed with parents (r = .24-.36), family affection (r = .18-.41), factors discouraging discussion with parents ($r = -.18-.41$), and the Attitudes to Sex Inventory ($r = -.41-.52$) for males and females; with the Sexual Knowledge Scale ($r = .50$) for males; and with recent sexual activity (Guttman-scaled score, $r = -.28$) for females (Bennett et al., 1980). Index and individual-item scores for rapport, discussion with parents, family affection, and permissiveness also vary significantly and meaningfully as a function of father's involvement in family work and discipline (Bennett, 1982, 1984, 1985). Recent sexual activity (Guttman-scaled score) correlates with traditionally masculine and feminine sex-role orientation ($r = .30-.34$) and the Attitudes to Sex Inventory ($r = .35-.56$) for males and females, and with sharing parents' attitudes ($r = -.28$ to $-.40$) for females (Bennett et al., 1980). Additional documentation of construct validity for SEI measures is available from the authors.

References

Allgeier, A. R. (1978, April). *The sex knowledge survey*. Paper presented at the eastern regional meeting of the Society for the Scientific Study of Sex, Atlantic City, NJ.

Bennett, S. M. (1982, May). *Family environment for sexual learning as a function of perceived paternal involvement in household care and discipline*. Paper presented at the meeting of the Midwestern Psychological Association, Minneapolis, MN. (ERIC Document Reproduction Service No. ED 225 070)

Bennett, S. M. (1984, August). *Fathers' roles in family work and discipline: Implications for their daughters' sexual development*. Paper presented at the Symposium on the Psychology of Women (Division 35), American Psychological Association, Toronto.

Bennett, S. M. (1985). Family environment for sexual learning as a function of fathers' involvement in family work and discipline. *Adolescence, 19*, 609-627.

Bennett, S. M., & Dickinson, W. B. (1980). Student-parent rapport and parent involvement in sex, birth control, and venereal disease education. *The Journal of Sex Research, 16*, 114-130.

Bennett, S. M., Dickinson, W. B., Price, E. P., & Karwoski, J. A. (1980, November). *Parental influences on sexual knowledge, activity, attitudes, and sex-role orientation of university students*. Paper presented at the meeting of the Society for the Scientific Study of Sex, Dallas, TX.

Eysenck, H. J. (1970). Personality and attitude to sex: A factorial study. *Personality, 1*, 353-376.

Reiss, I. L. (1967). *The social context of premarital sexual permissiveness*. New York: Holt, Rinehart & Winston.

Sorensen, R. C. (1973). *Adolescent sexuality in contemporary America*. New York: World Publishing.

Spanier, G. B. (1977). Sources of sex information and premarital sexual behavior. *The Journal of Sex Research, 13*, 73-88.

Exhibit

Sex Education Inventory

The statements and questions that follow ask you to indicate your attitudes and experiences regarding sex education and sexual activities. Please read each item carefully and respond as indicated on the basis of your own true beliefs. Your responses will remain anonymous.

1. Circle the *one letter* identifying the person or persons who should have primary responsibility for teaching young people about sexual matters.
    a.   No one special
    b.   Friends
    c.   Young people should find out on their own
    d.   Teachers (content of schoolwork)
    e.   Physicians and/or nurses
    f.   Parents
    g.   Professional sex educators or counselors
    h.   Ministers, priests, or other religious leaders
    i.   Other (Please specify) _____

Now complete Items 2 through 5 by using the list in Item 1. Write *one letter* to indicate who should have primary responsibility for teaching young people about each of the following:

2.   Birth control _____
3.   Recognizing and preventing venereal disease _____
4.   Moral and ethical questions related to sex _____
5.   Interpersonal relations and sexuality _____
6.   Circle the *letter* beside your *one main source* of information about sex in general.
    a.   No source
    b.   Female friends
    c.   Male friends
    d.   Father
    e.   Mother
    f.   Other family members
    g.   Physician and/or nurse
    h.   Professional sex educator or counselor (including personnel at family planning clinic)
    i.   Minister, priest, or other religious leader
    j.   Media (radio, TV)
    k.   Reading on my own
    l.   Teachers in school (content of schoolwork)
    m.   Other (Please specify) _____

Now complete Items 7 through 10 by using the list in Item 6. Write the *letter of the one main source* from which you learned most of what you know about each of the following:

7.   Birth control _____
8.   Recognizing and preventing venereal disease _____

9. Moral and ethical questions related to sex _____
10. Interpersonal relations and sexuality _____

11. Place an X next to all the following sex-related topics you have discussed with your parents at any time or studied in high school or college.

	Discussed with		Studied in	
	Father	Mother	High School	College
a. Personal hygiene	_____	_____	_____	_____
b. Menstruation	_____	_____	_____	_____
c. Pregnancy and delivery	_____	_____	_____	_____
d. Intercourse	_____	_____	_____	_____
e. Birth control	_____	_____	_____	_____
f. Specific methods of birth control	_____	_____	_____	_____
g. Venereal disease	_____	_____	_____	_____
h. Abortion	_____	_____	_____	_____
i. Orgasm	_____	_____	_____	_____
j. Masturbation	_____	_____	_____	_____
k. Homosexuality	_____	_____	_____	_____
l. What to do to prevent venereal disease (VD)	_____	_____	_____	_____
m. Where to go for help if you need birth control information	_____	_____	_____	_____
n. Where to go for help if you suspect VD	_____	_____	_____	_____
o. What to look for in a mate	_____	_____	_____	_____
p. "How far to go" on a date	_____	_____	_____	_____

Read each item and indicate how much it applies to you by circling the *one* most appropriate number.

Completely false	Mostly false	Partly true, partly false	Mostly true	Completely true
1	2	3	4	5

12. I have a lot of respect for my father.   1 2 3 4 5
*13. I have never really gotten to know my father.   1 2 3 4 5
14. My father has a lot of respect for me.   1 2 3 4 5
*15. My father doesn't understand what I want out of life.   1 2 3 4 5
16. When it comes to sex, my attitudes and my father's attitudes are pretty much the same.   1 2 3 4 5
*17. My father and I find it uncomfortable to talk about sex.   1 2 3 4 5
18. I often ask my father for advice about sexual matters.   1 2 3 4 5
19. My father probably would stand by me if I had a serious problem related to sex.   1 2 3 4 5
*20. When I talk about sex with my father, I tell him only what I think he can accept.   1 2 3 4 5
21. My father has very traditional ideas about a man's role in life.   1 2 3 4 5
22. My father hugged and kissed me a lot when I was a child.   1 2 3 4 5
23. I have often seen my parents show physical affection for each other.   1 2 3 4 5
24. As a child, I was encouraged to be affectionate with my parents and other family members.   1 2 3 4 5
25. My parents permitted me to see them nude after I was five or six years old.   1 2 3 4 5

26.-36. These items parallel Items 12-22, but refer to mother rather than father. They are excluded here to reduce the length of the exhibit.

37. Which parent have you discussed sex-related topics with most often? (Circle *one* letter.)
    a. Never discussed with either parent   d. Both parents equally often
    b. Father   e. Other (Please specify) _____
    c. Mother

38. When you discuss sex-related topics with your father, who usually starts the conversation? (Circle *one* letter.)
    a. We never discuss such things   d. Sometimes I do, sometimes he does
    b. I usually do   e. Other (Please specify) _____
    c. He usually does

39. About how old were you the last time you asked your father a question about human sexuality?
    a. Never asked   c. Other (Please specify) _____
    b. _____ years (Write number.)

40. Circle the letters next to all the factors which have discouraged you from discussing sex-related topics with your father.

a.   He was embarrassed when I asked
b.   He didn't know how to answer my questions
c.   He got angry when I asked
d.   He told me things that were not true
e.   He gave me a lecture instead of answering questions
f.   He asked me why I wanted to know

g.   He wasn't around when I had questions on my mind
h.   I seldom had a chance to talk to him without other people listening
i.   He never brought up sex-related subjects
j.   I was embarrassed to ask
k.   I was afraid of his reaction
l.   Other (Please specify) _____

41.-43. These items parallel Items 38-40, but refer to mother rather than father. They are excluded here to reduce the length of the exhibit.

44. Which parent should take a more active role in the sex education of children? (Circle *one* letter.)

a.   Both should share the responsibility equally
b.   The mother
c.   The father

d.   It depends on the sex of the children. The father should be more responsible for the boys, and the mother should be more responsible for the girls.
e.   Other (Please specify.) _____

Please indicate your reaction to the following statements by circling the *one* most appropriate number.

Very dissatisfied	Dissatisfied	Somewhat dissatisfied	Not sure	Somewhat satisfied	Satisfied	Very satisfied
1	2	3	4	5	6	7

45. How satisfied are you with the way(s) in which you found out most of what you know about things having to do with sex?   1   2   3   4   5   6   7

46. How satisfied are you with your current knowledge about things having to do with sex?   1   2   3   4   5   6   7

47. Would you handle your own children's sex education pretty much the same your was handled? (Check *one*.)

Yes _____   No _____   Can't say _____

Please explain why or why not. _____

_____

Please answer the following items by circling *T* for true, *F* for false, or ? for can't say.

48. My father or mother instructed me about situations in which boys and girls should *not* be together when I was a child or early teen.   T   F   ?

49. My father or mother warned me about "sex play" when I was a child.   T   F   ?

Male subjects only:

50. My father or mother cautioned me not to act like a "sissy" when I was a child or early teen.   T   F   ?

51. My father or mother cautioned me to be careful not to get some girl pregnant before marriage.   T   F   ?

Female subjects only:

52. My father or mother cautioned me not to act like a "tomboy" when I was a child or early teen .   T   F   ?

53. My father or mother cautioned me not to get pregnant before marriage.   T   F   ?

Sexual Activities Inventory

Indicate how much each of the following items applies to you by using the following format:

Never	Rarely	Sometimes	Frequently
1	2	3	4

54. Engaged in deep kissing (French kissing) in the past 2 years.   1   2   3   4

55. Engaged in light petting (fondling, or having breasts fondled) in the past 2 years.   1   2   3   4

56. Engaged in heavy petting (fondling partner's sex organs or being fondled) in the past 2 years.   1   2   3   4

57. Engaged in sexual intercourse in the past 2 years.   1   2   3   4

Please look back and make sure that you have not left out any items or pages of items.

_____

*These items are negative and should be reversed for scoring purposes.

Human Sexuality Education Concepts Scale

Valerie M. Chamberlain,[1] *University of Vermont*
Brenda B. Mendiola, *Mertzon High School, Mertzon, Texas*
Merrilyn N. Cummings, *New Mexico State University*

Perceptions of inservice educators regarding the importance of various human sexuality concepts can provide a critical basis for the planning, implementation, and evaluation of needs assessment programs and for general program development and evaluation. To provide a data collection instrument to meet this purpose, the Human Sexuality Education Concepts Scale (HSECS) was developed. Using this instrument, data can be collected regarding educators' feelings about the importance for inclusion of certain human sexuality concepts in secondary curricula. The HSECS can also be used to determine emphases actually being placed on human sexuality concepts in educational settings. Comparative data can be analyzed to determine similarities and differences between perceived importance and actual inclusion of human sexuality concepts in educational programs. Data generated using the HSECS can facilitate program evaluation for human sexuality education in secondary schools, community colleges, universities, teacher education programs, and community service endeavors such as human service delivery systems, youth groups, and family-oriented outreach projects.

Description

Concepts for the HSECS were derived from a review of scholarly literature and curriculum materials. The initial version of the instrument consisted of a list of 50 concepts related to human sexuality.

Face and content validity of the HSECS were established by a panel of 36 experts. The panel consisted of 6 university faculty members who taught home economics education, child development, and family relationships courses; 10 students enrolled in a graduate course titled "Evaluation in Home Economics"; and 20 home economics teachers who taught child development and/or family relationship courses at the secondary level.

Panel members were requested to critique the first version of the HSECS in terms of concepts that should be added and deleted, item construction, ease of answering, and clarity of content and instructions. Panel members were asked to indicate the degree of importance they thought should be placed on each of the 50 human sexuality con-

cepts for inclusion in secondary courses. The Likert-type scale categories used and the point values assigned to each response were *very important* = 4, *somewhat important* = 3, *of little importance* = 2, and *unimportant* = 1. The highest possible scoring using the responses of the 36 panel members was 144 for each individual item, and the lowest possible score for each item was 36. Individual item scores ranged from 139 to 69.

Three concepts receiving total scores of less than 103 were deleted from the initial version of the scale because they were judged least important in relation to the purposes of the study. The concepts omitted were causes of multiple births, nocturnal emissions during puberty, and the physical act of sexual intercourse.

Five concepts were added to the revised version of the HSECS based on the recommendations of panel members. The additional concepts were peer pressure affecting sexual activity, community services in human sexuality education, legal aspects of abortion, types of natural childbirth, and psychological effects of pregnancy on unmarried parents. The final version of the HSECS contains 52 concepts related to human sexuality.

Recommendations from the panel members on wording and format were incorporated into the final version of the instrument.

Response Mode and Timing

Respondents are asked to indicate the degree of importance of each concept using four response options (see above). Typically, about 15 minutes are required to complete the instrument.

Scoring

Using the same 4-point values described above, a total score can be computed for each respondent by adding the item scores. Individual item scores may also be looked at for specific purposes.

Reliability

The internal consistency statistic, coefficient alpha, was used to assess the reliability of the HSECS with a proportionate stratified random sample of 250, or 10%, of the secondary home economics teachers in Texas. The final revised version of the scale had an alpha coefficient of .93. Therefore, the instrument appears to be sound for needs assessment studies and program evaluation in a variety of situations.

[1]Address correspondence to Valerie M. Chamberlin, Family and Consumer Sciences Education and Nutrition Education, University of Vermont, Terrill Hall, Burlington, VT 05405-0148; email: vchamber@moose.uvm.edu.

Validity

There are no construct validity data for the HSECS. There have not been any other instruments developed to assess home economics teachers' feelings about the importance for inclusion and the emphasis placed on human sexuality education concepts in secondary curricula to use for construct validation purposes.

Other Information

The instrument was developed as part of Brenda Barrington's (1981) master's thesis research and is available through the library at Texas Tech University, Lubbock, TX 79409. More information can also be found in Chamberlain, Couch, Cummings, and Barrington (1983).

References

Barrington, B. J. (1981). *Development and analysis of a scale to measure human sexuality education concepts.* Unpublished master's thesis, Texas Tech University, Lubbock, TX.

Chamberlain, V. M., Couch, A. S., Cummings, M. N., & Barrington, B. J. (1983). Human sexuality education as perceived and taught by home economics teachers in Texas. *Texas Home Economist Research Issue, 50,* 6-7.

Exhibit

Human Sexuality Education Concepts Scale

For each concept, please place a check in the *box* to the *right* to indicate *how* important you think the concept is for inclusion in secondary home economics classes. In addition, please place a check in the *space* to the *right* of each concept to indicate *whether you teach* the concept in any of your home economics classes.[a]

1. Understanding adolescent male sexuality
2. Understanding adolescent female sexuality
3. Physical changes in the male during puberty
4. Physical change in the female during puberty
5. Menstruation during puberty
6. Emotions of males during puberty
7. Emotions of females during puberty
8. Community dating standards
9. Necking and petting in dating
10. Dating as preparation for mate selection
11. Premarital sexual behavior
12. Double standard in male-female relationships
13. Sex codes in dating
14. Peer pressure affecting sexual activity
15. Emotions involved in sex offenses
16. Preventing sex offenses
17. Types of contraceptives
18. How to use contraceptives
19. Community services in human sexuality education
20. Emotional effects of abortion
21. Physical effects of abortion
22. Legal aspects of abortion
23. Venereal diseases
24. Causes of venereal diseases
25. Treatment of venereal diseases
26. Emotions involved in sexual intercourse
27. Fertilization of the egg
28. Psychological effects of pregnancy on unmarried parents
29. Signs of pregnancy
30. Drugs, alcohol, and tobacco use in pregnancy
31. Nutrition during pregnancy
32. Infectious diseases during pregnancy
33. Rh-factor and pregnancy
34. Dominant and recessive traits
35. Genetics and sex determination
36. Purposes of genetic counseling
37. Effects of environment on birth defects
38. Effects of heredity on birth defects
39. Mother's emotional changes during pregnancy
40. Father's role during pregnancy
41. Physical change of mother during pregnancy
42. Three stages of prenatal development
43. Types of natural childbirth
44. Stages of birth
45. Problems with multiple births
46. Causes of premature births
47. Problems associated with premature births
48. Role of father during birth
49. Procedure during cesarean birth
50. Reasons for cesarean birth
51. Causes of miscarriages
52. Emotional concerns related to miscarriages

a. Each item has a box for the four response options and spaces to indicate whether or not the concept is taught. These are not shown in the exhibit.

Family Life Sex Education Goal Questionnaire

Steven Godin,[1] *East Stroudsburg University*
Susan Frank and Stacy Jacobson, *Michigan State University*

The Family Life Sex Education Goal Questionnaire (FLSE-GQ) is a measure designed to assess the attitudes of school personnel and community members toward the various goals of family life and sex education in the public schools. Kirby and Alter (1980), Kirby, Alter, and Scales (1979), and Kirkendall (1965) have argued that a comprehensive program ought to provide accurate information about sexuality, reduce sex-related fears and anxieties, facilitate informed and responsible sexual decision making, encourage students to develop more tolerant attitudes toward the sexual behavior of others, facilitate communication about sexuality with parents and peers, reduce sex-related problems such as unplanned pregnancies, and integrate sex into a balanced and purposeful pattern of living (see Chilman, 1983, p. 209). Obviously, these goals vary not only in content but also in the degree of controversy surrounding their implementation. Scales (1983) reported that many administrators shy away from including more controversial goals in their school programs for fear of negative community reactions or resistance from teachers or other school personnel; however, there is evidence that negative attitudes are found mostly among a small but vocal minority (Scales, 1983). The FLSE-GQ provides an empirical basis for determining the extent of school and community support for the various goals of sex education and offers a means of clarifying diverse attitudes and priorities.

Description, Response Mode, and Timing

The instrument has a long and a short form. The long form consists of 57 goal items, and the short form consists of 20 goal items. Items on both forms have a 5-point Likert-type response format with response options labeled from *very unimportant* to *very important*. Respondents circle the number indicating the relative importance of each goal item for a family life sex education program. The long form takes 40 minutes for the parents to complete, somewhat less for the teachers. Due to the length of the long form, the short form may be more appropriate for some parent groups. Researchers should consider the degree of literacy, interest, and so forth in the population to be sampled in determining which version to use.

The FLSE-GQ has been used with two major samples: 337 elementary and high school teachers and 248 parents of elementary and high school children. Separate factor analyses were carried out on the 57 goal items from the teacher and parent samples. These analyses identified five

goal dimensions or themes common to both samples: (a) facilitating sexual decision making, (b) teaching about male and female physical development, (c) encouraging respect for diversity, (d) providing secondary prevention (e.g., to help pregnant girls to stay in school), and (e) teaching about the family and integrating sexuality in personal growth. Sexual decision making was the largest factor (31% of the variance) in the parent sample, whereas family life and personal growth were the largest factors (30% of the variance) in the teacher sample. The remaining goal dimensions were minor goal dimensions in both samples (4% to 9% of the variance). The five scales of the short form correspond to each of the common goal dimensions and include items that had loadings of .5 or greater on corresponding factors in both the parent and teacher samples.

Scoring

Investigators working with large samples will probably want to score the long form of the FLSE-GQ by subjecting the importance ratings for all 57 items to a principal components analysis. This procedure avoids any a priori assumptions about the salient goal dimensions within a particular population. The investigators can then derive scores for each goal dimension either by using computer-generated factor scores or by adding the importance ratings for the items with the highest loadings on each factor. Investigators working with smaller samples and/or preferring the short form of the FLSE-GQ can derive scores for the Sexual Decision Making (Items 8, 10, 17, 18, 21, 43), Physical Development (Items 32, 33, 44), Respect for Diversity (Items 47, 48, 49), Secondary Prevention (Items 39, 45, 57), and Family Life and Personal Growth (Items 16, 20, 22, 23, 54) scales by adding responses for each scale item and dividing by the total number of scale items.

Reliability and Validity

Cronbach alphas for the five goal dimensions from the long form range from .69 to .79 for the sample of 337 teachers and from .65 to .85 for the sample of 278 parents. Cronbach alphas for the five scales from the short form range from .73 to .83 for the sample of 337 teachers and from .79 to .87 for the sample of 248 parents. Although the Cronbach alphas are slightly higher for the short form, researchers may want to use the longer form to assess whether new goal dimensions exist for their specific population. The questionnaire has been used to identify school personnel and community member goals for a Family Life Sex Education program in a large, midwestern urban center. Frank, Godin, Jacobson, and Sugrue (1982) and Godin, Frank, and Jacobson (1984) assessed relationships between

---

[1]Address correspondence to Steven Godin, Health Department, East Stroudsburg University, East Stroudsburg, PA 18301.

goal dimensions derived from the long form of the FLSE-GQ and the teachers' and parents' demographic characteristics (i.e., age, sex, race, and religiosity). Among the teachers, religiosity was the best predictor of differing attitudes toward the goals of family life sex education in the public schools, whereas among the parents, both religiosity and race contributed significantly to attitude differences. Both parents and teachers rated sexual decision-making goals as significantly less important than the other goal dimensions, contributing to the greater controversy surrounding this topic area in family life sex education (see Chilman, 1983, pp. 207-208, 221-223).

Other Information

The Family Life Sex Education Goal Questionnaire was copyrighted in 1985 and in 1994. Copies of the questionnaire, including an optional demographic questionnaire, are available for $1.50 (to cover printing and handling costs) from the senior author.

References

Chilman, C. S. (1983). *Adolescent sexuality in a changing American society.* New York: Wiley.

Frank, S., Godin, S., Jacobson, S., & Sugrue, J. (1982, August). *Respect for diversity: Teachers' goals for a family life sex education program.* Paper presented at the meeting of the American Psychological Association, Washington, DC.

Godin, S., Frank, S., & Jacobson, S. (1984, March). *Respect for diversity: Parents' goals for a family life sex education program.* Paper presented at the Midwestern Conference of the National Council on Family Relations, Des Moines, IA.

Kirby, D., & Alter, J. (1980). The experts rate important features and outcomes of sex education programs. *Journal of School Health, 50,* 497-502.

Kirby, D., Alter, J., & Scales, P. (1979). *An analysis of U.S. sex education programs and evaluation methods.* Springfield, VA: National Technical Information Service.

Kirkendall, L. A. (1965). *Sex education.* New York: Sex Information and Education Council of the United States.

Scales, P. (1983). The new opposition to sex education: A powerful threat to a democratic society. *Journal of School Health, 5,* 300-304.

Exhibit

Family Life and Sex Education Goal Questionnaire

This questionnaire lists goals which some people have described as important for a family life sex education program. Some goals may be of lesser importance than others. For each of the goals listed, we would like you to indicate (on the 5-point scale provided) whether or not you view the goal as *important for a family life sex education program* in the _____ (specify program, school, grade levels, etc.).

Instructions: In the column to the right of the goals listed on the pages which follow, indicate the importance of each goal by using the following scale:

1	2	3	4	5
Very unimportant	Somewhat unimportant	Neutral importance	Somewhat important	Very important

Here is an example of how to use the scale:

Example Items
A. To teach children about how to stay physically healthy as they grow.   1 2 3 4 5
B. To teach children how to play a musical instrument.   1 2 3 4 5

If, in your opinion, the first goal ("To teach children about how to stay physically healthy as they grow") is *somewhat important* (number "4" on the scale) for a family life sex education program, you would circle "4" next to the goal statement in the column on the right. If, in your opinion, the second goal ("To teach children how to play a musical instrument") is *very unimportant* for a family life sex education program, you would circle the number "1" in the column to the right.

Remember, you may see some goals as more important than others. Please circle *your opinion* by circling the number that best represents *your* views beside each goal statement.

1. To help adolescents feel good about their physical appearance.[a]
2. To help adolescents to appreciate their special qualities and personality as well as that of other boys and girls.
3. To reduce guilt and fear about sexuality.
4. To provide information about abnormal sexual development and behavior.
5. To help adolescents understand how sexual development affects other aspects of personal growth and development.
6. To provide complete information about male and female genitalia (sex organs) and other physical differences between men and women.

7. To involve parents in selecting instruction materials and planning the curriculum of the family life sex education program.
8. To provide information about abortion and its effects on the body.
9. To provide information about the biology of human reproduction and birth.
10. To discuss ways of coping with an unexpected pregnancy.
11. To help adolescents develop skills in getting along with members of the opposite sex.
12. To provide information about how to be good parents.
13. To help adolescents learn to understand and communicate with each other better.
14. To make youth aware of community services related to health and prenatal care.
15. To emphasize the importance of the family as the keystone of American life.
16. To help adolescents understand their responsibilities to self, family, and friends, as they grow up.
17. To inform youth of community services related to birth control and sexual decision making.
18. To counsel adolescents to make their own decisions about how far to go in their sexual activities.
19. To encourage adolescents to talk more openly with their parents about sexuality.
20. To discuss the role of the family in personal growth and development.
21. To encourage adolescents to use contraceptives if they decide to have sexual intercourse.
22. To discuss ways in which families work out conflicts and solve problems.
23. To help adolescents understand people's feelings and points of view.
24. To educate adolescents about peer pressure and how to deal with it.
25. To provide information about sexually transmitted diseases including HIV and AIDS.
26. To teach about abstention as a form of contraception.
27. To encourage discussion of personal family experiences in the classroom.
28. To provide special courses about family life and sexuality for disabled students.
29. To encourage adolescents to think about alternatives to abortion.
30. To bring in outside speakers to talk to youth about sexuality.
31. To counsel boys who are expectant fathers.
32. To correct myths and misinformation about the body.
33. To help adolescents to view the growth changes in their bodies as normal and healthy.
34. To discuss how the attitudes toward growth and development may be different for different ethnic groups and cultures in our society.
35. To provide information about alternative sexual behaviors and lifestyles, such as homosexuality.
36. To discuss abortion as a form of contraception.
37. To provide workshops to assist parents in talking more openly with their adolescent children about sexuality.
38. To encourage grooming and thoughtfulness about personal appearance.
39. To counsel girls who are pregnant.
40. To refer students with special needs to social service agencies.
41. To make adolescents aware of the negative effects of sex role stereotypes.
42. To provide information about good prenatal care.
43. To provide information about contraceptives and how they work, and describe their effects on the body.
44. To teach about biological changes during puberty, as well as other times of life.
45. To provide individual counseling to students with low self-esteem or those who feel embarrassed about their bodies.
46. To meet with parents about a child who is having difficulties with sexual issues and stresses.
47. To learn about different kinds of families in our society.
48. To teach about how families may differ in how they make rules and decisions.
49. To provide information about how different ethnic and cultural groups differ in sexual beliefs and behaviors.
50. To work with outside community agencies to provide rap groups about sexuality and sexual decision making.
51. To help adolescents to see that most young people are going through many of the same things as they grow toward maturity.
52. To help adolescents plan for and start working toward future goals.
53. To provide information about the roles and challenges that go along with reaching different ages in life.
54. To discuss ways to help families talk more openly and improve family communication.
55. To listen and respond to the opinions of outside community and local interest groups in making family life sex education goals.
56. To encourage personal hygiene.
57. To encourage pregnant girls to stay in school and to provide special classes for them in prenatal care.

a. The 5-point scale is provided after each item.

The Sexuality Education Program Feature/Program Outcome Inventory

Daniel Klein,[1] *Northern Illinois University*

The intent of this inventory is to evaluate the impact of a sexuality education program on students by examining self-reported changes in knowledge, attitudes, and behaviors. In addition, the inventory can be used to examine students' perceptions of several program characteristics and the extent to which curriculum topics were presented during a program.

Description

The inventory is an extension of the early research of Kirby, Alter, and Scales (1979). In their investigation of the effectiveness of sexuality education programs, a list of important program features and program outcomes was generated, based on a review of the existing sexuality education literature. Their review identified 147 potentially important program features and 92 potentially important program outcomes for sexuality education. The Delphi technique was used by Kirby et al. (1979) in the ranking of each identified feature and outcome to the two major goals for sexuality education: the reduction in unplanned adolescent pregnancies and the achievement of a positive and fulfilling sexuality.

Based on previous research, the Sexuality Education Program Feature/Program Outcome Inventory was developed. Selected from the original list of features and outcomes were 36 program features and 30 program outcomes. As a result of the process undertaken by Kirby et al. (1979), items were selected based on their ratings.

Sixty-nine items relating to sexuality education are contained in the inventory. Twelve items examine program characteristics and focus on classroom atmosphere, teacher encouragement to examine and to discuss one's values, and course activities. Changes in students are examined through 33 items focusing on the following important sexuality education outcomes: knowledge, understanding of self, values, interaction skills, reduction in the fear of sex-related activities, and improved self-esteem.

A Likert-type scale is used to examine student perceptions to the items relating to program characteristics and program outcomes. Response options range from *strongly agree* to *strongly disagree,* with an additional option of *don't know.*

Curriculum implementation of several important topics in sexuality education are examined with a nominal scale. Three levels of presentation, *formally, informally,* and *not at all,* are defined and identified for each of the 24 topics. Each topic on the inventory is a component of one of the

following areas: physiology; sexual myths; values; contraception; and skills related to decision making, communication, and conflict resolution.

Curriculum coverage is also included on the inventory. When evaluating program outcome achievement, it is essential to examine the manner in which content was presented to students. If a program outcome is not achieved, this may, in part, be related to the manner in which the topic was presented to students.

Response Mode and Timing

Respondents circle the response option indicating their answer to each item. Average completion time is 10 minutes.

Scoring

To facilitate scoring and data analysis, Items 1-45 are assigned the following values: *strongly agree* = 4, *agree* = 3, *disagree* = 2, *strongly disagree* = 1, and *don't know* = 0. Curriculum coverage items are assigned the following values: *not at all* = 0, *informally covered* = 1, *formally covered* = 2, and *don't know* = 3.

When a class completes the inventory, comparisons can be made by examining the number of students who indicated a specific response to each item. For example, it might be revealed that 75% of the students now strongly agree to having a greater understanding of the positive role of sexuality in their lives as a result of their course. Also, depending on the responses to each program outcome, an instructor may wish to examine how students perceived the classroom coverage of specific topics.

Reliability and Validity

Because the inventory is an extension of early research efforts, procedures to assess reliability and validity were undertaken. A review panel was used to assess the face validity of the inventory. Because the content was previously established (Kirby et al., 1979), the intent was to examine and refine the inventory's clarity.

The inventory was broken into subscales prior to assessing reliability. Program Characteristics include Items 1-12, and the subscale for Curriculum Topics includes Items 46-49. Changes in Knowledge subscale includes Items 13-24. Understanding of Self subscale contains Items 25-28, Changes in Values are Items 29-31 and 42-45, and Changes in Interaction Skills are Items 32-39.

Item 40 examines a reduction in the fear of sex-related activities, and Item 41 examines changes in self-esteem. Because these are single items, subscales were not developed. However, the two items were included when the reliability of the total inventory was assessed.

[1]Address correspondence Daniel Klein, Department of Physical Education, Northern Illinois University, DeKalb, IL 60115-2854; email: dklein@niu.edu.

Students who completed a sexuality education program were used to establish reliability. This population was selected from a high school previously identified as having an outstanding sexuality education program (Kirby et al., 1979). Reliability coefficients using Cronbach's alpha for each subscale and the total inventory are as follows: Program Characteristics, .50; Knowledge, .80; Understanding of Self, .89; Values, .79; Interaction skills, .53; Curriculum Topics, .83; and Total Inventory, .88.

References

Allgeier, E. R. (1983). Sexual values in the classroom. *SIECUS Report,* 9(4), 9-10.

Klein, D. (1984). Knowledge, attitude and behavioral changes as a result of sex education. *Journal of Sex Education and Therapy, 10,* 26-30.

Kirby, D., Alter, J., & Scales, P. (1979). *An analysis of U.S. sex education programs and evaluation methods* (CDC Report No. 2021-79-DK-FR). Atlanta, GA: Centers for Disease Control. (NTIS No. PB 80-201932 A02)

Exhibit

The Sexuality Education Program Feature/Program Outcome Inventory

Dear Student:

This survey is designed to gather important information about your feelings concerning the Human Sexuality Course you had in high school. Your responses are most important and we are hoping you will take a few moments to assist us. Thank you for your cooperation.

    A. Have you taken a Human Sexuality Course in high school? _____ Yes _____ No
        If yes, please complete the survey and return in the envelope provided.
        If no, please complete page 4 and return the survey in the envelope provided.
    B. If you have already returned a completed survey, there is no need to complete the survey again.
        Thank you for your cooperation.

Below is a list of statements about the Human Sexuality Course you had. Please respond to each statement by circling one response based on the following scale: SA—Strongly agree; A—Agree; D—Disagree; SD—Strongly disagree; DK—Don't know.

1. The teacher was enthusiastic about teaching the course.[a]
2. The teacher discussed topics in a way that made me feel comfortable.
3. The teacher encouraged me to talk about my opinions.
4. The teacher encouraged me to think about my own values concerning sexuality.
5. The teacher encouraged me to consider the use of birth control in order to avoid an unplanned pregnancy.
6. I was encouraged to ask questions about sexuality in class.
7. The teacher provided class activities aimed at improving decision-making skills.
8. I was permitted to express my own values in the class.
9. The teacher provided class activities aimed at improving factual knowledge.
10. The teacher was comfortable during class discussions concerning sexuality.
11. The teacher got along well with students in class.
12. The teacher encouraged me to think about the consequences of sexual relationships before I enter into them.

The following is a list of statements which relate to your high school's Human Sexuality Course. Please circle the response that best represents your feelings about each statement.

As a result of your high school's human sexuality course, do you feel you have a greater understanding of:

13. Physical changes during adolescence.
14. Human reproduction.
15. The emotional needs of adolescents.
16. The social needs of adolescents.
17. The emotional changes during adolescence.
18. The social changes during adolescence.
19. Abstinence as an alternative to sexual intercourse.
20. The effectiveness of different birth control methods.
21. The probability of becoming pregnant.
22. The problems associated with adolescent parenthood.
23. Sexually transmitted diseases.
24. Common myths concerning sexuality.
25. The positive role of sexuality in your life.
26. Your long-range life goals.

27. Your own emotional needs.
28. Your sexual feelings.
29. Being responsible for your own behavior.
30. Accepting your own body variation.
31. Accepting your own set of rules to guide your behavior.

As a result of your high school's human sexuality course, do you feel you have a greater ability to:

32. Make decisions.
33. Communicate your feelings verbally.
34. Discuss sexual behavior with your potential partner.
35. Express your desire to use birth control in order to avoid an unplanned pregnancy.
36. Express your desire not to be involved sexually if you don't wish to be.
37. Resolve conflicts that may exist between you and another person.
38. Respect the individual dignity of each person.
39. Feel comfortable when discussing sexual issues with friends.
40. Feel comfortable with your own bodily functions.
41. Be satisfied with who you are.
42. Form your own sex role standards.
43. Be responsible for your own behavior.
44. Accept your own body variations.
45. Accept your own set of rules to guide your behavior.

The following is a scale representing how topics in your school's Human Sexuality Course were (are) presented: 0—Not at all; 1—Informally covered; 2—Formally covered; DK—Don't know. *Not at all* means the topic was (is) not discussed. *Informally covered* means the topic was (is) discussed only if a student asks a question about the topic. *Formally covered* means the topic was (is) discussed in a class period or unit in which the teacher presented information through lecture, discussion, class activity, media, or guest speaker. *Don't know* means you do not have enough information to respond to the statement.

Please circle the response that best represents how you feel each topic was (is) covered in your school's human sexuality course.

46. Anatomy and physiology[b]
47. Biological aspects of human reproduction
48. The probability of becoming pregnant
49. Human sexuality as an aspect of one's total personality
50. The relationship between how one feels about oneself and one's behavior
51. The emotional needs during adolescence
52. The social needs during adolescence
53. Adolescent pregnancy
54. Students' attitudes about sexual activity
55. Students' feelings about sexual activity
56. The range of sexual behaviors
57. Sexually transmitted diseases
58. Common myths concerning sexuality
59. Students' attitudes about sex roles
60. Students' feelings about sex roles
61. Peer pressure and sexual behavior
62. Avoiding unwanted sexual experiences
63. Advantages of the various contraceptive methods
64. Disadvantages of the various contraceptive methods
65. The effectiveness of the various contraceptive methods
66. Improving decision-making skills
67. Improving problem-solving skills
68. Improving communication skills with peers
69. Improving communication skills with parents

---

a. For Items 1-45, the five options, *strongly agree-strongly disagree,* are provided next to the item.
b. For Items 46-69, the four options indicated in the instructions are provided next to the item.

Family Life and Sex Education Questionnaire

David Marini and Herb Jones,[1] *Ball State University*

The purpose of the Family Life and Sex Education Questionnaire is to measure the attitudes and beliefs about sex education held by local school policymakers (e.g., superintendent and school board members).

Description

The instrument was developed between October 1981 and April 1982. This development process included several revisions. Previously published questionnaires were searched to obtain items that had been field tested and that were related to the following topics: the public schools' responsibility for providing sex education, reasons for including sex education in the curriculum, barriers to sex education programming in the schools, desired outcomes for sex education, issues for inclusion in the curriculum, and opinions on selected issues with sex education programming. After the initial synthesis of items was undertaken, several revisions were made of the instrument based on comments of various research professionals. The instrument was then reviewed by representatives of the professional organizations for school boards and school superintendents, as well as representatives from the state departments of education and health. Input from these persons was used in further instrument refinement. The final step in development was a pilot test with one school corporation, its board, and its superintendent. Their input was incorporated into the final version of the instrument. The instrument consists of six parts and 115 items.

Response Mode and Timing

In some cases, the options are a simple *yes, no, don't know;* in other cases, the respondent must indicate his or her view on a Likert-type scale ranging from *very important* to *no importance,* or *strongly agree* to *strongly disagree.*

The maximum time needed for completion would be 30 minutes, with most completing the instrument in a much

shorter time period. Some respondents suggested that much more time would be necessary for those providing a thoughtful response.

Scoring

A simple tally of the responses, converted to percentages, indicates the agreement or disagreement with each of the issues.

Reliability

No reliability studies have been conducted on the instrument.

Validity

Face validity was determined in two ways. First, test construction professionals were involved in the original development. This was followed by having the executive directors of a state-level school board association and a state-level school superintendents association, as well as state-level health education and public health officials, check for content. Second, a pilot study was done with one local school board to check for clarity and purpose.

Other Information

Obtaining permission from the authors is requested before using the questionnaire. Copies of the instrument are not available for purchase, but a single copy will be provided for duplication by those wishing to use the instrument.

References

Jones, H., & Marini, D. (1984). The schools and sex education: A view from the top. *Eta Sigma Gamma, 16*(2), 25-29.

Marini, D., & Jones, H. (1983). Beliefs of Indiana school policy makers on the role of the school in education about sexuality. *Health Education, 14*(7), 4-7.

Marini, D., & Jones, H. (n.d.). *Beliefs of Indiana public school policy makers in the role of the school in education about sexuality: Its responsibility; its quality; its direction.* Unpublished monograph. (Available from the authors for $2.50 plus postage and handling)

[1]Address correspondence to Herb Jones, Department of Physiology and Health Science, Ball State University, Muncie, IN 47306.

Exhibit

Family Life and Sex Education Questionnaire (sample items only)

Part 1 (7 items; response options: *yes/no/don't know*)

1. Do you believe that the public school has a responsibility to teach about human sexuality?
   (Regardless of your answer to this question, please complete the questionnaire.)
2. Do you or would you approve of such an educational program in your school system?
3. Do you believe that the majority of members of your school board agree with you on the above question?

Part II (15 items; response options: *very important, important, no opinion, little importance, no importance*)

Following are some reasons which have been given for offering sex education in the schools. Please check how important you think the reasons might be in your schools.

1. Signs of inadequate teaching about sexuality are numerous: unhappy people, disorganized home, divorces, irresponsible behavior, and inability to discuss the subjects of sex and reproduction plainly and without embarrassment.
2. The best intentioned parents usually lack information, vocabulary, and naturalness to carry out the all important sex instruction of their children.
3. There is good evidence that uninformed children and adolescents most often obtain their sex education from the peer group.
4. Studies conducted in school and public health programs have, for a long time, revealed the ignorance and misinformation which prevails among teenagers and adults in regard to anatomy, human reproduction, and sexually transmitted diseases.
5. Most teenagers still believe in waiting for sexual fulfillment until they marry. But those who are chaste are increasingly pressed to defend their stand, especially by those who indicate virginity is a sign of immaturity.

Part III (10 items; response options: *very important, important, no opinion, little importance, no importance*)

Following are some reasons which have been given for not offering sex education in the schools. Please check how important you think the reasoning might be in your schools.

1. Concern over parental reaction.
2. Concern over church reaction.
3. Concern over community reaction.
4. Concern over encouraging youth to be sexually promiscuous.

Part IV (13 items; response options: *very important, important, no opinion, little importance, no importance*)

The outcomes of sex education programs are both numerous and varied. Below is a sampling of often cited outcomes. Please check how important you believe each of the following is as an outcome of sex education.

1. To provide accurate information about sexuality.
2. To facilitate insights into personal sexual behavior.
3. To reduce fears and anxieties about personal sexual development and feelings.
4. To help people make more informed choices.

Part V (42 items; response options: *should not be included, probably better not to include, undecided, probably should be included, essential to include*)

Please check, in the appropriate column, your view on the inclusion of the following topics in a school sex education program (assuming they are presented at the proper grade level by qualified persons).

1. Difference between sexes.
2. Structure and function of reproductive organs.
3. Changes at puberty.
4. Menstruation.
5. Menopause (change of life).
6. Masturbation.
7. Nocturnal emissions.
8. Contraception
9. Conception.
10. Pregnancy and fetal development.

Part VI (28 items; response options: *strongly disagree, agree, undecided, agree, strongly agree*)

Please react to the following statements which express a variety of views and comments found in the literature on sex education. Please check the box which reflects the extent of your agreement or disagreement with the statement.

1. "Experts" such as doctors, nurses, psychologists, or clergy, rather than classroom teachers, should be called on to handle sex instruction in the school.
2. A well-qualified teacher is the most important ingredient in an effective school sex education program.
3. Before a person is allowed to teach sex education, he/she should have met some established criteria.
4. Persons who are involved in school sex education programs, in most cases, need adequate training.
5. Administrative guidelines, clearly defined and written, and program supervision are more necessary in sex education programs than in other curricular areas.

Sex-Role Egalitarianism Scale

Lynda A. King[1] and Daniel W. King, *National Center for Post-Traumatic Stress Disorder, Boston Veterans Affairs Medical Center*

The Sex-Role Egalitarianism Scale (SRES; King & King, 1993) is a measure of gender role attitudes toward the equality of men and women. King and King described the egalitarianism construct, which the scale measures, as "bidirectional" (p. 2) in nature, going beyond many of the commonly used instruments that concentrate primarily on attitudes toward women in nontraditional roles. According to the construct's definition, a true sex role egalitarian is one who would neither negatively judge or discriminate against men exhibiting stereotypically female characteristics or behaviors, nor negatively judge or discriminate against women exhibiting stereotypically male characteristics or behaviors. The scale's content is drawn from five domains of adult living: marital roles, parental roles, employment roles, social-interpersonal-heterosexual roles, and educational roles. Also, items express several features of equality wherein egalitarian attitudes may be manifest: qualification or ability, obligation or duty, right, opportunity, and consequences.

Description

A multistage test development process yielded the four SRES forms that are available. An initial pool of 500 items was generated using a table of specifications framed by the five domain categories crossed with the features of equality. Also, items were generated to reflect both men and women engaging in possibly gender-incongruent role behaviors. Next, these items were subjected to a sorting task in which graduate students judged their clarity and content. A reduced pool of 204 items was administered to a sample of university students, item characteristics were computed, and two alternate 95-item forms (B and K) were constructed. The forms were administered to police officers, senior citizens, and students to estimate reliability and preliminary validity. A final stage of test development (King & King, 1990) involved the creation of two alternate 25-item abbreviated SRES forms (BB and KK). For all four versions of the instrument, items are declarative statements accompanied by a 5-point Likert-type response scale. The SRES is intended for adolescents and adults with at least a 6th- to 7th-grade reading level.

Response Mode and Timing

For each item, respondents are asked to judge their extent of agreement or disagreement (*strongly agree, agree,*

neutral, disagree, or *strongly disagree*) via a paper-and-pencil selection task. Completing the 95-item versions typically takes less than 20 minutes; the 25-item versions, about 5 minutes.

Scoring

Each item receives a score of 1 to 5, with 5 indicating the most egalitarian perspective. For each of the 95-item forms, a total score is obtained across all items (possible range = 95-495), and five domain scores (marital, parental, employment, social-interpersonal-heterosexual, and educational) may likewise be computed across the 19 items within each category (possible range = 19-95). For each of the 25-item abbreviated forms, only a total score is recommended (possible range = 25-125).

Reliability

Test development generated the following information about the SRES reliability. For the 95-item forms, internal consistency was .97 for total scores on both Forms B and K, with an average of .87 for the domain subscales; test-retest reliability (3- to 4-week interval) was .88 and .91 for Forms B and K, respectively, with an average of .85 for the domain subscales; and alternate forms reliability was .93 for total scores, with an average of .83 for the domain subscales. For abbreviated forms BB and KK, internal consistency was .94 and .92, respectively; test-retest reliability (3-week interval) was .88 for both; and the alternate forms coefficient was .87. King and King (1993) presented a table of internal consistency coefficients for another 14 samples; the values were quite comparable.

In addition to reliability estimates computed from a classical test theory perspective, the SRES has been subjected to a generalizability analysis (King & King, 1983), as well as an item response theory analysis (Vreven, King, & King, 1994).

Validity

Validity evidence for the SRES first may be found in expected group differences. For example, Beere, King, Beere, and King (1984) hypothesized and documented that women score significantly more egalitarian than men. In addition, expected group differences have been found between younger and older respondents, between police officers and college students, between students enrolled in business courses and those enrolled in psychology courses (Beere et al., 1984; Gaffney, 1990), and between feminist and nonfeminist women (Royse & Clawson, 1988). Scores on the scale are also related to other conceptually mean-

---

[1]Address correspondence to Lynda A. King, Women's Health Sciences Division (116B3), National Center for PTSD, Boston VAMC, 150 S. Huntington Avenue, Boston, MA 02130; email: king.lynda@boston.va.gov.

ingful variables, such as attitudes toward domestic violence (Crossman, Stith, & Bender, 1990; Stith, 1990), attitudes toward rape (Billingham & King, 1991), and marital adjustment (Li & Caldwell, 1987; Sparks, 1995).

Furthermore, there is support for the discriminant and convergent validity of the SRES. It does not appear to be contaminated by social desirability (Beere et al., 1984; Stith, 1986; Stith, Crossman, & Bischof, 1991). As expected (Archer, 1989; Spence, 1993), scores on the SRES share little variance with measures of gender-related traits (King, King, Carter, Surface, & Stepanski, 1994). Finally, a hypothesized curvilinear relationship between SRES scores and scores on measures of attitudes toward women has been demonstrated (King & King, 1986; King et al., 1994). As proposed, there was a positive linear relationship (representing an underlying shared traditional-nontraditional attitudinal dimension), but at the high end of the SRES continuum, the relationship "flattened out." These findings were interpreted in terms of the distinction between attitudes toward women and the bidirectional emphasis of the egalitarianism construct, that is, attitudes toward both men and women.

Other Information

All SRES forms are copyrighted and distributed by Sigma Assessment Systems, Inc., 1110 Military St., P.O. Box 610984, Port Huron, MI 48061-0984 (800-265-1285) in the United States and by Research Psychologists Press, Inc., 650 Waterloo St., Suite 100, P.O. Box 3292, Station B, London, ON N6A 4K3 (519-673-0833) in Canada.

References

Archer, J. (1989). The relationship between gender-role measures: A review. *British Journal of Social Psychology, 28,* 173-184.

Beere, C. A., King, D. W., Beere, D. B., & King, L. A. (1984). The Sex-Role Egalitarianism Scale: A measure of attitudes toward equality between the sexes. *Sex Roles, 10,* 563-576.

Billingham, P., & King, L. A. (1991, May). *Sex-role egalitarianism and heterosexual violence.* Paper presented at the annual meeting of the Midwestern Psychological Association, Chicago.

Crossman, R. K., Stith, S. M., & Bender, M. M. (1990). Sex role egalitarianism and marital violence. *Sex Roles, 22,* 293-304.

Gaffney, J. (1990). *The relationship between androgyny and sex-role egalitarianism.* Unpublished manuscript, Wilfred Laurier University.

King, D. W., & King, L. A. (1983). Measurement precision of the Sex-Role Egalitarianism Scale: A generalizability analysis. *Educational and Psychological Measurement, 43,* 435-447.

King, L. A. (1985). [Administration of Sex-Role Egalitarianism Scale]. Unpublished raw data, Central Michigan University.

King, L. A., & King, D. W. (1986). Validity of the Sex-Role Egalitarianism Scale: Discriminating egalitarianism from feminism. *Sex Roles, 15,* 207-213.

King, L. A., & King, D. W. (1990). Abbreviated measures of sex-role egalitarian attitudes. *Sex Roles, 23,* 659-673.

King, L. A., & King, D. W. (1993). *Manual for the Sex-Role Egalitarianism Scale: An instrument to measure attitudes toward gender-role equality.* Port Huron, MI: Sigma Assessment Systems.

King, L. A., King, D. W., Carter, D. B., Surface, C. R., & Stepanski, K. (1994). Validity of the Sex-Role Egalitarianism Scale: Two replication studies. *Sex Roles, 31,* 339-348.

Li, J. T., & Caldwell, R. A. (1987). Magnitude and directional effects of marital sex-role incongruence on marital adjustment. *Journal of Family Issues, 8,* 97-110.

Royse, D., & Clawson, D. (1988). Sex-role egalitarianism, feminism, and sexual identity. *Psychological Reports, 63,* 160-162.

Sparks, J. (1995). *Role incongruence and marital adjustment late in the transition to parenthood.* Unpublished doctoral dissertation, California School of Professional Psychology, Fresno.

Spence, J. T. (1993). Gender-related traits and gender ideology: Evidence for a multifactorial theory. *Journal of Personality and Social Psychology, 64,* 624-635.

Stith, S. M. (1986). *Police officer response to marital violence predicted from the officers; attitudes, stress, and marital experience: A path analysis.* Unpublished doctoral dissertation, Kansas State University, Manhattan.

Stith, S. M. (1990). Police response to domestic violence: The influence of individual and familial factors. *Violence and Victims, 5,* 37-49.

Stith, S. M., Crossman, R., & Bischof, G. (1991). Alcoholism and marital violence: A comparative study of men in alcohol treatment programs and batterer treatment programs. *Alcoholism Treatment Quarterly, 8,* 3-20.

Vreven, D. L., King, L. A., & King, D. W. (1994). *Item response theory-based information on the Sex-Role Egalitarianism Scale: A technical report to accompany the manual.* Mount Pleasant: Central Michigan University, Department of Psychology.

Exhibit

Sex-Role Egalitarianism Scale (sample items)

Marital Domain:

The husband should be the head of the family.
Things work out best in a marriage if a husband leaves his hands off domestic tasks.

Parental Domain:

It is more appropriate for a mother rather than a father to change their baby's diaper.
Keeping track of a child's out-of-school activities should be mostly the mother's responsibility.

Employment Domain:

It is wrong for a man to enter a traditionally female career.
Women can handle pressures from their jobs as well as men can.

Social-Interpersonal-Heterosexual Domain:

Women are more likely than men to gossip about their acquaintances.
A person should generally be more polite to a woman than to a man.

Educational Domain:

Home economics courses should be as acceptable for male students as for female students.
Choice of college is not as important for women as for men.

Source. Sample items are reprinted here with permission. All versions of the instrument are available from the publisher, Sigma Assessment Systems.

Female Sexual Response Patterns: Grafenberg Spot/Area and Ejaculation

Carol Anderson Darling,[1] *Florida State University*
J. Kenneth Davidson, Sr., *University of Wisconsin–Eau Claire*

Investigations of the physiological aspects of the Grafenberg spot/area have often been conducted in clinical settings; however, many social science researchers are also interested in this topic and may prefer to use a survey research design. Thus, women can be asked questions about their knowledge, attitudes, and feelings regarding their sexuality and experience with the Grafenberg spot/area and ejaculation. This survey instrument on female sexual response patterns was designed to obtain information about female sexuality with a special focus on experiences related to stimulation of the Grafenberg spot/area and female ejaculation. Various sections of the instrument contain questions concerning the Grafenburg spot/area and other related topics, such as experiencing orgasm and ejaculation through stimulation of the Grafenburg spot/area along with related urinary and bladder conditions.

Description

The entire instrument consists of 192 open-ended and closed-form items. Several variables were included concerning demographics, parent-child attachment, childhood/adolescence, socialization, partner relationships, sexual attitudes, sexual behaviors, and knowledge and/or

experience with the Grafenberg spot/area and female ejaculation. It was important to us to obtain accurate descriptions of the location of the Grafenburg spot/area and source of ejaculation. Thus, these questions were open ended and contained labeled diagrams of the female anatomy. Although these diagrams were used each time a question related to "location" was asked, the diagrams are included only once in this description.

We chose not to use the name "Grafenberg Spot," which had been familiarized in the popular press, because its use could possibly result in preformed notions, bias, or confusion for the respondents. Thus, the terminology used throughout the questionnaire refers to an "especially sensitive area in your vagina." There were four sections of questions pertinent to the "sensitive area," including sensitive area, sensitive area orgasm, sensitive area ejaculation, and sensitive area urination/pubococcygeus musculature. These sections are not identified in the actual questionnaire, although subtitles have been included to provide clarity in this condensed version of the instrument. Because the questions pertaining to the sensitive area were distributed throughout the instrument, they are not numbered within this description. Furthermore, if the question did not apply, the respondent was directed to another question by "if and go" statements.

The instrument was first pretested with female students enrolled in an upper-division human sexuality course. A revised questionnaire was pretested using acquaintances of

[1]Address correspondence to Carol Anderson Darling, Department of Family and Child Sciences, Florida State University, Tallahassee, FL 32306-2033; email: cdarling@mailer.fsu.edu.

professional colleagues in various academic settings. Finally, the questionnaire was reviewed by six female professionals involved in either teaching and/or research about human sexuality and/or sex education as part of the process of developing the final draft of the questionnaire. The actual investigation involved an anonymous survey of 2,350 professional women in health-related fields in the United States that yielded 1,289 completed questionnaires. A purposeful sample of women employed in the fields of nursing, sex education, sex therapy, and counseling was used. Given the nature of their academic training, it was assumed that these individuals would have a degree of familiarity with the anatomical structures and physiological processes associated with sexual responsiveness. The respondents were well educated, and their expertise was deemed important to reply in more precise language to a number of open-form items contained in the survey instrument.

This survey instrument is best suited for use with populations that contain women with 2 or more years of college education and who are at least 25 years of age. The level of language sophistication found in the instrument would appear to preclude its application to populations that have no college education. Furthermore, given the nature of the instrument, a woman would need to be sexually experienced to be able to respond in a meaningful way to a substantial number of the items. It is assumed that a greater opportunity for having considerable sexual experience will exist for women ages 25 years or older.

Response Mode and Timing

Respondents either check the appropriate answer category or answer the open-ended items in their own words within the space provided. Given the detailed personal information being sought regarding sexuality, the survey instrument should be completed in total privacy and anonymity. Thus, this instrument is ideally suited for distribution as a mail questionnaire using a business reply envelope.

Based on the pretest results and feedback from actual respondents, an average of 45 minutes is required to complete all segments of the survey instrument, whereas only 8 to 10 minutes are needed to complete the "sensitive area" portions of the survey.

Scoring

Although some Likert-type scale items were incorporated pertaining to the Grafenberg spot/area and ejaculation, it was not intended that such questions would constitute a scale that could stand alone. Moreover, the open-ended questions need to be coded and categorized accordingly.

Reliability

Reliability of the instrument has not been determined.

Validity

Content validity has been established through a review of the instrument by colleagues in the field.

Other Information

The entire instrument is available from the authors at a cost of $12.00. There is no charge for the use of the items included in this description.

References

Darling, C. A., Davidson, J. K., Sr., & Conway-Welch, C. (1990). Female ejaculation: Perceived origins, role of the Grafenberg spot/area, and sexual responsiveness. *Archives of Sexual Behavior, 19,* 29-47.

Darling, C. A., Davidson, J. K., Sr., & Conway-Welch, C. (1992). Shaping women's sexuality: The role of parental attachments. *Journal of Feminist Family Therapy, 4,* 61-90.

Davidson, J. K., Sr., & Darling, C. A. (1989). The role of the Grafenberg spot and female ejaculation in the female orgasmic response: An empirical analysis. *Journal of Sex & Marital Therapy, 15,* 102-120.

Exhibit

Grafenburg Spot/Area and Ejaculation Questionnaire

Sensitive Area

Is there any especially sensitive area in your vagina which, if stimulated, produces pleasurable feelings? (Circle number)

1. Yes, always produces pleasurable feelings
2. Yes, most of the time produces pleasurable feelings
3. Yes, sometimes produces pleasurable feelings
4. No

At what age did you *first* conclude that this sensitive area exists inside your vagina?

_____ years old

If no sensitive area exists in vagina, go to Question _____:

Under what bladder circumstances are the pleasurable sensations associated with this sensitive area in your vagina most easily detectable? (Circle number)

1. Bladder full
2. Bladder partially full
3. Bladder empty
4. Not associated with condition of bladder
5. Not aware of bladder condition when pleasurable sensations occur
6. Other

When during your menstrual cycle are the pleasurable sensations associated with this sensitive area in your vagina most easily detectable? (Circle number)

1. Just before menstrual period
2. During menstrual period
3. Just after menstrual period
4. Midway between menstrual periods
5. No difference during menstrual cycle
6. No difference, had hysterectomy with removal of uterus only
7. No difference, had hysterectomy with removal of ovaries and uterus
8. Not aware of difference in menstrual cycle when pleasurable sensations occur

When a speculum is inserted and opened in your vagina during a pelvic examination, does it ever stimulate this sensitive area in your vagina so that it produces pleasurable sensations? (Circle number)

1. Never
2. Rarely
3. Occasionally
4. Frequently
5. Very frequency
6. Always

Sensitive Area—Orgasm

In your opinion, does such a sensitive area exist inside the vagina which, if stimulated, can produce an orgasm without any clitoral contact and/or stimulation? (Circle number)

1. No
2. Yes, for all females
3. Yes, for some females
    If never had an orgasm go to Question _____:

Does stimulating this sensitive area in your vagina during sexual arousal produce an orgasm? (Circle number)

1. Yes, always
2. Yes, most of the time
3. Yes, sometimes
4. No
    If stimulated, sensitive area in vagina does not produce orgasm go to Question _____:

Is it possible for you and/or your sex partner to stimulate this sensitive area to produce an orgasm without causing clitoral contact to be made? (Circle number)

1. Yes
2. No
3. Never tried to stimulate sensitive area
4. Other _____ (Please specify)

If yes: Please describe how it is possible to stimulate this sensitive area to produce an orgasm independent of any clitoral stimulation.

   (Note: A larger space is necessary for open-ended response)

What is the location of this sensitive area inside your vagina which, if stimulated, will produce an orgasm?

Describe its specific, perceived location in relationship to the other genital and pelvic structures using the terminology from the diagram. Please do not just circle the terminology on the diagram and do not draw arrows.

   (Note: A larger space is necessary for the open-ended response)

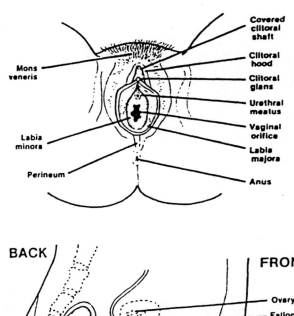

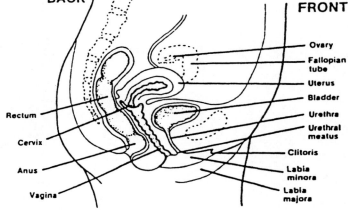

Which of the following factors play a role in whether this sensitive area in the vagina can be stimulated to produce an orgasm during sexual activity including masturbation, petting (mutual masturbation and/or oral-genital sex), or sexual intercourse. (Circle numbers for all applicable categories)

   1. Not using diaphragm as a contraceptive technique
   2. Long penis for vaginal penetration
   3. Long internal vibrator or dildo for vaginal penetration
   4. Large diameter penis for vaginal penetration
   5. Large diameter internal vibrator or dildo for vaginal penetration
   6. Degree of emotional involvement with sex partner
   7. Angle of entry of erect penis, dildo, or vibrator during vaginal penetration
   8. Use of your fingers to provide extra stimulation inside vagina
   9. Use of your partner's fingers to provide extra stimulation inside vagina
   10. Ability of partner to rotate pelvis during sexual activity
   11. Ability to rotate your pelvis during sexual activity
   12. Use of waterbed for sexual intercourse
   13. Position used for sexual intercourse
   14. Other _____ (Please specify)

Which position for sexual intercourse, if any, is most likely to result in stimulation of the sensitive area to produce orgasm? (Circle number)

1. Face-to-face/Male above
2. Face-to-face/Male above with legs of female over shoulders of male
3. Face-to-face/Female above
4. Face-to-face/Side
5. Prone (female lying face down)/Rear entry with vaginal penetration
6. Prone (female lying face down)/Rear entry with anal penetration
7. Kneeling/Rear entry with vaginal penetration
8. Kneeling/Rear entry with anal penetration
9. Sitting/Face-to-face
10. Sitting/Rear entry with vaginal penetration
11. Sitting/Rear entry with anal penetration
12. Standing/Face-to-face
13. Side/Rear entry with vaginal penetration
14. Supine (lying on back)/Male kneeling
15. Supine (lying on back/Male standing
16. Side/Rear entry with anal penetration
17. Rear entry with vaginal penetration/Male on back/Female above
18. Male on side/Female on back, with knees bent
19. Other _____ (Please specify)

Sensitive Area—Ejaculation

In your opinion, does the process of ejaculation (sudden spurt of fluid at the moment of orgasm) exist in some females? (Circle number)

1. No   2. Yes

   If yes: At what approximate age did you first conclude that ejaculation at the time or orgasm exists for some females? _____ years old

At the time that you experience orgasm, do you suddenly experience a spurt of fluid (i.e., ejaculation) in the genital area? (Circle number)

1. Never
2. Rarely
3. Sometimes
4. Almost always
5. Always

If never experience spurt of fluid during orgasm go to Question _____:

How does this spurt of fluid seem to be released at the time of your orgasm? (Please describe in your own words)

   (Note: A larger space is necessary for the open-ended response)

What do you believe to be the source of this spurt of fluid at the time of your orgasm? (Please describe)

   (Note: A larger space is necessary for the open-ended response)

In your own words, describe the difference, if any, between vaginal lubrication during your sexual arousal and the spurt of fluid at the moment of your orgasm.

   (Note: A larger space is necessary for the open-ended response)

During masturbation and/or sexual intercourse, are you able to consciously contract the muscles surrounding the vagina to grasp a phallic substitute (if utilized) or the penile shaft of your sex partner? (Circle number)

1. Yes   2. No

Sensitive Area—Urination/Pubococcygeus Musculature

Do you ever prolong the act of urination by starting and stopping the flow of urine because of pleasurable sensations associated with contracting of the muscles involved in bladder control? (Circle number)

1.   Yes   2.   No

Have you ever held back from experiencing an orgasm due to the fear of urinating? (Circle number)

1.   Yes   2.   No
      If never experienced orgasm go to Question _____:

Have you ever thought that you have urinated during your orgasm? (Circle number)

1.   Yes   2.   No
      If yes: How often do you think you have urinated during orgasm? (Circle number)
1. Very frequently
2. Frequently
3. Occasionally
4. Seldom

Are you aware of the existence of the pubococcygeus muscle located at the vaginal entrance? (Circle number)

1.   Yes   2.   No

Can you consciously identify your pubococcygeus muscle through voluntary contractions? (Circle number)

1.   Yes   2.   No
      If yes: Do you periodically exercise your pubococcygeus muscle through Kegel exercises or by another related method, such as starting and stopping the flow of urine? (Circle number)
1.   Yes   2.   No

The Sexual Opinion Survey

William A. Fisher,[1] *University of Western Ontario*

The personality dimension of erotophobia-erotophilia is conceptualized as the learned disposition to respond to sexual stimuli with negative-to-positive affect and evaluations and is believed to determine avoidance or approach

[1]Address correspondence to William A. Fisher, Department of Psychology and Department of Obstetrics and Gynaecology, Social Sciences Center, University of Western Ontario, London, Ontario N6A 5C2, Canada; email: fisher@sscl.uwo.ca.

responses to sexual stimuli. The Sexual Opinion Survey (SOS) is a measure of this trait disposition.

Description

A pool of 53 items intended to assess affective and evaluative responses to a range of sexual stimuli (autosexual, heterosexual, and homosexual behavior; sexual fantasy; and visual sexual stimuli) was developed by White, Fisher, Byrne, and Kingma (1977). Each item depicts a sexual situation in one of these domains and a negative or positive affective or evaluative response to it, and individuals are asked to indicate their degree of agreement or disagreement with the statement.

To determine which of the 53 items were valid measures of the construct, an external criterion item selection procedure was undertaken. White et al. (1977) asked 90 male and 105 female U.S. university undergraduates to respond to the 53-item pool and to a measure of social desirability responding (Crowne & Marlowe, 1964). The students then viewed 19 erotic slides depicting a variety of sexual activities (Levitt & Brady, 1965) and rated their positive and negative emotional responses to these stimuli on a self-report measure. Twenty-one of the 53 items were significantly correlated with emotional responses to the erotic stimuli for both men and women. Scores aggregated across the items were significantly correlated with emotional responses to the erotic stimuli for males, $r = .61$, and for females, $r = .72$, and scores were not significantly correlated with the measure of social desirability responding. Cross-validation research with an independent sample of undergraduate students showed that these 21 items are generally stable predictors of emotional responses to sexual stimuli for men and women, and they constitute the SOS.

The SOS items presented in the exhibit have been slightly updated since the time item selection was undertaken because several of the terms then used (e.g., *go-go dancer, pornography*) have become dated or have changed in meaning and were replaced with more current terms (e.g., *stripper, erotica*—defined as "sexually explicit books, movies, etc."). In comparative research conducted with undergraduates who completed the revised and original forms of the SOS and a measure of heterosexual experience, the revised form correlated with the original form of the SOS very highly, $r = .93$, the mean scores for the revised and original forms did not differ significantly, and the two were correlated similarly with the measure of heterosexual experience (Fisher, Byrne, White, & Kelley, 1988). The SOS has been used extensively in research in college student populations in the United States and Canada (see Fisher, Byrne, et al., 1988, and references in the following sections for reports of this research) and with nonstudent populations, including high school teachers (Yarber & McCabe, 1981), parents (Gilbert & Gamache, 1984; Yarber & Whitehill, 1981), pregnant and postpartum women and their husbands (Fisher & Gray, 1988), military wives (Hurlbert, Apt, & Rabehl, 1993), abusive and nonabusive but maritally distressed husbands (Hurlbert & Apt, 1991), and sexually transmitted disease (STD) clinic patients (Yarber & Fisher, 1983). The SOS has also been used extensively in cross-cultural research (see references). Translations of the SOS into Hebrew, French, Finnish, German, Portuguese, and Japanese are available from the author.

Response Mode and Timing

Research participants are given the scale and read instructions indicating that responses are confidential and asking participants to be as honest as they can. Completion of the SOS usually takes 10 minutes or less. If test participants are unfamiliar with the Likert-type response format employed (see exhibit), appropriate instructions for completion may be appended to the scale.

Scoring

Details for scoring the SOS are provided in the exhibit. Missing data may be handled by calculating a participant's average response to the positively or negatively worded items (for responses missing from positively or negatively worded items, respectively) and substituting this value for the missing data point, providing that the participant has responded to at least half of the positive or negative items on the scale. Sexual orientation will likely affect mean scores on the SOS because homosexual and bisexual individuals may respond more positively to homosexually oriented items than do heterosexuals, and there are more specifically homosexual than specifically heterosexual items on the scale. Sexual orientation, gender, and other factors that may affect mean scores on the SOS are not, according to theory, presumed to affect the nature of the relationship between individual differences in relative degree of erotophobia-erotophilia and avoidance or approach responses to sexuality.

A short form of the SOS was developed by Semph (1979). Regression analyses identified five items (4, 12, 13, 17, 21) that were good predictors of total scale scores for both men and women. Item presentation and scoring for the short form of the SOS appears in a footnote to the exhibit, and normative data for the short form of the SOS appear in Table 1.

Reliability

Test-retest reliability of the SOS over a 2-month period was studied among public school teachers in training to become sexuality educators and was found to be reasonably high for both males, $r(11) = .85$, and females, $r(55) = .80$. Test-retest reliability of .84 across 2 weeks for a sample of undergraduate student couples has been reported as well (Tanner & Pollack, 1988). Cronbach's alpha coefficient of internal consistency in the .82 to .90 range in undergraduate student samples has been reported (Fisher, Byrne, et al., 1988).

Although the SOS is a highly internally consistent scale, factor analytic research has been conducted in efforts to identify meaningful clusters of items within the scale. Gilbert and Gamache (1984) reported evidence of three factors within the SOS responses of a group of parents, including factors for Open Sexual Display, Sexual Variety, and Homoeroticism. More recently, Rise, Traeen, and Kraft (1994) factor analyzed the SOS responses of a large sample of Norwegian adolescents in the 17- to 19-year-old age range and reported evidence for the existence of factors for Erotophilia (positive responses to sexuality), Unconventional Sex (positive responses to unconventional sex), Erotophobia (negative responses to sexuality), and Homosexual Orientation (positive and negative responses to homosexuality). Further research is needed to demonstrate the generality and stability of these sets of factors and to clarify the potential utility of SOS factor-based subscale scores in

Table 1 Normative Data for the Sexual Opinion Survey (SOS)

	N	Mean	SD	Sample characteristics
Students				
United States				
Males	149	71.26_a	19.24	Volunteers for sex research from introductory psychology classes,
Females	118	53.74_b	19.60	midwestern university
Canada				
Males	54	78.22_a	14.28	Volunteers for sex research from introductory psychology classes,
Females	41	71.81_b	16.04	Ontario University
Adults				
United States				
Males	116	76.67_a	22.19	Parents who agreed to take part in sex education study at home
Females	210	65.88_b	23.91	(Gilbert & Gamache, 1984)
Canada				
Males	50	66.70_a	19.82	Couples in prenatal education classes
Females	50	57.54_b	25.85	
Samples from other nations				
India				
Males	33	70.21_a	4.92	The India, Hong Kong, Israel, and Brazil samples were composed of
Females	33	64.30_a	8.01	university undergraduates. The India and Hong Kong samples
Hong Kong				responded to the SOS in English; the Israeli sample responded to a
Males	69	59.17_a	12.63	Hebrew translation of the scale; and the Brazilian sample[a]
Females	114	47.89_b	15.87	responded to a Portuguese translation of the scale. The Japanese
Israel				sample was composed of female students in a Red Cross midwives
Males	52	70.77_a	12.79	school and responded to a Japanese translation of the SOS.
Females	49	58.84_b	21.69	
Brazil				
Males	190	79.99	17.59	
Females	190	67.57	20.55	
Japan				
Females	35	60.11	12.87	
Group comparisons				
Age				
34 or below	195	74.04_a	34.41	U.S.
35 or above	132	66.04_b	24.59	
Socioeconomic status				
55 or above	149	77.79_a	35.99	U.S. adults (Gilbert & Gamache, 1984)
54 or below	178	64.97_b	24.95	
Religion—males				
Agnostic	24	81.88_a	21.25	U.S.
Protestant	64	70.88_b	15.93	
Catholic	41	69.27_b	19.57	
Religion—females				
Agnostic	11	61.91_a	21.94	U.S.
Protestant	67	53.15_a	18.74	
Catholic	33	50.70_a	20.86	
Short form SOS				
Males	72	19.09_a	5.13	Canadian undergraduate students in a human sexuality course
Females	178	12.83_b	5.55	
Revised SOS				
Males	107	77.81_a	15.16	Canadian undergraduate students in a sexuality course
Females	216	67.11_b	18.59	

Note. Means with different subscripts differ at the .05 level by *t* tests. In comparison of religious affiliations, agnostic was assumed when respondents responded "none" when asked about their religious affiliation.

a. Data on the Brazilian students' SOS norms are from C. Hutz (personal communication, October 10, 1990).

comparison with SOS aggregate scores in efforts to predict and understand criterion measures.

Validity

The construct validity of the SOS has been developed in nearly a decade of research concerning the antecedents and consequents of erotophobia-erotophilia (see Fisher, Byrne, et al., 1988, for a review and specific studies cited below). With respect to antecedents of this disposition, erotophobic (compared to erotophilic) parents give relatively little sexual information to their children, and erotophobic individuals retrospectively report relatively punishing sexual socialization experiences during childhood and adolescence. With respect to consequents of this disposition, it has been found that erotophobia-erotophilia is linked with a variety of behaviors that reflect broad-based avoidance or approach of sexuality. Researchers have shown that erotophobic (compared to erotophilic) persons engage in less autosexual or heterosexual behavior; find it difficult to learn, talk, or teach about sexuality; engage in less sexual activity during pregnancy or postpartum; are less likely to acquire or to use contraception; and are less likely to engage in certain sex-related health care practices. Erotophobic individuals also report more negative attitudes about sexuality, produce briefer or less explicit sexual fantasies, and have seen less erotica.

Erotophobia-erotophilia has also been correlated with a variety of conceptually related personality dimensions: erotophobic persons score as more authoritarian, higher in sex guilt, more homophobic, more sex role traditional (vs. androgynous), and as more value orthodox on an omnibus personality measure.

Evidence of discriminant validity is provided by findings that show that the SOS is uncorrelated with a measure of social desirability, with achievement in neutral content (vs. sexual) coursework, and with responses to communicating a neutral content (vs. sexual) message (see Fisher, Byrne, et al., 1988, for a review).

Researchers have investigated the association of erotophobia-erotophilia and sexual behavior in a variety of samples and have determined that this personality dimension is associated with women's reports of their frequency of sexual activity, number of orgasms, sexual desire, sexual assertiveness, sexual excitability, and sexual satisfaction over a 21-day report period (Hurlbert et al., 1993), with the length of women's extramarital sexual involvements (Hurlbert, 1992), and with men's lifetime number of sexual partners and maximum number of sexual partners in any given month (Bogaert & Fisher, 1995). In related research, it has been has demonstrated that erotophobia-erotophilia is linked with the tendency to desire and to initiate condom use in a relationship (Freimuth, Hammond, Edgar, McDonald, & Fink, 1992), with the accuracy of women's perceptions of vulnerability to pregnancy (Gerrard & Luus, 1995), and with consistency of women's contraceptive use across four different university campuses (Kelley, Smeaton, Byrne, Przybyla, & Fisher, 1987; see Fisher, 1984, for a parallel finding for a relationship between erotophobia-erotophilia and condom use among university men across a month's

time, and see Wilson and Marindo, 1989, for findings linking erotophobia-erotophilia and contraception in a multiethnic sample of Zimbabwean university students). Researchers have also linked erotophobia-erotophilia with individual differences in sexual knowledge and with evidence concerning selective exposure to sex education and differential absorption of sex information as a function of erotophobia-erotophilia (Fisher, Grenier, et al., 1988; Gerrard, Kurylo, & Reis, 1991; Gerrard & Reis, 1989). Furthermore, erotophobia-erotophilia has been linked with individual difference measures of sexual preoccupation (Snell, Fisher, & Schuh, 1992); sensation seeking (Bogaert & Fisher, 1995); and sexual permissiveness, openness to diverse sex practices, sexual instrumentality, and sex guilt (Hendrick & Hendrick, 1987). Researchers have also examined the role of erotophobia-erotophilia in the development and maintenance of relationships and have determined that husband-wife similarity of erotophobia-erotophilia is considerable ($r = .58$; see also Fisher & Gray, 1988, for a parallel finding), that husband-wife discrepancies in erotophobia-erotophilia are associated with sexual dissatisfaction, and that the experimental manipulation of perceived similarity of erotophobia-erotophilia is a determinant of interpersonal attraction (Smith, Becker, Byrne, & Przybyla, 1993). Erotophobia-erotophilia has also been found to be associated with homophobia (Ficarrotto, 1990).

It should be noted that as with any construct, null findings have been reported for the relationship of erotophobia-erotophilia and theorized correlates (see references for examples). In interpreting these findings, it would seem important to clarify the psychological meaning of the criterion behavior under study, such as condom use, and to determine whether it reflects approach or avoidance of sexuality and may therefore be legitimately expected to correlate with erotophobia-erotophilia, and if so, in which direction. Some criterion behaviors may represent both approach and avoidance of sexuality for different members of a study population, and this complexity may result in the failure to observe expected relationships with erotophobia-erotophilia.

References

Baffi, C. R., Schroeder, K. K., Redican, K. J., & Lawrence, McCluskey, L. (1989). Factors influencing selected heterosexual male college students' condom use. *Journal of the American College Health Association, 38,* 137-141.

Bogaert, A. E., & Fisher, W. A. (1995). Predictors of university men's number of sexual partners. *The Journal of Sex Research, 32,* 119-130.

Byrne, D. (1977). Social psychology and the study of sexual behavior. *Personality and Social Psychology Bulletin, 1,* 3-30.

Caron, S. L., Davis, C. M., Halteman, W. A., & Stickle, M. (1993). Predictors of condom-related behaviors among first-year college students. *The Journal of Sex Research, 30,* 252-259.

Crowne, D. P., & Marlowe, D. (1964). *The approval motive: Studies in evaluative dependence.* New York: Wiley.

Ficarrotto, T. J. (1990). Racism, sexism, and erotophobia: Attitudes of heterosexuals toward homosexuals. *Journal of Homosexuality, 19,* 111-116.

Ficarrotto, T. J., & Braun-Munzinger, G. (1986, August). *Correlates of homophobia in Germany and the United States.* Paper presented at the annual meeting of the American Psychological Association, Washington, DC.

Fisher, W. A. (1984). Predicting contraceptive behavior among university men: The roles of emotions and behavioral intentions. *Journal of Applied Social Psychology, 14,* 104-123.

Fisher, W. A. (1986). A psychological approach to human sexuality: The Sexual Behavior Sequence. In D. Byrne & K. Kelley (Eds.), *Alternative approaches to the study of sexual behavior* (pp. 131-171). Hillsdale, NJ: Lawrence Erlbaum.

Fisher, W. A., Byrne, D., White, L. A., & Kelley, K. (1988). Erotophobia-erotophilia as a dimension of personality. *The Journal of Sex Research, 25,* 123-151.

Fisher, W. A., & Gray, J. (1988). Erotophobia-erotophilia and couples' sexual behavior during pregnancy and postpartum. *The Journal of Sex Research, 25,* 379-396.

Fisher, W. A., Grenier, G., Watters, W. W., Lamont, J., Cohen, M., & Askwith, J. (1988). Students' sexual knowledge, attitudes toward sex, and willingness to treat sexual concerns. *Journal of Medical Education, 63,* 379-385.

Freimuth, V. S., Hammond, S. L., Edgar, T., McDonald, D. A., & Fink, E. L. (1992). Factors explaining intent, discussion, and use of condoms in first-time sexual encounters. *Health Education Research, 7,* 203-215.

Gerrard, M., Kurylo, M., & Reis, T. (1991). Self-esteem, erotophobia, and retention of contraceptive and AIDS information in the classroom. *Journal of Applied Social Psychology, 21,* 368-379.

Gerrard, M., & Luus, C. A. E. (1995). Judgments of vulnerability to pregnancy: The role of risk factors and individual differences. *Personality and Social Psychology Bulletin, 21,* 160-171.

Gerrard, M., & Reis, T. J. (1989). Retention of contraceptive and AIDS information in the classroom. *The Journal of Sex Research, 26,* 315-323.

Gilbert, F. S., & Gamache, M. P. (1984). The Sexual Opinion Survey: Structure and use. *The Journal of Sex Research, 20,* 293-309.

Hendrick, S., & Hendrick, C. (1987). Multidimensionality of sexual attitudes. *The Journal of Sex Research, 23,* 502-526.

Hurlbert, D. F. (1992). Factors influencing a woman's decision to end an extramarital sexual relationship. *Journal of Sex & Marital Therapy, 18,* 104-113.

Hurlbert, D. F., & Apt, C. (1991). Sexual narcissism and the abusive male. *Journal of Sex & Marital Therapy, 17,* 279-292.

Hurlbert, D. F., Apt, C., & Rabehl, S. M. (1993). Key variables to understanding female sexual satisfaction: An examination of

women in nondistressed marriages. *Journal of Sex & Marital Therapy, 19,* 154-165.

Kelley, K., Smeaton, G., Byrne, D., Przybyla, D. P. J., & Fisher, W. A. (1987). Sexual attitudes and contraception among females across five college samples. *Human Relations, 40,* 237-254.

Levitt, E. E., & Brady, J. P. (1965). Sexual preferences in young adult males and some correlates. *Journal of Clinical Psychology, 21,* 347-359.

Rise, J., Traeen, B., & Kraft, P. (1993). The Sexual Opinion Survey scale: A study on dimensionality in Norwegian adolescents. *Health Education Research, 8,* 485-494.

Semph, M. E. (1979). *Emotional orientation towards sexuality: Its relation to expecting and perceiving contraceptive side effects.* Unpublished honours thesis, University of Western Ontario, Department of Psychology, London, Ontario, Canada.

Smith, E. R., Becker, M. A., Byrne, D., & Przybyla, D. P. J. (1993). Sexual attitudes of males and females as predictors of interpersonal attraction and marital compatibility. *Journal of Applied Social Psychology, 23,* 1011-1034.

Snell, W. E., Fisher, T. D., & Schuh, T. (1992). Reliability and validity of the Sexuality Scale: A measure of sexual-esteem, sexual-depression, and sexual-preoccupation. *The Journal of Sex Research, 29,* 261-273.

Tanner, W. M., & Pollack, R. H. (1988). The effect of condom use and erotic instructions on attitudes toward condoms. *The Journal of Sex Research, 25,* 537-541.

White, L. A., Fisher, W. A., Byrne, D., & Kingma, R. (1977, May). *Development and validation of a measure of affective orientation to erotic stimuli: The Sexual Opinion Survey.* Paper presented at the annual meeting of the Midwestern Psychological Association, Chicago.

Wilson, D., & Marindo, R. (1989). Erotophobia and contraception among Zimbabwean students. *Journal of Social Psychology, 129,* 721-723.

Yarber, W. L., & Fisher, W. A. (1983). Affective orientation to sexuality and venereal disease preventive behaviors. *Health Values, 7,* 19-23.

Yarber, W. L., & McCabe, G. P. (1981). Teacher characteristics and the inclusion of sex education topics in Grades 6-8 and 9-11. *Journal of School Health, 51,* 288-291.

Yarber, W. L., & Whitehill, L. L. (1981). The relationship between parental affective orientation toward sexuality and response to sex-related situations of preschool-age children. *Journal of Sex Education and Therapy, 7,* 36-39.

Exhibit

The Sexual Opinion Survey

Please respond to each item as honestly as you can. There are no right or wrong answers, and your answers will be completely anonymous.

1. I think it would be very entertaining to look at hard-core erotica (sexually explicit books, movies, etc.).
   I strongly agree   I strongly disagree[a]
2. Erotica is obviously filthy and people should not try to describe it as anything else.
3. Swimming in the nude with a member of the opposite sex would be an exciting experience.
4. Masturbation can be an exciting experience.
5. If I found that a close friend of mine was a homosexual, it would annoy me.
6. If people thought that I was interested in oral sex, I would be embarrassed.
7. Engaging in group sex is an entertaining idea.
8. I personally find that thinking about engaging in sexual intercourse is arousing.
9. Seeing a pornographic movie would be sexually arousing to me.

10. Thoughts that I may have homosexual tendencies would not worry me at all.
11. The idea of my being physically attracted to members of the same sex is not depressing.
12. Almost all pornographic material is nauseating.
13. It would be emotionally upsetting to me to see someone exposing themselves publicly.
14. Watching a stripper of the opposite sex would not be very exciting.
15. I would not enjoy seeing an erotic movie.
16. When I think about seeing pictures showing someone of the same sex as myself masturbating, it nauseates me.
17. The thought of engaging in unusual sex practices is highly arousing.
18. Manipulating my genitals would probably be an arousing experience.
19. I do not enjoy daydreaming about sexual matters.
20. I am not curious about explicit erotica.
21. The thought of having long-term sexual relations with more than one sex partner is not disgusting to me.

Source. This survey was originally published in *The Journal of Sex Research* (1988). Reprinted with permission.

Note. Score the survey as follows. First, score responses from 1 = *I strongly agree* to 7 = *I strongly disagree*. Second, add scores from Items 2, 5, 6, 12, 13, 14, 15, 16, 19, and 20. Third, subtract from this total the sum of Items 1, 3, 4, 7, 8, 9, 10, 11, 17, 18, and 21. Fourth, add 67 to this quantity. Scores range from 0 (most erotophobic) to 126 (most erotophilic). For the short form of the SOS, administer Items 12, 4, 13, 17, and 21 (in this order, renumbered 1-5) and score responses from 1 = *I strongly agree* to 7 = *I strongly disagree*.

a. The scale is repeated after each item.

Hurlbert Index of Sexual Excitability

David F. Hurlbert,[1] *Adult and Adolescent Counseling Center*

The Hurlbert Index of Sexual Excitability (HISE) is described by Hurlbert, Apt, and Rabehl (1993).

[1]Address correspondence to David F. Hurlbert, Adult and Adolescent Counseling Center, 619 North Main, Belton, TX 76513.

Reference

Hurlbert, D. F., Apt, C., & Rabehl, S. M. (1993). Key variables to understanding female sexual satisfaction: An examination of women in nondistressed marriages. *Journal of Sex & Marital Therapy, 19,* 154-165.

Exhibit

Hurlbert Index of Sexual Excitability

1. I quickly become sexually excited during foreplay. (R)
2. I find sex with my partner to be exciting. (R)
3. When it comes to having sex with my partner, I experience orgasms. (R)
4. It is difficult for me to become sexually aroused.
5. During sex, I seem to lose interest after initial level of sexual excitement.
6. I feel I take too long to get sexually aroused.
7. It is hard for me to become sexually excited.
8. Sex is boring.
9. I quickly become sexually excited when my partner performs oral sex on me. (R)

10. Just thinking about sex turns me on. (R)
11. I find anal sex to be exciting. (R)
12. When it comes to sex, I am easily aroused by my partner touching me. (R)
13. I find masturbation to be sexually stimulating. (R)
14. I seem to lose my sexual excitement too fast.
15. Kissing is sexually arousing for me. (R)
16. Even when I am in the mood, it is difficult for me to get excited about sex.
17. Sexual foreplay is exciting for me. (R)
18. When it comes to sex, it seems to take me a long time to get sexually aroused.
19. Pleasing my partner is sexually exciting for me. (R)
20. I have difficulty maintaining my sexual excitement.
21. I find sexual intercourse to be exciting. (R)
22. When it comes to sex, I think my level of sexual excitement is low.
23. Even when I desire sex, it seems hard for me to become excited.
24. Giving my partner oral sex is sexually exciting for me. (R)
25. In general, sex is satisfying for me. (R)

Source. This index was originally published in "Key Variables to Understanding Female Sexual Satisfaction: An Examination of Women in Nondistressed Marriages," by D. F. Hurlbert, C. Apt, and S. M. Rabehl, 1993, *Journal of Sex & Marital Therapy, 19,* 154-165. Reprinted with permission.

Note. (R) = reverse-scored items. Scoring system responses: *all of the time* = 0 points; *most of the time* = +1 point; *some of the time* = +2 points; *rarely* = +3 points; *never* = +4 points.

Extramarital Behavioral Intentions Scale

Bram Buunk,[1] *University of Nijmegen*

Several researchers have correlated the incidence of extramarital sex with variables such as dissatisfaction with the marital relationship, assuming that these factors could be viewed as *causes* for engaging in extramarital relationships (e.g., Bell, Turner, & Rosen, 1975). In this type of research, however, it is difficult to unravel the direction of causality (Buunk, 1980a). To better assess the factors that do indeed lead to extramarital sexual involvement, a scale assessing extramarital behavioral intentions was developed, based on Fishbein and Ajzen's (1975) theoretical perspective. From this perspective, a behavioral intention is defined as the subjective probability that someone will exhibit a certain behavior if the opportunity presents itself. As Fishbein and Ajzen have argued, and have shown in many studies, specific behavioral intentions correlate highly with actual

future behavior. Another assumption behind the construction of the scale was that there is a continuum of extramarital sexual involvement, varying from flirting to a long-term sexual relationship, and that such a continuum should be included in the scale.

Description, Response Mode, and Timing

The scale consists of five items. The format for each item is the same. The respondents are asked to indicate for each of the following behaviors the probability of engaging in it were an opportunity to present itself: flirting, light petting, falling in love, sexual intercourse, and a long-term sexual relationship with someone other than their partner. The seven response options range from *certainly no* to *certainly yes,* with a midpoint formulated as *uncertain.* Each of the possible answers is spelled out literally. The respondents circle the number corresponding with the answer that best fits the perceived likelihood under consideration. The scale

[1]Address correspondence to Bram Buunk, University of Nijmegen, Postbus 9104, 6500 HE Nijmegen, The Netherlands.

usually requires no more than 1 or 2 minutes for completion.

Scoring

The items can simply be summed. No reverse scoring is necessary. Higher scores indicate a higher intention to engage in extramarital sexual behaviors.

Reliability

Although there are slight variations across samples, the Cronbach alpha of the scale is rather high: .91 in a sample more or less representing the general Dutch population and consisting of people with diverse levels of sexual permissiveness (Buunk, 1980a); .73 in a study of people who had all been involved in extramarital relationships (Buunk, 1982); .75 in a sample of people in sexually open marriages (Buunk, 1980b), and .87 in a sample of undergraduate students. Over a 3-month period, test-retest reliability in the open-marriage sample was $r(100) = .70, p < .001$. Furthermore, the scale fulfills the requirements of a Guttman scale, with a coefficient of scalability of .78 and a coefficient of reproducibility of .92. The order of the items in the Guttman scale is flirting, falling in love, light petting, sexual intercourse, and a long-term sexual relationship (Buunk, 1980a).

Validity

There is considerable evidence for the concurrent validity of the scale. In the sample from the average population, it was found that the more extensive the extramarital experience had been during the previous year, the higher the scores on the Extramarital Behavioral Intentions Scale, $r(250) = .74, p < .001$. The scale particularly differentiates between persons high and low in sexual permissiveness. Individuals from the open-marriage sample scored much higher on the scale than a sample more or less representative of the average population, $t(348) = 22.46, p < .001$, and also much higher than a sample of undergraduate students, $t(478) = 15.16, p < .001$. Also, the Extramarital Behavioral Intentions Scale clearly discriminates between those whose reference group accepts extramarital sex and those who socialize with others disapproving of such behavior: The scale correlated highly with one's friends' approval of extramarital sex and the perceived opportunity for extramarital sex (Buunk, 1980a).

Construct validity of the scale has been established in several studies showing positive correlations with scales indicating permissive attitudes toward extramarital sex, and negative correlations with scales measuring the opposite. Thus, in the sample of individuals from the average population, a negative correlation was established with a scale measuring the desire for an exclusive relationship, $r(250) = -.54, p < .001$, and positive correlations were found with scales reflecting needs for intimacy outside marriage and for relational variety (see Buunk, 1980a). In the same sample, the Extramarital Behavioral Intentions Scale correlated highly and negatively with a scale measuring moral disapproval of extramarital sex, $r(250) = -.65, p < .001$ (cf. Buunk, 1981). Furthermore, in three samples strong negative correlations were found between the scale and a scale for anticipated sexual jealousy (Buunk, 1982). Also, in the sample of persons who had been involved in extramarital relationships, a positive correlation was found between the Extramarital Behavioral Intentions Scale and a scale for Psychosexual Stimulation developed by Frenken (1976), $r(250) = .21, p < .001$. This last scale measures the tendency to allow sexual perceptions and fantasizing about sexuality versus the tendency to suppress such perceptions and fantasies.

Final evidence for the validity of the Extramarital Behavioral Intentions Scale comes from the open-marriage study. Here, among women, a high correlation was found between the scale and their extramarital intentions as perceived by their husbands, $r(50) = .53, p < .001$. The same correlation among men was somewhat lower, but also significant, $r(50) = .42, p < .001$.

References

Bell, R. R., Turner, S., & Rosen, L. (1975). A multivariate analysis of female extramarital coitus. *Journal of Marriage and the Family, 37,* 375-384.

Buunk, B. (1980a). Extramarital sex in the Netherlands: Motivations in social and marital context. *Alternative Lifestyles, 3,* 11-39.

Buunk, B. (1980b). Sexually open marriages. Ground rules for countering potential threats to marriage. *Alternative Lifestyles, 3,* 312-328.

Buunk, B. (1981). De samenhang van attitudes en sociale normen met de intentie tot buitenechtelijke sex [The relationships between extramarital behavioral intentions and attitudes and social norms]. *Nederlands Tidschrift voor de Psychologie, 36,* 165-170.

Buunk, B. (1982). Anticipated sexual jealousy: Its relationships to self-esteem, dependency and reciprocity. *Personality and Social Psychology Bulletin, 8,* 310-316.

Fishbein, M., & Ajzen, I. (1975). *Belief, attitude, intention, and behavior.* Reading, MA: Addison-Wesley.

Frenken, J. (1976). *Afkeer van seksualiteit* [Aversion to sexuality]. Beventer: Van Loghum Slaterus.

Exhibit

Extramarital Behavioral Intentions Scale

Would you engage in the following behavior with another man/woman if the opportunity were to present itself?

1. Flirting
   a. certainly not
   b. probably not
   c. maybe not
   d. uncertain
   e. maybe yes
   f. probably yes
   g. certainly yes

2. Sexual intercourse[a]
3. Light petting
4. A long-term sexual relationship
5. Falling in love

Source. This scale is reprinted with permission of the author.
a. The seven response options are repeated for each item.

Reiss Extramarital Sexual Permissiveness Scale

Ira L. Reiss,[1] *University of Minnesota*

The scale measures the degree to which people accept extramarital coitus for themselves under several culturally relevant conditions. There are two sets of four questions each that can be used as measures of the conditions, if any, under which one would accept extramarital coitus, when in a happy marriage and when in an unhappy marriage.

Description

The questions ask about the acceptability to the respondent of extramarital coitus under the following specific conditions: (a) The extramarital relationship emphasizes a love relationship; (b) the extramarital relationship emphasizes physical pleasure; (c) your spouse does not accept your having that type of physical or love-focused extramarital

relationship; and (d) your spouse accepts your having that type of physical or love-focused extramarital relationship. The resultant four questions are asked separately with reference to being in a happy marriage and for being in an unhappy marriage.

These four conditions and the happiness of the marriage are assumed to be the key decision bases for people in Western culture when judging the acceptability of extramarital coitus. In addition, because the Western world generally grants greater sexual rights to men, it may be helpful also to ask respondents if they would accept from their mates the same responses they themselves gave. To make this instrument relevant to as wide a range of populations as possible, the format asks people to assume they are in a happy marriage on four questions and then to assume they are in an unhappy marriage and answer the same four questions. That format makes the instrument relevant even to unmarried people and does not force married people to globally and permanently define their own marital state as either happy or unhappy.

[1]Address correspondence to Ira L. Reiss, Department of Sociology, University of Minnesota, 267 19th Avenue South, Minneapolis, MN 55455-0412; email: reiss001@atlas.socsci.umm.edu.

Early forms of the scales were used in doctoral dissertations (Dunn, 1980; Raschke, 1972). Other researchers compared our questions to their own formulations and afforded us many insights (Glass & Wright, 1992; Sponaugle, 1993). Together with two colleagues, I analyzed four national samples to help examine the key determinants involved in extramarital sexual attitudes (Reiss, Anderson, & Sponaugle, 1980). The final version of the scales presented here grew out of these many research endeavors.

Response Mode and Timing

Respondents are given a choice between acceptance or rejection on each of the questions in terms of their personal values about marriage. For simplicity, I would combine the responses *definitely* and *probably* as acceptance responses and combine *unlikely* and *never* as rejection. If researchers wish to measure degree of acceptance or rejection, they can analyze all four responses separately. Most respondents answer all eight questions in 4 or 5 minutes.

Scoring

Each set of four questions can be treated separately and 1 point assigned for each affirmative response. One could also apply Guttman scaling techniques and compose two 4-item Guttman scales. Regardless of the scaling method used, the responses to all eight questions can be combined into one overall score. In addition, comparisons can be made between the "happy marriage" and "unhappy marriage" scores on the relative endorsement of the four extramarital conditions. Responses can also be checked for differences when answered by wives or by husbands. Special checks can be made on currently married respondents. Married respondents can be asked to rate their current marriage and differences in responses examined between those who rate their current marriage happy or unhappy. Egalitarianism can be measured by asking the respondents if they would accept their partners, or potential partners, if they gave the same responses as they themselves gave. A great deal of theoretical value, helpful in building an explanation of attitudes toward extramarital coitus, can be obtained in all these types of analyses.

Reliability

The scales meet general Guttman criteria concerning the coefficient of reproducibility and coefficient of scalability.

Validity

My colleagues and I analyzed four different national samples from four different years to find the best predictors of extramarital sexual permissiveness attitudes (Reiss et al., 1980). All these analyses supported very similar findings as to key predictors of extramarital attitudes. All four national samples used the same variables and were all carried out by the National Opinion Research Center.

Construct validity was established by finding the expected differences between religiously devout and nondevout groups of people and between men and women (Dunn, 1980; Raschke, 1972; Sponaugle, 1993). Other researchers reported finding dimensions, duplicative of those in my four questions, as important in measuring extramarital acceptance within their own formats (Glass & Wright, 1992; Sponaugle, 1993).

Other Information

I would be interested in being sent a summary of your research results if the scale is used.

References

Dunn, M. E. (1980). *Women's perceptions of male's sexual attractiveness: The role of male eye contact.* Unpublished doctoral dissertation, Institute for Advanced Study in Human Sexuality, San Francisco.

Glass, S. P., & Wright, T. L. (1992). Justifications for extramarital relationships: The association between attitudes, behaviors, and gender. *The Journal of Sex Research, 29,* 361-387.

Raschke, V. J., (1972). *Religiosity and sexual permissiveness.* Unpublished doctoral dissertation, University of Minnesota, Minneapolis.

Reiss, I. L., Anderson, R., & Sponaugle, G. C. (1980). A multivariate model of the determinants of extramarital sexual permissiveness. *Journal of Marriage and the Family, 42,* 395-411.

Sponaugle, G. C. (1993). *A study of attitudes toward extramarital relations.* Unpublished doctoral dissertation, University of Minnesota, Minneapolis.

Exhibit

Reiss Extramarital Sexual Permissiveness Scale (revised, 1995)

Answer in terms of your personal values concerning what you would accept in your marriage under the conditions stated. (If you are not currently married answer in terms of a possible future marriage.)

Assume you are in a happy marriage and answer the following four questions:

1. Would you accept an extramarital relationship in which physical pleasure is your focus even though your mate would not accept your having such a relationship?
   a) Definitely   b) Probably   c) Unlikely   d) Never[a]
2. Would you accept an extramarital relationship in which physical pleasure is your focus if your mate would accept your having this type of relationship?

3. Would you accept an extramarital relationship in which love is emphasized even though your mate would not accept your having such a relationship?
4. Would you accept an extramarital relationship in which love is emphasized if your mate would accept your having this type of relationship?

Assume you are in an unhappy marriage and answer the following four questions:[b]

Source. This scale is reprinted with permission of the author.
a. These same four choices follow every question.
b. The four questions are repeated.

Interview Schedule for Couples Involved in Sexually Open Marriages

The Editors

This instrument was originally created by Knapp (1976) as an interview schedule for couples with sexually open marriages. She subsequently converted it into a self-report questionnaire (Schechter, 1981). Many items are open ended; others are Likert type or forced choice.

Additional information and the instrument may be obtained from the first editor.

References

Knapp, J. (1976). An exploratory study of seventeen sexually open marriages. *The Journal of Sex Research, 12,* 206-219.
Schechter, J. (1981). *Personality and sexually open marriage.* Unpublished manuscript.

Attitudes Toward Marital Exclusivity Scale

David L. Weis,[1] *Bowling Green State University*

In recent years, researchers have given increasing attention to the investigation of extramarital relationships. Most of this research has focused on extramarital sexuality (ES). Prominent concerns of researchers have included the incidence of ES, the association between ES and marital happiness, the phenomenon of swinging, the social-psychological correlates of ES attitudes, and the dynamics of ES relationships.

Relatively little research has studied nonsexual extramarital relationships (NERs). This is unfortunate in at least two respects. First, it is obvious that virtually all married persons form relationships of various types and intensity outside their marriages. Little is known about the social networks surrounding married couples or how NERs serve as a source of support/rewards or of conflict/costs for married persons. In fact, cross-sex NERs are frequently cited as a source of marital conflict and jealousy (Clanton & Smith, 1977; Gagnon & Greenblat, 1978; Neubeck, 1969), and there is some evidence that the potential for such conflict is quite high (Weis & Felton, 1987; Weis & Slosnerick, 1981). Second, it seems reasonable to suggest that cross-sex NERs may serve as the social context for subsequent ES involvement. In other words, opportunities for ES are likely to arise in ostensibly nonsexual extramarital interactions (Johnson, 1970; Neubeck, 1969; Weis, 1983).

Viewed in this fashion, marital exclusivity can be seen as a concept determining what married individuals can and cannot share or experience with persons outside their marriages. Moreover, it can be suggested that exclusivity is an issue in all marriages regardless of attitudinal orientation toward ES itself and that it is a much broader issue than ES alone. The Attitudes Toward Marital Exclusivity Scale was designed to measure the extent to which an individual accepts or rejects opportunities for cross-sex interaction when the spouse is not present.

Description

The scale consists of seven 5-point Likert-type items (see the exhibit). The Attitudes Toward Marital Exclusivity Scale was adapted from similar scales used in previous research (Johnson, 1970; Neubeck & Schletzer, 1962). Both studies had employed the "spouse is out of town" scenario to assess projective extramarital involvement. For purposes of the present scale, the scenario was modified; additional extramarital behaviors were added, and the Likert-type scoring was employed. At this time, the scale has been tested with five separate samples of undergraduate students drawn from four American universities.

[1]Address correspondence to David L. Weis, Department of Family and Consumer Sciences, Bowling Green State University, Bowling Green, OH 43403; email: weis@bgnet.bgsu.edu.

The scale was originally included in a questionnaire anonymously administered to 321 undergraduates at a state university in New England (Weis & Slosnerick, 1981). In a subsequent study, the scale was included in a questionnaire anonymously administered to 835 undergraduates at three state universities: one each in the Northeast, Northwest, and Southwest (Weis, Slosnerick, Cate, & Sollie, 1986).

Response Mode, Timing, and Scoring

Respondents are asked to indicate the degree to which they accept or reject each of the behaviors in the scenario presented by writing their response in the appropriate blank. Response options range from *total rejection* to *total acceptance*. The scale can be completed in a few minutes; thus, it is well suited for inclusion in questionnaires assessing additional variables.

For purposes of scoring, responses to individual items are coded as follows: *total rejection* = 1, *moderate rejection* = 2, *no feelings either way* = 3, *moderate acceptance* = 4, and *total acceptance* = 5. A single score for exclusivity attitude is derived for each respondent by summing the responses to each individual item. In this sense, the scale is scored to correspond to the concept of acceptability or permissiveness (Reiss, Anderson, & Sponaugle, 1980). Thus, the greatest degree of acceptance would be represented by a score of 35 (a coding of 5 for each item), and the lowest degree would be represented by a score of 7 (a coding of 1 for each item).

Reliability and Validity

The reliability of the scale with the first sample tested was .87, as indicated by Cronbach's alpha. Initial data concerning the construct validity of the scale were also obtained. Exclusivity attitudes were found to be significantly related to two separate measures of ES attitude and to sex-love-marriage association. Students who tended to accept the various extramarital situations were more likely to approve ES and were less likely to cognitively associate sex, love, and marriage.

Reliability coefficients for each of the three university samples tested in the second phase ranged from .85 to .88. This data set also allowed a fuller examination of the construct validity of the scale. Persons who tend to find the extramarital situations acceptable were found to be significantly more likely to have had multilateral sexual and dating experiences, to have participated in a greater range of sexual behaviors, and to believe that they could form intimate relationships with a number of alternative partners. They were also less likely to cognitively associate sex, love, and marriage or to be currently involved in an exclusive relationship.

Weis and Felton (1987) have used the scale in a study of 379 unmarried, female students at a state university in the Northeast. They reported a reliability coefficient of .81 and found the scale to be significantly related to a separate measure of ES attitude, jealousy, sex-love association, and intimacy diffusion (belief that persons in love maintain interest in other possible partners).

In a more recent investigation, Weis and his associates (Moore-Hirschl, Parra, Weis, & Laflin, 1995) used the scale in a study of 1,372 female college students matriculating at a state university between 1980 and 1988. They found little change in attitudes toward sexual and nonsexual involvements during this time period. The scale exhibited sound measurement properties for all years of the study. Cronbach's alphas ranged from .74 to .83. Moreover, the scale met a series of criteria for Guttman scaling. Comparable analyses with male samples remain to be conducted.

References

Clanton, G., & Smith, L. G. (Eds.). (1977). *Jealousy*. Englewood Cliffs, NJ: Prentice Hall.

Gagnon, J. H., & Greenblat, C. S. (1978). *Life designs: individuals, marriages, and families*. Glenview, IL: Scott, Foresman.

Johnson, R. D. (1970). Extramarital sexual intercourse: A methodological note. *Journal of Marriage and the Family, 32*, 279-282.

Moore-Hirschl, S., Parra, L. F., Weis, D. L., & Laflin, M. T. (1995). Attitudes of college females toward marital exclusivity over a nine-year period. *Journal of Psychology & Human Sexuality, 7*, 61-75.

Neubeck, G. (Ed.). (1969). *Extramarital relations*. Englewood Cliffs, NJ: Prentice Hall.

Neubeck, G., & Schletzer, V. (1962). A study of extramarital relationships. *Marriage and Family Living, 24*, 279-281.

Reiss, I. L., Anderson, R. E., & Sponaugle, G. C. (1980). A multivariate model of the determinants of extramarital sexual permissiveness. *Journal of Marriage and the Family, 42*, 395-411.

Weis, D. L. (1983, March 6). *Extramarital sex scripts at professional conventions*. Paper presented at Philadelphia Chapter of the Society for the Scientific Study of Sex, Philadelphia.

Weis, D. L., & Felton, J. R. (1987). Attitudes toward marital exclusivity among female college students: The potential for future marital conflict. *Social Work, 32*(1), 45-49.

Weis, D. L., & Slosnerick, M. (1981). Attitudes toward sexual and nonsexual extramarital involvements among a sample of college students. *Journal of Marriage and the Family, 43*, 349-358.

Weis, D. L., Slosnerick, M., Cate, R. M., & Sollie, D. L. (1986). A survey instrument for assessing the cognitive association of sex, love, and marriage. *The Journal of Sex Research, 22*, 206-220.

Exhibit

Attitudes Toward Marital Exclusivity Scale

Indicate the extent to which you would reject or accept each of the following situations by writing your answer in the blank. To answer, use these responses:

1. Total rejection
2. Moderate rejection
3. No feelings either way
4. Moderate acceptance
5. Total acceptance

(If you are single, answer as you would if were married.)

Suppose that you were very close friends with several married couples in the _____ area. As it happened, your husband (wife) had gone on an extended trip, leaving you home alone. A similar thing happens to some of your close friends. That is, the wife (husband) of one of these acquaintances left the state of _____ to visit relatives, leaving her husband (wife) home alone.

How would you feel about:
_____ 1. Spending an evening or evenings with him (her) in his (her) living room?
_____ 2. Going to the movies or theater together?
_____ 3. Going out to dinner with him (her) at a secluded place?
_____ 4. Dancing with him (her) to the stereo?
_____ 5. Spending a couple of days at a secluded cabin with him (her) near a beautiful lake where no one would find out?
_____ 6. Harmless necking or petting?
_____ 7. Becoming sexually involved?

Source. This scale is reprinted with permission of the author.

Population Policy Questionnaire

The Editors

The Population Policy Questionnaire (PPQ) is designed to assess five attitudinal aspects of population policy: contraception, abortion, family planning, population management, and modernity or progressivism. Each of the five scales in the PPQ contains eight items. Details concerning the development and use of the test were described in Gough (1975). An Italian standardization is presented in Lazzari and Gough (1977). It takes about 20 minutes to complete the questionnaire.

Additional information and a copy of the instrument may be obtained from the first editor.

References

Gough, H. G. (1975). An attitude profile for studies of population psychology. *Journal of Research in Personality, 9,* 122-135.

Gough, H. G. (1976). A measure of individual modernity. *Journal of Personality Assessment, 40,* 3-9.

Gough, H. G. (1977). Further validation of a measure of individual modernity. *Journal of Personality Assessment, 41,* 49-57.

Gough, H. G., Gendre, F., & Lazzari, R. (1976). Attitudes toward the number of children wanted and expected by college students in three countries. *Journal of Cross-Cultural Psychology, 7,* 413-424.

Lazzari, R., & Gough, H. G. (1977). Primi risultati di una ricerca per la misura degli atteggiamenti verso l'aborto, il controllo delle nascite, la painficazione familiare e la politica demografica. *Aggiornamenti in Ostetricia e Ginecologia, 10,* 375-383.

Child-Timing Questionnaire and Childbearing Questionnaire

Warren B. Miller,[1] *Transnational Family Research Institute*

The purpose of the Child-Timing Questionnaire (CTQ) is to measure attitudes and beliefs relevant to when or how soon the respondent would like to have a child. The purpose of the Childbearing Questionnaire (CBQ) is to measure general and specific motives of the respondent for having children. These questionnaires derive from a theoretical framework (Miller, 1994; Miller & Pasta, 1994) in which motives, attitudes, and beliefs are proposed to contribute to conscious desires, which in turn influence intentions and, ultimately, behaviors. The CBQ and CTQ assess

childbearing motives and child-timing attitudes and beliefs, which form part of the basis for childbearing, child-timing, and child-number desires. These desires ultimately lead to reproductive behaviors, both proceptive (intended to increase fertility) and contraceptive.

Description

CTQ. Respondents indicate how desirable it is that the timing of the first (or next) child fit with 14 aspects of the respondent's life, such as health and career, with each aspect referred to as a "consequence." They then indicate their belief about how soon each of the 14 consequences is likely to apply to them. One item is open ended, allowing respondents to indicate relevant consequences omitted from the

[1]Address correspondence to Warren B. Miller, Director, Transnational Family Research Institute, 355 West Olive Avenue, Suite 207, Sunnyvale, CA 94086.

previous items. Male and female versions of the CTQ are almost identical, except for a single item about physical readiness for childbearing ("having a child when I am physically ready" for the female version was altered to "having a child when my wife is physically ready" for the male version).

CTQ items may then be divided into two scales. The Child-Timing Index (CTI) includes all items related to the respondent's own readiness, and the Child-Timing Index–Spouse (CTIS) includes all items related to the perceived readiness of the respondent's spouse. Two additional indexes, the Don't Know Index and the Don't Know Index–Spouse, are calculated from the proportion of relevant items answered "don't know" by the respondent.

CBQ. The CBQ includes two parts, related to (a) desirable and (b) undesirable consequences of having a child. In Part 1, respondents indicate on a 4-point scale how desirable each of 28 consequences is. In Part 2, they indicate how undesirable 21 consequences are, using the same 4-point scale. Male and female versions are nearly identical except for appropriate changes in item wording (e.g., substituting "wife" for "husband") or item structure (e.g., substituting "seeing my wife experiencing the pain of childbirth" for "experiencing the pain of childbirth").

Scores for the desirable and undesirable consequences form two main scales for the CBQ: positive childbearing motivation (PCM) and negative childbearing motivation (NCM). In addition, factor analysis (Miller, 1995) derived five subscales for the PCM and four for the NCM, describing more discrete components of each type of motivation (e.g., "satisfactions of childrearing" and "negatives of childcare").

Although both questionnaires are worded so as to apply to married heterosexual couples, it would be possible to modify the wording so as to apply to unmarried couples or to homosexual couples (such as lesbian partners) seeking to have a child.

Response Mode and Timing

For the CTQ attitude (desirability) items, respondents indicate, using a 4-point scale, how desirable each consequence of child timing is (from *very* to *moderately* to *slightly* to *not*). For beliefs about when each consequence will apply to them, respondents indicate either a specific number of years and months or fill in *now, never, DNA (does not apply),* or *DK (don't know)*. On the CBQ, respondents circle the term indicating how desirable or undesirable they find each consequence of childbearing, with the same four response options used in the CTQ.

There are no specific times for completion. The CTQ generally takes 8 to 10 minutes to complete. The CBQ requires about 10 to 12 minutes to complete.

Reliability and Validity

For the CTQ, 2-week test-retest correlations ranged from .67 to .89 with a sample of husbands and wives with one child (Miller & Pasta, 1994). For the CBQ, Cronbach's alpha ranged from .83 to .94 for a similar sample of both husbands and wives with either one or no child. Two-week test-retest correlations for the CBQ ranged from .81 to .93.

Evidence of validity for the CTQ comes from its relationship to respondent ratings of both intentions and desires to have a first (or second) child (Miller & Pasta, 1994). In regression analyses including the CTQ and additional variables such as childbearing desires, marital duration, and marital problems, the CTI of the CTQ emerged as the most important predictor of both child-timing desires and child-timing intentions.

Evidence for validity of the CBQ comes from respondents' information on childbearing desires and intentions, number of children desired, and reported efforts to conceive at follow-up interviews conducted 1, 2, and 3.5 years after initial data collection (Miller, 1995). Both the PCM and NCM scales were significantly correlated in predicted directions with respondents' ratings of their desire to have children and their childbearing intentions. In addition, PCM was significantly correlated in the predicted direction with actual efforts to conceive (proceptive sexual behaviors), and NCM was also correlated as predicted with proceptive behaviors, although this relationship was significant only for men and women who were still childless.

Other Information

The questionnaires are available from Warren B. Miller, Director, Transnational Family Research Institute, 355 West Olive Avenue, Suite 207, Sunnyvale, CA 94086.

References

Miller, W. B. (1994). Childbearing motivations, desires, and intentions: A theoretical framework. *Genetic, Social, and General Psychology Monographs, 120*(2), 223-258.

Miller, W. B. (1995). Childbearing motivation and its measurement. *Journal of Biosocial Science, 27,* 473-487.

Miller, W. B., & Pasta, D. J. (1994). The psychology of child-timing: A measurement instrument and a model. *Journal of Applied Social Psychology, 24,* 218-250.

Exhibit

Child-Timing Questionnaire (sample items)

Wife/One Child Version

Section I

In planning the timing of your second child, how desirable are each of the following consequences—circle the word "not" if the consequence does not apply to you or if you feel neutral about the consequence.

	How Desirable			
1. Having a child when I am physically ready	Very	Moderately	Slightly	Not
3. Having a child when it fits best with my career or work	Very	Moderately	Slightly	Not

Section II

Complete each statement below by indicating as well as you can in years and months how soon each one is likely to be true. For example, if a statement will be true for you in about a year and a half, write:

... in 1 years and 6 months.

1. I will be physically ready for a child in _____ years and _____ months.
9. My husband will feel personally ready for a child in _____ years and _____ months.

Childbearing Questionnaire (sample items)

Male version

Part I

Below are listed some consequences of having children. Read over the list and indicate how desirable each one is to you by circling one of the four answers in the column on the right. If you feel that a consequence is very desirable, then circle the word "very."

Desirable Consequences	How Desirable			
1. Knowing that I am fertile.	Very	Moderately	Slightly	Not
4. Giving my wife/partner the satisfaction of motherhood.	Very	Moderately	Slightly	Not

Part II

In this part of the questionnaire we have listed some of the consequences of having children that can be undesirable. Use the same way of answering as in Part I, except remember that this time "very" means very undesirable, "moderately" means moderately undesirable, etc. Thus, if you feel that an item is very undesirable, circle the word "very."

Undesirable Consequences	How Undesirable			
1. Seeing my wife/partner experience the discomforts of pregnancy.	Very	Moderately	Slightly	Not
5. Being responsible for a needy and demanding baby.	Very	Moderately	Slightly	Not

Source. These sample items from the questionnaires are reprinted with permission of the author.

Sexual Daydreaming Scale of the Imaginal Processes Inventory

Leonard M. Giambra,[1] *National Institute on Aging*
Jerome L. Singer, *Yale University*

The Imaginal Processes Inventory (IPI) was developed to measure the various aspects of daydreaming and related mental processes, such as attention, distractibility, and curiosity. The IPI is intended to be taken by normally functioning persons and is meant to measure the range of normal functioning. The Sexual Daydreaming Scale (SDS) was constructed to reveal the extent to which a person has daydreams of a sexual or erotic nature.

Description

The SDS consists of 12 items selected initially by requesting a large sample of "normal" adults to record their recurrent fantasies. An additional sample of respondents reviewed these fantasies and checked off those they had experienced by indicating the degree of frequency on a Likert-type scale. Those items bearing specifically on sexuality and showing reasonable intercorrelations as well as relatively normal distributions on the 5-point scale were employed for further refinement in the procedure used for generating the 12-item scales of the IPI (Singer & Antrobus, 1963, 1972). In general, this scale has not been used to any degree independently of the other 27 scales that make up the IPI because it loads on at least two of the three second-order factors that consistently emerge from the larger questionnaire.

Response Mode and Scoring

Each of the 12 items has the same five optional responses: *definitely not true for me, usually not true for me, usually true for me, true for me,* and *very true for me.* These options, in the order given, are assigned increasing larger integer values, either 0 to 4 or 1 to 5, depending on the study cited. All items are scored directly, and a scale score consists of the sum of the values of the responses to the 12 items. Using this scoring method, the SDS can range from a minimum of zero to a maximum of 48 (or from 12 to 60). Higher scale scores indicate a greater likelihood of sexual daydreaming. An alternate method of scoring based on a factor analysis of the IPI items is available in Giambra (1980).

Reliability

The internal consistency of the SDS as measured by Cronbach's alpha has been reported to be quite high: .87 (Singer & Antrobus, 1972), .93 (Giambra, 1977-1978), .93 (Giambra, 1979-1980). Test-retest reliability over a 1- to 3-year period based on 45 men was .58, and no significant difference was observed between the first and second testing, $t < 1$.

Validity

In a sample of 565 men and 745 women from 17 to 92 years of age, it was found that the SDS correlated –.56 for men and –.52 for women with age; the partial correlation holding daydreaming frequency constant was –.41 for men and –.40 for women (Giambra, 1979-1980). For a life-span sample of men, Giambra and Martin (1977) determined that men who reported having a greater number of coital partners, who had a greater frequency of coitus during the first year or two of marriage, or who had a higher number of sexual events per week between ages 20 and 40 had significantly higher SDS values. For a sample of 477 women aged 40 to 60 years, the SDS was found to be significantly related to menopausal state, a menopausal symptom index, frequency of masturbation, interest in sexual relations relative to partner, and level of moodiness prior to menstrual period (Giambra, 1983a, 1983b); however, age did interact with these variables.

An extensive study of masturbatory fantasy in college students conducted by Campagna (1975) included a factor analysis of self-reports of sexual behavior as well as the scales of two factors of the IPI. One factor, reflecting a generally positive and constructive acceptance and use of daydreaming, included positive loadings for the SDS. Higher frequency and variability of sexual behavior of a relatively conventional heterosexual type was associated with higher scale scores for sexual fantasy. Those respondents who reported more elaborate, "storylike" masturbation fantasies were also more likely to report more general fantasies and more sexual daydreams on the IPI.

Other Information

A revised, restandardized short form of the IPI (SIPI) has been developed by Huba, Aneshensel, and Singer (1981). This 45-item inventory taps the three second-order factors emerging from the longer IPI. The three scales are Poor Attentional Control (mindwandering and distractibility), Positive-Constructive Daydreaming, and Guilty-Dysphoric

[1]Address correspondence to Leonard M. Giambra, Box 03, Laboratory of Personality and Cognition, NIA/NIH, Johns Hopkins Bayview Campus, 4940 Eastern Avenue, Baltimore, MD 21224; email: leonard-giambra@nih.gov.

Daydreaming. In a study conducted by Rosenberg (1983) examining sexual fantasy and overt behavior in young male adults, there were indications that the Poor Attentional Control pattern characterized men who had more homosexual and less heterosexual fantasies or less masturbatory fantasies involving past sexual experiences. The Guilty Daydreaming Scale was more associated with masturbatory fantasies of beating or domination in masturbatory imagination ($r = .34$). The data suggested positive general daydreaming is associated with a more accepting attitude toward sexual behavior and sexual fantasies.

The longer form of the IPI is copyrighted by Singer and Antrobus and is available at cost from the Test Collection Service of the Educational Testing Service, Princeton, NJ 08540. Persons using the instrument should acknowledge its origin. A copy of any resulting publication would be appreciated by the authors. The SIPI is published by Research Psychologists Press, P.O. Box 984, Port Huron, MI 48060, and specimen copies and manual are available only through the publisher. It has not been studied for clinical application.

References

Campagna, A. F. (1975). *The function of men's erotic fantasies during masturbation.* Unpublished doctoral dissertation, Yale University, New Haven, CT.

Giambra, L. M. (1977-1978). Adult male daydreaming across the lifespan: A replication, further analyses, and tentative norms based upon retrospective reports. *International Journal of Aging and Human Development, 8,* 197-228.

Giambra, L. M. (1979-1980). Sex differences in daydreaming and related mental activity from the late teens to the early nineties. *International Journal of Aging and Human Development, 10,* 1-34.

Giambra, L. M. (1980). A factor analysis of the items for the Imaginal Processes Inventory. *Journal of Clinical Psychology, 36,* 383-409.

Giambra, L. M. (1983a). Daydreaming in 40- to 60-year-old women: Menopause, health, values, and sexuality. *Journal of Clinical Psychology, 39,* 11-21.

Giambra, L. M. (1983b). Sexual daydreams in 40- to 60-year-old women: The influence of menopause, sexual activity, and health. In J. E. Shorr, G. Gobel-Whittington, P. Robin, & J. Connella (Eds.), *Imagery: Theoretical and clinical applications* (Vol. 3, pp. 297-302). New York: Plenum.

Giambra, L. M., & Martin, C. E. (1977). Sexual daydreams and quantitative aspects of sexual activity: Some relations for males across adulthood. *Archives of Sexual Behavior, 6,* 497-505.

Huba, G. J., Aneshensel, C. S., & Singer, J. L. (1981). Development of scales for three second-order factors of inner experience. *Multivariate Behavioral Research, 16,* 181-206.

Rosenberg, L. G. (1983). *Sex-role identification, erotic fantasy and sexual behavior: A study of heterosexual, bisexual and homosexual males.* Unpublished predissertation research, Yale University, New Haven, CT.

Singer, J. L., & Antrobus, J. S. (1963). A factor analytic study of daydreaming and conceptually related cognitive and personality variables [Monograph]. *Perceptual and Motor Skills, 17*(Suppl. 3-V17), 187-209.

Singer, J. L., & Antrobus, J. S. (1972). Daydreaming, imaginal processes, and personality: A normative study. In P. Sheehan (Ed.), *The function and nature of imagery* (pp. 175-202). New York: Academic Press.

Exhibit

Sexual Daydreaming Scale

1. My daydreams about love are so vivid, I actually feel they are occurring.
2. I imagine myself to be physically attractive to people of the opposite sex.
3. While working intently at a job, my mind will wander to thoughts about sex.
4. Sometimes on my way to work, I imagine myself making love to an attractive person of the opposite sex.
5. My sexual daydreams are very vivid and clear in my mind.
6. While reading, I often slip into daydreams about sex or making love to someone.
7. While traveling on a train or bus [or airplane], my idle thoughts turn to love.
8. Whenever I am bored, I daydream about the opposite sex.
9. Sometimes in the middle of the day, I will daydream of having sexual relations with someone I am fond of.
10. In my fantasies, I arouse great desire in someone I admire.
11. Before going to sleep, my idle thoughts turn to lovemaking.
12. My daydreams tend to arouse me physically.

Note. Item 7 has been modified from the original by addition of the material in brackets.

Hurlbert Index of Sexual Fantasy

David F. Hurlbert,[1] *Adult and Adolescent Counseling Center*

The Hurlbert Index of Sexual Fantasy is described by Hurlbert and Apt (1993).

[1]Address correspondence to David F. Hurlbert, Adult and Adolescent Counseling Center, 619 North Main, Belton, TX 76513.

Reference

Hurlbert, D. F., & Apt, C. (1993). Female sexuality: A comparative study between women in homosexual and heterosexual relationships. *Journal of Sex & Marital Therapy, 19*, 315-327.

Exhibit

Hurlbert Index of Sexual Fantasy

1. I think sexual fantasies are healthy. (R)
2. I enjoy fantasizing about sex. (R)
3. I feel comfortable sharing my sexual fantasies with my partner. (R)
4. I enjoy using my sexual fantasies during masturbation. (R)
5. I am easily aroused by thoughts of sex. (R)
6. Even when I am in the mood for sex, it is difficult for me to think about sexual things.
7. I enjoy hearing my partner's sexual fantasies. (R)
8. It is hard for me to focus or concentrate on my sexual fantasies during sex.
9. I find my sexual fantasies to be boring.
10. My memories of past sexual experiences are negative.
11. It is difficult for me to think about sexual things during sex with my partner.
12. Thoughts about sex enter my mind without much effort. (R)
13. I believe sexual fantasy enhances sex. (R)
14. I feel uncomfortable discussing my sexual fantasies with my partner.
15. I don't like thinking about sex.
16. I feel uncomfortable telling my partner my sexual thoughts.
17. I feel guilty about my sexual fantasies.
18. I find my sexual fantasies to be simulating. (R)
19. When it comes to my past sexual experiences, my memories are negative.
20. It is hard for me to daydream about sex.
21. I find my partner's sexual fantasies to be exciting. (R)
22. I enjoy using my sexual fantasies during sex. (R)
23. I feel guilty when I think about sex.
24. I have negative thoughts about my past sexual experiences.
25. I experience negative feelings just thinking about sex.

Source. This index was published in *Canadian Journal of Human Sexuality,* Vol. 4, No. 1, 1995, and is reprinted with permission of SIECCAN.

Note. (R) = Reverse-scored items as indicated by the responses: *all of the time* = 0 points; *most of the time* = +1 point; *some of the time* = +2 points; *rarely* = +3 points; *never* = +4 points.

Women's Sexuality Questionnaire

Dianne L. Chambless,[1] *Center for Psychotherapy Research*
Diane DeMarco, *American University*

The Women's Sexuality Questionnaire (WSQ) is a structured interview with rating scales devised to assess the frequency and subjective experience of female orgasm and activities leading to orgasm.

Description

To allow for rapport to be established, as well as to collect information on potentially confounding variables, the WSQ begins with 16 questions concerning demographics and the respondent's reproductive and genital health. The second section is devoted to a brief sexual history concerning masturbation and noncoital and coital sex with a partner. Information collected includes the respondent's age when beginning to engage in the activity under question, frequency, and techniques of stimulation. The third section is the heart of the questionnaire. Questions concern the frequency of orgasm during various sexual activities in addition to scales asking respondents to rate the subjective quality of the orgasmic experience and of the stimulation leading to orgasm. Information obtained in the first two sections allows the interviewer to screen for variables that would reduce the probability of orgasm, such as drugs, dyspareunia, or inadequate stimulation. Although there are a variety of question formats, the major questions in Sections II and III are on ordinal scales.

Response Mode and Timing

The WSQ is designed to be administered in a private interview of approximately 45-60 minutes duration. The interview format allows the experimenter to develop rapport and to explore answers so as to yield more careful, thoughtful answers. Experience with the interview has shown that many women are confused by sexual terms and need explanations to give valid responses. Interviewers can also provide education about sexuality in the context so that the respondent truly benefits from taking part in research.

Scoring

Items are used as single-item scores with 1-5 or 1-7 ordinal scales, or as simple ages or frequencies. Items 22-25 are reverse scored.

Reliability

Test-retest reliability was established on a sample of 38 women reinterviewed by a second interviewer from 6 to 8

[1]Address correspondence to Dianne L. Chambless, Center for Psychotherapy Research, Science Center, Seventh Floor, 3600 Market Street, Philadelphia, PA 19104-2648.

weeks after the first interview (median = 6 weeks). Space limitations preclude the listing of the reliability coefficient for each item. These are available from the authors. Items concerning personal history, such as the respondents' age when first having intercourse and the frequency of sexual behaviors, were highly reliable. Pearson correlations ranged from .80 to .98, with the exception of the item concerning noncoital genital sex play with a partner, $r = .37, p < .03$.

Reliability of the remaining (ordinal) items was assessed by Kendall's tau. Taus for frequency of orgasm with clitoral stimulation by partner or self, coitus accompanied by clitoral stimulation, and coitus not accompanied by clitoral stimulation were .42, .74, and .61, respectively. Based on respondents' feedback, the item for clitoral stimulation has subsequently been rewritten to yield two items: orgasm through masturbation and orgasm through partner stimulation. Additional reliability data have yet to be collected. Although the reliability of the other two items is somewhat lower than would be desirable, we believe the responses largely reflect true variance due to the reactive nature of the interview itself rather than mostly measurement error. Interviewers provided information and reassurance on the basis of which, according to respondents' reports on retesting, the respondents made changes, often substantial ones, in their sexual behavior. Taus on items concerning the respondents' perception of the intensity and pleasurability of coitus and the orgasmic experience generally reflected good reliability, ranging from .57 to .87 (median tau = .78).

Validity

The WSQ items possess high face validity and have been examined for construct validity through a series of correlational analyses. Using a community sample of 90 heterosexual women, Chambless and Lifshitz (1984) found that, as predicted, frequency of orgasm on the WSQ was related to higher arousal on the previously validated Sexual Arousability Inventory (Hoon, Hoon, & Wincze, 1976) (tau = .18, $p < .03$). In further research with these 90 women, plus 12 lesbians, we have found predictable relationships among WSQ items. For example, higher frequency of coital orgasm was related to greater emphasis on vaginal stimulation in reaching orgasm (tau = .50, $p < .001$) and the higher ratings on the pleasurability of vaginal sensations during the nonorgasmic phase of coitus (tau = .28, $p < .01$). Higher frequency of orgasm through clitoral stimulation was related to a greater emphasis on clitoral stimulation in reaching orgasm (tau = −.29, $p < .005$). Additional information concerning WSQ item correlations is available from the authors. Although further validation work is desirable, data collected to date support the construct validity of the items.

Other Information

The WSQ, as well as accompanying information on reliability and validity, is available at no charge from Dianne Chambless.

References

Chambless, D. L., & Lifshitz, J. (1984). Self-reported sexual anxiety and arousal: The Expanded Sexual Arousability Inventory. *The Journal of Sex Research, 20,* 241-254.

Hoon, E. F., Hoon, P. W., & Wincze, J. P. (1976). An inventory for the measurement of female sexual arousability: The SAI. *Archives of Sexual Behavior, 5,* 291-300.

Exhibit

Women's Sexuality Questionnaire

Section I

1. Date of interview _____
2. Assessment No. _____
   Interviewer _____
3. S.S. No. _____ 4. D.O.B. _____
5. Occupation (do not inquire about place of employment) _____
6. Highest grade completed _____
7. Affiliative status:
   single   married   divorced   separated   cohabiting
8. Steady sexual partner: YES   NO
9. Looking over your whole life, would you say your primary sexual orientation is:
   bisexual   heterosexual   lesbian?
10. What drugs do you usually take (including alcohol, caffeine, street drugs, prescribed drugs)? In what amount and how often do you take these?

   _____

   Are any of these taken at times you plan on having sex? If so, in what way?

   _____

11. What is your present method of contraception? Do you have any problems with it?

   _____

12. Have you ever been pregnant? YES   NO
    a. No. of full-term deliveries _____
        how long ago was each? _____
        No. vaginal _____   No. caesarean _____
    b. No. of premature deliveries _____
        how long ago was each? _____
        No. vaginal _____   No. caesarean _____
    c. No. of spontaneous or induced abortions _____
        how long ago was each? _____
        how many weeks pregnant with each? _____
13. Have you ever undergone any surgery involving the vagina, other sexual organs, or organs closely related to sexual organs (i.e., anus, urethra, kidneys, bladder)?   YES   NO   If so, please describe:

   _____

14. Do you have any physical problems which interfere with your sexual functioning or pleasure?   YES   NO
    If so, please explain (including chronic illnesses, infections, vaginal tears)

   _____

   Specifically, do you get a lot of vaginal infections, and if so, how long do they usually last?

   _____

15. Have you ever done exercises for the vaginal muscle? (Show a diagram) If so, explain and describe.

   _____

16. When not pregnant, do you ever leak urine when you cough or sneeze?

   _____

Section II

17. Masturbation:
    a. How long ago did you begin to masturbate regularly? _____
    b. On an average over the last 6 months, how often have you masturbated? _____
    c. How many times would you estimate you've masturbated?
       _____ under ten times
       _____ 10-25
       _____ 26-100
       _____ 101-500
       _____ over 500
    d. How do you usually masturbate?
       _____ by inserting object into vagina
       _____ by using vibrator on external genitalia
       _____ by stimulating clitoral area with fingers, etc.
       _____ by manipulating the mons (define if necessary)
       _____ by pressure against object or pressure from thighs
       _____ by stimulating the entrance of the vagina (introitus)
       _____ other (please describe unless it makes you uncomfortable)
       _____

       Do you need to be in one particular position to reach orgasm? YES   NO
       If so, please describe:
       _____

18. Sex with partner excluding intercourse:
    a. At what age did you begin having genital sex with another person excluding intercourse (including manual, oral stimulation, etc.)? _____
    b. How often do you do so now? _____
    c. Roughly how many times have you done so? _____
19. Intercourse (defined according to woman's orientation as insertion & thrusting of penis, fingers, or objects by partner):
    a. At what age did you begin having intercourse? _____
    b. How often do you do so now? _____
    c. How many times, roughly, have you done so? _____
    d. What positions do you usually use? _____
       Do you generally get simultaneous clitoral stimulation while in this/these positions? If so, how?
       _____

20. On the average, what is the duration of sex play (defined as prior to intercourse if you have intercourse)?
    _____ no sex play   _____ 11-19 minutes
    _____ less than 5 minutes   _____ 20 or more minutes
    _____ 5-10 minutes
21. If you have intercourse, are you sufficiently lubricated at the time of insertion so that no artificial lubricant is needed for your comfort?   YES NO   If not, to what does this seem due? Likely factors are anxiety, insufficient stimulation, irritation from local contraceptives, menopause, infections, vaginal deodorant sprays, overwiping after diaphragm insertion, unlubricated condoms, postpartum estrogen imbalance (particularly likely if nursing), and oral contraceptives. In addition, intercourse may be uncomfortable despite lubrication during early experiences due to tightness of the vaginal entrance.
    _____

Section III

22. If you have intercourse, how long does it last on the average from the beginning of thrusting until thrusting stops? (Counts as one occasion if intercourse disrupted only long enough to change position or pause to prevent ejaculation)
    _____
    Out of all occasions of intercourse how often do you come to an orgasm, with simultaneous clitoral stimulation?
    _____ almost always 90-100%   _____ sometimes 1-29%
    _____ most of the time 60-89%   _____ never have 0%
    _____ often 30-59%

23. Out of all occasions of intercourse how often do you come to an orgasm, *without* simultaneous clitoral stimulation (defined as pressure or manipulation)?
    _____ almost always 90-100%   _____ sometimes 1-29%
    _____ most of the time 60-89%   _____ never have 0%
    _____ often 30-59%

24. Out of all occasions of clitoral stimulation during masturbation, how often do you come to orgasm?
    _____ almost always 90-100%   _____ sometimes 1-29%
    _____ most of the time 60-89%   _____ never have 0%
    _____ often 30-59%

25. If after having an orgasm you continue to receive stimulation, how often do you have sequential orgasms (a series of peaks and releases of tension)?
    a. During stimulation of clitoris (exclusively)?
       _____ almost always 90-100%   _____ sometimes 1-29%
       _____ most of the time 60-89%   _____ never have 0%
       _____ often 30-59%
    b. During intervaginal stimulation (intercourse) with clitoral stimulation?
       _____ almost always 90-100%   _____ sometimes 1-29%
       _____ most of the time 60-89%   _____ never have 0%
       _____ often 30-59%
    c. During intervaginal stimulation (intercourse) exclusively?
       _____ almost always 90-100%   _____ sometimes 1-29%
       _____ most of the time 60-89%   _____ never have 0%
       _____ often 30-59%

26. Out of all occasions of clitoral stimulation by your partner (manual or oral, but excluding intercourse), how often do you come to orgasm?
    _____ almost always 90-100%   _____ sometimes 1-29%
    _____ most of the time 60-89%   _____ never have 0%
    _____ often 30-59%

27. In attaining orgasm for you, what is the most accurate statement:
    _____ 1. Clitoral stimulation contributes *much more* than vaginal stimulation.
    _____ 2. Clitoral stimulation contributes *somewhat more* than vaginal stimulation.
    _____ 3. Clitoral and vaginal stimulation are *about equal* in contribution.
    _____ 4. Vaginal stimulation contributes *somewhat more* than clitoral stimulation.
    _____ 5. Vaginal stimulation contributes *much more* than clitoral stimulation.

28. (If you have orgasms) which statement best describes your physical sensations during orgasm with intercourse *with clitoral stimulation:*
    _____ 1. A slight pulsating feeling in the vagina.
    _____ 2. A distinct pulsating feeling in the vagina.
    _____ 3. A very strong pulsating feeling in the vagina with sensation spreading to the legs.
    _____ 4. An intense feeling throughout the abdomen and legs with rhythmic contractions in the vagina.
    _____ 5. An intense feeling traveling throughout the entire body.
    _____ 6. Other, specify: _____

29. For me, having an orgasm during intercourse (with clitoral stimulation) is:
       1   2   3   4   5   6   7
       blah   most intense
       experience   experience possible

30. What kind of feeling do you typically experience in the vagina during intercourse *without* direct clitoral stimulation?
    _____ 1. Experience an unpleasant feeling the entire time
    _____ 2. Experience an unpleasant feeling which eventually changes to no particular feeling at all
    _____ 3. Experience an unpleasant feeling which eventually increases to a pleasant feeling
    _____ 4. Experience no particular feeling the entire time
    _____ 5. Experience no particular feeling which eventually increases to a pleasant feeling
    _____ 6. Experience a pleasant feeling the entire time
    _____ 7. Experience a pleasant feeling which eventually increases to a more pleasant feeling
    _____ 8. Other, specify: _____

31. (If you have orgasms) which statement best describes your physical sensations during orgasm with intercourse *without* direct clitoral stimulation? (include pressure, manual manipulation, etc. as clitoral stimulation)
    _____ 1. a slight pulsating feeling in the vagina
    _____ 2. a distinct pulsating feeling in the vagina
    _____ 3. a very strong pulsating feeling in the vagina with a sensation spreading to the legs

_____ 4. an intense feeling throughout the abdomen and legs with rhythmic contractions in the vagina
_____ 5. an intense feeling traveling throughout the entire body with rhythmic contractions in the vagina
_____ 6. Other, specify: _____

32. For me, having an orgasm during intercourse (without clitoral stimulation) is:

   1   2   3   4   5   6   7
   blah   most intense
   experience   experience possible

33. (If you have orgasms) when a partner stimulates your clitoris to orgasm (no entry into the vagina) which statement best describes your feelings?
_____ 1. a slight pulsating feeling in the vagina
_____ 2. a distinct pulsating feeling in the vagina
_____ 3. a very strong pulsating feeling in the vagina with a sensation spreading to the legs
_____ 4. an intense feeling throughout the abdomen and legs with rhythmic contractions in the vagina
_____ 5. an intense feeling traveling throughout the entire body with rhythmic contractions in the vagina
_____ 6. Other, specify: _____

34. For me, having an orgasm when a partner stimulates my clitoris (no entry into vagina) is:

   1   2   3   4   5   6   7
   blah   most intense
   experience   experience possible

35. If you have orgasms when you stimulate your clitoris (masturbate) (nothing in vagina) what best describes your physical sensations?
_____ 1. a slight pulsating feeling in the vagina
_____ 2. a distinct pulsating feeling in the vagina
_____ 3. a very strong pulsating feeling in the vagina with a sensation spreading to the legs
_____ 4. an intense feeling throughout the abdomen and legs with rhythmic contractions in the vagina
_____ 5. an intense feeling traveling throughout the entire body with rhythmic contractions in the vagina
_____ 6. Other, specify: _____

36. For me, having an orgasm through masturbation (nothing in vagina) is:

   1   2   3   4   5   6   7
   blah   most intense
   experience   experience possible

Source. This scale is reprinted with permission of the authors.

Sexual Self-Schema Scale–Women's Version

Jill M. Cyranowski and Barbara L. Andersen,[1] *Ohio State University*

The Sexual Self-Schema Scale is a cognitive measure of a woman's sexual self-view. Sexual self-views, or sexual self-schemas, are cognitive representations (or thoughts) about

[1]Address correspondence to Barbara L. Andersen, Department of Psychology, Ohio State University, 202 Townsend Hall, Columbus, OH 43210-1222; email: banderse@magnus.acs.ohio-state.edu.

sexual aspects of the self. They are derived from past experience, manifest in current experiences, influential in the processing of social information, and they guide sexual behavior. If the self-concept is multifaceted, there may be certain aspects that are more central or pervasive than others. Sexual self-schema represents one such aspect. Specifically, one's sexual self-view may function to interpret and to organize sexually relevant actions and experiences; to provide standards or scripts for sexual behaviors; and to guide future judgments, decisions, inferences, or predictions about the self within sexual or social domains (Andersen & Cyranowski, 1994, 1995; Cyranowski, 1993). In short, sexual self-schema represents a cognitive individual difference in women's sexuality.

Description

The Sexual Self-Schema Scale (titled "Describe Yourself" for respondent use) is a 50-item (26 scored and 24 filler items) measure that taps individual differences in sexual self-schema. The classic approach of using trait adjectives as markers of important personality dispositions was used to identify a semantic representation of a "sexual woman." Conceptual ratings of respondents, facts of discriminant and convergent validity, and studies of internal structure were considered and incorporated into scale construction. Moreover, the scale is uncorrelated with measures of negative affect and social desirability. The majority of developmental and validity studies were conducted with samples of undergraduate women; however, the scale has been cross-validated with samples of older women (i.e., with mean ages between 34 and 49). Factor analytic research (N = 387) indicates that the scale includes two positive factors, passionate/romantic self-views (Factor 1) and directness/openness (Factor 2), and one negative factor, embarrassment or conservatism (Factor 3), which may be a deterrent to sexual or romantic affects and behaviors (Andersen & Cyranowski, 1994).

Women who obtain high total scale scores, or "positive" sexual self-schemas, view themselves as emotionally romantic or passionate and behaviorally open while reporting low levels of embarrassment or conservatism in sexual contexts. In contrast, women obtaining low total scale scores, or "negative" sexual self-schemas, report experiencing lower levels of romantic or passionate emotions and describe themselves as behaviorally inhibited in their sexual and romantic relationships. These women tend to espouse conservative and, at times, negative, attitudes about sexual matters, and they may describe themselves as self-conscious, embarrassed, or not confident in a variety of sexual contexts.

Response Mode and Timing

Respondents rate the 50 trait adjectives on a 7-point Likert-type scale, ranging from 0 = *not at all descriptive of me* to 6 = *very much descriptive of me*. The scale takes 5-10 minutes to complete.

Scoring

There are 26 scored sexual self-schema items and 24 filler items. Individual factor scores are calculated by summing respondent ratings on the items listed as follows: (Item 45 is reverse keyed.) Factor 1 = Items 5, 11, 20, 35, 37, 39, 44, 45, 48, and 50; Factor 2 = Items 2, 5, 9, 13, 16, 18, 24, 25, and 32; Factor 3 = Items 3, 8, 22, 28, 31, 38, and 41. Total sexual self-schema scores = (Factor 1 + Factor 2) – Factor 3. Total sexual self-schema scores can range from –42 to 114. Means and standard deviations of factor

and total sexual self-schema scores reported for a sample of college-aged women (N = 387) are as follows: Factor 1: 47.44 (6.45); Factor 2: 36.26 (7.15); Factor 3: 23.22 (5.91); total score: 60.47 (14.15) (Andersen & Cyranowski, 1994; Cyranowski, 1993).

This bipolar scoring system describes women who vary along a continuum from low to high total schema scorers. Alternatively, the Sexual Self-Schema Scale can be scored using a two-dimensional, or bivariate, model. Advantages of the latter measurement model are (a) it enables both positive and negative schema dimensions to have some functional independence, and (b) it allows for the examination of those women who fall in the middle of the total schema score distribution. The bivariate scoring procedure uses simple median-split cutoffs of the positive (sum of Factors 1 and 2) and negative (Factor 3) dimensions to delineate four types of schematic representations: positive (high on positive/low on negative schema dimensions), negative (low on positive/high on negative schema dimensions), aschematic (low on both positive and negative schema dimensions) and co-schematic (or "conflicted," i.e., high on both positive and negative schema dimensions) (see Andersen & Cyranowski, 1994, Part III).

Women who are aschematic report weak endorsements of both positive and negative schema items. These women appear to lack a coherent or accessible cognitive framework from which to guide sexually relevant perceptions, cognitions, and behaviors. Alternatively, co-schematic individuals are those with a schematic framework of their sexuality, yet one that is, in a sense, conflicted. Individuals in this group provide simultaneously strong endorsements of both positive and negative schema aspects: They view themselves as romantic, passionate, and open, yet experience concomitant embarrassment, conservatism, or anxiety in social or sexual situations. The bivariate conceptualization has received preliminary empirical support (Andersen & Cyranowski, 1994, Part III), and further psychometric studies are in progress.

Reliability

Test-retest reliabilities for the Sexual Self-Schema Scale have been obtained for both 2- and 9-week intervals. The total score reliability values for these intervals were similar, at .89 (N = 20) and .88 (N = 172), respectively. Cronbach's alpha values for the total score and individual factors are as follows: Full scale, .82; Factor 1, .81; Factor 2, .77; and Factor 8, .66 (N = 387) (Andersen & Cyranowski, 1994; Cyranowski, 1993).

Validity

The Sexual Self-Schema Scale predicts a wide range of sexual cognitions, behaviors, and responses. Convergent validity data (N = 220) indicate significant correlations of total sexual self-schema scores with measures of sexual affects (e.g., sex guilt, r = –.16), sexual behaviors (e.g., lifetime sexual activities, r = .30; number of sexual partners, r = .36), sexual arousal (e.g., the Sexual Arousability Inventory, r = .25), and romantic relationships (e.g., number of love relationships, r = .32; passionate love, r = .14)

(Andersen & Cyranowski, 1994). Convergent validity data with a sample of older women ($N = 21$) indicate significant schema score correlations with the sexual response cycle: sexual desire ($r = .47$), sexual excitement ($r = .66$), orgasm ($r = .46$) and resolution ($r = .59$). Moreover, the Sexual Self-Schema Scale has been shown to account for significant increments of variance in sexual behaviors, cognitions, and other responses, in addition to the variance accounted for by other sexuality measures and measures of extroversion and self-esteem. Finally, studies of process confirm the unobtrusive quality of the measure: Respondents are unaware that a sexuality construct is being assessed, which represents a methodological advantage given the levels of respondent bias and method error that plague many sexuality measures.

Contrast group data comparing positive and negative sexual self-schema groups ($N = 171$) indicate that women with positive sexual self-schema evaluate sexual experiences more positively (i.e., the Sexual Opinion Survey), report higher levels of arousability across sexual experiences (i.e., the Sexual Arousability Inventory), are more willing to engage in uncommitted sexual relationships (i.e., the Sociosexual Orientation Inventory), and generally rate themselves as "more sexual" than negative schema women. Positive schema women also report experiencing more sex-

ual activities and more previous sexual partners, and they anticipate more future sexual partners than their low-schema counterparts. Finally, despite this seemingly unrestricted view of sexuality, it is important to note that affects and behaviors indicative of romantic, loving, and intimate attachments are also central to women with positive sexual schemas, as they report more extensive histories of romantic relationships and higher levels of passionate love within relationships (Andersen & Cyranowski, 1994).

References

Andersen, B. L., & Cyranowski, J. M. (1994). Women's sexual self-schema. *Journal of Personality and Social Psychology, 67,* 1079-1100.

Andersen, B. L., & Cyranowski, J. M. (1995). Women's sexuality: Behaviors, responses, and individual differences. *Journal of Consulting and Clinical Psychology, 63,* 891-906.

Andersen, B. L., Woods, X., & Cyranowski, J. M. (1994). Sexual self-schema and sexual morbidity following cancer. *Canadian Journal of Human Sexuality, 3,* 165-170.

Cyranowski, J. M. (1993). *Sexual self-schema: Mapping women's cognitive representations of their sexual selves.* Unpublished master's thesis, Ohio State University, Columbus.

Exhibit

Sexual Self-Schema Scale

Describe Yourself

Directions: Below is a listing of 50 trait adjectives. For each word, consider whether or not the term describes you. Each adjective is to be rated on a 7-point scale, ranging from 0 = *not at all descriptive of me* to 6 = *very much descriptive of me.* For each item, fill in the appropriate circle on your computer answer sheet. Please be thoughtful and honest.

Question: To what extent does the term _____ describe me?

Rating Scale:

Not at all descriptive of me	0	1	2	3	4	5	6	Very much descriptive of me

(1) generous	(26) disagreeable
(2) uninhibited	(27) serious
(3) cautious	(28) prudent
(4) helpful	(29) humorous
(5) loving	(30) sensible
(6) open-minded	(31) embarrassed
(7) shallow	(32) outspoken
(8) timid	(33) level-headed
(9) frank	(34) responsible
(10) clean-cut	(35) romantic
(11) stimulating	(36) polite
(12) unpleasant	(37) sympathetic
(13) experienced	(38) conservative
(14) short-tempered	(39) passionate
(15) irresponsible	(40) wise
(16) direct	(41) inexperienced
(17) logical	(42) stingy

Not at all	0	1	2	3	4	5	6	Very much
descriptive of me								descriptive of me

(18) broad-minded
(19) kind
(20) arousable
(21) practical
(22) self-conscious
(23) dull
(24) straightforward
(25) casual

(43) superficial
(44) warm
(45) unromantic
(46) good-natured
(47) rude
(48) revealing
(49) bossy
(50) feeling

Source. This scale was originally published in "Women's Sexual Self-Schema," by B. L. Andersen and J. M. Cyranowski, 1994, *Journal of Personality and Social Psychology, 67,* 1079-1100. Copyright © 1994 by the American Psychological Association. Reprinted with permission.

Self-Perceptions of Female Sexuality Survey Instrument

J. Kenneth Davidson, Sr.,[1] *University of Wisconsin–Eau Claire*
Carol A. Darling, *Florida State University*

The Self-Perceptions of Female Sexuality Survey Instrument covers a wide range of beliefs, attitudes, feelings, and responses about a woman's own sexuality and, to a lesser extent, that of her partners. The instrument was developed for the primary purpose of providing further clarification of the apparently inseparable nature of clitoral and vaginal orgasms. More specifically, the instrument ascertains whether perceived differences exist with regard to experiencing orgasm via masturbation, petting, and sexual intercourse in terms of physiological and psychological sexual satisfaction.

Description

The complete instrument consists of 123 open-ended and closed-form questions concerning sexual attitudes, sexual behavior, and the female sexual response. The following categories of items appear in the instrument:

1. Demographic variables, including age, marital status, dating status, formal education, religious preference, and religiosity.

2. Physiological and psychological sexual satisfaction variables, including early knowledge about the pleasurable sensations of the clitoris, level of sexual adjustment, perceived levels of current physiological and psychological sexual satisfaction, and desired changes in sex life.

3. Peer communication and mass media variables, including sources of information about female orgasm, sources of information about any differences between orgasmic responses, discussion with peers regarding different kinds and/or types of orgasms, and ages at various stages of opinion formation regarding perceived differences in orgasmic responses.

4. Masturbatory attitude variables, including perceived acceptance of masturbation of self, acceptance of masturbation by acquaintances, and the relationship of masturbation to marital sexual adjustment.

5. Sexual history variables, including masturbatory, petting, and sexual intercourse experience; frequency of masturbation, petting, and sexual intercourse; experience with pretending orgasm; relationships with past and current sex

[1]Address correspondence to J. Kenneth Davidson, Sr., Department of Sociology and Anthropology, University of Wisconsin–Eau Claire, Eau Claire, WI 54701; email: davidsj@uwec.edu.

partners; and frequency and preference for various sexual intercourse positions for achieving orgasm.

6. Orgasmic quality variables, including perceived differences, if any, in experiencing orgasm via masturbation, petting, and sexual intercourse; the relative contribution of clitoral versus vaginal stimulation in achieving orgasm during masturbation, petting, and sexual intercourse; and the degree of physiological and psychological satisfaction associated with orgasms achieved via masturbation, petting, and sexual intercourse.

The survey instrument was first pretested with students enrolled in upper-division marriage/family and human sexuality courses. After appropriate revisions, the instrument was pretested a second time using the nursing staff of a large midwestern family planning organization. After making additional changes, the instrument was then critically reviewed by 10 female professionals involved in either teaching and/or research about human sexuality or the delivery of community-based family planning services. The recommendations received from these reviewers were incorporated into the final version of the instrument.

The survey instrument is best suited for use with populations containing women with 2 or more years of college education and who are at least 25 years of age. The level of language sophistication found in the instrument would appear to preclude its application to populations having no college education. Furthermore, given the nature of the instrument, a woman would need to have had considerable sexual experience to be able to respond in a meaningful way to a substantial number of the items. It is assumed that a greater opportunity for having experienced substantial sexual activity will exist for women aged 25 years or older. To date, this survey instrument has been used for data collection from professional nurses holding at least an associate degree/diploma in nursing and from professional women in academia holding at least a baccalaureate degree.

Response Mode and Timing

Respondents either check the appropriate answer category or answer the open-ended items in their own words within the space provided. Given the detailed personal information being sought regarding sexuality, the survey instrument should be completed in total privacy and anonymity. Thus, this instrument is ideally suited for distribution as a mail questionnaire using a business reply envelope.

Based on the pretest results and feedback received from actual respondents, an average of 45 minutes is required to complete all segments of the survey instrument.

Scoring

Although some attitudinal items do appear, it is not intended for this survey instrument to be employed as a scale that can stand alone. It is recommended, however, that all attitudinal items selected for use be arranged in a reverse/nonreverse response pattern to help ensure that respondents give sufficient concentration to the completion of the survey instrument.

Reliability

The test-retest reliability of the instrument has not been established.

Validity

Construct validity has been established by reviewing pretest data for the various measures that suggest the same relationship between the variables associated with perceived differences in orgasm achieved during masturbation, petting, and sexual intercourse. The instrument has successfully delineated perceived differences in orgasmic responses between orgasms achieved via masturbation, petting, and sexual intercourse; the influence of multiple sex partners on sexual satisfaction; factors associated with pretending orgasm; and levels of sexual satisfaction and desired changes in the sexual lives of single professional women (see references).

Other Information

The entire survey instrument can be purchased at a cost of $8 by writing to the authors.

References

Darling, C. A., & Davidson, J. K., Sr. (1985, November). *Enhancing relationships: Understanding the feminine mystique of pretending orgasm.* Paper presented at the annual meeting of the National Council on Family Relations, Dallas, TX.

Davidson, J. K., Sr., & Darling, C. A. (1983, October). *The stereotype of single women revisited: Sexual behavior and sexual satisfaction among professional women.* Paper presented at the annual meeting of the Mid-South Sociological Association, Birmingham, AL.

Davidson, J. K., Sr., & Darling, C. A. (1984, November). *Perceived differences in the female orgasmic response: New meanings for sexual satisfaction.* Paper presented at the annual meeting of the National Council on Family Relations, San Francisco.

Davidson, J. K., Sr., & Darling, C. A. (1985, August). *The sexually experienced female: The influence of multiple sex partners.* Paper presented at the annual meeting of the Society for the Study of Social Problems, Washington, DC.

Exhibit

Self-Perceptions of Female Sexuality[a]

1. How would you rate your current level of sexual adjustment? (*Very much adjusted-Very unadjusted;* 6 point)
2. At what age did you first *become aware* of possible pleasurable sensations of the clitoris? (PLEASE SPECIFY)
3. It is necessary for a female to achieve an orgasm in a majority of the instances when she experiences masturbation, petting (mutual masturbation), and/or sexual intercourse in order to be classified as sexually adjusted. (*Strongly agree-Strongly disagree;* 4 point)

4. Do you feel that most of your female friends believe that a female must experience an orgasm in order to be sexually adjusted? (*Yes/No*)

5. What has been your *most* important source of information about the female orgasm? (15 options)

6. Have you ever consciously considered the possibility that orgasms reached through masturbation while alone and/or sexual intercourse might be different? (*Yes/No*)

7. Have you ever read any material about different kinds and/or types of orgasms? (*Yes/No*)

8. *If ever read materials about different kinds and/or types of orgasm:*
   From the material that you have read, what conclusions, if any, did the authors reach regarding different kinds and/or types of orgasm?

9. Have your ever discussed with a friend, relative, and/or acquaintance whether different kinds and/or types of orgasms exist for the female during sexual intercourse and/or masturbation while alone? (*Yes/No*)

10. *If ever discussed different kinds and/or types of orgasm:*
    With whom have you ever discussed different kinds and/or types of orgasm? (15 categories)

11. *If ever discussed different kinds and/or types of orgasm:*
    At what age did you *first* discuss different kinds and/or types of orgasms with another person?

12. In your opinion, do different kinds and/or types of orgasm exist for the human female (*Yes/No/Uncertain*)

13. *If yes, or uncertain that different kinds and/or types of orgasm exist:*
    Would you please describe in your own words, the different kinds and/or types of orgasm that can be achieved through masturbation while alone, petting, and/or sexual intercourse.

14. Have you ever masturbated while alone? (*Yes/No*)

15. Have you ever achieved an orgasm? (*Yes/No/Uncertain*)

16. Have you ever experienced sexual intercourse? (*Yes/No*)

17. *If ever had orgasm:*
    How did you first experience orgasm?
    _____ 1. Masturbation while alone
    _____ 2. Petting (mutual masturbation)
    _____ 3. Sexual intercourse
    _____ 4. Other _____

18. *If ever had orgasm:*
    At what age did you experience your first orgasm?

19. *If ever had orgasm:*
    Under which of the following circumstances have you *ever* experienced an orgasm? (Check all applicable categories) (32 options)

20. *If ever had orgasm through masturbating while alone:*
    At what age did you experience your first orgasm through masturbating while alone?

21. *If ever had orgasm through petting:*
    At what age did you experience your first orgasm through petting?

22. *If ever had orgasm through sexual intercourse:*
    At what age did you experience your first orgasm through sexual intercourse?

23. *If ever masturbated while alone:*
    How old were you the first time that you masturbated while alone?

24. *If ever masturbated while alone:*
    How often do you experience an orgasm through masturbating while alone? (*Always-Never; 5 point*)

25. *If ever masturbated while alone:*
    How many orgasms do you usually experience during a single episode of masturbating alone?

26. *If masturbated while alone within the past two years:*
    During the past two years, about how many times per week, month, or year have you averaged masturbating while alone?
    (Choose only one category and do not use range of times or check the category)
    _____ 1. Times per week   _____ 2. Times per month   _____ 3. Times per year

27. *If ever had orgasm while masturbating alone:*
    In what specific area of your genital region do you most feel the sensation of orgasm occurring during masturbating while alone?

28. *If ever masturbated alone:*
    How would you rate your *physiological* reaction from masturbating while alone?
    (*Intense satisfaction-No satisfaction; 5 point*)

29. *If ever masturbated alone:*
    How would you rate your *psychological* reaction from masturbating while alone?
    (*No satisfaction-Intense satisfaction; 5 point*)

30. *If ever petted:*
    How often do you experience an orgasm while petting? (*Always-Never;* 5 point)
31. *If ever had orgasm during petting:*
    How many orgasms do you usually experience during a single episode of petting?
32. *If ever had orgasm during petting:*
    In what specific area of your genital region do you most feel the sensation of orgasm occurring during petting?
33. *If ever had orgasm:*
    Do you experience a *physiological* need in yourself to have an orgasm prior to any sexual arousal and/or sexual activity? (*Never-Always;* 5 point)
34. *If ever had orgasm:*
    Do you experience a *physiological* need in yourself to have more than one orgasm while engaging in masturbating while alone, petting, and/or sexual intercourse? (*Never-Always;* 5 point)
35. *If ever had orgasm:*
    Do you experience a *psychological* need in yourself to have an orgasm prior to any sexual arousal and/or sexual activity? (*Never-Always;* 5 point)
36. *If ever had orgasm:*
    Do you experience a *psychological* need in yourself to have more than one orgasm while engaging in masturbating while alone, petting, and/or sexual intercourse? (*Never-Always;* 5 point)
37. *If ever experienced more than one orgasm during a single sexual experience, including masturbation while alone:*
    Do successive orgasms during a single sexual experience become stronger or weaker? (10 options)
38. *If ever had sexual intercourse:*
    At what age did you first experience sexual intercourse?
39. *If had sexual intercourse within the past two years:*
    During the past two years, about how many times per week, month, or year have you averaged having sexual intercourse?
    (Choose only one category and do not use a range of times or check the category)
    _____ 1. Times per week   _____ 2. Times per month   _____ 3. Times per year
40. *If ever had sexual intercourse:*
    With how many different partners have you ever had sexual intercourse?
41. *If ever had sexual intercourse:*
    During sexual intercourse, at what point does your most recent male sex partner usually achieve his first orgasm? (6 options)
42. *If ever had sexual intercourse:*
    Would you please indicate the most frequent position that you utilize for sexual intercourse. You are to rank the sexual intercourse positions with regard to frequency of occurrence with 1-most often, 2-second most often, and 3-third most often only. (12 options)
43. *If ever had sexual intercourse:*
    How often do you experience an orgasm during sexual intercourse? (*Always-Never;* 5 point)
44. *If rarely or never have orgasm during sexual intercourse:*
    Why do you believe that you experience difficulty in achieving orgasm during sexual intercourse?
45. *If ever had orgasm during sexual intercourse:*
    How many orgasms do you usually experience during a single vaginal penetration while having sexual intercourse?
46. *If ever had orgasm during sexual intercourse:*
    After having experienced orgasm during sexual intercourse, what is the typical extent of your *physiological* reaction? (*Intense satisfaction-No satisfaction;* 5 point)
47. *If ever had orgasm during sexual intercourse:*
    After having experienced orgasm during sexual intercourse, what is the typical extent of your *psychological* reaction? (*Intense satisfaction-No satisfaction;* 5 point)
48. *If ever masturbated to orgasm while alone and had sexual intercourse:*
    Do you prefer to masturbate to orgasm while alone rather than having sexual intercourse? (*Always-Never;* 5 point)
49. *If ever had orgasm:*
    Would you please indicate the *most frequent* techniques that you use to achieve orgasm? You are to rank the following techniques with regard to frequency of occurrence with 1-most often, 2-second most often, and 3-third most often only. (32 options)
50. *If ever masturbated while alone, petted, had sexual intercourse, and experienced orgasm:*
    Do you experience a difference between an orgasm reached during masturbating while alone, during petting, and during sexual intercourse with vaginal penetration? (*Yes/No*)
51. *If yes, differences exist between orgasm achieved during masturbation while alone, petting, and sexual intercourse:*
    In your own words, please describe the difference between orgasms achieved during masturbation while alone, petting, and sexual intercourse with vaginal penetration.

52. *If ever had orgasm during sexual intercourse:*
    In what specific area of your genital region do you most feel the sensation of orgasm occurring during sexual intercourse with vaginal penetration?

53. *If ever had orgasm during sexual intercourse:*
    What is the relative contribution of clitoral versus vaginal stimulation in helping you to achieve orgasm *during sexual intercourse*? (7 options)

54. *If ever had orgasm during masturbation:*
    What is the relative contribution of clitoral versus vaginal stimulation in helping you to achieve orgasm *during masturbating while alone:* (7 options)

55. *If ever had orgasm during petting:*
    What is the relative contribution of clitoral versus vaginal stimulation in helping you to achieve orgasm *during petting*? (7 options)

56. Which of the following changes, if any, would you like to have in your current sex life? (44 options)

57. How would you rate your overall personal *physiological* level of sexual satisfaction? (*Very much satisfied-Very much dissatisfied;* 6 point)

58. How would you rate your overall personal *psychological* level of sexual satisfaction? (*Very much satisfied-Very much dissatisfied;* 6 point)

Source. The items from the instrument are reprinted with permission of the author.

a. In the interest of brevity, only select items specifically related to the orgasmic response have been included in this exhibit. Additional demographic, attitudinal, and behavioral items/variables that are critical to appropriate analyses and understanding of the perceived differences have been omitted because of space limitations.

Sexuality of Women Survey

The Editors

This is an extensive questionnaire that was developed to collect data for a book on female sexuality by Ellison (in preparation). It contains both open-ended and closed-ended questions pertaining to many aspects of women's sexuality. The database contains 2,632 respondents from throughout the United States born between 1905 and 1977. This questionnaire and the database are available from Carol Rinkleib Ellison, 1957 Oak View Drive, Oakland, CA 94602-1945.

McCoy Female Sexuality Questionnaire

Norma L. McCoy[1] and Joseph R. Matyas, *San Francisco State University*

The intent of the McCoy Female Sexuality Questionnaire (MFSQ) is to assess a woman's general level of sexual interest and response at or near the time of questioning. It may be used to map changes in sexual functioning over time or as an information source to aid in diagnosis.

Description

The basic form of the MFSQ consists of 19 questions; 18 answered on a 7-point scale ranging from *very low* or

[1]Address correspondence to Norma L. McCoy, Department of Psychology, San Francisco State University, 1600 Holloway Ave., San Francisco, CA 94132; email: mccoy@sfsu.edu.

absent to *extremely high,* and a 19th question requesting an overall frequency of heterosexual coitus during the preceding 4-week period. The first 11 questions explore general elements of sexual enjoyment, arousal, interest, satisfaction with partner as lover or friend, and feelings of attractiveness. The next eight questions focus on heterosexual coitus, including coital frequency, enjoyment, orgasm frequency and pleasurability, lubrication, and the incidence of decreased satisfaction due to partner's erectile difficulties. The content areas are shown in Table 1.

Three optional sections increase the MFSQ to 33 items providing information on masturbation, partnered sexual activity without heterosexual coitus, and heterosexual anal intercourse.

Table 1 McCoy Female Sexuality Questionnaire Content

Questionnaire items	*7-point scales, labels for 1 and 7*
General sexuality/sexual interest	
Enjoyment of sexual activity	*Not at all enjoyable* to *Extremely enjoyable*
Frequency of sexual activity	*Too infrequent* to *Too frequent*
Frequency of sexual thoughts, fantasies	*Never* to *More than 10 times a day*
Excitement/arousal during sexual activity	*Not at all excited* to *Extremely excited*
Level of sexual interest	*Extremely low* to *Extremely high*
Vaginal lubrication	*Absent* to *Excessive*
Decreased satisfaction due to partner's disinterest	*Every time* to *Never*
Satisfaction with partner as lover	*Not at all satisfied* to *Extremely satisfied*
Satisfaction with partner as friend	*Not at all satisfied* to *Extremely satisfied*
Sexually attractive, generally	*Not at all sexually attractive* to *Extremely sexually attractive*
Sexually attractive, to partner	*Not at all sexually attractive* to *Extremely sexually attractive*
Sexual intercourse	
Frequency (past 4 weeks)	(Reported frequency)
Enjoyment	*Not at all enjoyable* to *Extremely enjoyable*
Frequency of orgasm	*Never* to *Every time*
Pleasure of orgasm	*Slightly pleasurable* to *Extremely pleasurable*
Additional stimulation needed to reach orgasm	*Never* to *Every time*
Insufficient lubrication	*Every time* to *Never*
Painful sexual intercourse	*Every time* to *Never*
Erectile problems of partner	*Every time* to *Never*
Sexual activity with a partner, no sexual intercourse (petting)	
Frequency (past 4 weeks)	(Reported frequency)
Enjoyment	*Not at all enjoyable* to *Extremely enjoyable*
Frequency of orgasm	*Never* to *Every time*
Pleasure of orgasm	*Slightly pleasurable* to *Extremely pleasurable*
Sexual activity without a partner (masturbation)	
Frequency (past 4 weeks)	(Reported frequency)
Enjoyment	*Not at all enjoyable* to *Extremely enjoyable*
Frequency of orgasm	*Never* to *Every time*
Pleasure of orgasm	*Slightly pleasurable* to *Extremely pleasurable*
Anal intercourse	
Frequency (past 4 weeks)	(Reported frequency)
Enjoyment	*Not at all enjoyable* to *Extremely enjoyable*
Frequency of orgasm	*Never* to *Every time*
Pleasure of orgasm	*Slightly pleasurable* to *Extremely pleasurable*

The MFSQ was originally designed in English, but it is available in French and Swedish. McCoy and Matyas (1996) used an additional section that requests general demographic information, as well as other, more detailed, information on reproductive health history and medication usage.

The MFSQ may be used with heterosexual and/or bisexual female populations and is adaptable to lesbian populations by deleting heterosexual coitus questions.

Response Mode and Timing

Respondents mark a printed form, choosing one of seven choices per question or supplying frequencies for specified sexual activities. Depending on respondent's reading skills and comfort level with question content, completion of the basic 19-item questionnaire should average 5-10 minutes, and completion of the 33-item questionnaire should average 10-15 minutes.

Scoring

Summary scores may be computed for the entire 19-item question set or for subsets of questions. Frequencies of sex activities may be converted into 7-point categories on a percentage-wise basis. Higher summary scores are interpreted as representing higher, more complete, or better-integrated levels of female sexual function occurring at or near the time of questioning. McCoy and Matyas (1996) used a 17-item MFSQ, minus 2 items that deal with sexual attractiveness (Beach, 1976). They reported five factors, labeled sexual interest, satisfaction, vaginal lubrication, orgasm, and sex partner. Information concerning factor score weightings and factor interpretations may be obtained by referring to the above publication or by contacting the authors.

Reliability

McCoy and Matyas (1996) used 17 items of the 19-item MFSQ with a sample of 364 university women ages 18-26. They reported an internal consistency alpha of .77. Test-retest correlations, following a 2-week time interval, for individual items ranged from .69 to .95, with an average test-retest correlation of .83.

Validity

The MFSQ has been successfully employed to estimate changes in general sexual functioning in clinical and non-clinical samples of menopausal-aged women. In a longitudinal study, McCoy and Davidson (1985) found significant within-subject differences prior to and following the last menstrual cycle on MFSQ items relating to the frequency of sexual thoughts and fantasies, vaginal lubrication, and diminished satisfaction with partner as lover. In a study (McCoy, 1990) using a subsample from the same longitudinal study, data for each respondent were divided on the basis of low or normal estradiol levels. When estrogen was low, women reported significantly more dyspareunia, lack of vaginal lubrication, decreased satisfaction with sex because of their partner's level of sexual interest, fewer sexual thoughts, and decreased satisfaction with their partners as lovers. Limouzin-Lamothe, Mairon, Joyce, and Le Gal (1994) used a French-language translation of nine items selected from the MFSQ that deal with sexual satisfaction, enjoyment, arousal, orgasm, lubrication, and dyspareunia. These authors found that global scores on these MFSQ items were significantly higher among menopausal women given estrogen replacement therapy (ERT) compared with menopausal women given symptomatic treatment. They found convergent validity for the MFSQ items with the Women's Health Questionnaire sex life subscale (Hunter, 1990; Hunter, Battersby, & Whitehead, 1986), reproducing the same direction and magnitude of significance. Nathorst-Böös, Wiklund, Mattsson, Sandin, and von Schoultz (1993) and Nathorst-Böös, von Schoultz, and Carlström (1993) used a Swedish translation of the same nine-item MFSQ subscale. In the first study, the authors found significant differences between postmenopausal women given ERT compared with those on placebo for MFSQ items relating to sexual fantasies, satisfaction, sexual enjoyment, vaginal lubrication, and dyspareunia. In the second study, ovariectomized women using ERT reported a significantly greater frequency of sexual thoughts and fantasies than untreated ovariectomized women, yet reported significantly less vaginal lubrication and pleasure with intercourse than intact women. The MFSQ has also been used with a sample of university women to assess the effects of oral contraceptive (OC) usage and type of OC used on sexual functioning in sexually active women. Significant differences were noted on MFSQ items relating to sexual interest, enjoyment, sexual fantasies, satisfaction, and vaginal lubrication as well as for a Sexual Interest factor (McCoy & Matyas, 1996). Given that the pattern of MFSQ findings in these studies is consistent with predictions of greater or lesser degrees of overall female sexual functioning, the MFSQ possesses good construct and content validity.

Other Information

Researchers may use the MFSQ for noncommercial purposes without charge. Otherwise, an honorarium must be paid. Interested parties should contact Norma L. McCoy.

References

Beach, F. A. (1976). Sexual attractivity, proceptivity, and receptivity in female mammals. *Hormones and Behavior, 7,* 105-138.

Hunter M. (1990). Emotional well-being, sexual behavior and hormone replacement therapy. *Maturitas, 12,* 299-314.

Hunter, M., Battersby, R., & Whitehead, M. (1986). Relationships between psychological symptoms, somatic complaints and menopausal status. *Maturitas, 8,* 217-228.

Limouzin-Lamothe, M., Mairon, N., Joyce, C. R. B., & Le Gal, M. (1994). Quality of life after menopause: Influence of hormonal replacement therapy. *American Journal of Obstetrics and Gynecology, 170,* 618-624.

McCoy, N. L. (1990). Estrogen levels in relation to self-reported symptoms and sexuality in perimenopausal women. [Summary]. In M. Flint, F. Kronenberg, & W. Utian (Eds.), *Multidisciplinary perspectives in menopause. Annals of the New York Academy of Sciences, 592,* 450-452.

McCoy, N. L., & Davidson, J. M. (1985). A longitudinal study of the effects of menopause on sexuality. *Maturitas, 7,* 203-210.

McCoy, N. L., & Matyas, J. R. (1996). Oral contraceptives and sexuality in university women. *Archives of Sexual Behavior, 25,* 73-90.

Nathorst-Böös, J., von Schoultz, B., & Carlström, K. (1993) Elective ovarian removal and estrogen replacement therapy—Effects on

sexual life, psychological well-being and androgen status. *Journal of Psychosomatic Obstetrics and Gynaecology, 14,* 283-293.

Nathorst-Böös, J., Wiklund, I., Mattsson, L., Sandin, K., & von Schoultz, B. (1993). Is sexual life influenced by transdermal estrogen therapy? A double blind placebo controlled study in postmenopausal women. *Acta Obstetrica et Gynecologica Scandinavica, 72,* 656-660.

Exhibit

McCoy Female Sexuality Questionnaire (sample items)

Please answer the following questions in terms of your present experience—roughly the last 4 weeks. For some questions, you are asked to fill in the blank with a number. For others, circle the number or NA for "not applicable," meaning that you have not had a partner and/or sexual activity during that time period.

1. How enjoyable has sexual activity been for you?
4. How excited or aroused have you been during sexual activity (for instance, increased heartbeat/flushing/ heavy breathing, etc.)?
8. How sexually attractive do you feel you are to your primary sexual partner?
12. During the past 4 weeks, how often have you had sexual intercourse (penis inserted in the vagina)?
19. How often have you been prevented from having sexual intercourse because your partner could not achieve or maintain an erection?

Brief Index of Sexual Functioning for Women

Raymond C. Rosen,[1] Jennifer F. Taylor, and Sandra R. Leiblum, *University of Medicine and Dentistry of New Jersey, Robert Wood Johnson Medical School*

The Brief Index of Sexual Functioning for Women (BISF-W) was developed in response to the lack of a brief, standardized self-report measure of overall sexual function in women. Previous self-report measures have been either overly restrictive or inappropriate for use in large-scale clinical trials. None of the self-report measures to date provides a comprehensive, reliable assessment of key dimensions of sexual function in women, including sexual desire, orgasm, and satisfaction. Reynolds et al. (1988) have described the Brief Sexual Function Questionnaire (BSFQ) for men, a 21-item self-report inventory of sexual inter-

est, activity, satisfaction, and preference. The BSFQ has been found to be highly reliable and to discriminate between depressed, sexually dysfunctional, and healthy males (Howell et al., 1987; Reynolds et al., 1988). Surprisingly, no corresponding measures to the BSFQ for self-report assessment of female sexual function are available. The present questionnaire was developed to provide a comparable, brief, self-report measure of sexual function for women.

Description

The BISF-W consists of 22 items, assessing the major dimensions of sexual desire, arousal, orgasm, and satisfaction. Several items were adapted from the BSFQ, particularly those assessing frequency of sexual behavior, fantasy,

[1]Address correspondence to Raymond C. Rosen, Center for Sexual and Marital Health, Department of Psychiatry, Robert Wood Johnson Medical School, UMDNJ, 675 Hoes Lane, Piscataway, NJ 08854-5635; email: rosen@umdnj.edu.

masturbation, and sexual preference. Additional items were included to address specific issues believed to affect women's sexual functioning and satisfaction, such as body image, partner satisfaction, and sexual anxiety. Several items were designed to evaluate sexual performance difficulties in women, such as diminished arousal or lubrication, pain or tightness during intercourse, and difficulties in reaching orgasm. Items assessing the impact of health problems on sexual functioning are also included. Most items are arranged in Likert-type format to rate the frequency of occurrence of sexual desire, arousal, or satisfaction associated with common sexual behaviors. Based on a principal components analysis, three major factors were identified, which were labeled Sexual Desire, Sexual Activity, and Sexual Satisfaction.

Response Mode and Timing

Respondents circle the single best answer to each question. An automated scoring system is not available at the present time. The inventory takes approximately 10-15 minutes to complete.

Scoring

Individual items are scored, and the aggregate scores for each of the three major factors are computed. Items for the Sexual Desire factor are 3, 6, 8, 14, and 20. Items for the Sexual Activity factor are 3, 4, 5, 7, 9, 10, 11, 17, and 20. Items for the Sexual Satisfaction factor are 6, 9, 10, 15, 18, and 19. Item 16 is used independently as a measure of body image. Items 1, 2, 21, and 22 assess the presence of a sexual partner, sexual activity during the past month, and the respondent's sexual orientation, in terms of both experience and desire. These items are individually scored.

Reliability

In a sample of 269 women, aged 20-73, test-retest reliability was assessed by means of repeated administration of the questionnaire over a 1-month interval. Reliability was determined by means of a Pearson correlation coefficient between factor scores at the baseline and 1-month retest interval. Internal consistency was evaluated by means of

Cronbach alpha coefficients for each of the factor scales. The test-retest reliability of factor scores ranged from .68 to .78. The internal consistency of the instrument ranged from .39 for Factor 1 to .83 for Factor 2. The relatively low consistency for Factor 1 was attributed to the split loading of several items with other factors.

Validity

No significant correlations were observed between the BISF-W factor scores and the Crowne and Marlowe (1964) Social Desirability Scale. This indicates that responses to the BISF-W were not biased by the effects of social desirability. Concurrent validity was assessed by means of comparison of specific factor scores with the corresponding scales of the Derogatis Sexual Function Inventory (DSFI), a comprehensive, 261-item measure of sexual information, attitudes, experience, drive, body image, sex roles, and sexual satisfaction. Correlations between BISF-W factors and subscales of the DSFI were all in a positive direction, ranging from .59 to .69. Item 16, which assesses body image, was significantly correlated with the DSFI Body Image Scale ($r = .62$; $p < .001$). The scale has been used for assessment of sexual functioning in a community-based sample of 329 adult women (Rosen, Taylor, Leiblum, & Bachmann, 1993).

References

Crowne, D. P., & Marlowe, D. (1964). The approval motive: Studies in evaluative dependence. New York: Wiley.

Howell, J. R., Reynolds, C. F., Thase, M. E., Frank, E., Jennings, J. R., Houck, P. R., Berman, S., Jacobs, E., & Kupfer, D. J. (1987). Assessment of sexual function, interest, and activity in depressed men. *Journal of Affective Disorders, 13*, 61-66.

Reynolds, C. F., Frank, E., Thase, M. E., Houck, P. R., Jennings, J. R., Howell, J. R., Lilienfeld, S. O., & Kupfer, D. J. (1988). Assessment of sexual function in depressed, impotent, and healthy men: Factor analysis of a Brief Sexual Function Questionnaire for men. *Psychiatric Research, 24*, 231-250.

Rosen, R. C., Taylor, J. F., Leiblum, S. R., & Bachmann, G. A. (1993). Prevalence of sexual dysfunction in women: Results of a survey study of 329 women in an outpatient gynecological clinic. *Journal of Sex & Marital Therapy, 19*, 171-188.

Exhibit

Brief Index of Sexual Functioning for Women

ID# _____ Date _____

This index covers material that is sensitive and personal. Your responses will be kept completely confidential. If you are unable or do not wish to answer any question, you may leave it blank.

Answer the following questions by choosing the most accurate response <u>*for the past month.*</u>

   1. Do you currently have a sex partner? _____ Yes _____ No
   2. Have you been sexually active during the past month? _____ Yes _____ No

3. During the past month, how frequently have you had sexual thoughts, fantasies, or erotic dreams?
   (*Please circle the most appropriate response.*)
   (0) Not at all
   (1) Once
   (2) 2 or 3 times
   (3) Once a week
   (4) 2 or 3 times per week
   (5) Once a day
   (6) More than once a day
4. Using the scale to the right, indicate how frequently you have felt a desire to engage in the following activities during
   the past month? (*An answer is required for each, even if it may not apply to you.*)
   Kissing   _____   (0) Not at all
   Masturbation   _____   (1) Once
   Mutual masturbation   _____   (2) 2 or 3 times
   Petting and foreplay   _____   (3) Once a week
   Oral sex   _____   (4) 2 or 3 times per week
   Vaginal penetration or intercourse   _____   (5) Once a day
   Anal sex   _____   (6) More than once a day
5. Using the scale to the right, indicate how frequently you have become aroused by the following sexual experiences
   during the past month. (*An answer is required for each, even if it may not apply to you.*)
   Kissing   _____   (0) Have not engaged in this activity
   Masturbation alone   _____   (1) Not at all
   Mutual masturbation   _____   (2) Seldom, less than 25% of the time
   Petting and foreplay   _____   (3) Sometimes, about 50% of the time
   Oral sex   _____   (4) Usually, about 75% of the time
   Vaginal penetration or intercourse   _____   (5) Always became aroused
   Anal sex   _____
6. Overall, during the past month, how frequently have you become anxious or inhibited during sexual activity with
   a partner? (*Please circle the most appropriate response.*)
   (0) I have not had a partner
   (1) Not at all anxious or inhibited
   (2) Seldom, less than 25% of the time
   (3) Sometimes, about 50% of the time
   (4) Usually, about 75% of the time
   (5) Always became anxious or inhibited
7. Using the scale to the right, indicate how frequently you have engaged in the following sexual experiences during the
   past month. (*An answer is required for each, even if it may not apply to you.*)
   Kissing   _____   (0) Not at all
   Masturbation   _____   (1) Once
   Mutual masturbation   _____   (2) 2 or 3 times
   Petting and foreplay   _____   (3) Once a week
   Oral sex   _____   (4) 2 or 3 times per week
   Vaginal penetration or intercourse   _____   (5) Once a day
   Anal sex   _____   (6) More than once a day
8. During the past month, who has usually initiated sexual activity? (*Please circle the most appropriate response.*)
   (0) I have not had a partner
   (1) I have not had sex with a partner during the past month
   (2) I usually have initiated activity
   (3) My partner and I have equally initiated activity
   (4) My partner usually has initiated activity
9. During the past month, how have you usually responded to your partner's sexual advances? (*Please circle the most
   appropriate response.*)
   (0) I have not had a partner
   (1) Has not happened during the past month
   (2) Usually refused
   (3) Sometimes refused
   (4) Accepted reluctantly
   (5) Accepted, but not necessarily with pleasure
   (6) Usually accepted with pleasure
   (7) Always accepted with pleasure

10. During the past month, have you felt pleasure from any forms of sexual experience?
    (*Please circle the most appropriate response.*)
    (0) I have not had a partner
    (1) Have had no sexual experience during the past month
    (2) Have not felt any pleasure
    (3) Seldom, less than 25% of the time
    (4) Sometimes, about 50% of the time
    (5) Usually, about 75% of the time
    (6) Always felt pleasure

11. Using the scale to the right, indicate how often you have reached orgasm during the past month with the following activities. (*An answer is required for each, even if it may not apply to you.*)

    In dreams or fantasy   _____   (0) I have not had a partner
    Kissing   _____   (1) Have not engaged in this activity
    Masturbation alone   _____   (2) Not at all
    Mutual masturbation   _____   (3) Seldom, less than 25% of the time
    Petting and foreplay   _____   (4) Sometimes, about 50% of the time
    Oral sex   _____   (5) Usually, about 75% of the time
    Vaginal penetration or intercourse _____   (6) Always reached orgasm
    Anal sex   _____

12. During the past month, has the frequency of your sexual activity with a partner been: (*Please circle the most appropriate response.*)
    (0) I have not had a partner
    (1) Less than you desired
    (2) As much as you desired
    (3) More than you desired

13. Using the scale to the right, indicate the level of change, if any, in the following areas during the past month. (*An answer is required for each, even if it may not apply to you.*)

    Sexual interest   _____   (0) Not applicable
    Sexual arousal   _____   (1) Much lower level
    Sexual activity   _____   (2) Somewhat lower level
    Sexual satisfaction   _____   (3) No change
    Sexual anxiety   _____   (4) Somewhat higher level
                                                 (5) Much higher level

14. During the past month, how frequently have you experienced the following? (*An answer is required for each, even if it may not apply to you.*)

    Bleeding or irritation after vaginal
        penetration or intercourse _____   (0) Not at all
    Lack of vaginal lubrication   _____   (1) Seldom, less than 25% of the time
    Painful penetration or intercourse _____   (2) Sometimes, about 50% of the time
    Difficulty reaching orgasm   _____   (3) Usually, about 75% of the time
    Vaginal tightness   _____   (4) Always
    Involuntary urination   _____
    Headaches after sexual activity _____
    Vaginal infection   _____

15. Using the scale to the right, indicate the frequency with which the following factors have influenced your level of sexual activity during the past month. (*An answer is required for each, even if it may not apply to you.*)

    My own health problems
        (for example, infection, illness) _____   (0) I have not had a partner
    My partner's health problems   _____   (1) Not at all
    Conflict in the relationship   _____   (2) Seldom, less than 25% of the time
    Lack of privacy   _____   (3) Sometimes, about 50% of the time
    Other (please specify):   _____   (4) Usually, about 75% of the time
    _____   _____   (5) Always

16. How satisfied are you with the overall appearance of your body? (*Please circle the most appropriate response.*)
    (0) Very satisfied
    (1) Somewhat satisfied
    (2) Neither satisfied nor dissatisfied
    (3) Somewhat dissatisfied
    (4) Very dissatisfied

17. During the past month, how frequently have you been able to communicate your sexual desires or preferences to your partner? (*Please circle the most appropriate response.*)
    (0) I have not had a partner
    (1) I have been unable to communicate my desires or preferences
    (2) Seldom, about 25% of the time
    (3) Sometimes, about 50% of the time
    (4) Usually, about 75% of the time
    (5) I was always able to communicate my desires or preferences
18. Overall, how satisfied have you been with your sexual relationship with your partner? (*Please circle the most appropriate response.*)
    (0) I have not had a partner
    (1) Very satisfied
    (2) Somewhat satisfied
    (3) Neither satisfied nor dissatisfied
    (4) Somewhat dissatisfied
    (5) Very dissatisfied
19. Overall, how satisfied do you think your partner has been with your sexual relationship? (*Please circle the most appropriate response.*)
    (0) I have not had a partner
    (1) Very satisfied
    (2) Somewhat satisfied
    (3) Neither satisfied nor dissatisfied
    (4) Somewhat dissatisfied
    (5) Very dissatisfied
20. Overall, how important a part of your life is your sexual activity? (*Please circle the most appropriate response.*)
    (0) Not at all important
    (1) Somewhat unimportant
    (2) Neither important nor unimportant
    (3) Somewhat important
    (4) Very important
21. Circle the number that corresponds to the statement that best describes your sexual experience.
    (1) Entirely heterosexual
    (2) Largely heterosexual, but some homosexual experience
    (3) Largely heterosexual, but considerable homosexual experience
    (4) Equally heterosexual and homosexual
    (5) Largely homosexual, but considerable heterosexual experience
    (6) Largely homosexual, but some heterosexual experience
    (7) Entirely homosexual
22. Circle the number that corresponds to the statement that best describes your sexual desires.
    (1) Entirely heterosexual
    (2) Largely heterosexual, but some homosexual experience
    (3) Largely heterosexual, but considerable homosexual experience
    (4) Equally heterosexual and homosexual
    (5) Largely homosexual, but considerable heterosexual experience
    (6) Largely homosexual, but some heterosexual experience
    (7) Entirely homosexual

Source. This index was originally published in J. F. Taylor, R. C. Rosen, & S. R. Leiblum, "Self-Report Assessment of Female Sexual Function," 1994, *Archives of Sexual Behavior, 23,* 627-643. Reprinted with permission of Plenum Publishers and the authors.

Peak of Sexual Response Questionnaire

Jeanne Warner,[1] *Dimensions Research and Development, Inc.*

The Peak of Sexual Response Questionnaire (PSRQ) is a quantified self-report measure of the qualitative experience at the physical peak of sexual response and of the emotional reactions to the physical response. It also inquires about sites, modes, and effectiveness of stimulation.

Individuals can respond to the PSRQ regardless of how they define orgasm or whether they experience one. The factor-analytically derived scales provide interval data; specific stimuli and sites as multiple response items yield dichotomous data; both kinds are suitable for the multivariate analyses necessary to examine the complex interactions involved in sexual experience. The four parallel measures permit comparison of male and female and of partner-related and solitary masturbation responses. The comparison of the PSRQ scores of a normative sample to those of respondents for whom concurrent physiologic measures are obtained could serve as an indication of the generalizability of the physiologic data. Repeated administrations of the PSRQ can be used in longitudinal studies, such as evaluating group outcomes with pre-, during-, and post-therapy measures, and obtaining profiles of intraindividual variation. As an educational tool, it is a means of increasing a respondent's awareness of the possible range of feelings.

Description, Response Mode, and Timing

My initial interest in measuring "orgasm" and "sexual satisfaction" and the relationship between them led to the development of the PSRQ and to the identification of (a) six dimensions of the physical reactions and sensations experienced at peak of sexual response, (b) four dimensions of the emotional reaction to the physical peak, and (c) the relationships of those dimensions to self-defined orgasm (Warner, 1981). *Dimension* is used in the psychometric sense, as an independent source of variation common to or underlying, in this case, a group of descriptive phrases (Rummel, 1970).

The 1981 study was delimited to the experience of women in partner-related sexual activity. The original 76 phrases describing physical sensations and reactions were generated to represent the gamut of conceptual, operational, clinical, impressionistic, and subjective definitions and descriptions of levels of arousal and of orgasm as release or climax, as pelvic muscle contractions, and as types. In 1982, four parallel forms were produced: for men and women, in solitary masturbation and partner-related activity. In the new forms, 16 items were added, including phrases to describe physical reactions and sensations associated with "G spot" stimulation and fluid expulsion. In

items that refer to sex-specific anatomic structure, embryologically derived homologues are used.

The PSRQ is in booklet form, $7 \times 8\frac{1}{2}$ inches. Part 1 consists of 92 items to describe physical reactions and sensations experienced. The exhibit illustrates instructions and six of the descriptive items. Part 2 consists of 59 items, in the same format, to describe how the respondents felt about the physical peak described in Part 1, not to describe the circumstances of the activity or the partner. Part 3 pertains primarily to stimulus variables and Part 4 to background characteristics of the respondent. The entire PSRQ requires an average of 25 minutes to complete.

The term *physical peak* is used rather than *orgasm* to permit a respondent to describe an experience irrespective of any definition or occurrence of orgasm. *Partner-related sexual activity* (vs. *intercourse*) includes any of the variety of sexual interactions that may take place with any partner, male or female. For the purpose of factor analyses, one specific experience (the most recent one) is used as the point of reference in answering the questionnaire. This allows for greater precision and, it is hoped, for less confusion and less social desirability.

Scoring, Reliability, and Validity

The 1981 study sample was composed of 318 women, a usable response rate of 74%, ranging in age from 15 to 60 years, with a mean of 33.1 years ($SD = 9.44$) and a median of 32.7 years. The sample was geographically diverse and approximated the population of U.S. women (U.S. Bureau of the Census, 1979, pp. xix, xxi, 9, 144, 415) on age, race, and marital status, with a slight upward skew on education and occupation.

The 76 physical items were subjected to a principal axes factor analysis with iteration and varimax orthogonal rotation, using the squared multiple correlation of each item with all other items in the main diagonal as the initial estimate of communality (Nie, Hull, Jenkins, Steinbrenner, & Bent, 1975, p. 480). Rotation yielded six factors of three or more items with a loading of .35 or greater.

Dimensions were named according to the content of their strongest loading items. Release is characterized by descriptions of release, relaxation, feelings of moderate arousal, and suspension. Throbbing reflects perceptions of throbbing, pulling, pulsating, and other internal or external pelvic sensations. These factors suggest that feelings of release are not the same entity as the reactions and sensations associated with the involuntary contractions of the pelvic muscles. Continued Arousal represents a not uncomfortable arousal remaining after a multiple/mild/indefinite peak. Genital Sensation suggests the vasocongestion of the labia and outer third of the vagina. Sudden Cessation suggests some ambiguity regarding ceasing of excitement and

[1] Address correspondence to Jeanne Warner, 307 West 136th Street, New York, NY 10030; email: jw162@inibara.cc.columbia.edu.

relief of tension. Nongenital is an assortment of vocal, breathing, and body reactions. Four affective dimensions were identified: Evaluative, Depressed, Unresponsive, and Almost.

A respondent's score for each factor-derived scale is computed by dividing the sum of the item responses on that scale by the number of items scored. Presented in Table 1 are the number of items, coefficient of reliability as internal consistency (Cronbach's alpha), mean, and standard deviation for each scale.

Table 1 Statistics for 10 Scales of the Peak of Sexual Response Questionnaire

Scale	No. of items	Cronbach's alpha	M	SD
Physical				
Release	11	.86	3.7	0.78
Throbbing	14	.87	2.8	0.80
Continued arousal	10	.71	2.9	0.68
Genital sensation	3	.71	2.8	1.05
Sudden cessation	4	.59	2.3	0.84
Nongenital	7	.61	2.9	0.94
Affective				
Evaluative	13	.94	3.4	1.06
Depressed	6	.87	1.4	0.64
Unresponsive	5	.80	1.3	0.57
Almost	3	.65	2.0	0.99

Note. Possible range of scale scores is 1 to 5.

In research on the four parallel forms, preliminary analyses of data from 219 women and 118 men have resulted in similar reliability coefficients for the 10 scales.

In Part 3, respondents answer the question "Was your physical peak an orgasm?" (*yes* = 78%, *uncertain* = 8%, *no* = 15%). When dimension scores were dichotomized at 3.0, the scale midpoint, 93% of the group who answered yes had high scores on the Release dimension; only 47% had high scores on the Throbbing dimension. These data

suggest that report of self-defined orgasm reflects release rather than pelvic contractions and that perhaps nearly half of women who report orgasm do not experience reactions and sensations associated with pelvic contractions.

Arbitrary but mutually exclusive and exhaustive types of perceived physical peak were created using the 64 possible combinations of greater and lesser degrees of the six physical dimensions; 43 of these occurred in 318 women. Each of 13 patterns occurred in 3% to 8% of the sample; each of the remaining 30 patterns occurred in less than 3% of the women. The Warner-Bohlen matrix (Warner, Bohlen, Clifford, & Graber, 1983) represents the conceptualization of orgasm as being constituted of numerous discrete phenomena and experiences, which, until empirically demonstrated otherwise, should be considered to vary independently.

Other Information

Permission to use the PSRQ and copies of it may be requested from Jeanne Warner. I gratefully acknowledge the invaluable assistance of Joseph G. Bohlen in preparing the four parallel forms of this instrument. Research in progress on the PSRQ was supported, in part, by the Mary and Milton Rosenback Foundation Postdoctoral Fellowship in Health Education, Teachers College, Columbia University.

References

Nie, H. H., Hull, C. H., Jenkins, J. G., Steinbrenner, K., & Bent, D. N. (1975). *SPSS: Statistical package for the social sciences* (2nd ed.). New York: McGraw-Hill.

Rummel, R. J. (1970). *Applied factor analysis.* Evanston, IL: Northwestern University Press.

U.S. Bureau of the Census. (1979). *Statistical abstract of the United States: 1978* (100th ed.). Washington, DC: Author.

Warner, J. (1981). A factor analytic study of the physical and affective dimensions of peak of female sexual response in partner-related sexual activity (Doctoral dissertation, Teachers College, Columbia University, 1981). *Dissertation Abstracts International, 42,* 1967A–1968A. (University Microfilms No. DDJ81-22996)

Warner, J., Bohlen, J. G., Clifford, R., & Graber, B. (1983, November). *What do we mean by "orgasm"? A multidimensional view.* Symposium presented at the annual meeting of the Society for the Scientific Study of Sex, Chicago.

Exhibit

Peak of Sexual Response Questionnaire (sample page)

Part 1: Physical Reactions and Sensations

In this section, I am interested in what *physical* reactions and sensations you experienced in your one *most recent* situation of *partner-related* sexual activity (heterosexual or homosexual).

More specifically, I want to learn *only* about those reactions and sensations you had *at the physical peak* (the point of the most intense physical feeling) and *immediately after* that peak. (I do not want you to answer about feelings that occurred while building up to that peak.) If you had *two or more peaks of equal intensity* in that one situation, answer the items based on the *last* peak.

For each item in this section please *circle one answer* based on how well that item describes your own *physical* reactions or sensations *during and immediately after your physical peak* of that experience. Use the following scale:

1—*Not at all* like what I experienced
2—*Very little* like what I experienced
3—*Somewhat* like what I experienced
4—*Very much* like what I experienced
5—*Exactly* like what I experienced

Remember to base your answer to each item on:

—your *most recent partner-related* sexual experience.
—your *physical* reactions and sensations.
—*Only* the physical *peak*, and *immediately after*.
—*What you really* felt, *not* what you think you *should* have felt. Be as open and as careful as you can be, but don't spend a lot of time on any one item.

It is very important that you answer every item. If a particular description doesn't mean anything to you, then it is probably "not at all" or "very little" like what you experienced.

			Describes my *physical peak*			
	Not at all	Very little	Somewhat	Very much	Exactly	(For office use)
1. Floating sensation	1	2	3	4	5	(15)
2. Involuntarily hold breath then explosively exhale	1	2	3	4	5	(16)
3. Strenuous pelvic movements	1	2	3	4	5	(17)
4. Body, arms and legs tend to curl up	1	2	3	4	5	(18)
5. No definite beginning and ending	1	2	3	4	5	(19)
6. A pulling deep inside pelvis	1	2	3	4	5	(20)

Please be sure you have answered every item on this page.

Source. These sample items are reprinted with permission of the author.

The Hyperfemininity Scale

Sarah K. Murnen,[1] *Kenyon College*

The personality dimension of *hyperfemininity* was defined by Murnen and Byrne (1991) as an exaggerated attitudinal adherence to a stereotypic feminine gender role, particularly as it applies to heterosexual sexual relationships. It

[1]Address correspondence to Sarah K. Murnen, Department of Psychology, Kenyon College, Gambier, OH 43022; email: murnen@kenyon.edu.

was proposed that hyperfeminine women believe that their success is determined by developing and maintaining a relationship with a man and that their primary value in a romantic relationship is their sexuality. Hyperfeminine women endorse beliefs that sexuality can be used to obtain the goal of relationship maintenance. It has been proposed that hyperfemininity is likely to develop in a patriarchal society that subordinates women and rewards them for being sexual objects (Murnen, 1990). Women in North

American culture are sometimes rewarded for defining themselves as sexual objects. Unfortunately, it is proposed by some that this sexual objectification, combined with other societal forces, such as sexual aggression against women, perpetuates women's lower status (e.g., Sheffield, 1987).

Description

Twenty-six items representing one internally consistent dimension (as determined by principal components analysis) were selected for inclusion on the scale based on an item analysis from a group of 145 Caucasian college women from an Eastern state university (Murnen & Byrne, 1991).

Response Mode and Timing

The scale uses a forced-choice format similar to that used by the Hypermasculinity Inventory (Mosher & Sirkin, 1984). Respondents are asked to "choose the statement that is more characteristic of you."

Scoring

Each hyperfeminine choice receives a score of 1, and a total score is computing by summing the number of hyperfeminine responses. It generally takes between 10 and 15 minutes to complete the scale.

Reliability

The internal consistency of the scale in the original sample was .76, and was in the .80 to .90 range in subsequent samples. A test-retest coefficient was computed for a sample of 30 women who completed the scale at two different time periods, separated by 2 weeks. This temporal reliability coefficient was .89 (Murnen & Byrne, 1991).

Validity

Murnen and Byrne (1991) reported that hyperfeminine women advocated more agreement with attitudes that support a subordinate societal position for women. Hyperfeminine women reported more negative attitudes toward women and a greater endorsement of a traditional family ideology. They indicated that they thought marriage was more important for them than a career, although they rated it more important for a potential spouse to have an economically successful, prestigious job. Also, job competitiveness and job concern were negatively related to hyperfemininity scores.

It was also expected that hyperfeminine women would be conditioned to be more accepting of women's lower status as it applies to sexual subordination and be more accepting of sexual aggression against women. Hyperfemininity scores were correlated with advocating less "harsh" reactions to a sexual coercion scenario (Murnen & Byrne, 1991) and more self-blame when women were victims of sexual coercion (Murnen, Perot, & Byrne, 1989).

Hyperfemininity scores were positively correlated with endorsement of myths about rape (Murnen & Byrne, 1991).

Future work is exploring the societal acceptance of women's sexual objectification. Matschiner and Murnen (1995) found that women college students who described themselves as hyperfeminine prior to a speech they gave influenced men to a greater extent than did women who described themselves as less hyperfeminine, despite the fact that the high-hyperfeminine woman was perceived as less competent than the low-hyperfeminine woman. The high-hyperfeminine speaker was less influential with women participants than the low-hyperfeminine speaker. Consistent with these findings on the social acceptability of hyperfeminine responses, college women who were led to believe that they would be interacting with a man who endorsed many hypermasculine attitudes subsequently reported higher hyperfemininity scores than a group of women led to believe they would interact with a man who endorsed only a moderate amount of hypermasculine attitudes, provided that the man was liked (Matschiner & Murnen, 1995).

McKelvie and Gold (1994) found that hyperfeminine women were more likely to report being alienated from themselves and others and to suffer from psychological symptoms, such as anxiety and high levels of interpersonal sensitivity. They also found that in some scenarios that they presented to their participants, hyperfemininity scores were positively associated with justifying male sexual coercion of females. Similarly, Maybach and Gold (1994) found that women low in hyperfemininity reported less attraction to a description of a hypermasculine man than did high-hyperfeminine women.

There is information available concerning the discriminant validity of the scale as well. In one set of analyses, Murnen and Byrne (1991) found that endorsement of hyperfeminine items was negatively related to the tendency to report socially desirable responses. That is, it was socially undesirable to report hyperfeminine responses. When variation between social desirability was statistically partialed out of relationships between hyperfemininity and other nonsocially desirable variables, the relationships generally became stronger. This suggests that endorsing hyperfeminine attitudes is not a mere matter of reporting a socially desirable response (in fact, it seems to be that the opposite is true); social desirability might have a suppressing effect on some of the associations between hyperfemininity and other variables.

In addition, this dimension is not measuring adherence to socially acceptable feminine traits, as indicated by the fact that scores on the Hyperfemininity Scale were unrelated to scores on a scale of endorsement of socially desirable feminine traits (Murnen & Byrne, 1991). Apparently, the scale is measuring an aspect of femininity that is not as socially desirable as femininity measured by other scales. However, as indicated by Matschiner and Murnen's (1995) data, hyperfeminine behavior appears to be a successful influence strategy to use with some college men, and this finding indicates that there is some societal reward for this behavior. Along with numerous other variables, women's "acceptance" of their own sexual subordination might serve to support the status quo.

References

Matschiner, M., & Murnen, S. K. (1995). *Hyperfemininity as an effective social influence strategy.* Manuscript submitted for publication.

Maybach, K. L., & Gold, S. R. (1994). Hyperfemininity and attraction to macho and non-macho men. *The Journal of Sex Research, 31,* 91-98.

McKelvie, M., & Gold, S. R. (1994). Hyperfemininity: Further definitions of the construct. *The Journal of Sex Research, 31,* 219-228.

Mosher, D. L., & Sirkin, M. (1984). Measuring a macho personality constellation. *Journal of Research in Personality, 18,* 150-163.

Murnen, S. K. (1990, November). *The social control model and women's reactions to unwanted sexual activity.* Paper presented at the annual meeting of the Society for the Scientific Study of Sex, Minneapolis, MN.

Murnen, S. K., & Byrne, D. (1991). Hyperfemininity: Measurement and initial validation of the construct. *The Journal of Sex Research, 28,* 479-489.

Murnen, S. K., Perot, A., & Byrne, D. (1989). Coping with unwanted sexual activity: Normative responses, situational determinants, and individual differences. *The Journal of Sex Research, 26,* 85-106.

Sheffield, C. J. (1987). Sexual terrorism: The social control of women. In B. B. Hess & M. M. Ferree (Eds.), *Analyzing gender: A handbook of social science research* (pp. 171-189). Newbury Park, CA: Sage.

Exhibit

The Hyperfemininity Scale

Choose the response that is more characteristic of you.

1. a. These days men and women should each pay for their own expenses on a date.
   b. Men should always be ready to accept the financial responsibility for a date.*
2. a. I would rather be a famous scientist than a famous fashion model.
   b. I would rather be a famous fashion model than a famous scientist.*
3. a. I like a man who has some sexual experience.*
   b. Sexual experience is not a relevant factor in my choice of a male partner.
4. a. Women should never break up a friendship due to interest in the same man.
   b. Sometimes women have to compete with one another for men.*
5. a. I like to play hard-to-get.*
   b. I don't like to play games in a relationship.
6. a. I would agree to have sex with a man if I thought I could get him to do what I want.*
   b. I never use sex as a way to manipulate a man.
7. a. I try to state my sexual needs clearly and concisely.
   b. I sometimes say "no" but really mean "yes."*
8. a. I like to flirt with men.*
   b. I enjoy an interesting conversation with a man.
9. a. I seldom consider a relationship with a man as more important than my friendship with women.
   b. I have broken dates with female friends when a guy has asked me out.*
10. a. I usually pay for my expenses on a date.
    b. I expect the men I date to take care of my expenses.*
11. a. Sometimes I cry to influence a man.*
    b. I prefer to use logical rather than emotional means of persuasion when necessary.
12. a. Men need sex more than women do.*
    b. In general, there is no difference between the sexual needs of men and women.
13. a. I never use my sexuality to manipulate men.
    b. I sometimes act sexy to get what I want from a man.*
14. a. I feel anger when men whistle at me.
    b. I feel a little flattered when men whistle at me.*
15. a. It's okay for a man to be a little forceful to get sex.*
    b. Any force used during sex is sexual coercion and should not be tolerated.
16. a. Effeminate men deserve to be ridiculed.*
    b. So-called effeminate men are very attractive.
17. a. Women who are good at sports probably turn men off.*
    b. Men like women who are good at sports because of their competence.
18. a. A "real" man is one who can get any woman to have sex with him.*
    b. Masculinity is not determined by sexual success.
19. a. I would rather be president of the U.S. than the wife of the president.
    b. I would rather be the wife of the president of the U.S. than the president.*

20. a.   Sometimes I care more about my boyfriend's feelings than my own.*
    b.   It is important to me that I am as satisfied with a relationship as my partner is.
21. a.   Most women need a man in their lives.*
    b.   I believe some women lead happy lives without male partners.
22. a.   When a man I'm with gets really sexually excited, it's no use trying to stop him from getting what he wants.*
    b.   Men should be able to control their sexual excitement.
23. a.   I like to have a man "wrapped around my finger."*
    b.   I like relationships in which both partners are equal.
24. a.   I try to avoid jealousy in a relationship.
    b.   Sometimes women need to make men feel jealous so they will be more appreciative.*
25. a.   I sometimes promise to have sex with a man to make sure he stays interested in me.*
    b.   I usually state my sexual intentions honestly and openly.
26. a.   I like to feel tipsy so I have an excuse to do anything with a man.*
    b.   I don't like getting too drunk around a man I don't know very well.

Source. This scale was originally published in "Hyperfemininity: Measurement and Initial Validation of the Construct," by S. K. Murnen and D. Byrne, 1991, *The Journal of Sex Research, 28,* 479-489. Reprinted with permission.
*Indicates the hyperfeminine choice.

Global Sexual Functioning: A Single Summary Score for Nowinski and LoPiccolo's Sexual History Form (SHF)

Laura Creti,[1] *SMBD-Jewish General Hospital and Concordia University*
Catherine S. Fichten, *SMBD-Jewish General Hospital and Dawson College*
Rhonda Amsel, *McGill University*
William Brender, *SMBD-Jewish General Hospital and Concordia University*
Leslie R. Schover, *Cleveland Clinic Foundation*
Dennis Kalogeropoulos, *SMBD-Jewish General Hospital*
Eva Libman, *SMBD-Jewish General Hospital and Concordia University*

The Sexual History Form (SHF; Nowinski & LoPiccolo, 1979; Schover & Jensen, 1988) is a widely used multiple-choice questionnaire evaluating the frequency of sexual activity; sexual function relating to desire, arousal, orgasm, and pain; and overall sexual satisfaction for men and women. Originally developed for clinical use and to provide standardized data for diagnosis and research (Schover, Friedman, Weiler, Heiman, & LoPiccolo, 1982), the SHF has been widely used in sex therapy clinics, in clinical studies of sex therapy outcome (Fichten, Libman, Takefman, & Brender, 1988; Schover & LoPiccolo, 1982; Trudel, Ravart, & Matte, 1993), and in longitudinal assessments of the impact of chronic illness on sexuality (Schover, Fife,

[1]Address correspondence to Laura Creti, Behavior and Sex Therapy Services—ICFP, SMBD-Jewish General Hospital, 4333 Cote Ste. Catherine, Montreal, Quebec H3T 1E4, Canada.

& Gershenson, 1989; Schover, Novick, Steinmuller, & Goormastic, 1990; Schover et al., 1995).

In its present format, the SHF provides a very detailed self-report assessment of sexual behavior and function. It has been used in an item-by-item fashion to describe sexual problems in a particular population or to compare sexual function before and after a medical intervention. A limitation of the SHF for research has been the lack of a reliable and valid global score that could measure differences in overall sexual function between groups or across time.

To enhance the utility of the SHF, we developed a new scoring system that generates a single summary score: global sexual functioning (Creti, Fichten, Libman, Amsel, & Brender, 1988; Creti, Fichten, Libman, Kalogeropoulos, & Brender, 1987). The global sexual functioning score is easy to calculate, and concisely and accurately reflects overall level of sexual functioning. The single score also permits results from different investigations to be more readily compared.

Description

The SHF is a self-report sexual history measure. The original version consisted of 28 items; the latest version has 46. The format of the measure is multiple choice; items have variable numbers of response options and different response scales (e.g., Item 1 has nine options, with 1 = *more than once a day* and 9 = *not at all;* Item 18 has six options, with 1 = *never* and 6 = *nearly always [over 90% of the time]*). Response options are numbered from 1 to 4, 1 to 5, 1 to 6, or 1 to 9 and have a verbal descriptor corresponding to each number. The measure is typically scored on an item-by-item basis, resulting in 46 variables. Normative data for most items are presented in Schover and Jensen (1988); these are based on 92 couples in stable relationships who responded to an advertisement in New York in 1980. The mean age of the sample was in the early 30s, and they were predominantly Caucasian and middle class. Comparative item data from other samples can be found in Libman, Fichten, Creti, Amsel, and Brender (1986), LoPiccolo (1981), Nowinski and LoPiccolo (1979), and Weinstein et al. (1989).

Response Mode and Timing

Respondents circle the number that corresponds to the single most appropriate response for each question. The measure requires approximately 15 minutes to complete.

Scoring

The global sexual functioning score is calculated using 12 of the original 28 items (items have been renumbered in the current 46-item version). Because certain items are relevant only for males, whereas others are relevant only for females, the items used to calculate the male and female global sexual functioning score are somewhat different. The 12 items were selected as representative of various domains of sexual functioning: frequency of sexual activities, sexual desire, arousal, orgasmic, and erectile abilities.

To arrive at the single summary score, SHF items are grouped into a 12-item scale; this reflects either male or female global sexual functioning. The single summary score is derived by (a) converting the scores on each of the 12 items to a proportion of the maximum possible value, for example, if on Item 1, where response options are numbered 1 to 9, the respondent answers "(4) twice a week," this is converted to 4/9 = .44; (b) summing the 12 proportions; and (c) calculating the mean by dividing the total by the number of items which the respondent is deemed to have answered (usually 12). The resulting mean value, which is the global sexual functioning score, will be greater than 0 and less than 1. The calculation can be easily carried out using a calculator.

Specified in Table 1 are the items included in the calculation of the global sexual functioning score. For items with an asterisk, responses equaling 6 are considered missing because this response option is *have never tried;* in this case, the summed proportions are divided not by 12 but by the number of items that are deemed to have been answered (i.e., not missing). The scoring system is summarized in Table 1. Lower scores indicate better functioning.

Table 1 Calculating the Global Sexual Functioning Score

Male		Female	
Item no.	Divide by	Item no.	Divide by
1	9	1	9
2	9	2	9
6	9	6	9
7	9	7	9
10	6	16	5
16	5	23*	5
18	6	24*	5
19	6	25*	5
22	6	26*	5
23*	5	27*	5
24*	5	29	6
25*	5	37*	5

Note. Score as follows: (a) convert scores to proportions, (b) sum proportions, and (c) divide by number of items. Although all items included in the global sexual functioning score are present in the original 28-item version, items have been renumbered in the current 46-item version.

*Responses equaling 6 are considered missing.

Reliability

The global sexual functioning scores have excellent temporal stability. For example, in a sample of 27 older married women (mean age = 59), 2-week test-retest reliability was .92 (Creti et al., 1988). Temporal stability of the male global sexual functioning score, based on a sample of older married men described by Libman et al. (1989) (*n* = 45, mean age = 65), was .98.

Evaluation of internal consistency also shows acceptable psychometric properties for the global sexual functioning scores. For example, Cronbach's alpha for the male global sexual functioning was .65. Good internal consistency is reported for the female global sexual functioning score; item-total correlation coefficients presented by Creti et al. (1988) show *r* values ranging from .18 to .85, with the majority of values between .50 and .70.

Validity

Male global sexual functioning. Data indicate that, first, the global sexual functioning score can differentiate sexually well-functioning from poorly functioning men, and it is responsive to changes with therapy: Creti et al. (1987) reported that men with diagnosed sexual dysfunction had significantly ($p < .05$) worse scores ($M = .66$, $SD = .14$) than well-functioning men ($M = .37$, $SD = .08$), and Kalogeropoulos (1991) found scores to significantly improve in a sample of 53 males who had undergone vasoactive intracavernous pharmacotherapy for erectile dysfunction. Second, the global sexual functioning score is significantly related to other sexual functioning measures: Creti et al. (1987) found that men with higher sexual self-efficacy scored significantly better ($M = .48$, $SD = .07$) than men with lower sexual self-efficacy ($M = .59$, $SD = .10$), and global sexual functioning scores were found to be logically and significantly related to scores on measures of sexual satisfaction, sexual repertoire, sexual self-efficacy and sexual drive (Creti et al., 1987; Creti & Libman, 1989). Third, the global sexual functioning score is sensitive to age differences in sexual functioning: Libman et al. (1989) and Libman et al. (1991) showed that older married men (age 65+) had significantly worse scores ($M = .50$) than middle-aged married men (age = 50-64, $M = .46$), and Creti et al. (1987) and Creti and Libman (1989) found the score to be logically and significantly correlated with age. In addition, Libman et al. (1989) and Libman et al. (1991) showed that there is a small but significant deterioration in middle-aged and older men who have undergone surgery for benign prostatic enlargement (change from presurgery $M = .43$, $SD = .08$, to postsurgery $M = .48$, $SD = .11$).

Female global sexual functioning. Data reported by Creti et al. (1988) indicate that (a) women with diagnosed sexual dysfunction had worse scores ($M = .68$, $SD = .17$) than women who were functioning well ($M = .49$, $SD = .14$); (b) female global sexual functioning scores were logically and significantly correlated with sexual harmony, sexual satisfaction, diversity of sexual repertoire, and sexual drive; and (c) younger women (age 21-46) had better scores ($M = .46$, $SD = .03$) than older women (age greater than 64) ($M = .62$, $SD = .16$). Global sexual functioning scores were also found to be related to the females' sexual efficacy expectations for her male partner (Creti & Libman, 1989).

Other Information

The 28-item version of the SHF is also available in French (*Formulaire d'Histoire Sexuelle*).

References

Creti, L., Fichten, C. S., Libman, E., Amsel, R., & Brender, W. (1988, June). *Female sexual functioning: A global score for Nowinski and LoPiccolo's Sexual History Form.* Paper presented at the annual convention of the Canadian Psychological Association, Montreal, Quebec. (Abstracted in *Canadian Psychology, 29*[2a], Abstract 164)

Creti, L., Fichten, C. S., Libman, E., Kalogeropoulos, D., & Brender, W. (1987, November). *A global score for the "Sexual History Form" and its effectiveness.* Paper presented at the 21st annual convention of the Association for Advancement of Behavior Therapy, Boston.

Creti, L., & Libman, E. (1989). Cognitions and sexual expression in the aging. *Journal of Sex & Marital Therapy, 15*, 83-101.

Fichten, C. S., Libman, E., Takefman, J., & Brender, W. (1988). Self-monitoring and self-focus in erectile dysfunction. *Journal of Sex & Marital Therapy, 14*, 120-128.

Kalogeropoulos, D. (1991). *Vasoactive intracavernous pharmacotherapy for erectile dysfunction: Its effects on sexual, interpersonal, and psychological functioning.* Unpublished doctoral dissertation, Concordia University, Montreal, Quebec.

Libman, E., Fichten, C. S., Creti, L., Amsel, R., & Brender, W. (1986, June). *Aspects of sexual functioning in an aging population.* Paper presented at the Canadian Psychological Association, Toronto. (Abstracted in *Canadian Psychology, 27*, Abstract 354)

Libman, E., Fichten, C. S., Creti, L., Weinstein, N., Amsel, R., & Brender, W. (1989). Transurethral prostatectomy: Differential effects of age category and presurgery sexual functioning on postprostatectomy sexual adjustment. *Journal of Behavioral Medicine, 12*, 469-485.

Libman, E., Fichten, C. S., Rothenberg, P., Creti, L., Weinstein, N., Amsel, R., Liederman, G., & Brender, W. (1991). Prostatectomy and inguinal hernia repair: A comparison of the sexual consequences. *Journal of Sex & Marital Therapy, 17*, 27-34.

Libman, E., Rothenberg, I., Fichten, C. S., & Amsel, R. (1985). The SSES-E: A measure of sexual self-efficacy in erectile functioning. *Journal of Sex & Marital Therapy, 11*, 233-244.

LoPiccolo, J. (1981). *Norms for Sex History Form (male and female).* Unpublished manuscript, Texas A&M University, College Station.

Nowinski, J. K., & LoPiccolo, J. (1979). Assessing sexual behaviors in couples. *Journal of Sex & Marital Therapy, 5*, 225-243.

Schover, L. R., Fife, M., & Gershenson, D. M. (1989). Sexual dysfunction and treatment for early stage cervical cancer. *Cancer, 63*, 204-212.

Schover, L. R., Friedman, J. M., Weiler, J., Heiman, J. R., & LoPiccolo, J. (1982). Multiaxial problem-oriented system for sexual dysfunctions: An alternative to DSM-III. *Archives of General Psychiatry, 39*, 614-619.

Schover, L. R., & Jensen, S. B. (1988). *Sexuality and chronic illness: A comprehensive approach.* New York: Guilford.

Schover, L. R., & LoPiccolo, J. (1982). Treatment effectiveness for dysfunctions of sexual desire. *Journal of Sex & Marital Therapy, 8*, 179-197.

Schover, L. R., Novick, A. C., Steinmuller, D. R., & Goormastic, M. (1990). Sexuality, fertility, and renal transplantation: A study of survivors. *Journal of Sex & Marital Therapy, 16*, 3-14.

Schover, L. R., Yetman, R. J., Tuason L. J., Meisler, E., Esselstyn, C. B., Hermann, R. E., Grundfest-Broniatowski, S., & Dowden, R. V. (1995). Comparison of partial mastectomy with breast reconstruction on psychosocial adjustment, body image, and sexuality. *Cancer, 75*, 54-64.

Trudel, G., Ravart, G., & Matte, B. (1993). The use of the multiaxial diagnostic system for sexual dysfunctions in the assessment of hypoactive sexual desire. *Journal of Sex & Marital Therapy, 19*, 123-130.

Weinstein, N., Pencer, I., Libman, E., Fichten, C. S., Creti, L., Rothenberg, P., Liederman, G., Amsel, R., & Brender, W. (1989, October). *Does aging affect sexual expression?* Paper presented at the annual convention of the Société Québecoise pour la Recherche en Psychologie, Montreal, Quebec. (Abstracted in *XIIième congrès annuel: Programme et résumés des communication, 177.* Montreal: Société Québecoise pour la Recherche en Psychologie)

Exhibit

Sexual History Form

Please circle the most appropriate response to each question.

1. How frequently do you and your mate have sexual intercourse or activity?
   1) More than once a day
   2) Once a day
   3) 3 or 4 times a week
   4) Twice a week
   5) Once a week
   6) Once every 2 weeks
   7) Once a month
   8) Less than once a month
   9) Not at all

2. How frequently would you like to have sexual intercourse or activity?
   1) More than once a day
   2) Once a day
   3) 3 or 4 times a week
   4) Twice a week
   5) Once a week
   6) Once every 2 weeks
   7) Once a month
   8) Less than once a month
   9) Not at all

3. Who usually initiates sexual intercourse or activity?
   1) I always do
   2) I usually do
   3) My mate and I initiate about equally often
   4) My mate usually does
   5) My mate always does

4. Who would you ideally like to initiate sexual intercourse or activity?
   1) Myself, always
   2) Myself, usually
   3) My mate and I equally often
   4) My mate, usually
   5) My mate always

5. When your mate makes sexual advances, how do you usually respond?
   1) I usually accept with pleasure
   2) Accept reluctantly
   3) Often refuse
   4) Usually refuse

6. How often do you experience sexual *desire* (this may include wanting to have sex, planning to have sex, feeling frustrated due to lack of sex, etc.)?
   1) More than once a day
   2) Once a day
   3) 3 or 4 times a week
   4) Twice a week
   5) Once a week
   6) Once every 2 weeks
   7) Once a month
   8) Less than once a month
   9) Not at all

7. How often do you masturbate (bring yourself to orgasm in private)?
   1) More than once a day
   2) Once a day
   3) 3 or 4 times a week
   4) Twice a week
   5) Once a week
   6) Once every 2 weeks
   7) Once a month
   8) Less than once a month
   9) Not at all

8. For how long do you and your mate usually engage in sexual foreplay (kissing, petting, etc.) before having intercourse?
   1) Less than 1 minute
   2) 1 to 3 minutes
   3) 4 to 6 minutes
   4) 7 to 10 minutes
   5) 11 to 15 minutes
   6) 16 to 30 minutes
   7) 30 minutes to one hour

9. How long does intercourse usually last, from entry of the penis to the male's orgasm/climax?
   1) Less than 1 minute
   2) 1 to 2 minutes
   3) 2 to 4 minutes
   4) 4 to 7 minutes
   5) 7 to 10 minutes
   6) 11 to 15 minutes
   7) 15 to 20 minutes
   9) More than 30 minutes

10. Does the male ever reach orgasm while he is trying to enter the vagina with his penis?
    1) Never
    2) Rarely (less than 10% of the time)
    3) Seldom (less than 25% of the time)
    4) Sometimes (50% of the time)
    5) Usually (75% of the time)
    6) Nearly always (over 90% of the time)

11. Do you feel that premature ejaculation (rapid climax) is a problem in your sexual relationship?
    1) Yes
    2) No

12. How satisfied are you with the *variety of sexual activities* in your current sex life? (This includes the different types of kissing and caressing with a partner, different positions for intercourse, etc.)
    1) Extremely satisfied
    2) Moderately satisfied
    3) Slightly satisfied
    4) Slightly *un*satisfied
    5) Moderately *un*satisfied
    6) Extremely *un*satisfied
13. Would you like your lovemaking to include *more:*
    Breast caressing   1) Yes   2) No
    Hand caressing of your genital area   1) Yes   2) No
    Oral caressing (kissing) of your genital area   1) Yes   2) No
    Different positions for intercourse   1) Yes   2) No
14. If you would like a certain kind of sexual caress or activity, which way do you *typically* let your partner know?
    1) I wait to see if my partner will do what I like without my asking
    2) I show my partner what I would like by moving their hand or changing my own position
    3) I tell my partner exactly what I would like
15. How have you *typically* learned about your partner's sexual likes and dislikes?
    1) From my partner telling me exactly what they want
    2) From my partner moving my hand or changing their position to signal what they would like me to do
    3) From watching my partner's reactions during sex
    4) From intuition
16. When you have sex with your mate do you feel sexually aroused (e.g., feeling "turned on," pleasure, excitement)?
    1) Nearly always (over 90% of the time)
    2) Usually (about 75% of the time)
    3) Sometimes (about 50% of the time)
    4) Seldom (about 25% of the time)
    5) Never
17. When you have sex with your mate, do you have negative emotional reactions (e.g., fear, disgust, shame, or guilt)?
    1) Never
    2) Rarely (less than 10% of the time)
    3) Seldom (less than 25% of the time)
    4) Sometimes (50% of the time)
    5) Usually (75% of the time)
    6) Nearly always (over 90% of the time)
18. Does the male have any trouble getting an erection before intercourse begins?
    1) Never
    2) Rarely (less than 10% of the time)
    3) Seldom (less than 25% of the time
    4) Sometimes (50% of the time)
    5) Usually (75% of the time)
    6) Nearly always (over 90% of the time)
19. Does the male have any trouble keeping an erection once intercourse has begun?
    1) Never
    2) Rarely (less than 10% of the time)
    3) Seldom (less than 25% of the time
    4) Sometimes (50% of the time)
    5) Usually (75% of the time)
    6) Nearly always (over 90% of the time)
20. If the male loses an erection, when does that usually happen?
    1) Before penetrating to start intercourse
    2) While trying to penetrate
    3) After penetration, during the thrusting of intercourse
    4) Not applicable, losing erections is not a problem
21. What is the male's *typical* degree of erection during sexual activity?
    1) 0% to 20% of a full erection
    2) 20% to 40% of a full erection
    3) 40% to 60% of a full erection
    4) 60% to 80% of a full erection
    5) 80% to 100% of a full erection
22. Does the male ejaculate (climax) without having a full, hard erection?
    1) Never
    2) Rarely (less than 10% of the time)
    3) Seldom (less than 25% of the time
    4) Sometimes (50% of the time)
    5) Usually (75% of the time)
    6) Nearly always (over 90% of the time)
23. If you try, is it possible to reach orgasm (sensation of climax) through masturbation?
    1) Nearly always (over 90% of the time)
    2) Usually (about 75% of the time)
    3) Sometimes (about 50% of the time)
    4) Seldom (about 25% of the time)
    5) Never
    6) Have never tried to
24. If you try, is it possible for you to reach orgasm (sensation of climax) through having your genitals caressed by your mate?
    1) Nearly always (over 90% of the time)
    2) Usually (about 75% of the time)
    3) Sometimes (about 50% of the time)
    4) Seldom (about 25% of the time)
    5) Never
    6) Have never tried to
25. If you try, is it possible for you to reach orgasm (sensation of climax) through sexual intercourse?
    1) Nearly always (over 90% of the time)
    2) Usually (about 75% of the time)
    3) Sometimes (about 50% of the time)
    4) Seldom (about 25% of the time)
    5) Never
    6) Have never tried to

26. Can you reach orgasm (sensation of climax) through stimulation of your genitals by an electric vibrator or any other means (i.e., running water, rubbing with some object, etc.)?
    1) Nearly always (over 90% of the time)
    2) Usually (about 75% of the time)
    3) Sometimes (about 50% of the time)
    4) Seldom (about 25% of the time)
    5) Never
    6) Have never tried to
27. (Women only) Can you reach orgasm during sexual intercourse if, at the same time, your genitals are being caressed (by yourself or your mate with a vibrator, etc.)?
    1) Nearly always (over 90% of the time)
    2) Usually (about 75% of the time)
    3) Sometimes (about 50% of the time)
    4) Seldom (about 25% of the time)
    5) Never
    6) Have never tried to
28. Have you noticed a change in the intensity and pleasure of your orgasm?
    1) Much more intense and pleasurable than in the past
    2) Somewhat more intense and pleasurable than in the past
    3) The same as in the past
    4) Somewhat less intense and pleasurable than in the past
    5) Much less intense and pleasurable than in the past
29. Is the female's vagina so "dry" or "tight" that intercourse cannot occur?
    1) Never
    2) Rarely (less than 10% of the time)
    3) Seldom (less than 25% of the time
    4) Sometimes (50% of the time)
    5) Usually (75% of the time)
    6) Nearly always (over 90% of the time)
30. Do you feel pain in your genitals (sexual parts) during intercourse?
    1) Never
    2) Rarely (less than 10% of the time)
    3) Seldom (less than 25% of the time
    4) Sometimes (50% of the time)
    5) Usually (75% of the time)
    6) Nearly always (over 90% of the time)
31. How often does pain (genital or nongenital) interfere with your ability to feel sexual pleasure?
    1) Never
    2) Rarely (less than 10% of the time)
    3) Seldom (less than 25% of the time
    4) Sometimes (50% of the time)
    5) Usually (75% of the time)
    6) Nearly always (over 90% of the time)
32. Have you noticed a change in the sensitivity to touch of your genitals?
    1) Much more sensitive than in the past
    2) Somewhat more sensitive than in the past
    3) About as sensitive as in the past
    4) Somewhat less sensitive than in the past
    5) Much less sensitive than in the past
33. Overall, how satisfactory to you is your sexual relationship with your mate?
    1) Extremely unsatisfactory
    2) Moderately unsatisfactory
    3) Slightly unsatisfactory
    4) Slightly satisfactory
    5) Moderately satisfactory
    6) Extremely satisfactory
34. Overall, how satisfactory do you think your sexual relationship is to your mate?
    1) Extremely unsatisfactory
    2) Moderately unsatisfactory
    3) Slightly unsatisfactory
    4) Slightly satisfactory
    5) Moderately satisfactory
    6) Extremely satisfactory
35. Do you feel that your partner plays a part in causing a problem in your sex life?
    1) Yes
    2) No
36. If your lovemaking does not go well, how does your partner usually react?
    1) Accepting and understanding
    2) Frustrated or annoyed
    3) Anxious and blaming self
    4) Neutral or uncaring
37. (Women only, men go on to Question 38) When you have sex with your mate (including foreplay and intercourse) do you notice some of these things happening: your breathing and pulse speed up, wetness in your vagina, pleasurable sensations in your breasts and genitals?
    1) Nearly always (over 90% of the time)
    2) Usually (about 75% of the time)
    3) Sometimes (about 50% of the time)
    4) Seldom (about 25% of the time)
    5) Never
    6) Have never tried to
38. (Men only) How often do you wake from sleep with a firm erection (including times when you wake up needing to urinate)?
    1) Daily
    2) 3-4 times a week
    3) 1-2 times a week
    4) Once every 2 weeks
    5) Once a month
    6) Less than once a month
    7) Never
39. (Men only) How often do you wake from sleep with a partial (semisoft) erection?
    1) Daily
    2) 3-4 times a week
    3) 1-2 times a week
    4) Once every 2 weeks
    5) Once a month
    6) Less than once a month
    7) Never

40. *(Men only)* How often are you able to get and keep a firm erection in your own masturbation (self-touch in private)?
    1) Nearly always, over 90% of the time
    2) Usually, 75% of the time
    3) Sometimes, 50% of the time
    4) Seldom, less than 25% of the time
    5) Rarely, less than 10% of the time
    6) Never
    7) Have not tried masturbation in the past 6 months
41. *(Men only)* What is your *typical* degree of erection during masturbation (self-touch in private)?
    1) 0% to 20% of a full erection
    2) 20% to 40% of a full erection
    3) 40% to 60% of a full erection
    4) 60% to 80% of a full erection
    5) 80% to 100% of a full erection
42. *(Men only)* Do you feel your erect penis has an abnormal curve to it, or have you noticed a lump or "knot" on your penis?
    1) Yes
    2) No
43. *(Men only)* Do you believe your penis is abnormally small?
    1) Yes
    2) No
44. *(Men only)* How does the amount of ejaculate (liquid or semen) now compare to the amount you ejaculated in the past?
    1) Much greater than in the past
    2) Somewhat greater than in the past
    3) About the same as in the past
    4) Somewhat less than in the past
    5) Much less than in the past
    6) I do not know
45. *(Men only)* Do you ever have the sensation of orgasm (climax) without any ejaculation of fluid?
    1) Never
    2) Rarely, less than 10% of the time
    3) Seldom, less than 25% of the time
    4) Sometimes, about 50% of the time
    5) Usually, about 75% of the time
    6) Nearly always, over 90% of the time
46. *(Men only)* Do you ever have pain and/or burning during or after ejaculation?
    1) Never
    2) Rarely, less than 10% of the time
    3) Seldom, less than 25% of the time
    4) Sometimes, about 50% of the time
    5) Usually, about 75% of the time
    6) Nearly always, over 90% of the time
    7) I do not ejaculate

Note. Items 1, 2, 6, 7, 10, 16, 18, 19, 22, 23, 24, 25, 26, 27, 29, and 37 are used to compute the global sexual functioning score.

The Derogatis Interview for Sexual Functioning

Leonard R. Derogatis,[1] *Clinical Psychometric Research, Inc.*

Description

The Derogatis Interview for Sexual Functioning (DISF) is a brief semistructured interview designed to provide an estimate of the quality of an individual's current sexual functioning in quantitative terms. The DISF represents quality of current sexual functioning in a multidomain format, which to some degree parallels the phases of the sexual response cycle (Masters & Johnson, 1966). The 26 interview items of the DISF are arranged into five domains of sexual functioning: I. Sexual Cognition/Fantasy, II. Sexual Arousal, III. Sexual Behavior/Experience, IV. Orgasm, and V. Sexual Drive/Relationship. In addition, the DISF total score is computed, summarizing quality of sexual functioning

[1]Address correspondence to Leonard R. Derogatis, Clinical Psychometric Research, Inc., Suite 302, 100 W. Pennsylvania Avenue, Towson, MD 21204.

across the five primary DISF domains. There are distinct gender-keyed versions for men and women.

In addition to the DISF interview, there is a distinct self-report version of the test known as the DISF-SR. The DISF-SR is also composed of 26 items and was designed to be as comparable to the DISF interview as possible. With slight modifications in format, the DISF-SR may also be used to gain evaluations of the patient's sexual performance by the patient's spouse.

The DISF and DISF-SR were developed to address the unmet need for a set of brief, gender-keyed, multidimensional outcome measures that would represent the status of an individual's current sexual functioning, and do so at multiple levels of interpretation. The DISF and DISF-SR are designed to be interpreted at three distinct levels: the *discrete item* level (e.g., "A full erection upon awakening," "Your ability to have an orgasm,") the *functional domain* level (e.g., sexual arousal score), and the *global summary* level (e.g., DISF/DISF-SR total score). Because the DISF interview and the DISF-SR self-report inventory are matched on an almost item-for-item basis, clinician and patient assessments of the patient's quality of sexual functioning may be obtained in both raw and standardized score formats. Both instruments may be used repeatedly throughout efficacy or effectiveness trials, or may be implemented solely at pre- and postintervention without significant "practice" effects or loss of validity.

Norms have been developed for both the DISF and the DISF-SR, based in each case on several hundred nonpatient community respondents. The norms are gender keyed (i.e., separate norms for men and women) and are represented as standardized scores in terms of area *t* scores. The area standardized score possesses distinct advantages over the simple linear transformation in that the former provides accurate percentile equivalents (i.e., *t* score of 30 = 2nd centile; *t* score of 40 = 16th centile; *t* score of 50 = 50th centile; *t* score of 60 = 84th centile; *t* score of 70 = 98th centile, etc.). This important characteristic is not true of linear *t* scores except when the underlying raw-score distribution is perfectly normal. In addition to enabling accurate comparisons across respondents, area *t* scores also facilitate meaningful comparisons of strengths and weaknesses *within* a respondent's profile of sexual functioning. A patient may reveal a relatively unremarkable profile with the exception of a profound decrement in a single functional domain, or may show a low-grade degradation of performance across multiple areas of functioning. Because DISF/DISF-SR domain scores are available in an equivalent standardized metric, such evaluations can help pinpoint the nature and extent of sexual dysfunctions.

Response Mode and Timing

The DISF and DISF-SR are each composed of 26 items. In the case of the former, items are cast in the format of a semistructured interview, structured via 4-point Likert-type scales. The items of the DISF-SR are also represented as 4-point Likert-type scales.

The DISF interview requires between 15 and 20 minutes to complete. Time requirements for the DISF-SR are similar to the DISF; however, in most contexts the self-report version typically requires a few minutes less than the interview. Time requirements drop noticeably for both versions on successive administrations, such as in clinical efficacy or effectiveness trials, in which the test is administered sequentially.

Reliability and Validity

The DISF and DISF-SR have both demonstrated favorable profiles of psychometric characteristics. Internal consistency coefficients for the subscales range from .74 to .80. Test-retest correlations over a 1-week interval are all above .80, and interrater correlations range from .84 to .92.

An important validity demonstration for multidimensional or multidomain psychological outcome measures concerns the subtest intercorrelation matrix, and domain score-total score correlation vector. The pattern of these correlations represents a central psychometric characteristic of the test that relates to almost all discernible aspects of construct validity (Messick, 1995). If correlations between dimension scores are high, concerns may be raised that operational definitions of the domain constructs are redundant. If domain scores do not correlate at least moderately with the total score, then the possibility exists that the domain constructs (e.g., Sexual Arousal, Orgasm), as operationally defined by the test items, are not valid components of the higher-order, more general construct (e.g., Quality of Sexual Functioning). A theoretical optimum would find correlations between domains near zero, with each domain score showing a moderately high correlation with the total score. In such an ideal design, each domain would contribute independent true variance to the total score, with minimum redundancy or overlap.

Subtest intercorrelation matrices of the DISF/DISF-SR have been constructed based on two normal samples and one sexually dysfunctional sample. In all cases, the mean interdomain correlation coefficients are relatively low (i.e., .23 to .39), whereas the average domain-total correlations for the three samples range from .60 to .71. This pattern of subtest correlations begins to approach optimal and strongly confirms that DISF domains are contributing relatively independent variance to the DISF total score.

The DISF and DISF-SR have been introduced only recently, and much of the clinical research done with the tests has primarily involved corporate-sponsored clinical drug trials. Although preliminary data from these studies indicate that the tests are highly sensitive to sexual dysfunction and to a broad range of therapeutic agents, most of the data are proprietary and have not yet been made generally available. In two studies that have been published (Zinreich et al., 1990a, 1990b), the DISF was used with males suffering from prostate cancer about to undergo a course of radiation therapy. At time of initial cancer diagnosis, the DISF was used in a logistic regression model as a screen for impotence, with detailed clinical evaluation as the ultimate criterion. In this study, sensitivity was found to be 86%, specificity was 80%, and the predictive value of a positive was 86%. Subsequent to treatment, patients were assigned to three functional categories on the basis of clinical evaluation: (a) totally functional, (b) marginally functional, and (c) impotent. Scores on the five domains of the DSFI were significantly different across the three groups, with mean DISF total scores being 48.2, 21.5, and 14.0, respectively. In this study, with a complex sample of patients, the DISF did a superior job of identifying those individuals who were dysfunctional prior to treatment, and it validly reflected differences in quality of sexual functioning subsequent to therapeutic intervention.

Currently, other studies using the DISF and DISF-SR are in the process of submission and review for publication, and several new norms (e.g., geriatric, gay men) are in the process of being developed.

Other Information

The instruments are available in English, French, Italian, Spanish, Dutch, Danish, and Norwegian. The DISF and DISF-SR are distributed exclusively by Clinical Psychometric Research, Inc., Suite 302, 100 W. Pennsylvania Avenue, Towson, MD 21204; phone: 1-800-245-0277 or (410) 321-6165; fax: (410) 321-6341.

References

Derogatis, L. R. (1996). *Derogatis Interview for Sexual Functioning (DISF/DISF-SR): Preliminary scoring, procedures & administration manual.* Baltimore, MD: Clinical Psychometric Research.

Masters, W. H., & Johnson, V. E. (1966). *Human sexual response.* Boston: Little, Brown.

Messick, S. (1995). Validity of psychological assessment: Validation of inferences from person's responses and performances as scientific inquiry into score meaning. *American Psychologist, 50,* 741-749.

Zinreich, E. Derogatis, L. R., Herpst, J., Auvil, G., Piantodosi, S., & Order, S. E. (1990a). Pre- and posttreatment evaluation of sexual function in patients with adenocarcinoma of the prostate. *International Journal of Radiation Oncology & Biological Physics, 19,* 729-732.

Zinreich, E., Derogatis, L. R., Herpst, J., Auvil, G., Piantodosi, S., & Order, S. E. (1990b). Pretreatment evaluation of sexual function in patients with adenocarcinoma of the prostate. *International Journal of Radiation Oncology & Biological Physics, 19,* 1001-1004.

The Derogatis Sexual Functioning Inventory

Leonard R. Derogatis,[1] *Clinical Psychometric Research, Inc.*

The Derogatis Sexual Functioning Inventory (DSFI) measures constructs believed to be fundamental to successful sexual functioning (e.g., drive, body image, sexual satisfaction) and in addition, measures several basic indicators of general well-being (e.g., affects balance and psychological distress).

Description

The DSFI is an "omnibus" self-report inventory designed to measure the quality of the *current sexual functioning* of an individual. The DSFI is multidimensional in nature because the comprehensive study of sexual functioning has revealed it to be a highly multidetermined behavior. Although apparently straightforward, successful human sexual functioning rests on a complex interplay of endocrine, emotional, cognitive, and experiential factors that preclude the simple enumeration of sexual episodes, or orgasms, as meaningful forms of measuring the quality of sexual functioning.

The individual respondent is the basis for evaluation by the DSFI in part because it represents the most parsimonious and straightforward unit to work with, and also because, regardless of context, quality of sexual functioning is ultimately appreciated by the individual. *Current sexual functioning* is the conceptual continuum for the DSFI because it comes closest to the central evaluative question in the clinical assessment of sexual disorder: "What is the current level and nature of the patient's sexual functioning?" By quantifying the principal dimensions of the

[1]Address correspondence to Leonard R. Derogatis, Clinical Psychometric Research, Inc., 100 W. Pennsylvania Avenue, Suite 302, Towson, MD 21204.

patient's sexual experience in profile form, an insight is gained into both the nature and magnitude of the individual's sexual dysfunction.

The DSFI is composed of 10 substantive dimensions that are judged to reflect the principal components of sexual behavior. The conceptual basis for the DSFI was outlined by Derogatis in 1976, and several subsequent monographs have been published on the instrument (Derogatis, 1980; Derogatis & Melisaratos, 1979). Of the 10 subtests constituting the DSFI, two of them, Psychological Symptoms and Affects, are themselves complete, multidimensional tests. The Brief Symptom Inventory (BSI; Derogatis, 1993) and the Derogatis Affects Balance Scale (ABS; Derogatis, 1975; Derogatis & Rutigliano, 1996) provide measurement of psychological distress and mood and affects, respectively.

Since its introduction in the mid-1970s, the DSFI has been used as an outcome measure in approximately 50 empirical studies of sexual functioning (see references). In most instances, dimension or global score measures from the instrument have proven sufficiently sensitive to discriminate differences in the groups under study. Discriminations have ranged from relatively large effect sizes (e.g., comparisons of gender-dysphoric patients with normal heterosexuals) to much more demanding discriminations (e.g., sexual functioning in diabetic vs. normal women, inflatable vs. noninflatable prostheses in penile implant surgery).

Response Mode

The DSFI is composed of 254 items, arranged into 10 subtests. Formats vary from simple endorsements of *yes* or *no* to multiple-point Likert-type scales.

DSFI Dimensions and Global Score Descriptions

Information. The Information subtest consists of 26 items in true-false format that measure the level of accurate information possessed by the respondent concerning the physiology, anatomy, and other aspects of sexual functioning. A single information score is determined as the sum of the number of correct responses.

Experiences. The Experiences subtest consists of a list of 24 sexual behaviors ranging from very fundamental behaviors to various forms of sexual intercourse and oral-genital activities. The respondent indicates which behaviors he or she has experienced lifetime, and which experiences have occurred during the past 60 days. The Experiences score is the sum of lifetime experiences.

Drive. The Drive subtest is a composite summary measure of libidinal erotic interests expressed in the five behavioral domains of sexual intercourse, masturbation, kissing and petting, sexual fantasy, and ideal frequency of intercourse. The respondent indicates the frequencies of these behaviors during the current period. A single Drive score is developed by summing across domains.

Attitudes. Based on work showing liberal and conservative sexual attitudes to be predictive of quality of sexual functioning, this subtest is composed of 30 items (15 liberal items and 15 conservative items) represented on 5-point Likert-type scales. The respondent indicates the degree to which he or she is in agreement with each item. Liberal, conservative, and total attitude scores are generated.

Psychological Symptoms. Psychological distress is measured by the 53 items of the Brief Symptom Inventory (BSI). Each symptom of the BSI is represented on a 5-point scale from *not at all* (0) to *extremely* (4). Scores are summed across items to achieve a single Symptoms score. The BSI may optionally be scored for the nine dimensions (e.g., Depression, Anxiety) and global scores that underlie the items of the BSI.

Affects. The Affects subtest is also a complete multidimensional test termed the Derogatis Affects Balance Scale (DABS). The DABS measures affect and mood through 40 adjective items endorsed by the respondent. Twenty items represent positive affects, and 20 items reflect negative affects. Scores include a Positive Affects total, a Negative Affects total and the overall Affects Balance Index. The latter is used as the affects measure for the DSFI.

Gender Role Definition. Consistent with the concept that masculinity and femininity are components of all individuals' gender role definitions, the two primary components of gender role are each measured in terms of 15 adjective items that the respondent endorses in varying degrees. A Masculinity score, a Femininity score, and a Gender Role Definition score are determined.

Fantasy. This subtest consists of 20 major sexual themes that have been culled from research on normal sexual fantasies as well as fantasies arising from clinical variations on routine sexual behaviors. The Fantasy score consists of a simple summation of the items endorsed.

Body Image. Body image has been demonstrated to be an integral aspect of self-concept and, as such, is an important determinant of successful sexual functioning. It is measured in the DSFI in terms of 15 items, 10 common and 5 gender keyed, that reflect the individual's level of appreciation of his or her body. A single Body Image score is developed.

Sexual Satisfaction. The Sexual Satisfaction subtest is itself multidimensional in nature, being composed of a number of distinct components (e.g., frequency of intercourse, quality of communication, quality of orgasm). Ten true-false items comprise the Satisfaction subtest, each reflecting whether the respondent is satisfied with that specific aspect of his or her sexual functioning. A single Satisfaction score is calculated as a sum of endorsements indicating satisfaction with a particular component.

SFI: The DSFI total score. The Sexual Functioning Index (SFI) is the total or global summary score of the DSFI. It is calculated as a direct unweighted linear combination of the 10 subtest or principal dimension scores. Because subtest scores are calculated along very different score continua, and some are gender keyed (i.e., distinct for men and women), subtest scores are first transformed to area t scores ($\mu = 50$, $SD = 10$) before being summed to achieve the SFI. Because the transformation is a normalizing, area (under the curve) type, the actuarial characteristics of the resulting standardized distribution are retained.

The Global Sexual Satisfaction Index (GSSI). The GSSI is the second global measure of the DSFI, and it is quite different in nature from the SFI or DSFI total score.

Whereas the DSFI total score reveals the respondent's quality of sexual functioning in psychometric terms, the GSSI reflects the individual's *subjective* perception of his or her sexual behavior. The GSSI represents quality of sexual functioning on a 9-point scale anchored at the lower extreme by 0 (*could not be worse*) to 8 (*could not be better*) at the upper limit. Each scale point is characterized by a descriptive phrase, and the respondent is provided an opportunity to globally summarize his or her perception of the quality of sexual behavior in straightforward terms.

Normative population. Norms for the DSFI were developed based on a sample of 230 individuals in attendance at university continuing education classes. The majority of the sample were White (80%) and middle aged (M = 32) with some college education. Approximately 60% of the sample were married at the time of assessment, with the majority (75%) coming from middle-class and upper-middle-class backgrounds.

Reliability and Validity

Published studies by both the author of the scale and numerous other investigators suggest the DSFI is highly reliable and is a valid measure of the construct of sexual functioning. Derogatis and Melisaratos (1979) reported internal consistency reliability coefficients based on an N of 325 between .60 and .97, and test-retest coefficients across a 14-day interval ranging predominantly from the high .70s to the low .90s. Howell et al. (1987) also reported test-retest coefficients over a 14-day period, and all coefficients were $\geq$ .70. Over four dozen published studies currently exist using the DSFI as a measure of functional discrimination and outcomes in a broad variety of medical treatment populations (see references). The majority show the DSFI to be highly sensitive to naturally occurring and disease-induced interference with sexual functioning, as well as positive treatment effects.

Other Information

The DSFI is available in Arabic, Chinese, English, French, French Canadian, Indian, Korean, Norwegian, Spanish, and Turkish. The DSFI is distributed exclusively by Clinical Psychometric Research, Inc., Suite 302, 100 W. Pennsylvania Avenue, Towson, MD 21204; phone: 1-800-245-0277 or (410) 321-6165; fax: (410) 321-6341.

References

Conte, H. R. (1989). Development and use of self-report techniques for assessing sexual function: A review and critique. *Archives of Sexual Behavior, 12*, 555-576.

Derogatis, L. R. (1975). *Derogatis Sexual Functioning Inventory (DSFI): Preliminary scoring manual.* Baltimore: Clinical Psychometric Research.

Derogatis, L. R. (1976). Psychological assessment of sexual disabilities. In J. K. Meyer (Ed.), *Clinical management of sexual disorders* (pp. 35-73). Baltimore: Williams and Wilkins.

Derogatis, L. R. (1980). Psychological assessment of psychosexual functioning. In J. K. Meyer (Ed.), *The Psychiatric Clinics of North America Symposium on Sexuality* (pp. 113-131). Philadelphia: Saunders.

Derogatis, L. R. (1993). *Brief Symptom Inventory: Administration, scoring, and procedures manual* (3rd ed.). Minneapolis, MN: National Computer Systems.

Derogatis, L. R., Lopez, M. C., & Zinzeletta, E. M. (1988). Clinical applications of the DSFI in the assessment of sexual dysfunctions. In R. Brown & E. Roberts (Eds.), *Advances in the understanding and treatment of sexual disorders*. New York: PNA.

Derogatis, L. R., & Melisaratos, N. (1979). The DSFI: A multidimensional measure of sexual functioning. *Journal of Sex & Marital Therapy, 5*, 244-281.

Derogatis, L. R., & Rutigliano, P. J. (1996). Derogatis Affects Balance Scale. In B. Spiker (Ed.), *Quality of life and pharmacoeconomics in clinical trials* (2nd ed., pp. 160-177). Philadelphia: Lippincott-Raven.

Derogatis, L. R., Schmidt, C. W., Fagan, P. J., & Wise, T. N. (1989). Subtypes of anorgasmia via mathematical taxonomy. *Psychosomatics, 30*, 166-173.

Howell, J. R., Reynolds, C. F., Thase, M. E., Frank, E., Jennings, J. R., Houck, P. R., Berman, S., Jacobs, N., & Kupfer, D. J. (1987). Assessment of sexual function, interest, and activity in depressed men. *Journal of Affective Disorders, 13*, 61-66.

Jewish General Hospital (JGH) Sexual Self-Monitoring Form: Diary Evaluation of Sexual Behavior and Satisfaction

Eva Libman,[1] *SMBD-Jewish General Hospital and Concordia University*
Ilana Spector, *Douglas Hospital and McGill University*
Yitzchak Binik, *McGill University and Royal Victoria Hospital*
William Brender, *SMBD-Jewish General Hospital and Concordia University*
Catherine S. Fichten, *SMBD-Jewish General Hospital and Dawson College*

Self-monitoring represents a systematic, low-cost method of assessing a target behavior from the client's own perspective across a wide range of situations in the client's natural environment. These features are helpful in the assessment of sexual behavior when it is not appropriate for the therapist to observe directly and when it is important to measure the nature and frequency of sexual interactions.

When evaluating the frequency and the range of sexual behaviors, researchers and clinicians are often obliged to use retrospective questionnaires, which are subject to memory distortions and estimation errors. Researchers have shown that both retrospective and prospective measurement of sexual behaviors are useful because they do not always yield the same results (Binik, Meana, & Sand, 1994; McLaws, Oldenburg, Ross, & Cooper, 1990; Reading, 1983). Sexual diaries have been used in a number of studies. Even though some have been shown to have excellent temporal stability (e.g., White, Case, McWhirter, & Mattison, 1990), no widely accepted structured forms exist to systematically self-monitor frequency, variability, or satisfaction with sexual activity.

The Jewish General Hospital (JGH) Sexual Self-Monitoring Form provides information about the frequency and quality of a range of individual and couple sexual behaviors on a daily basis. Initially a clinical instrument designed to assess sexual and affectional activities on an ongoing basis in a population presenting with inhibited female orgasm, the JGH Sexual Self-Monitoring Form was modified so that it can evaluate outcome in sex therapy research. The measure can also be used in process studies of sex therapy to assess the impact of various therapeutic interventions and to monitor compliance with the treatment program. It can be completed by nonproblematic populations of single individuals or couples to obtain descriptive and normative information.

Description

This measure consists of eight questions asking respondents to indicate, on a daily basis, whether they engaged in each of 18 individual or interpersonal sexual activities, whether they experienced orgasm (and during which activities), how they felt about their partner and their sexual experience, and how satisfied they were with the amount of affection received.

Response Mode and Timing

Respondents complete the form on a daily basis, regardless of whether any sexual activity has taken place. Partners are told not to discuss their answers and to complete the forms individually. The measure takes less than 5 minutes to complete. Self-Monitoring Forms should be collected at least once per week (at the time of therapy session, by mail, or by telephone contact).

Scoring

Daily responses should each be examined and scored individually. For clinical purposes, scoring is optional; a qualitative evaluation of responses may be more appropriate for monitoring therapeutic progress and tailoring therapy to specific clients. For research purposes, the JGH Sexual Self-Monitoring Form can be scored as follows: For Question 1, item scores can be summed for 7-day periods to provide weekly measures of frequency for each sexual activity; other sexual activities may be added to this list. Enjoyment ratings (Question 2) can also be summed for each sexual activity and divided by the number of times that the activity occurred during the week. This yields a mean enjoyment score for each sexual activity. Responses to Questions 3, 6, and 7 are also summed and divided by 7 to provide a weekly estimate of feelings about one's sexual experience, satisfaction with affection received, and feelings toward one's partner.

Questions 4 and 5 examine the experience of orgasm. The weekly frequency of orgasms during each sexual activity can be counted to determine the percentage of times that the sexual activity in question resulted in orgasm (suc-

---

[1]Address correspondence to Eva Libman, Behavior and Sex Therapy Services–ICFP, SMBD-Jewish General Hospital, 4333 Cote Ste. Catherine, Montreal, Quebec H3T 1E4, Canada.

cess/experience ratio: cf. Auerbach & Kilmann, 1977). For example, if a woman engaged in masturbation three times during the week and experienced orgasm with masturbation once, her percentage orgasm score would be 1/3 = 33%. If the focus of interest is not orgasmic experience but erection quality, speed of ejaculation, and so forth, Questions 4 and 5 may be replaced as needed.

To simplify scoring, activities may be clustered. Our method involves the following groupings: Individual Sexual Activities (dreams, fantasies, masturbation, reading and viewing erotica), Affectional Display (hugging, kissing, and receiving and giving nongenital manual or oral caresses), Couple Sexual Noncoital Activities (receiving and giving genital manual or oral stimulation, and anal activities), and Intercourse. Using these clusters, we calculate frequency of type of activity cluster per week, orgasm ratio (%), and enjoyment ratings (cf. Fichten, Libman, & Brender, 1983). Averaging these data over a month is recommended to eliminate the effects of weekly variability in sexual encounters.

Reliability and Validity

Because this measure was originally developed as a clinical instrument (Burstein et al., 1985) rather than a research tool, reliability and validity information have not been systematically obtained. However, the JGH Sexual Self-Monitoring Form has been used in several studies.

An empirical question about sexual self-monitoring concerns whether it adds useful information to traditional retrospective methods of measurement. To explore this issue, Fichten, Libman, and Brender (1986) examined 23 married couples presenting for treatment of female orgasmic disorder. Respondents completed traditional, retrospective questionnaires and the JGH Sexual Self-Monitoring Forms. Results indicated that on cognitive/affective ratings (e.g., enjoyment of specific sexual activities; satisfaction with affection), there were no differences between the two types of measurement. On behavioral variables, such as frequency of specific sexual activities and percentage of orgasmic success, however, the two types of measurement diverged. Retrospective methods yielded more frequent (and therefore more positive) behavioral and orgasmic counts than did self-monitoring, indicating that self-monitoring is not redundant with questionnaire methods.

Another question concerns the possibility that completing self-monitoring forms is reactive. Findings of an investigation of 16 couples with male erectile disorder who, using a modified version of the JGH Sexual Self-Monitoring Form, self-monitored during a baseline period as well as during and after treatment, showed no significant differences on any of the behavioral or cognitive ratings from pre- to postbaseline self-monitoring, although there was significant improvement pre- to posttreatment (Fichten, Libman, Takefman, & Brender, 1988; Takefman & Brender, 1984). These findings provide preliminary evidence for the nonreactivity of sexual self-monitoring with this instrument. Findings using other sexual self-monitoring measures, however, do suggest the existence of reactivity (Ochs, Meana, Mah, & Binik, 1993). Therefore, the pos-

sible reactivity of sexual self-monitoring should be assessed in future studies.

The JGH Sexual Self-Monitoring Form has also been used in treatment-outcome studies to verify compliance and to examine changes in sexual behavior frequency and satisfaction (Fichten et al., 1983, 1986; Libman, Fichten, & Brender, 1984; Takefman & Brender, 1984). Findings indicating high degrees of concordance between partners on behavioral frequency ratings provide preliminary evidence for interrater reliability. Results also show that (a) the JGH Sexual Self-Monitoring Form is effective in determining differences in treatment compliance that predict successful therapy outcome, (b) pretreatment scores on several self-monitoring variables predict posttreatment findings, and (c) the Sexual Self-Monitoring Form can highlight differences between treatments and show pre- to posttherapy changes.

Other Information

The JGH Sexual Self-Monitoring Form is also available in French (*Hôpital Géneral Juif [HG] Formulaire d'Enregistrement Quotidien des Activités Sexuelles*). This measure was developed with research funding from the Conseil Québécois de la Recherche Sociale.

References

Auerbach, R., & Kilmann, P. R. (1977). The effects of group systematic desensitization on secondary erectile failure. *Behavior Therapy, 8*, 330-339.

Binik, Y. M., Meana, M., & Sand, N. (1994). Interaction with a sex-expert system changes attitudes and may modify sexual behavior. *Computers in Human Behavior, 10*, 395-410.

Burstein, R., Libman, E., Binik, Y., Fichten, C. S., Cohen, J., & Brender, W. (1985). A short-term treatment program for secondary orgasmic dysfunction. *Psychological Documents, 15*, 9. (Ms. No. 2688)

Fichten, C. S., Libman, E., & Brender, W. (1983). Methodological issues in the study of sex therapy: Effective components in the treatment of secondary orgasmic dysfunction. *Journal of Sex & Marital Therapy, 9*, 191-202.

Fichten, C. S., Libman, E., & Brender, W. (1986). Measurement of therapy outcome and maintenance of gains in the behavioral treatment of secondary orgasmic dysfunction. *Journal of Sex & Marital Therapy, 12*, 22-33.

Fichten, C. S., Libman, E., Takefman, J., & Brender, W. (1988). Self-monitoring and self-focus in erectile dysfunction. *Journal of Sex & Marital Therapy, 14*, 120-128.

Libman, E., Fichten, C. S., & Brender, W. (1984). Prognostic factors and classification issues in the treatment of secondary orgasmic dysfunction. *Personality and Individual Differences, 5*, 1-10.

McLaws, M. L., Oldenburg, B., Ross, M. W., & Cooper, D. A. (1990). Sexual behavior in AIDS-related research: Reliability and validity of recall and diary measures. *The Journal of Sex Research, 27*, 265-281.

Ochs, E. P., Meana, M., Mah, K., & Binik, Y. M. (1993). The effects of exposure to different sources of sexual information on sexual behavior: Comparing a "sex-expert system" to other educational material. *Behavior Research Methods, Instruments and Computers, 25*, 189-194.

Reading, A. E. (1983). A comparison of the accuracy and reactivity of methods of monitoring male sexual behavior. *Journal of Behavioral Assessment, 5*, 11-23.

Takefman, J., & Brender, W. (1984). An analysis of the effectiveness of two components in the treatment of erectile dysfunction. *Archives of Sexual Behavior, 13,* 321-340.

White, J. R., Case, D. A., McWhirter, D., & Mattison, A. M. (1990). Enhanced sexual behavior in exercising men. *Archives of Sexual Behavior, 19,* 193-209.

Exhibit

Jewish General Hospital (JGH) Sexual Self-Monitoring Form

(please fill out alone)

Name: _____   Date: _____

(1)   Sexual activities (please *check* (✓) in *column 1* if the activity occurred)

	1 ✓ Check if activity occurred	2 Rate according to Scale A (1-10)			1 ✓ Check if activity occurred	2 Rate according to Scale A (1-10)
Individual activities						
a) fantasies (daydreams)	_____	_____	j)	breast caressing	_____	_____
b) dreams	_____	_____	k)	genital touching (giving)	_____	_____
c) masturbation	_____	_____	l)	genital touching (receiving)	_____	_____
d) reading erotica	_____	_____	m)	oral stimulation (giving)	_____	_____
e) seeing erotica	_____	_____	n)	oral stimulation (receiving)	_____	_____
f) other (specify below)	_____	_____	o)	anal stimulation (giving)	_____	_____
Interpersonal activities			p)	anal stimulation (receiving)	_____	_____
g) kissing	_____	_____	q)	mutual masturbation	_____	_____
h) caressing—non genital (giving)	_____	_____	r)	intercourse	_____	_____
i) caressing—non genital (receiving)	_____	_____	s)	other (specify below)	_____	_____

(2)   Please look at Scale A below and then rate each activity checked (✓) above. Write the *rating in column 2* above.

Scale A

Very unenjoyable									Very enjoyable
1	2	3	4	5	6	7	8	9	10

(3)   How did you feel about your sexual experience today? (Put X in box)

Very negative   Very positive

| 1 | 2 | 3 | 4 | 5 |

(4)   Did you experience any orgasms? _____
(5)   If yes, during which activity? _____
(6)   How satisfied are you with the amount of affection you received today?

Very dissatisfied   Very satisfied

| 1 | 2 | 3 | 4 | 5 |

(7)   In general, how did you feel about your partner today?

Very negative   Very positive

| 1 | 2 | 3 | 4 | 5 |

(8)   Please add, in your own words, any important information or feelings concerning *yourself,* your *marriage,* your *sex life, or any other issues* you'd like to bring up in your session with your therapist.

Sexual Function Scale: History and Current Factors

Marita P. McCabe,[1] *Deakin University*

The Sexual Function Scale (SFS) is designed to evaluate the contribution of attitudes and experiences from the family of origin, the period of adolescence, and current individual and relationship factors to a person's sexual functioning. It may be completed by people who are sexually functional or sexually dysfunctional. For people who are sexually dysfunctional, it can be used as a clinical measure to evaluate the factors that need to be addressed in therapy.

Description

The SFS consists of three major sections: childhood, puberty and adolescence, and current attitudes and behavior. There are subsections within these three sections. These are summarized in Table 1.

Table 1 Subscales of the Sexual Function Scale

	Coefficient alpha	Test-retest
Childhood		
A. Attitudes Toward Sex in the Home (10 items)	Distinct items	
B. Emerging Sexuality (6 items)	Distinct items	
Puberty and adolescence		
A. Sexual Education (6 items)	Distinct items	
B. Dating Behavior (2 items)	Distinct items	
C. Petting Behavior (7 items)	Distinct items	
D. Coital Experiences During Adolescence	Distinct items (2 items)	
E. (a) Homosexual Experiences (3 items)	Distinct items	
(b) Unpleasant Experiences (3 items)	.36	.71
F. Depth of Relationship (3 items)	.43	.76
Current attitudes and behavior		
A. Current Attitudes Towards Sex (32 items)	.85	.89
B. Sexual Identity (3 items)	Distinct items	
C. Lifestyle (6 items)	Distinct items	
D. Types of Sexual Activity		
E. (a) Range of Sexual Activity (16 items)	.72	.88
(b) Response to Sexual Activity and Nature of Extra Stimulation (22 items)	.78	.92
E. Sexual Communication (9 items)	.80	.90
F. Sexual Satisfaction (3 items)	.63	.98
G. Other Relationships (9 items)	.60	.88
H. Communication (10 items)	.68	.91
I. Quality of Relationship (12 items)	.80	.98
J. Performance Anxiety (10 items)	.85	.97

The SFS was originally developed as a measure to evaluate the factors that are associated with sexual dysfunction in males and females. The original questions were drawn from the literature that assessed the etiology of sexual dysfunction. This material was used to generate a guided-interview measure, with open-ended responses. This measure was used to assess the sexuality of 55 respondents with sexual dysfunction and 58 respondents who were sexually functional. The responses of these participants allowed scales to be created for each question. Some items were removed from the scale as analyses indicated that they had no impact on their sexual functioning. The modified scales were administered to a further sample of clinical sexually dysfunctional, nonclinical sexually dysfunctional, and sexually functional respondents (McCabe, 1994a, 1994b). The results of this study allowed the scale to be reorganized and modified to produce the present measure.

Response Mode and Timing

Respondents complete the scale as a questionnaire. Some items in the scale are categorical (e.g., What type of contraception do you use?), some are *yes/no* responses (e.g., Did you have any unpleasant sexual experiences during adolescence?), and some are on a 5-point Likert-type scale (e.g., How often do you feel highly aroused before you have intercourse?). The questionnaire takes about 1 hour to complete.

Scoring

Items are scored in the same direction so that a total score is obtained for each subsection. Some items are categorical and so do not contribute to a total score for the subsection. Because there are different numbers of items in each subsection, the highest possible score varies from one section to another.

Reliability and Validity

Coefficient alpha has been calculated for a number of the subscales. These alphas are reported in Table 1. Some of the items in the scales tap very separate aspects of a particular construct or result in categorical responses, and so it is not appropriate to add responses or expect that respondents will answer in any consistent manner. The alphas have been calculated on a sample size of 171 cases. Of these, 82 respondents (50 females, 32 males) were

[1]Address correspondence to Marita P. McCabe, School of Psychology, Deakin University, 221 Burwood Highway, Burwood, Victoria 3125, Australia; email: maritam@deakin.edu.au.

sexually functional, 51 respondents (27 females, 24 males) were sexually dysfunctional and not seeking treatment, and 38 respondents (20 females, 18 males) were clinical dysfunctional. The scale was also completed by 30 sexually functional and 30 sexually dysfunctional respondents on two occasions 6 weeks apart. The test-retest reliability coefficients for each subscale are reported in Table 1. The method of scale construction has ensured some level of construct validity. The scale needs to be administered along with other psychometrically sound measures of the subscales to further demonstrate the level of construct validity of the scale.

Other Information

The scale, along with the scoring code, can be purchased from the author for a cost of U.S.$10.

References

McCabe, M. P. (1994a). Childhood, adolescent and current psychological factors associated with sexual dysfunction. *Sexual and Marital Therapy, 9,* 267-276.

McCabe, M. P. (1994b). The influence of the quality of relationship on sexual dysfunction. *Australian Journal of Marriage and the Family, 15,* 2-8.

Personal Sentence Completion Inventory

L. C. Miccio-Fonseca,[1] *Clinic for the Sexualities*

The Personal Sentence Completion Inventory (PSCI) was designed to obtain information regarding the erotic development of the person. The PSCI is a versatile tool that can be used in a variety of ways (e.g., a supplement in psychological evaluations, in forensic evaluations of sex offenders, as a therapeutic tool in individual therapy assisting in exploring sexual performance, or in identifying sexual dysfunctions or sexual trauma). Another use of the PSCI is in group therapy, where it provides a list of topics to assist people in exploring their sexuality in a nonthreatening way. The inventory can also be used by researchers exploring the application of theories of erotic development.

Description

The PSCI is a 50-item sentence stem inventory with 10 content factors: Family, Sex Education, Love Relationships, Sexual Dreams, Sexual Fantasy, Sexual Experiences, Erotic Pleasures, Sexual Discomforts, Sexual Dysfunctions, and Paraphilias. The inventory provides the professional with historical and current information of the psycho/socio/sexual experience of the person. The incomplete sentence stems elicit specific information about the individual's "lovemap" (Money, 1986, 1988), the love ideal the person has, and his or her erotic bonding. It does not ask for

opinion, and it is nonevaluative. The PSCI is open ended, allowing an almost unlimited variety of possible completions.

Response Mode and Timing

The PSCI can be administered to individuals who have a minimum of fifth-grade education. For younger individuals (ages 7 to 11), the PSCI should be given verbally, and only some items are appropriate.

The inventory is to be completed with a pen, not a pencil. Commonly seen with the PSCI is what Freud referred to as "slips of the pen." Using a pencil for completion offers the individual the opportunity to erase these slips-of-the-pen responses. Such slips are opportunities for the clinician to explore these responses.

Completion time varies but generally is approximately 15 minutes.

The PSCI can be given either individually or in a group format; there is a different set of instructions for each setting. Whether the PSCI is given individually or in groups, all items given are to be completed. The utmost privacy must be afforded the individual in either setting.

Scoring

The PSCI provides qualitative data. The PSCI relies on the professional skills and sophistication of the examiner administering the instrument. During the inquiry, the examiner brings out the individual and attempts to explore

[1]Address correspondence to L. C. Miccio-Fonseca, Clinic Director, Clinic for the Sexualities, 591 Camino de la Reina, Suite 533, San Diego, CA 92108.

the individual's sexual development. The inquiry affords the examiner an opportunity to see how the individual communicates, the individual's styles of interactions, and his or her verbal and social skills level. It also indicates how the individual handles the topic of human sexuality, as well as discussing his or her own sexual history. During the inquiry, the exploration of individual responses not only gives unique information about the individual but also what things the individual would not write down. This kind of information is often lost in the standard psychometric measures where the individual is usually forced to make choices. For this reason, there is no scoring scheme for the PSCI.

In the manual, each item on the PSCI is presented and accompanied by common responses and suggestions for further probes by the clinician. The manual provides a glossary of terms and cites current sex research in the content areas covered. Although the PSCI is not a normative instrument, there are patterns of common responses to several of the items. For most items, however, there is no clear pattern of responses. The PSCI user needs to follow up with oral questioning regarding unusual or unclear responses. The responses presented in the manual were abstracted from a variety of interviewees over a 4-year period.

Reliability and Validity

A pilot study was done with 185 people, ages 12-57. The subject sample was a sample of convenience; that is, the subject sample is composed mainly of individuals who received psychological evaluations and individual and group therapy. The respondent was either a sex offender, victim, or an individual who was not in either category. In the sample on which the inventory was developed, there were 173 males and only 12 females. The gender ratio is clearly biased as a result. Individuals were either self-referred or referred by a law enforcement official (probation, attorney, judge), or referred by Child Protective Services for either treatment, assessment, or consultation. Each completed PSCI was reviewed, and clarification was sought during qualitative interviews; those sentence stems that appeared to cause ambiguity and confusion were edited and revised.

The items were rewritten for clarification and a revised version of the PSCI was formulated. It has been administered to 155 individuals: 135 males and 20 females, ages 7 to 61 years. Individuals were of a variety of ethnic groups and different socioeconomic levels. The PSCI has been used extensively in court-ordered psychological evaluations of sex offenders.

References

Money, J. (1986). *Lovemaps*. New York: Irvington.

Money, J. (1988). *Gay, straight, and in between: The sexology of erotic orientation*. Baltimore: Johns Hopkins University Press.

Exhibit

Personal Sentence Completion Inventory (sample items)

Sexual Dreams

19. My sex dreams are usually about

Erotic Pleasures

32. What turns me on sexually is

Sexual Discomforts

40. The thing I tried sexually once but wouldn't do again is

Source. These items from the scale are reprinted with permission of the author.

Sexual Function Questionnaire for Heterosexuals

The Editors

The Sexual Function Questionnaire (SFQ) can be used as an adjunct to sexual dysfunction assessment interviews. It is a self-report instrument containing six sections, five of which examine aspects of normal and dysfunctional sexual behavior including present sexual experiences, past sexual experiences, intrapersonal factors, interpersonal factors, and medical history. The sixth section deals with the individual's medical history. It takes approximately 25 minutes to complete the SFQ.

Additional information may be obtained from the first editor.

References

Miller, G. D., McLoughlin, C. S., & Murphy, N. C. (1982). Personality correlates of college students reporting sexual dysfunction. *Psychological Reports, 51*, 1075-1082.
Ridgeway, D. M. C. (1978). *Sex dysfunction in female alcoholics.* Unpublished master's thesis, University of Utah.

The Sexual Interaction Inventory

Robert N. Reinhardt,[1] *Texas A&M University*

The Sexual Interaction Inventory (SII), developed by LoPiccolo and Steger (1974), is a paper-and-pencil self-report instrument for differentiating dysfunctional from nondysfunctional couples, and for the diagnosis of sexual dysfunctions. Useful in measuring treatment outcome, it reflects the current nature of a couple's sexual relationship with regard to both satisfaction and level of functioning.

Description

Developed as a revision of the Oregon Sex Inventory, the current format includes illustrations of each sexual activity (except intercourse). The inventory asks each member of a couple to provide information about 17 different sexual behaviors covering a fairly comprehensive range of heterosexual behaviors. For each behavior, the inventory collects data about (a) current frequency, (b) desired frequency, (c) current level of satisfaction, (d) estimate of partner's current level of satisfaction, (e) desired level of satisfaction in "ideal" self, and (f) desired level of satisfaction in an "ideal" partner. For each of the 17 behaviors, respondents are asked to rate Items 1 and 2 on a 6-point scale with labels of *never,*

rarely, occasionally (< 50%), fairly often (50%), usually (75%), and *always.* Items 4 to 6 are also rated on a 6-point scale; however, the labels here are (1) *extremely,* (2) *moderately,* or (3) *slightly unpleasant* and (4) *slightly,* (5) *moderately,* or (6) *extremely pleasant.*

Response Mode and Timing

Respondents indicate their response to the 102 questions by filling in circles on a sheet designed to be scored by an optical character reader. Respondents are asked to answer *every* item even if it requires imagining themselves engaging in an activity in which they have never participated. The inventory requires an average of 15 to 30 minutes to complete.

Scoring

The SII can be scored by hand in approximately 10 to 15 minutes and requires no special training. A computer program is available to assist in scoring (see Other Information). Scoring yields raw scores for 11 scales, which are converted to scale scores and plotted on forms provided. Each scale has a mean of 50 and a standard deviation of 10 with higher scores indicating greater pathology. The raw

[1]Address correspondence to Joseph LoPiccolo, Department of Psychology, University of Missouri, Columbia, MO 65211.

scores for each scale are obtained by the following procedure:

Scale 1: Frequency Dissatisfaction–Male. The sum across all 17 behaviors of the absolute differences between the responses given for Items 1 and 2 (i.e., questions [1 – 2] + [7 – 8] + . . . + [97 – 98]).

Scale 2: Self Acceptance–Male. The sum across all 17 behaviors of the absolute difference between Items 3 and 5 (i.e., questions [3 – 5] + [9 – 11] + . . . + [99 – 101]).

Scale 3: Pleasure Mean–Male. The sum across all 17 behaviors of the responses to Item 3, divided by 17 (i.e., questions [3 + 9 + . . . + 99]/17).

Scale 4: Perceptual Accuracy–Male of Female. The sum across all 17 behaviors of the absolute differences between the response on the 4th item from the male respondent's form and the 3rd item from the female respondent's form (i.e., questions [4m – 3f] + [10m – 9f] + . . . + [100m – 99f]).

Scale 5: Mate Acceptance–Male of Female. The sum across all 17 behaviors of the absolute difference between the responses to Item 4 and Item 6 (i.e., questions [4 – 6] + [10 – 12] + . . . + [100 – 102]).

Scale 6: Total Disagreement. The total of the raw scores obtained for Scale 1, 2, 4, 5, 7, 8, 10, and 11.

Scale 7: Frequency Dissatisfaction–Female. Follow procedures for Scale 1 using responses from female respondent's form.

Scale 8: Self Acceptance–Female. Follow procedures for Scale 2 using responses from female respondent's form.

Scale 9: Pleasure Mean–Female. Follow procedures for Scale 3 using responses from female respondent's form.

Scale 10: Perceptual Accuracy–Female of Male. Follow procedures for Scale 4; however, reverse the references to male and female responses (i.e., questions [4f – 3m] + [10f – 9m] + . . . + [100f – 99m]).

Scale 11: Mate Acceptance–Female of Male. Follow procedures for Scale 5 using responses from female respondent's form.

Reliability

LoPiccolo and Steger (1974) reported test-retest reliability over a 2-week period to be between .53 and .90 on the 11 scales with all the correlations significant at $p < .05$. The Cronbach alpha for each scale ranged between .79 and .93 indicating good internal consistency.

Validity

LoPiccolo and Steger (1974) tested convergent validity between the separate SII scales and an overall rating of sexual satisfaction. Nine of the scales (7 and 10 excluded) had correlations that were significant at $p < .05$ or better. However, the absolute magnitude of the correlations was low, indicating that the traits measured by the separate scales do not have a strong relationship to overall self-ratings of sexual satisfaction. Discriminant validity tests by the same authors indicated 9 of 11 (5 and 10 excluded) do discriminate client applicants from sexually satisfied couples.

Other Information

The SII and copyright permission is available from Joseph LoPiccolo, Department of Psychology, University of Missouri, Columbia, MO 65211. Included for the $10 fee are two reusable SII booklets, administration and scoring instructions, and answer forms and charts for plotting scaled scores for five couples. For those who have access to computer facilities, a scoring program, written in FORTRAN IV, is available. Information about this program can also be obtained from LoPiccolo.

References

LoPiccolo, J., & Steger, J. C. (1974). The Sexual Interaction Inventory: A new instrument for assessment of sexual dysfunction. *Archives of Sexual Behavior, 3,* 585-595.

Nowinski, J. K., & LoPiccolo, J. (1979). Assessing sexual behavior in couples. *Journal of Sex & Marital Therapy, 5,* 225-243.

Exhibit

Behaviors on Inventory

1. The male seeing the female when she is nude.
2. The female seeing the male when he is nude.
3. The male and the female kissing for one minute continuously.
4. The male giving the female a body massage, not touching her breasts or genitals.
5. The female giving the male a body massage, not touching his breasts or genitals.
6. The male caressing the female's breasts with his hands.
7. The male caressing the female's breasts with his mouth.
8. The male caressing the female's genitals with his hands.
9. The male caressing the female's genitals with his hands until she reaches orgasm.
10. The female caressing the male's genitals with her hands.
11. The female caressing the male's genitals with her hands until he ejaculates.
12. The male caressing the female's genitals with his mouth.
13. The male caressing the female's genitals with his mouth until she reaches orgasm.
14. The female caressing the male's genitals with her mouth.

15. The female caressing the male's genitals with her mouth until he ejaculates.
16. The male and female having intercourse.
17. The male and female having intercourse with both of them having an orgasm.

Sample Booklet Page

When you and your mate engage in sexual behavior, does this particular activity usually occur? How often would you like this activity to occur? ("Sexual behavior" refers to any type of physical contact which is intended to be sexual by either you or your mate.)

31. Currently occurs:
    1) Never
    2) Rarely (10% of the time)
    3) Occasionally (25% of the time)
    4) Fairly often (50% of the time)
    5) Usually (75% of the time)
    6) Always

32. I would like it to occur:
    1) Never
    2) Rarely (10% of the time)
    3) Occasionally (25% of the time)
    4) Fairly often (50% of the time)
    5) Usually (75% of the time)
    6) Always

How pleasant do you currently find this activity to be? How pleasant do you think your mate finds this activity to be?

33. I find this activity:
    1) Extremely unpleasant
    2) Moderately unpleasant
    3) Slightly unpleasant
    4) Slightly pleasant
    5) Moderately pleasant
    6) Extremely pleasant

34. I think my mate finds this activity:
    1) Extremely unpleasant
    2) Moderately unpleasant
    3) Slightly unpleasant
    4) Slightly pleasant
    5) Moderately pleasant
    6) Extremely pleasant

How would you like to respond to this activity? How would you like your mate to respond? (In other words, how pleasant do you think this activity ideally should be for you and your mate?)

35. I find this activity:
    1) Extremely unpleasant
    2) Moderately unpleasant
    3) Slightly unpleasant
    4) Slightly pleasant
    5) Moderately pleasant
    6) Extremely pleasant

36. I think my mate finds this activity:
    1) Extremely unpleasant
    2) Moderately unpleasant
    3) Slightly unpleasant
    4) Slightly pleasant
    5) Moderately pleasant
    6) Extremely pleasant

Sexual Interaction System Scale

Jane D. Woody[1] and Henry J. D'Souza, *University of Nebraska at Omaha*

The Sexual Interaction System Scale (SISS) is a self-report instrument designed to measure the quality of a heterosexual couple's sexual interaction, including specific sexual dysfunctions. It provides a measure of each partner's perception (i.e., individual's scores), which may then be added for a total couple score. The SISS measures five factors believed to interact during a given sexual encounter.

1. Sexual Functioning encompasses the *DSM* (American Psychiatric Association, 1987) classification of sexual dysfunctions; the subfactors are Desire, Arousal, Orgasm (and a fourth subfactor for females, Pain Dysfunctions). In systemic terms, sexual responses at each phase of the sexual response cycle, including physiological responses, constitute communication to which the partners are constantly reacting, in part, with their own physiological responses.

2. Attitudinal Set refers to each individual's attitudes about the purpose and focus of sexual intimacy and the level of maturity that these attitudes reflect—whether self-focused, role focused, or individual connected.

3. Nonsexual Interaction refers to the presence of interactions around territoriality, ranking, attachment, and exploratory/sensory patterns that may either promote or interfere with desired sexual arousal and satisfaction. This factor taps patterns that a couple has established for dealing with these issues in their overall relationship and that may emerge and be communicated during the sexual encounter.

4. Interaction Coordination refers to the partners' action language that serves to coordinate all aspects of the sexual encounter so as to lead to the desired outcome—arousal and satisfaction. It encompasses verbal and nonverbal behaviors that serve as communication exchanges that may move the couple's sexual interaction in the desired direction.

5. Postsexual Interaction refers to the emotional tenor of the relationship following sex. It consists of each partner's evaluation of the sexual encounter relative to feelings and behaviors of distance versus closeness toward the partner as a result of the sex. These feelings, and behaviors too, constitute communication that is assumed to carry over and affect the couple's next sexual encounter.

Description

The SISS is distinct from prior sexual functioning inventories in that it focuses on the interaction taking place during the couple's actual sexual encounters. Even though the couple is typically the preferred unit of treatment for sexual dysfunctions, a systemic understanding of a couple's sexual relationship is a fairly recent development (Schnarch,

1991; Woody, 1992). The five factors were derived in part from Verhulst and Heiman's (1979) systemic explanation of sexual functioning as an interactional communication process. The SISS consists of 48 statements with responses to be made on a 6-point scale (0 = *none, never, does not occur in our relationship* to 5 = *high, always, always occurs in our relationship*). Ten items deal with Sexual Functioning, 7 with Attitudinal Set, 12 with Nonsexual Interaction, 6 with Interaction Coordination, and 10 with Postsexual Interaction. Three items do not load on any of the five factors. The SISS is appropriate for use with heterosexual couples in clinical practice involving sexual distress, sexual dysfunction, or general relationship problems, and for use in couple premarital and enrichment programs.

Response Mode and Timing

Partners are to complete the SISS independently, preferably on the same day, so that they have a common frame of reference (i.e., their most recent two or three sexual encounters with each other). Completion time is approximately 10 minutes. Responses, for hand scoring, are placed on the line in front of each item.

Scoring

Directions appear on the Male and Female Scoring/Profile Sheets. These directions indicate the items for which the response must be reversed in value before totaling the items within each factor to obtain the subfactor, factor, and individual scores. Reversed values are placed on the inventory, and these can be totaled on the inventory itself and then transferred to the Scoring/Profile Sheets. The couple score is the sum of both partners' total individual scores. Individual scores can range from 0 to 225, with higher scores indicating more positive sexual interaction. Maximum scores possible for the factors are Sexual Functioning (50), Attitudinal Set (35), Nonsexual Interaction (60), Interaction Coordination (30), and Postsexual Interaction (50). Plotting scores on the profile allows comparison of the individual's scores to a nonclinical sample (*N* = 58) and to a sexual dysfunction sample (males, *N* = 20; females, *N* = 24). The profiles show mean scores for the nonclinical sample placed at *t* score = 50 and the mean scores of the sexual dysfunction sample circled; the latter suggests a cutoff score that may be seen as clinically significant.

Reliability

In a sample of 143 couples, internal consistency, analyzed by the five SISS factors, resulted in Cronbach's alpha = .90 (Woody & D'Souza, 1994). This coefficient was chosen because, theoretically, a systemic explanation of the sexual encounter holds that the five factors would be correlated.

---
[1]Address correspondence to Jane D. Woody, School of Social Work, University of Nebraska at Omaha, Omaha, NE 68182-0293; email: jwoody@fa-cpucs.unomaha.edu.

Validity

Validity was supported by several methods. Face validity was supported by the ratings of six experts on the content of the items of the scale. In addition, in a sample of 143 couples, significant differences were found on the t test between known groups: the sexual dysfunction group and the nonclinical group ($t = 7.14, p < .001$); and the sexual dysfunction group and other-problems group ($t = 2.05, p = .045$). Criterion validity was supported by a Pearson's correlation coefficient ($r = .80; p < .001$) between the SISS couple score and the couple score on a criterion question dealing with sexual satisfaction. Finally, as expected, a moderate correlation was found between the SISS couple score and the overall couple relationship as measured by the Dyadic Adjustment Scale ($r = 0.61, p < .001$) (Woody & D'Souza, 1994).

Other Information

Copyright is held by Jane D. Woody and Henry J. D'Souza (a transfer of copyright is pending). Address correspondence to the first author.

References

American Psychiatric Association. (1987). *Diagnostic and statistical manual of mental disorders* (3rd ed., rev.). Washington, DC: Author.

Schnarch, D. M. (1991). *Constructing the sexual crucible*. New York: Norton.

Verhulst, J., & Heiman, J. (1979). An interactional approach to sexual dysfunction. *American Journal of Family Therapy, 7*(4), 19-36.

Woody, J. D. (1992). *Treatment for sexual distress: Integrative systems therapy*. Newbury Park, CA: Sage.

Woody, J. D., & D'Souza, H. J. (1994). The Sexual Interaction System Scale: A new inventory for assessing sexual dysfunction and sexual distress. *Journal of Sex & Marital Therapy, 20*, 210-228.

Exhibit

Sexual Interaction System Scale (sample items)

Directions: The items in this scale deal with your current sexual relationship with your spouse or regular partner. In answering each item, think of the last few times you engaged in sex with your partner.

For each of the statements, you are to answer for yourself, that is, give a response choice that reflects your own experience, your own opinion, or your own impression. You will answer each item according to a response scale of 0 to 5, which is explained below. Put your answers on the line in front of each item. Please answer all items. See the sample answers, explanations, and directions below.

Response choices

For rating your experience or your opinion, select a rating from 0 to 5. The meanings of the ratings are as follows:

0	1	2	3	4	5

None or never on
the characteristic described.
Does not occur in the
relationship.

Extremely high or always on
the characteristic described.
Always occurs in our
relationship.

Sample Answers and Explanations

__0__   I express complaints or negative feelings during sex. This answer means that you gave a rating of 0 because you believe that you never express complaints or negative feelings during sex.

__1__   I worry about the success of my sexual performance. This answer means that you gave a rating of 1 because only rarely do you worry about the success of your performance.

__2__   Female has consistent or recurring genital pain with intercourse. (Males, respond as NA, not applicable). If you are a female, this answer means that you gave a rating of 2 because you occasionally have pain during intercourse. If you are a male, your answer in the response column will be NA, not applicable to you.

If an item describes a behavior that you *never engage* in or a reaction that you *never have* in *your relationship,* remember to look at the scale, as a rating of 0 means *none or never,* or *does not* occur in the relationship. The scale makes it possible for you *to answer all questions.*

Before starting to answer, take a minute to imagine yourself and your partner *during the most recent few times you engaged in sex.* This should be your frame of reference for answering the questions.

SISS Factors	Sample Items
Sexual Functioning	I am interested in sex—willing to get involved, either initiating or responding to partner's initiating.
Attitudinal Set	I worry about the success of my sexual performance.
Nonsexual Interaction	I feel my partner is too possessive of my body during sex.
Interaction Coordination	With actions and/or words, I do what it takes to make sex pleasurable for both of us.
Postsexual Interaction	I feel withdrawn and distant from my partner as a result of sex.

Masculine Gender Identity Scale for Females

Ray Blanchard,[1] *Clarke Institute of Psychiatry*

The Masculine Gender Identity Scale for Females (MGIS; Blanchard & Freund, 1983) was developed to measure "masculinity" occurring in homosexual females. Masculine gender identity in females was conceived as a continuous variable, inferable from the extent of an individual's departure from the usual female pattern of behavior toward the pattern typical of female-to-male transsexuals.

The MGIS was developed as a companion instrument to the Feminine Gender Identity Scale for Males (FGIS; Freund, Langevin, Satterberg, & Steiner, 1977; Freund, Nagler, Langevin, Zajac, & Steiner, 1974). The FGIS is presented elsewhere in this volume in the article by Freund and Blanchard; differences between the gender identity scales and conventional masculinity-femininity scales are also discussed there.

Description

The MGIS is a self-administered, multiple-choice questionnaire measure. It includes two subscales. The 20 items of Part A mainly concern the examinee's childhood preference for female versus male playmates, games, and toys; the predilection for stereotypically masculine household chores; childhood fantasies of adult pursuits commonly associated with the male or female sex; and the frequency of frank cross-gender wishes at various ages. Part A may be administered to any female older than age 17. Part B consists mostly of items concerning cross-dressing and erotic preferences presupposing homosexuality. This subscale, which includes nine items, is appropriate only for homosexual females.

Scale development for both parts was conducted using all-female samples. The initial item pool for Part A was administered to 236 heterosexuals, 44 homosexuals who did not desire sex-change surgery (simple homosexuals), and 50 homosexuals who did (female-to-male transsexuals). From an initial pool of 25 items, those 20 were retained whose part-remainder correlations were greater than or equal to .30. The item pool for Part B was administered only to the 94 homosexual subjects. Because none of the nine items in the pool had a part-remainder correlation less than .30, all were retained.

Response Mode and Timing

Examinees may check or circle the response option of their choice. They are instructed to endorse one and only one response option per item. Part A of the scale should take no longer than 10 minutes to complete, and Part B should take no longer than 5.

Scoring

The scoring weight for each response option is shown in parentheses in the accompanying exhibit. The total score for each subscale is simply the sum of scores of its individual

---

[1]Address correspondence to Ray Blanchard, Gender Identity Clinic, Clarke Institute of Psychiatry, 250 College Street, Toronto, Ontario M5T 1R8, Canada; email: blanchardr@cs.clarke-inst.on.ca.

items; the full scale score is the sum of the two subscale scores. Higher scores indicate more masculine gender identity.

Reliability

Blanchard and Freund (1983) found an alpha reliability coefficient for Part A of .89. The alpha reliability of Part B was .92.

Validity

Blanchard and Freund (1983) found that factor analysis of Part A revealed three weak factors (each accounting for less than 6% of the total variance), and one strong factor, accounting for 31% of the total variance and 70% of the common variance. Factor loadings of the 20 items of Part A may be found in their Table 2 (p. 208). Factor analysis of Part B revealed only one factor, accounting to 57% of the total variance.

The construct validity of Part A was supported by its reliable discrimination among three groups of females expected to show different degrees of masculine gender identity: heterosexuals, homosexuals, and female-to-male transsexuals (in ascending order). The homosexuals ob-tained higher scores than the heterosexuals, and the transsexuals obtained higher scores than the homosexuals. Part B, which is administered only to homosexual females (simple or transsexual), discriminated reliably between the homosexuals and the female-to-male transsexuals.

Age was not significantly correlated with Part A scores for heterosexuals, homosexuals, or transsexuals. Correlations between education and Part A scores ranged from .12 to .15, indicating that education accounts for only about 2% of the variance in Part A scores. Part B did not correlate with age or education for the homosexual or the transsexual group.

References

Blanchard, R., & Freund, K. (1983). Measuring masculine gender identity in females. *Journal of Consulting and Clinical Psychology, 51,* 205-214.

Freund, K., Langevin, R., Satterberg, J., & Steiner, B. W. (1977). Extension of the Gender Identity Scale for Males. *Archives of Sexual Behavior, 6,* 507-519.

Freund, K., Nagler, E., Langevin, R., Zajac, A., & Steiner, B. W. (1974). Measuring feminine gender identity in homosexual males. *Archives of Sexual Behavior, 3,* 249-260.

Exhibit

Masculine Gender Identity Scale for Females

Instructions to Subjects

The following questions ask what sex role you have preferred at different times of your life, what were your childhood fantasies and activities, and how you felt about being born a female. Try to answer questions pertaining to childhood in terms of the way you felt then and not the way you see things now.

Please circle one and only one answer to each question. If you are not sure of the meaning of a question, you may ask the person giving the questionnaire to explain it to you. There is no time limit for answering these questions.

Part A: *Items Administered to All Females*

1. Between the ages of 6 and 12, did you prefer:
   a. to play with boys (2)
   b. to play with girls (0)
   c. didn't make any difference (1)
   d. not to play with other children (1)
   e. don't remember (1)
2. Between the ages of 6 and 12, did you:
   a. prefer boys' games and toys (soldiers, football, etc.) (2)
   b. prefer girls' games and toys (dolls, cooking, sewing, etc.) (0)
   c. like or dislike both about equally (1)
   d. had no opportunity to play games or with toys (1)
3. In childhood, were you very interested in the work of a garage mechanic? Was this:
   a. prior to age 6 (1)
   b. between ages 6 and 12 (1)
   c. probably in both periods (1)
   d. do not remember that I was very interested in the work of a garage mechanic (0)
4. Between ages 6 and 14, which did you like more: romantic stories or adventure stories?
   a. liked romantic stories more (0)
   b. liked adventure stories more (2)
   c. it did not make any difference (1)
5. Between the ages of 6 and 12, did you like to do jobs or chores which are usually done by men?
   a. yes (2)
   b. no (0)
   c. don't remember (1)

6. Between the ages of 13 and 16, did you like to do jobs or chores which are usually done by men?
   a. yes (2)
   b. no (0)
   c. don't remember (1)
7. Between the ages of 6 and 12, when you read a story did you imagine that you were:
   a. the male in the story (cowboy; detective, soldier, explorer, etc.) (2)
   b. the female in the story (the girl being saved, etc.) (0)
   c. the male sometimes and the female other times (1)
   d. neither the male nor the female (1)
   e. did not read stories (1)
8. In childhood or at puberty, did you like mechanics magazines? Was this:
   a. between ages 6 and 12 (1)
   b. between ages 12 and 14 (1)
   c. probably in both periods (1)
   d. do not remember that I liked mechanics magazines (0)
9. Between the ages of 6 and 12, did you sometimes imagine yourself as being the courageous leader of others?
   a. yes (2)
   b. no (0)
   c. unsure (1)
10. Between the ages of 6 and 12, did you wish you had been born a boy instead of a girl?
    a. often (2)
    b. occasionally (1)
    c. never (0)
11. Between the ages of 13 and 16, did you wish you had been born a boy instead of a girl?
    a. often (2)
    b. occasionally (1)
    c. never (0)
12. Since the age of 17, have you wished you had been born a boy instead of a girl?
    a. often (2)
    b. occasionally (1)
    c. never (0)
13. Do you think your appearance is:
    a. very feminine (0)
    b. feminine (0)
    c. a little masculine (1)
    d. quite masculine (2)
14. Between ages 6 and 12, did you sometimes imagine, in your fantasies, yourself physically defending someone against a monster, a dangerous animal, or "evil" people?
    a. prior to age 6 (1)
    b. between ages 6 and 12 (1)
    c. probably in both periods (1)
    d. do not remember such fantasies (0)
15. In childhood fantasies, did you sometimes wish you could go hunting big game? Was this:
    a. prior to age 6 (1)
    b. between ages 6 and 12 (1)
    c. probably in both periods (1)
    d. do not remember such fantasies (0)
16. In childhood, did you wish you would become very strong physically? Was this:
    a. prior to age 6 (1)
    b. between ages 6 and 12 (1)
    c. probably in both periods (1)
    d. do not remember the desire to become very strong physically (0)
17. In childhood, was there ever a period in which you wished you would, when adult, become a dressmaker or dress designer? Was this:
    a. prior to age 6 (0)
    b. between ages 6 and 12 (0)
    c. probably in both periods (0)
    d. do not remember having this desire (1)
18. In childhood fantasies, did you sometimes imagine yourself driving a racing car? Was this:
    a. prior to age 6 (1)
    b. between ages 6 and 12 (1)
    c. probably in both periods (1)
    d. do not remember having this fantasy (0)
19. In childhood, did you ever wish to become a dancer? Was this:
    a. prior to age 6 (0)
    b. between ages 6 and 12 (0)
    c. probably in both periods (0)
    d. do not remember having this desire (1)
20. In childhood, did you ever wish to become a pilot, or did you fantasize yourself being a pilot? Was this:
    a. prior to age 6 (1)
    b. between ages 6 and 12 (1)
    c. probably in both periods (1)
    d. do not remember having such a desire (0)

Part B: *Items Administered Only to Homosexual Females*
     (Transsexual or Nontranssexual)

21. Between the ages of 6 and 12, did you put on men's underwear or clothing?
    a. once a month or more, for about a year or more (2)
    b. (less often, but) several times a year for about 3 years or more (1)
    c. very seldom did this during this period (0)
    d. never did this during this period (0)
    e. don't remember (0)

22. Between the ages of 13 and 16, did you put on men's underwear or clothing?
    a. once a month or more, for a least a year (2)
    b. (less often, but) several times a year for at least 2 years (1)
    c. very seldom did this during this period (0)
    d. never did this during this period (0)

23. Since the age of 17, have you put on men's underwear or clothing?
    a. once a month or more, for at least a year (2)
    b. (less often, but) several times a year for at least 2 years (1)
    c. very seldom did this during this period (0)
    d. never did this during this period (0)

24. If you have ever wished to have a male body rather than a female one, was this:
    a. mainly to please females but also for your own satisfaction (2)
    b. mainly for your own satisfaction but also to please females (2)
    c. entirely for your own satisfaction (2)
    d. entirely to please females (1)
    e. about equally to please females and for your own satisfaction (2)
    f. have never wanted to have a male body (0)

25. Have you ever felt like a man?
    a. only if you were wearing a least one piece of male underwear or clothing (1)
    b. while wearing at least one piece of male underwear or clothing and only occasionally at other times also (1)
    c. at all times and for at least one year (2)
    d. never felt like a man (0)

26. When completely dressed in female clothing (underwear, etc.), would you:
    a. have a feeling of anxiety because of this (2)
    b. have no feeling of anxiety but have another kind of unpleasant feeling because of this (2)
    c. have no unpleasant feelings to do with above (0)

27. What kind of sexual contact with a female would you have preferred on the whole, even though you may not have done it?
    a. touching your partner's privates with your hands (1)
    b. touching your partner's privates with your mouth (1)
    c. you would have preferred one of those two modes but you cannot decide which one (1)
    d. your partner touching your privates with her hands (0)
    e. your partner touching your privates with her mouth (0)
    f. you would have preferred one of those two latter modes but you cannot decide which one (0)
    g. you would have like all four modes equally well (0)
    h. you would have preferred some other mode of sexual contact (1)

28. What qualities did you like in females to whom you were sexually attracted?
    a. slightly masculine behavior (0)
    b. slightly feminine behavior (1)
    c. very feminine behavior (2)

29. Would you have preferred a partner:
    a. who was willing to have you lead her (2)
    b. who was willing to lead you (0)
    c. you didn't care (1)

Source. This scale was originally published in "Measuring Masculine Gender Identity in Females," by R. Blanchard and K. Freund, 1983, *Journal of Consulting and Clinical Psychology, 51,* 205-214. Copyright © 1983 by the American Psychological Association. Reprinted with permission.

Hypergender Ideology Scale

Merle E. Hamburger,[1] *Georgia College*
Matthew Hogben and Stephanie McGowan, *University at Albany,*
   State University of New York
Lori J. Dawson, *Worcester State College*

The Hypergender Ideology Scale (HGIS; Hamburger, Hogben, McGowan, & Dawson, 1996) is a dispositional measure that was developed to assess extreme gender role adherence in both men and women. Much of the research in this area to date has used the Hypermasculinity Inventory (HMI; Mosher & Sirkin, 1984) when studying males or the Hyperfemininity Scale (HFS; Murnen & Byrne, 1991) when studying females. Relying on gender-specific measures, however, precludes one's ability to directly compare men and women. The HGIS is a gender-neutral measure that identifies a broad constellation of attitudes that encompasses many of the attitudes assessed by the HMI (e.g., flirtation with danger, holding calloused sexual attitudes) and the HFS (e.g., primacy of relationships, using one's sexuality as a commodity).

Description

The HGIS is a 57-item dispositional measure (there is also a 19-item short form: HGIS-S). Respondents answer each survey item using a 6-point Likert-type scale anchored by *strongly disagree* (1) at one extreme and *strongly agree* (6) at the other. Exploratory principal components analysis, as well as confirmatory factor analysis via LISREL 8 (Jöreskog & Sörbom, 1993), extracted a one-factor and a five-factor solution. Further analyses by Hamburger et al. (1996), however, suggested that it is most parsimonious to view the HGIS as a unidimensional scale.

Response Mode and Timing

Participants indicate their responses by writing the number, in a space to the left of each statement, indicating the extent of their agreement with the statement. The response scale is printed at the top of each page of the questionnaire. Most participants respond to all 57 items in under 10 minutes.

Scoring

Before one can score the HGIS, Items 1, 2, 4, 5, 7, 13, 17, 18, 22, 26, 27, 30, 36, 37, 38, 45, 49, 51, 55, and 57 must be reverse scored. A total HGIS score is then computed by summing the responses to all 57 items. To calculate the

score for the HGIS-S, Items 10, 12, 16, 18, 21, 23, 24, 28, 31, 32, 34, 35, 36, 38, 39, 42, 44, 48, and 57 are summed.

Reliability

In a sample of 297 participants (150 men, 147 women), Hamburger et al. (1996) calculated a coefficient alpha for the HGIS of .96 for the entire sample, .94 for the male sample, and .92 the female sample. In an additional, independent sample of 235 participants (108 men, 127 women), they calculated a coefficient alpha for the HGIS of .96 in the overall sample, .96 for the male sample, and .94 for the female sample. Regarding the HGIS-S, Hamburger et al. (1996) computed a coefficient alpha of .93 for the overall sample, Hamburger (1995) computed a coefficient alpha of .88 in a sample of 242 men, and Hamburger (1996) computed a coefficient alpha of .95 for the HGIS-S in an independent sample of 111 participants (44 men, 67 women). To assess temporal stability, Hamburger et al. (1996) computed a 21-day test-retest reliability of $r(119)$ = .95 in an independent sample of 121 undergraduates (58 men, 63 women).

Validity

Hamburger et al. (1996) found that scores on the both the long and short versions of the HGIS were significantly and positively correlated with the HMI in men, $r(148)$ = .76 and $r(106)$ = .60, in two independent samples, and the HFS in women, $r(145)$ = .54 and $r(125)$ = .60, in two independent samples. Moreover, they found that both the long and short versions of the HGIS were significantly and positively correlated—correlation coefficients ranging from $r(233)$ = .28 to $r(233)$ = .77—with scores on the Traditional Family Ideology Scale (Levinson & Huffman, 1955), the Adversarial Sexual Beliefs Scale and the Rape Myth Acceptance Scale (Burt, 1980), the Attitudes Towards Women Scale (Spence & Helmrich, 1972; Spence, Helmreich, & Stapp, 1973), and the use of sexual aggression as assessed by a revised version of the Sexual Experiences Questionnaire (Hogben, Byrne, & Hamburger, 1996; Ross & Allgeier, 1991). In addition, Hamburger (1995) found that the HGIS-S was significantly and positively correlated with a number of variables including the consumption of alcohol, $r(240)$ = .23; having a psychopathic personality, $r(240)$ = .35; use of sexual coercion, $r(240)$ = .37; rape proclivity, $r(240)$ = .45; feelings of anger, $r(240)$ = .36, and hostility toward women, $r(240)$ = .39; acceptance of interpersonal violence, $r(240)$ = .49, and legitimate forms

---

[1]Address correspondence to Merle E. Hamburger, Department of Psychology, Georgia College, Milledgeville, GA 31601; email: mhambur@mail.gac.peachnet.edu.

of aggression, $r(240) = .52$; and dispositional impulsivity, $r(240) = .23$. Finally, Hamburger (1996) found that the HGIS-S was significantly and positively correlated with holding authoritarian beliefs, $r(109) = .39$.

References

Burt, M. R. (1980). Cultural myths and supports for rape. *Journal of Personality and Social Psychology, 38*, 217-230.

Hamburger, M. E. (1996). *Is hypergender ideology the same as hypertraditionality?* Unpublished manuscript, University of Pittsburgh at Johnstown, Johnstown, PA.

Hamburger, M. E. (1995). *Assessing the validity of a multidimensional model of sexual coercion in college men.* Unpublished doctoral dissertation, University at Albany, State University of New York, Albany.

Hamburger, M. E., Hogben, M., McGowan, S., & Dawson, L. J. (1996). Assessing hypergender ideology: Development and initial validation of a gender-neutral measure of adherence to extreme gender-role beliefs. *Journal of Research in Personality, 30*, 157-178.

Hogben, M., Byrne, D., & Hamburger, M. E. (1996). Coercive heterosexual sexuality in dating relationships of college students: Implications of differential male-female experiences. *Journal of Psychology & Human Sexuality, 8*(1/2), 69-78.

Jöoreskog, K. G., & Sörbom, D. (1993). *LISREL 8 user's reference guide.* Chicago: Scientific Software International.

Levinson, D. J., & Huffman, P. E. (1955). Traditional family ideology and its relation to personality. *Journal of Personality, 23*, 251-275.

Mosher, D. L., & Sirkin, M. (1984). Measuring a macho personality constellation. *Journal of Research in Personality, 18*, 150-163.

Murnen, S. K., & Byrne, D. (1991). The Hyperfemininity Scale: Measurement and initial validation of the construct. *The Journal of Sex Research, 28*, 479-489.

Ross, R. R., & Allgeier, E. R. (1991, August). *Correlates of males' femininity with sexually coercive attitudes and behavior.* Paper presented at the annual meeting of the American Psychological Association, San Francisco.

Spence, J. T., & Helmreich, R. L. (1972). The Attitudes Towards Women Scale: An objective instrument to measure attitudes towards the rights and roles of women in contemporary society. *JSAS Catalog of Selected Documents in Psychology, 2*, 66-67.

Spence, J. T., Helmreich, R. L., & Stapp, J. (1973). A short version of the Attitudes Towards Women Scale (AWS). *Bulletin of the Psychonomic Society, 2*, 219-220.

Exhibit

Hypergender Ideology Survey

The following survey contains various statements about attitudes concerning the relationships between men and women. Please read each statement carefully and indicate, in the space to the left of the item, the extent you agree with the statement. Please note, however, that some of the statements may not completely apply to you. In such cases, please try to imagine what your response would be if it DID apply to you, and answer accordingly. Please use the following scale to make your responses.

1	2	3	4	5	6
Strongly disagree	Disagree	Slightly disagree	Slightly agree	Agree	Strongly agree

_____ 1) I think it's gross and unfair for a man to use alcohol and drugs to convince a woman to have sex with him.

_____ 2) Physical violence never solves an issue.

_____ 3) Most women need a man in their lives.

_____ 4) I like to see a relationship in which the man and woman have equal power.

_____ 5) Using alcohol or drugs to convince someone to have sex is wrong.

_____ 6) Gays sicken me because they are not real men.

_____ 7) Sex should never be used as a bargaining tool.

_____ 8) A real man fights to win.

_____ 9) Real men look for fast cars and fast women.

_____ 10) A true man knows how to command others.

_____ 11) When a man spends a lot of money on a date, he should expect to get sex for it.

_____ 12) The only thing a lesbian needs is a good, stiff, cock.

_____ 13) I like relationships in which both partners are equals.

_____ 14) Sometimes it doesn't matter what you do to get sex.

_____ 15) Women should show off their bodies.

_____ 16) Men should be ready to take any risk, if the payoff is large enough.

_____ 17) A woman can be complete with or without a partner.

_____ 18) No wife is obliged to provide sex for anybody, even her husband.

_____ 19) Most women use their sexuality to get men to do what they want.

_____ 20) Most women play hard-to-get.

_____ 21) Women should break dates with female friends when guys ask them out.

_____ 22) Lesbians have chosen a particular life style and should be respected for it.

_____ 23) Men have to expect that most women will be something of a prick-tease.

_____ 24) A real man can get any woman to have sex with him.
_____ 25) Women should be flattered when men whistle at them.
_____ 26) It is important that my partner and I are equally satisfied with our relationship.
_____ 27) Some gay men are good people, and some are not, but it has nothing to do with their sexual orientation.
_____ 28) Women instinctively try to manipulate men.
_____ 29) Most women will lie to get something they want.
_____ 30) Men shouldn't measure their self-worth by their sexual conquests.
_____ 31) Get a woman drunk, high, or hot and she'll let you do whatever you want.
_____ 32) Men should be in charge during sex.
_____ 33) If you've not prepared to fight for what's yours, then be prepared to lose it.
_____ 34) It's okay for a man to be a little forceful to get sex.
_____ 35) Women don't mind a little force in sex sometimes because they know it means they must be attractive.
_____ 36) Homosexuals can be just as good at parenting as heterosexuals.
_____ 37) Any man who is a man can do without sex.
_____ 38) Gays and lesbians are generally just like everybody else.
_____ 39) Pick-ups should expect to put out.
_____ 40) Some women are good for only one thing.
_____ 41) Women often dress provocatively to get men to do them favors.
_____ 42) If men pay for a date, they deserve something in return.
_____ 43) It's natural for men to get into fights.
_____ 44) Effeminate men deserve to be ridiculed.
_____ 45) All women, even feminists, are worthy of respect.
_____ 46) If a woman goes out to a bar for some drinks, she's looking for a real good time.
_____ 47) I do what I have to do to get sex.
_____ 48) Any man who is a man needs to have sex regularly.
_____ 49) Masculinity is not determined by sexual success.
_____ 50) Homosexuality is probably the result of a mental imbalance.
_____ 51) Nobody should be in charge in a romantic relationship.
_____ 52) Real men look for danger and face it head on.
_____ 53) A gay man is an affront to real men.
_____ 54) He who can, fights; he who can't, runs away.
_____ 55) Gay men often have masculine traits.
_____ 56) Women sometimes say "no" but really mean "yes."
_____ 57) I believe some women lead happy lives without having male partners.

Source. This scale is reprinted with permission of the authors.

Revised Mosher Guilt Inventory

Donald L. Mosher,[1] *University of Connecticut*

The Mosher Guilt Inventories measure three aspects of the personality disposition of guilt: Sex-Guilt, Hostility-Guilt, and Morality-Conscience. Multitrait-multimethod matrices have provided evidence for the discriminant validity of the three guilt subscales (Mosher, 1966, 1968). Sex guilt is psychologically magnified (Tomkins, 1979) in scenes involving awareness of sexual arousal; the discrete affects of interest-excitement and enjoyment-joy; and the discrete affect of shame, which appears in consciousness as guilt due to its associations with moral cognitions about sexual conduct. Hostility guilt is psychologically magnified in scenes involving the discrete affects of anger-rage and guilty affect and cognition about the immorality of aggressive behavior or cognitions. Conscience is psychologically magnified in scenes involving moral temptations and/or guilty affect about the self. The inventory is measuring three aspects of guilt conceived as a *script*, which is defined by Tomkins as a set of rules for the interpretation, prediction, production, control, and evaluation of a co-assembled set of scenes that has been further amplified by affect. The Mosher Guilt Inventories, as measures of these guilty scripts, have a considerable body of evidence supporting their construct validity.

Description

The Mosher Guilt Inventories (Mosher, 1961, 1966, 1968) were developed from responses given to sentence completion stems in 1960. The weights used in scoring the sentence completion were assigned to items from the scoring manual to construct true-false and forced-choice inventories for men and women, because the scoring manual had been developed to score each sex separately. O'Grady and Janda (1979) demonstrated there was no need to use weights because a 1 or 0 scoring procedure for guilty and nonguilty responses was correlated .99 with the weighted system. To compare the sexes, it was necessary either to transform the raw scores to standard scores or to give the same inventory to both sexes, which seemed to create no problems. During the past 30+ years, the range of guilt scores has been truncated as the means have dropped, particularly for sex guilt (Mosher & O'Grady, 1979). The 39 items in the female form of the forced-choice sex guilt inventory, in comparison to 28 for men, have continued to be a successful predictor of a broad range of sexually related behavior, cognitions, and affects in spite of containing items drawing 100% nonguilty choices.

Given the unusually strong evidence of construct validity for the inventories, I was reluctant to generate a new set of

items that might be conceptually better but that would limit generalization from past research. Instead, I submitted the nonoverlapping items contained in both male and female versions of the true-false (233 items) and the forced-choice (151 items) inventory to a sample of 187 male and 221 female University of Connecticut undergraduates for an updated item analysis. As suspected, many guilty-true items and guilty-forced-choice alternatives were uniformly rejected in the current sample. The resulting Revised Mosher Guilt Inventory continues to measure Sex-Guilt, Hostility-Guilt, and Morality-Conscience, but it is now in a limited-comparison format that was selected to increase the range of response and to eliminate complaints about the forced-choice format.

The Revised Mosher Guilt Inventory consists of 114 items, arranged in pairs of responses to the same sentence completion stem, in 7-point Likert-type format to measure (a) Sex-Guilt, 50 items; (b) Hostility-Guilt, 42 items; and (c) Guilty-Conscience, 22 items. Items were selected from an item analysis of the 151 forced-choice items in the original inventories. For the selected items, the correlations of the items with the subscale totals ranged from .32 to .62 with a median of .46. In addition, to ensure discriminant validity between the subscales, 90% of the items had a correlation with its own subscale that was significantly different from the correlation of the item with the other subscale totals. Several Morality-Conscience items were too highly correlated with Sex-Guilt, and thus were eliminated. This subscale was renamed Guilty-Conscience to reflect more adequately the retained items. The inventory is suited for adult populations.

Response Mode and Timing

Respondents answer by rating their response on a 7-point subscale where 0 means *not at all true of (for) me* and 6 means *extremely true of (for) me*. Items are arranged in sets of two different completions to a single stem, the limited-comparison format, to permit respondents to compare the intensity of *trueness* for them because people generally find one alternative is more or less *true* for them. The inventory can be completed in approximately 20 minutes. Subscales can be omitted or given separately. Answers are usually recorded on machine-scorable answer sheets.

Scoring

Scores are summed for each subscale by reversing the nonguilty alternatives (nonitalicized item numbers in the following keys). The items for Sex-Guilt are 5, 6, 7, 8, 11, *12, 13,* 14, 15, *16,* 17, *18,* 25, 26, *31,* 32, 35, 36, 41, 42, *51, 52, 53, 54, 61, 62, 63, 64, 67,* 78, *71, 72, 75, 76, 81, 82, 83,* 84, 87, *88, 93,* 94, 101, *102, 103,* 104, 107, *108,* 111, and *112.*

[1]Address correspondence to Donald L. Mosher, 5051 North A1A, PH1-1, North Hutchinson Island, FL 34949; email: dlmosher@aol.com.

The items for Hostility-Guilt are 3, *4, 19,* 20, 21, 22, 23, 24, 29, *30, 33,* 34, 37, *38, 39,* 40, 43, *44, 45,* 46, *55,* 56, 69, 70, 77, 78, 79, 80, *85,* 86, *91,* 92, *95,* 96, 97, 98, 99, *100, 109,* 110, *113,* and 114.

The items for Guilty-Conscience are 1, *2,* 9, *10,* 27, *28,* 47, *48, 49,* 50, *57, 58, 59,* 60, *65,* 66, *73, 74,* 89, 90, *105,* and 106. Higher scores indicate more scripted guilt.

Reliability

Because the Revised Mosher Guilt Inventory was constructed for inclusion in this volume,[2] reliabilities in the new format have yet to be assessed. In past research, split-half or alpha coefficients have averaged around .90 (Mosher, 1966, 1968; Mosher & Vonderheide, 1985).

Validity

Mosher (1979) reviewed approximately 100 studies appearing by 1977 that consistently supported the construct validity of the Mosher Guilt Inventories. Recent research continues to add the construct validity of the inventory as a valid measure of guilt as a personality disposition (Green & Mosher, 1985; Kelley, 1985; Mosher & Vonderheide, 1985).

---

[2]This refers to the first edition of this volume.

References

Green, S. E., & Mosher, D. L. (1985). A causal model of sexual arousal to erotic fantasies. *The Journal of Sex Research, 21,* 1-23.

Kelley, K. (1985). Sex, sex guilt, and authoritarianism: Differences in responses to explicit heterosexual and masturbatory slides. *The Journal of Sex Research, 21,* 68-85.

Mosher, D. L. (1961). *The development and validation of a sentence completion measure of guilt.* Unpublished doctoral dissertation, Ohio State University, Columbus.

Mosher, D. L. (1966). The development and multitrait-multimethod matrix analysis of three measures of three aspects of guilt. *Journal of Consulting Psychology, 30,* 35-39.

Mosher, D. L. (1968). Measurement of guilt in females by self-report inventories. *Journal of Consulting and Clinical Psychology, 32,* 690-695.

Mosher, D. L. (1979). The meaning and measurement of guilt. In C. E. Izard (Ed.), *Emotions in personality and psychopathology.* New York: Plenum.

Mosher, D. L., & O'Grady, K. E. (1979). Sex guilt, trait anxiety, and females' subjective sexual arousal to erotica. *Motivation and Emotion, 3,* 235-249.

Mosher, D. L., & Vonderheide, S. G. (1985). Contributions of sex guilt and masturbation guilt to women's contraceptive attitudes and use. *The Journal of Sex Research, 21,* 24-39.

O'Grady, K. E., & Janda, L. H. (1979). Factor analysis of the Mosher Forced-Choice Guilt Inventory. *Journal of Consulting and Clinical Psychology, 47,* 1131-1133.

Tomkins, S. S. (1979). Script theory: Differential magnification of affects. In H. E. Howe, Jr., & R. A. Dienstbier (Eds.), *Nebraska Symposium on Motivation* (Vol. 26, pp. 201-236). Lincoln: University of Nebraska Press.

Exhibit

Revised Mosher Guilt Inventory

Instructions: This inventory consists of 114 items arranged in pairs of responses written by college students in response to sentence completion stems such as "When I have sexual dreams. . . ." You are to respond to each item as honestly as you can by rating your response on a 7-point scale from 0, which means *not at all true of (for) me* to 6, which means *extremely true of (for) me.* Ratings of 1 to 5 represent ratings of agreement-disagreement that are intermediate between the extreme anchors of *not at all true* and *extremely true* for you. The items are arranged in pairs of two to permit you to compare the intensity of a *trueness* for you. This limited comparison is often useful since people frequently agree with only one item in a pair. In some instances, it may be the case that both items or neither item is true for you, but you will usually be able to distinguish between items in a pair by using different ratings from the 7-point range for each item.

Rate each of the 114 items from 0 to 6 as you keep in mind the value of comparing items within pairs. Record your answer on the machine scorable answer sheet by filling in the blank opposite the item number with your rating from 0 to 6. Please do not omit any items; 0s must be filled in to be read by the computer.

I punish myself . . .
   1. very infrequently.
   2. when I do wrong and don't get caught.
When anger builds inside me . . .
   3. I let people know how I feel.
   4. I'm angry myself.
"Dirty" jokes in mixed company . . .
   5. do not bother me.
   6. are something that make me very uncomfortable.

Masturbation . . .
   7. is wrong and will ruin you.
   8. helps one feel eased and relaxed.
I detest myself for . . .
   9. nothing, I love life.
   10. for my sins and failures.
Sex relations before marriage . . .
   11. should be permitted.
   12. are wrong and immoral.

Sex relations before marriage . . .
    13. ruin many a happy couple.
    14. are good in my opinion.
Unusual sex practices . . .
    15. might be interesting.
    16. don't interest me.
When I have sexual dreams . . .
    17. I sometimes wake up feeling excited.
    18. I try to forget them.
After an outburst of anger . . .
    19. I am sorry and say so.
    20. I usually feel quite a bit better.
When I was younger, fighting . . .
    21. didn't bother me.
    22. never appealed to me.
Arguments leave me feeling . . .
    23. depressed and disgusted.
    24. elated at winning.
"Dirty" jokes in mixed company . . .
    25. are in bad taste.
    26. can be funny depending on the company.
I detest myself for . . .
    27. nothing at present.
    28. being so self-centered.
When someone swears at me . . .
    29. I swear back.
    30. it usually bothers me even if I don't show it.
Petting . . .
    31. I am sorry to say is becoming an accepted practice.
    32. is an expression of affection which is satisfying.
When I was younger, fighting . . .
    33. disgusted me.
    34. was always a thrill.
Unusual sex practices . . .
    35. are not so unusual.
    36. don't interest me.
After a childhood fight, I felt . . .
    37. good if I won, bad otherwise.
    38. hurt and alarmed.
After an argument . . .
    39. I am sorry for my actions.
    40. I feel mean.
Sex . . .
    41. is good and enjoyable.
    42. should be saved for wedlock and childbearing.
After an outburst of anger . . .
    43. I usually feel quite a bit better.
    44. I feel ridiculous and sorry that I showed my emotions.
After an argument . . .
    45. I wish that I hadn't argued.
    46. I feel proud in victory, understanding in defeat.
I detest myself for . . .
    47. nothing, I love life.
    48. not being more nearly perfect.
A guilty conscience . . .
    49. is worse than a sickness to me.
    50. does not bother me too much.
"Dirty jokes" in mixed company . . .
    51. are coarse to say the least.
    52. are lots of fun.

When I have sexual desires . . .
    53. I enjoy it like all healthy human beings.
    54. I fight them for I must have complete control of my body.
After an argument . . .
    55. I am disgusted that I allowed myself to become involved.
    56. I usually feel better.
Obscene literature . . .
    57. helps people become sexual partners.
    58. should be freely published.
One should not . . .
    59. lose his temper.
    60. say "one should not."
Unusual sex practices . . .
    61. are unwise and lead only to trouble.
    62. are all in how you look at it.
Unusual sex practices . . .
    63. are OK as long as they're heterosexual.
    64. Usually aren't pleasurable because you have preconceived feelings about their being wrong.
I regret . . .
    65. all of my sins.
    66. getting caught, but nothing else.
Sex relations before marriage . . .
    67. in my opinion, should not be practiced.
    68. are practiced too much to be wrong.
After an outburst of anger . . .
    69. my tensions are relieved.
    70. I am jittery and all keyed up.
As a child, sex play . . .
    71. is immature and ridiculous.
    72. was indulged in.
I punish myself . . .
    73. by denying myself a privilege.
    74. for very few things.
Unusual sex practices . . .
    75. are dangerous to one's health and mental condition.
    76. are the business of those who carry them out and no one else's.
Arguments leave me feeling . . .
    77. depressed and disgusted.
    78. proud, they certainly are worthwhile.
After an argument . . .
    79. I am disgusted that I let myself become involved.
    80. I feel happy if I won or still stick to my own views if I lose.
When I have sexual desires . . .
    81. I attempt to repress them.
    82. they are quite strong.
Petting . . .
    83. is not a good practice until after marriage.
    84. is justified with love.
After a childhood fight I felt . . .
    85. as if I had done wrong.
    86. like I was a hero.
Sex relations before marriage . . .
    87. help people adjust.
    88. should not be recommended.
If I robbed a bank . . .
    89. I should get caught.
    90. I would live like a king.

After an argument . . .
91. I am sorry and see no reason to stay mad.
92. I feel proud in victory and understanding in defeat.
Masturbation . . .
93. is wrong and a sin.
94. is a normal outlet for sexual desire.
After an argument . . .
95. I am sorry for my actions.
96. if I have won, I feel great.
When anger builds inside me . . .
97. I always express it.
98. I usually take it out on myself.
After a fight, I felt . . .
99. relieved.
100. it should have been avoided for nothing was accomplished.
Masturbation . . .
101. is all right.
102. is a form of self-destruction.

Unusual sex practices . . .
103. are awful and unthinkable.
104. are all right if both partners agree.
I detest myself for . . .
105. thoughts I sometimes have.
106. nothing, and only rarely dislike myself.
If I had sex relations, I would feel . . .
107. all right, I think.
108. I was being used not loved.
Arguments leave me feeling . . .
109. exhausted.
110. satisfied usually.
Masturbation . . .
111. is all right.
112. should not be practiced.
After an argument . . .
113. it is best to apologize to clear the air.
114. I usually feel good if I won.

Index of Sexual Harassment

Adrienne L. Decker
Walter W. Hudson,[1] *WALMYR Publishing Co.*

The Index of Sexual Harassment (ISH) is a short-form scale designed to measure sexual harassment.

Description

The ISH contains 19 category partition (Likert-type) items, each of which represents behavior that is illegal. Each item is scored on a relative frequency scale as shown in the scoring key of the instrument. Obtained scores range from 0 to 100, where higher scores indicate greater degrees of sexual harassment. The ISH can be used with all English-speaking populations aged 12 or older.

Response Mode and Timing

The ISH is a self-report scale that is normally completed in 5-7 minutes.

Scoring

The total score for the ISH is computed as $S = (\Sigma X_i - N)(100) / [(K - 1)N]$, where X is an item response, i is item, K is the number of response categories, and N is the number of properly completed items. Total scores remain valid in the face of missing values (omitted items) provided the respondent completes at least 80% of the items. The effect of the scoring formula is to replace missing values with the mean item response value so that scores range from 0 to 100 regardless of the value of N.

Reliability

Cronbach's alpha = .90, and *SEM* = 2.97. Test-retest reliability is not available.

Validity

Known-groups validity is not available for the ISH. Detailed information about content, factorial, and construct

[1]Address correspondence to Walter W. Hudson, WALMYR Publishing Co., P.O. Box 6229, Tallahassee, FL 32314-6229; email: walmyr@syspac.com.

validity are reported in Hudson and Decker (1994), which is available from the publisher.

Other Information

The ISH is a copyrighted commercial assessment scale and may not be copied, reproduced, altered, or translated into other languages. It may be obtained in tear-off pads of 50 copies per pad at $0.30 per copy ($15.00 per pad) by writing the WALMYR Publishing Co., P.O. Box 6229, Tallahassee, FL 32314-6229; phone and fax: (850) 656-2787; email: walmyr@syspak.com.

Reference

Hudson, W. W., & Decker, A. L. (1994). The Index of Sexual Harassment: A partial validation. *The WALMYR Monograph Series.* Tempe, AZ: WALMYR.

Exhibit

INDEX OF SEXUAL HARASSMENT (ISH)

Name: _____ Today's Date: _____

This questionnaire is designed to measure the level of sexual harassment in the workplace. It is not a test, so there are no right or wrong answers. Answer each item as carefully and as accurately as you can by placing a number beside each one as follows.

1 = None of the time
2 = Very rarely
3 = A little of the time
4 = Some of the time
5 = A good part of the time
6 = Most of the time
7 = All of the time

1. ____ My peer or supervisor tells sexually explicit jokes at work.
2. ____ My peer or supervisor describes me or a coworker using sexually explicit terminology.
3. ____ My peer or supervisor creates offensive rumors concerning the appearance or sexual behavior of me or a coworker.
4. ____ My peer or supervisor uses subtle questioning to determine my or my coworker's sexual behavior or availability.
5. ____ My peer or supervisor repeatedly asks me or a coworker for a date.
6. ____ My peer or supervisor asks me or a coworker for sexual favors.
7. ____ My peer or supervisor places obscene phone calls to me or a coworker.
8. ____ My peer or supervisor offers me or a coworker compensation or work benefits in exchange for sexual favors.
9. ____ My peer or supervisor demands sexual favors from me or a coworker to maintain job security.
10. ____ My peer or supervisor displays sexually explicit photographs and pictures at work.
11. ____ My peer or supervisor produces sexually explicit graffiti for display at work.
12. ____ My peer or supervisor shows pornographic videotapes at work.
13. ____ My peer or supervisor sends sexually explicit letters, cards or other written material to me or a coworker.
14. ____ My peer or supervisor uses gestures or staring considered sexually offensive by me or a coworker.
15. ____ My peer or supervisor stalks me or a coworker to pressure a personal relationship.
16. ____ My peer or supervisor blocks my or a coworker's pathway to force physical contact.
17. ____ My peer or supervisor touches self sexually in the presence of me or a coworker.
18. ____ My peer or supervisor touches me or a coworker in a sexually offensive manner.
19. ____ My peer or supervisor initiates unwelcome sexual activity with me or a coworker.

Source. This scale is reprinted with permission of WALMYR Publishing Co.

The Likelihood to Sexually Harass Scale

John B. Pryor,[1] *Illinois State University*

The Likelihood to Sexually Harass (LSH) scale was developed to measure men's proclivities to sexually harass women (Pryor, 1987). Current theory on sexual harassment recognizes that there are at least four different types of sexually harassing behavior with different social psychological bases (Pryor & Whalen, in press): sexual exploitation, sexual attraction/miscommunication, misogyny (the treatment of women as an outgroup), and homo-anathema (hostile reactions to people perceived as homosexual). The LSH scale measures a readiness for the first type, sexual exploitation. This is theorized to be the tendency to use social power for sexual access or gain. Pryor, Giedd, and Williams (1995) suggest that men's tendency to behave in a sexually exploitative manner toward women may be predicted by the LSH scale in combination with certain social normative factors that permit or condone such behavior.

Description

The LSH scale consists of 10 brief scenarios describing social situations in which a male protagonist has the power to sexually exploit a female with impunity. Male respondents are asked to imagine themselves in the role of the protagonist in each scenario. Following each scenario, respondents are asked to rate the likelihood that they would perform an act of quid pro quo sexual harassment. Ratings are made on a 5-point Likert-type scale with the anchors *not at all likely* (1) and *very likely* (5). Key items are embedded between two additional filler items that follow each scenario. From the responses of 100 college men, a varimax factor analysis extracted a single factor accounting for 63% of the variance. Thus, the LSH scale seems to measure a unidimensional construct.

Response Mode and Timing

Respondents typically complete the LSH scale in a group setting under conditions of anonymity. Responses are made by circling the number 1 to 5 on the items beneath each scenario or marking answers on a separate machine-scorable sheet. The LSH scale takes about 15 minutes to complete.

Scoring

The likelihood ratings from the key items (see the exhibit) are summed to form an LSH scale score. Scores range from 10 to 50. In a sample of 100 Illinois State University college men, the median was 17, 25% of the sample had scores of 25 and above, and 25% had scores 11 and below.

[1]Address correspondence to John B. Pryor, Department of Psychology, Illinois State University, Normal, IL 61790-4620; email: pryor@rs6000.cmp.ilstu.edu.

Reliability

Across several studies reviewed by Pryor et al. (1995), the Cronbach alpha for the LSH scale always exceeded .90. It is recommended that the summed score of the 10 items be viewed as a homogeneous measure of men's proclivity for sexual exploitation.

Validity

Pryor et al. (1995) reviewed studies examining the correlations between various individual difference measures and the LSH scale. They divided these into three categories: scales related to sexual violence, scales related to gender roles, and scales related to sexuality. Some example correlations include the following (all $ps < .05$): The LSH scale was correlated significantly with Malamuth's (1989) Attraction to Sexual Aggression Scale ($r = .38$) and the Greendlinger and Byrne (1987) Coercive Sexual Fantasy Scale ($r = .44$) (sample = 250 college men). The LSH scale was correlated significantly with the undesirable masculinity subscale from the Spence and Helmreich (1978) Personal Attributes Scale ($r = .42$) (sample = 130 college men) and three scales developed by Brannon and Junni (1984) to measure endorsement of a stereotypic male sex role norm: Antifemininity ($r = .32$), Status ($r = .39$), and Toughness ($r = .38$) (sample = 84 college men). The LSH scale was correlated significantly with Nelson's (1979) Dominance as a Sexual Function Scale ($r = .45$) (sample = 117 college men). Pryor (1987) also examined the discriminant validity of the LSH scale. For example, he found a relatively low correlation between the LSH scale and the Crowne and Marlowe (1964) Social Desirability Scale ($r = -.13$) (sample = 185 college men). Several researchers have examined the connection between the LSH scale and social cognitive processes. In these studies, researchers typically pretest with the LSH scale and then compare upper and lower quartiles. For example, using an illusory correlation methodology, Pryor and Stoller (1994) found that high-LSH men manifest evidence of a strong cognitive link between concepts concerning sexuality and concepts concerning social dominance. Such links are not manifested by low-LSH men (see also, Bargh, Raymond, Pryor, & Strack, 1995). Finally, several researchers have found that high-LSH men behave in a sexually harassing manner toward women in laboratory settings when the men are exposed to social norms accepting or condoning sexual harassment (Pryor et al. 1995; Pryor, LaVite, & Stoller, 1993). Pryor and Whalen (in press) also reviewed studies showing that men who are higher on the LSH scale tend to report having engaged in actual sexually harassing behavior in the past.

References

Bargh, J. A., Raymond, P., Pryor, J. B., & Strack, F. (1995). The attractiveness of the underling: An automatic power sex association and its consequences for sexual harassment. *Journal of Personality and Social Psychology, 68,* 768-781.

Brannon, R., & Junni, S. (1984). A scale for measuring attitudes about masculinity. *Psychological Documents, 14,* 6-7.

Crowne, D. P., & Marlowe, D. (1964). *The approval motive: Studies in evaluative dependence.* New York: Wiley.

Greendlinger, V., & Byrne, D. (1987). Coercive sexual fantasies of college men as predictors of self-reported likelihood to rape and overt aggression. *The Journal of Sex Research, 23,* 1-11.

Malamuth, N. M. (1989). The Attraction to Sexual Aggression Scale: Part one. *The Journal of Sex Research, 26,* 26-49.

Nelson, P. A. (1979). *A sexual functions inventory.* Unpublished doctoral dissertation, University of Florida, Gainesville.

Pryor, J. B. (1987). Sexual harassment proclivities in men. *Sex Roles, 17,* 269-290.

Pryor, J. B., Giedd, J. L., & Williams, K. B. (1995). A social psychological model for predicting sexual harassment. *Journal of Social Issues, 51*(1), 69-84.

Pryor, J. B., LaVite, C., & Stoller, L. (1993). A social psychological analysis of sexual harassment: The person/situation interaction. *Journal of Vocational Behavior, 42,* 68-83.

Pryor, J. B., & Stoller, L. (1994). Sexual cognition processes in men who are high in the likelihood to sexually harass. *Personality and Social Psychology Bulletin, 20,* 163-169.

Pryor, J. B., & Whalen, N. J. (in press). A typology of sexual harassment: Characteristics of harassers and the social circumstances under which sexual harassment occurs. In W. O'Donohue (Ed.), *Sexual harassment: Theory, research, and treatment.* Needham Heights, MA: Allyn & Bacon.

Spence, J. T., & Helmreich, R. (1978). *Masculinity and femininity: Their psychological dimensions, correlates, and antecedents.* Austin: University of Texas Press.

Exhibit

The Likelihood to Sexually Harass Scale

Instructions: On the sheets that follow you will find 10 brief scenarios that describe 10 different interactions between males and females. In each case you will be asked to imagine that you are the main male character in the scenario. Then you will be asked to rate how likely it is that you would perform each of several different behaviors in the described social context. Assume in each scenario that no matter what you choose to do, nothing bad would be likely to happen to you as a result of your action. Try to answer each question as honestly as you can. Your answers will be completely anonymous. No one will ever try to discover your identity, no matter what you say on the questionnaire.

Scenario 1

Imagine that you are an executive in a large corporation. You are 42 years old. Your income is above average for people at your job level. You have had numerous job offers from other companies. You feel very secure in your job. One day your personal secretary decides to quit her job and you have the task of replacing her. The personnel department sends several applicants over for you to interview. All seem to be equally qualified for the job. One of the applicants, Michelle S., explains during her interview that she desperately needs the job. She is 23 years old, single and has been job hunting for about a month. You find yourself very attracted to her. She looks at you in a way that possibly conveys she is also attracted to you. How likely are you to do the following things in this situation?

a. Would you give her the job over the other applicants? (Circle a number to indicate your response.)[a]

       1   2   3   4   5
    Not at all likely   Very likely

b. Assuming that you are secure enough in your job that no possible reprisals could happen to you, would you offer her the job in exchange for sexual favors? (Circle a number to indicate your response.)

c. Assuming that you fear no reprisals on your job, would you ask her to meet you later for dinner to discuss her possible employment?

Scenario 2

Imagine that you are the owner and manager of an expensive restaurant. One day, while going over the receipts, you discover that one of the waitresses has made some errors in her checks. She has undercharged several customers. The mistake costs you $100. In talking to some of the other employees, you find that the particular customers involved were friends of the waitress. You call her into your office and ask her to explain her behavior. The waitress confesses to having intentionally undercharged her friends. She promises that she will never repeat this dishonest act and tells you that she will do anything to keep her job. The waitress is someone you have always found particularly attractive. She is a divorcee and about 25 years old. How likely are you to do the following things in this situation?

a. Would you let her keep her job?
b. Would you let her keep her job in exchange for sexual favors?
c. Would you ask her to meet you for dinner after work to discuss the problem?

Scenario 3

Imagine that you are the manager of a shipping company. One day your supervisor asks you to study the possibility of buying several computers for the office. You call up several competing companies that sell computers. Each company sends a sales representative over to your office who describes the company's products. A salesperson from company "A" calls you and asks to come to your office. You agree and the next day a very attractive woman shows up. She can offer no real reason for buying her company's products over those of the other companies. However, she seems very sexy. How likely are you to do the following things in this situation?

a. Would you recommend her line of computers?
b. Assuming that you are secure enough in your job that no possible reprisals could happen to you, would you agree to recommend her line of computers in exchange for sexual favors?
c. Given the same assumptions as the last question above, would you ask her to meet you later for dinner to discuss the choice of computers?

Scenario 4

Imagine that you are a Hollywood film director. You are casting for a minor role in a film you are planning. The role calls for a particularly stunning actress, one with a lot of sex appeal. How likely are you to do the following things in this situation?

a. Would you give the role to the actress whom you personally found sexiest?
b. Would give the role to an actress who agreed to have sex with you?
c. Would ask the actress to whom you were most personally attracted to talk with you about the role over dinner?

Scenario 5

Imagine that you are the owner of a modeling agency. Your agency specializes in sexy female models used in television commercials. One of your models, Amy T., is a particularly ravishing brunette. You stop her after work one day and ask her to have dinner with you. She coldly declines your offer and tells you that she would like to keep your relationship with her "strictly business." A few months later you find that business is slack and you have to lay off some of your employees. You can choose to lay off Amy or one of four other women. All are good models, but someone has to go. How likely are you to do the following things in this situation?

a. Would you fire Amy?
b. Assuming that you are unafraid of possible reprisals, would you offer to let Amy keep her job in return for sexual favors?
c. Would you ask Amy to dinner so that you could talk over her future employment?

Scenario 6

Imagine that you are a college professor. You are 38 years old. You teach in a large Midwestern university. You are a full professor with tenure. You are renowned in your field (Abnormal Psychology) and have numerous offers for other jobs. One day following the return of an examination to a class, a female student stops in your office. She tells you that her score is one point away from an "A" and asks you if she can do some extra credit project to raise her score. She tells you that she may not have a sufficient grade to get into graduate school without the "A." Several other students have asked you to do extra credit assignments and you have declined to let them. This particular woman is a stunning blonde. She sits in the front row of the class every day and always wears short skirts. You find her extremely sexy. How likely are you to do the following things in this situation?

a. Would you let her carry out a project for extra credit (e.g., write a paper)?
b. Assuming that you are very secure in your job and the university has always tolerated professors who make passes at students, would you offer the student a chance to earn extra credit in return for sexual favors?
c. Given the same assumptions as in the question above, would you ask her to join you for dinner to discuss the possible extra credit assignments?

Scenario 7

Imagine that you are a college student at a large Midwestern university. You are a junior who just transferred from another school on the East coast. One night at a bar you meet an attractive female student named Rhonda. Rhonda laments to you that she is failing a course in English poetry. She tells you that she has a paper due next week on the poet Shelley, and fears that she will fail since she has not begun to write it. You remark that you wrote a paper last year on Shelley at your former school. Your paper was given an A+. She asks you if you will let her use your paper in her course. She wants to just retype it and put her name on it. How likely are you to do the following things in this situation?

a. Would you let Rhonda use your paper?
b. Would you let Rhonda use your paper in exchange for sexual favors?
c. Would you ask Rhonda to come to your apartment to discuss the matter?

Scenario 8

Imagine that you are the editor for a major publishing company. It is your job to read new manuscripts of novels and decide whether they are worthy of publication. You receive literally hundreds of manuscripts per week from aspiring novelists. Most of them are screened by your subordinates and thrown in the trash. You end up accepting about one in a thousand for publication. One night you go to a party. There you meet a very attractive woman named Betsy. Betsy tells you that she has written a novel and would like to check into getting it published. This is her first novel. She is a dental assistant. She asks you to read her novel. How likely are you to do the following things in this situation.

a. Would you agree to read Betsy's novel?
b. Would you agree to reading Betsy's novel in exchange for sexual favors?
c. Would you ask Betsy to have dinner with you the next night to discuss your reading her novel?

Scenario 9

Imagine that you are a physician. You go over to the hospital one day to make your rounds visiting your patients. In looking over the records of one of your patients, you discover that one of the attending nurses on the previous night shift made an error in administering drugs to your patient. She gave the wrong dosage of a drug. You examine the patient and discover that no harm was actually done. He seems fine. However, you realize that the ramifications of the error could have been catastrophic under other circumstances. You pull the files and find out who made the error. It turns out that a new young nurse named Wendy H. was responsible. You have noticed Wendy in some of your visits to the hospital and have thought of asking her out to dinner. You realize that she could lose her job if you report this incident. How likely are you to do each of the following things?

a. Would you report Wendy to the hospital administration?
b. Assuming that you fear no reprisals, would you tell Wendy in private that you will not report her if she will have sex with you?
c. Assuming that you fear no reprisals, would you ask Wendy to join you for dinner to discuss the incident?

Scenario 10

Imagine that you are the news director for a local television station. Due to some personnel changes you have to replace the anchor woman for the evening news. Your policy has always been to promote reporters from within your organization when an anchor woman vacancy occurs. There are several female reporters from which to choose. All are young, attractive, and apparently qualified for the job. One reporter, Loretta W., is someone whom you personally find very sexy. You initially hired her, giving her a first break in the TV news business. How likely are you to do the following things in this situation?

a. Would you give Loretta the job?
b. Assuming that you fear no reprisals in your job, would you offer Loretta the job in exchange for sexual favors?
c. Assuming that you fear no reprisals in your job, would you ask her to meet you after work for dinner to discuss the job?

Note. Scoring the LSH: The key items are respondents' answers to the "b" item for each scenario. Ratings for these items are simply summed to produce an overall LSH score.
a. The following scale is reproduced after each response option.

Sexual Harassment Attitudes Questionnaire

Jayne E. Stake[1] and Natalie J. Malovich, *University of Missouri–St. Louis*

Description

The incidence of sexual harassment in educational settings is well documented, yet the psychological dynamics that underlie the perpetuation of sexual harassment are still only partially understood. The Sexual Harassment Attitudes Questionnaire was developed as a research tool to explore psychological factors associated with sexual harassment in educational settings. The questionnaire measures respondents' attitudes regarding (a) responsibility for harassment behaviors, (b) appropriate responses to sexual harassment, and (c) effects of sexual harassment on victims. Respondents first read two scenarios that depict clear-cut incidents of sexual harassment in a college setting. After each scenario, they indicate to whom they attribute responsibility for the incident. Two questions pertain to victim blame, two to perpetrator blame, and two to no blame. A second set of six questions taps respondents' attitudes about appropriate responses to sexual harassment. Two questions refer to confronting the harassing behavior, two to complying with the harasser, and two to ignoring the harassment. Finally, a set of eight questions measures expectations of the effects of the harassment. Two questions refer to educational effects and six to emotional effects. All questions have 6-point Likert-type scales except for the questions regarding emotional effects, which have 7-point Likert-type scales.

Validity

Based on responses of 113 female and 111 male college undergraduates, the questionnaire shows evidence of construct validity (Malovich & Stake, 1990). Perpetrator blame scores in this sample were negatively related to victim blame (–.36) and no blame (–.57) scores. Victim blame was positively related to recommendations for compliance (+.47) and expectations for positive educational effects (+.32), and negatively related to recommendations for confrontive action (–.30), expectations for negative emotional effects (–.44), and liberal sex role attitudes (Attitudes Toward Women scores and victim blame: –.22). In contrast, perpetrator blame was positively related to recommendations for confrontive action (+.45), expectations for negative emotional effects (+.54), and liberal sex role attitudes (+.22), and negatively related to recommendations for compliance (–.45) and expectations for positive educational effects (–.37).

Reference

Malovich, N. J., & Stake, J. E. (1990). Sexual harassment on campus: Individual differences in attitudes and beliefs. *Psychology of Women Quarterly, 14,* 63-81.

[1]Address correspondence to Jayne E. Stake, Department of Psychology, University of Missouri–St. Louis, St. Louis, MO 63121; email: c4869@umslvma.umsl.edu.

Exhibit

Sexual Harassment Attitudes Questionnaire

The purpose of this questionnaire is to examine relationships between instructors and students. You will read two scenarios involving instructors and students. Each will be followed by a set of questions consisting of statements about the scenario you have read. You will be asked to imagine that you or a close woman friend of yours is the student in the situation presented. There are no right or wrong answers, only opinions. If you are unsure about an answer, just indicate the response that best fits your own opinion.

Scenario 1

Suppose that you or a close woman friend of yours is attending classes on this campus. After class one day, a professor asks that you come to his office to discuss your grade with him. When you get there he notes that you barely passed the last exam and are in danger of receiving a D for the course. He then tells you at length how much he enjoys having you in the class, leading up to a dinner invitation. He states that if you "get to know each other better" he might be able to work things out so that you can get a better grade.

The following are a number of statements about the situation that might help to explain why the above incident occurred. Rate your agreement with each of the following comments. Mark the number on your answer sheet that best describes your feeling. Use the following key:

0 = Strongly disagree
1 = Moderately disagree
2 = Somewhat disagree
3 = Somewhat agree
4 = Moderately agree
5 = Strongly agree

1. The student is probably hoping that getting to know the professor personally will help her get a better grade in the course.
2. The professor probably meant no harm so it should not be taken too seriously.
3. The professor is using his status unfairly to pressure the student into dating him.
4. The professor is responding to normal sexual attraction and cannot really be blamed for his actions in the situation.
5. The professor's actions were unethical and could he harmful to his students.
6. The student is most likely a flirtatious type who enjoys getting special attention from her professors.

The following are a number of statements describing possible ways that you could deal with the situation. Rate your agreement with each of the following statements. Mark the number on your answer sheet that best describes your feelings. Use the following key:

0 = Strongly disagree
1 = Moderately disagree
2 = Somewhat disagree
3 = Somewhat agree
4 = Moderately agree
5 = Strongly agree

7. Change the subject and try to forget about the conversation.
8. Go to dinner with the professor and talk over the problems you are having in the class.
9. Continue to work hard in the class and avoid any individual conversations with the professor.
10. Tell the professor that you are not interested in a personal relationship and that this should have nothing to do with your grade in the course.
11. See the professor on a social basis if he is interested as it may help your grade.
12. Go to the department head and tell him/her about the professor's actions.

Below is a set of word pairs that describe how you or a close woman friend might feel about this experience. The two feelings in each pair are separated by a 7-point scale, with one word on each side on the scale. For each word pair, mark the number on your answer sheet that is closest to how you think you or your friend might feel.

13.	Insulted	0	1	2	3	4	5	6	Flattered
14.	Pleased	0	1	2	3	4	5	6	Angry
15.	Comfortable	0	1	2	3	4	5	6	Uncomfortable
16.	Relaxed	0	1	2	3	4	5	6	Nervous
17.	Intimidated	0	1	2	3	4	5	6	Powerful
18.	Embarrassed	0	1	2	3	4	5	6	Proud

Scenario 2

Suppose that you or a close woman friend of yours is attending this campus. Through the course of the semester you notice that a professor in one of your classes frequently seems to be staring at you. When talking with him after class one day about an upcoming essay exam, he puts his arm around you (or the woman friend) and touches your hair. He then suggests that you come to his office at the end of the day so that the exam can be discussed further. He adds that if you fail to do so, you will probably not do as well on the exam as expected.[a]

Source. This questionnaire was originally published in "Sexual Harassment on Campus: Individual Differences in Attitudes and Beliefs," by N. J. Malovich and J. E. Stake, 1990, *Psychology of Women Quarterly, 14,* 63-81. Reprinted with permission.
a. Questions 19-36 are identical to Questions 1-18.

Herpes Attitude Scale

Katherine Bruce,[1] *University of North Carolina at Wilmington*
Judith McLaughlin, *University of Georgia*

The Herpes Attitude Scale (HAS) assesses beliefs and feelings about genital herpes. Subject areas include feelings about self, feelings about others who have herpes, communication about herpes, intimate relationships, friendship relationships, perceived coping abilities, and myths. People who have positive attitudes about herpes can be discriminated from those who have negative attitudes.

Description

This scale is a 40-item Likert-type scale (5 points) with response options labeled *strongly agree, agree, neither agree nor disagree, disagree,* and *strongly disagree.* The items on the scale were selected from an initial pool of 65 opinion statements about herpes. They were judged for readability by five undergraduate students and for acceptability for inclusion in the scale by a panel of five expert judges. The judges agreed on 45 of the original items for inclusion in the scale. The scale was administered to 250 undergraduate students in introductory psychology courses, and an item analysis was conducted to identify the statements that could best discriminate high and low scorers. Forty items had statistically significant item-total correlations ($p < .001$). These items were arranged in random order, and the scale was tested for reliability. This scale was designed to measure students' attitudes about herpes, but could be used for other populations.

Response Mode and Timing

Respondents circle or blacken one response option for each item on a separate labeled answer sheet. Most respondents complete the scale within 15 minutes.

[1]Address correspondence to Katherine Bruce, Department of Psychology, UNC-Wilmington, Wilmington, NC 28403; email: bruce@uncwil.edu.

Scoring

The 20 positive items (2, 3, 4, 6, 9, 11, 12, 15, 17, 18, 19, 20, 21, 24, 25, 26, 27, 28, 38, and 40) are scored such that *strongly agree* has a value of 5, *agree* a value of 4, and so forth. For the negative items (1, 5, 7, 8, 10, 13, 14, 16, 22, 23, 29, 30, 31, 32, 33, 34, 35, 36, 37, and 39), reverse scoring is used. The total attitude score is obtained by the following formula: HAS score = $(X - N)$ (100)/(N) (4), where X is the total of the scored responses and N is the number of items properly complete. Scores may range from 0 to 100; higher scores indicate a more positive attitude about genital herpes and coping with genital herpes.

Reliability

To measure internal consistency (split-half reliability), 148 undergraduates students in psychology and health education classes completed the scale. Reliability was high (Cronbach's alpha = .91; Bruce & McLaughlin, 1986).

Validity

Content and face validity were evaluated by a panel of five expert judges: a physician, a registered nurse, two health educators, and a graduate student with herpes. The judges assessed the relevance and importance of each item, as well as the comprehensiveness of the entire scale (Bruce & McLaughlin, 1986).

References

Bruce, K., & McLaughlin, J. (1986). The development of scales to assess knowledge and attitudes about genital herpes. *The Journal of Sex Research, 22,* 73-84.

Bruce, K. E. M., & Bullins, C. G. (1989). Students' attitudes and knowledge about genital herpes. *Journal of Sex Education and Therapy, 15,* 257-270.

Exhibit

Herpes Attitude Scale

Instructions: For each of the following 40 statements, please note on the answer sheet whether you agree or disagree with the statements. Use the following scale:

SA: Strongly agree with the statement
A: Agree with the statement
N: Neither agree nor disagree with the statement
D: Disagree with the statement
SD: Strongly disagree with the statement

Each statement is numbered. Be sure to match the statement's number with the number on the answer sheet. Please respond to all items on the questionnaire. There are NO right or wrong answers.

1. The thought of genital herpes is disgusting.
2. I would not feel dirty if I got genital herpes.
3. Genital herpes is not as scary as most people believe.
4. There are a lot of diseases that are worse than genital herpes.
5. People give genital herpes to others for revenge.
6. I could cope with having genital herpes.
7. If I had a roommate with genital herpes, I would move out.
8. Only bad people catch genital herpes.
9. I feel comfortable around friends who have genital herpes.
10. You can tell that someone has genital herpes just by looking at them.
11. I am pretty sure that I could handle having genital herpes if I caught it.
12. Having genital herpes is really no worse than having cold sores.
13. People who have genital herpes are looked down on.
14. I do not like to use public restrooms because I might catch genital herpes there.
15. I could remain calm if I found out that I had gotten genital herpes.
16. A person who has genital herpes got what s/he deserves.
17. If I had genital herpes, I would tell a potential sex partner.
18. There is more to a person who has genital herpes than the fact that s/he has genital herpes.
19. I would not avoid a friend if I found out that s/he had genital herpes.
20. I would consider marrying someone who has genital herpes.
21. People who have genital herpes should be treated the same as anyone else.
22. I would feel self-conscious if I got genital herpes.
23. If I found out that my sexual partner had genital herpes, I would never speak to him/her again.
24. The "new sexual leprosy" is an inappropriate term for genital herpes.
25. Catching genital herpes would not be the worst thing that could happen to me.
26. I would not be ashamed if I got genital herpes.
27. People who have genital herpes are worth getting to know.
28. Genital herpes is a manageable disease.
29. I think that people who have genital herpes are too sexually active.
30. If I caught genital herpes, I would consider suicide.
31. People who have genital herpes should never have sex again.
32. I would be embarrassed to tell anyone if I had genital herpes.
33. Only unclean people catch genital herpes.
34. If I got genital herpes, no one would want to marry me.
35. If I got genital herpes, I would not want to have children.
36. Everyone would know if I got genital herpes.
37. People who have genital herpes are promiscuous.
38. I could discuss genital herpes with my parents.
39. If I asked a friend a question about genital herpes, s/he would think that I had genital herpes.
40. I would date a person known to have genital herpes.

Herpes Knowledge Scale

Katherine Bruce,[1] *University of North Carolina at Wilmington*
Judith McLaughlin, *University of Georgia*

The Herpes Knowledge Scale (HKS) assesses general knowledge about genital herpes. Subject areas include cause, symptoms, treatment, contagion, recurrences, prevalence, complications, myths, and the relationship between oral and genital herpes. People who have high knowledge about these areas can be discriminated from those who have low knowledge.

Description

This scale is a 54-item true-false test with response options labeled *true, false,* and *don't know.* The items on the scale were selected from an initial pool of 64 rationally field-derived statements about herpes. They were judged for readability by five undergraduate students and for their relevance and importance for inclusion in the scale by a panel of five expert judges. The judges agreed on 57 of the original items for inclusion. The scale was administered to 250 undergraduate students in introductory psychology courses, and an item analysis was conducted to identify the statements that could best discriminate high and low scorers. Fifty-four items had statistically significant item-total correlations ($p < .0007$). These items were arranged in random order, and the scale was tested for reliability. This scale was designed to measure students' knowledge about herpes, but it could be used for other populations.

Response Mode and Timing

Respondents circle or blacken one response option for each item on a separate labeled answer sheet. Most respondents complete the scale within 15 minutes.

---
[1]Address correspondence to Katherine Bruce, Department of Psychology, UNC-Wilmington, Wilmington, NC 28403; email: bruce@uncwil.edu.

Scoring

The response to each item is scored as correct or incorrect. *Don't know* is scored as an incorrect response. Items 1, 2, 4, 7, 9, 10, 14, 15, 19, 20, 24, 25, 26, 27, 28, 29, 31, 32, 33, 34, 35, 36, 40, 41, 46, 48, and 49 are true. Items 3, 5, 6, 8, 11, 12, 13, 16, 17, 18, 21, 22, 23, 30, 37, 38, 39, 42, 43, 44, 45, 47, 50, 51, 52, 53, and 54 are false. The total score is obtained by summing the number of correct responses, dividing this by 54, and multiplying this fraction by 100 so that scores are expressed as percentage correct (0-100%).

Reliability

To measure internal consistency (split-half reliability), 148 undergraduate students in psychology and health education classes completed the scale. Reliability was high (Cronbach's alpha = .88; Bruce & McLaughlin, 1986).

Validity

Content and face validity were evaluated by a panel of five expert judges: a physician, a registered nurse, two health educators, and a graduate student with herpes. The judges assessed the relevance and importance of each item, as well as the comprehensiveness of the entire scale (Bruce & McLaughlin, 1986).

References

Bruce, K., & McLaughlin, J. (1986). The development of scales to assess knowledge and attitudes about genital herpes. *The Journal of Sex Research, 22,* 73-84.

Bruce, K. E. M., & Bullins, C. G. (1989). Students' attitudes and knowledge about genital herpes. *Journal of Sex Education and Therapy, 15,* 257-270.

Exhibit

Herpes Knowledge Scale

Instructions: For each of the following 54 statements, please note on the answer sheet whether you think the statement is true or false. If you do not have any idea whether or not the statement is true or false, please note that you don't know. Use the following code for your responses:

T: The statement is true
F: The statement is false
DK: I don't know whether the statement is true or false

Each statement is numbered. Be sure to match the statement's number with the number on the answer sheet. Please respond to all statements on the questionnaire.

1. The length and severity of genital herpes outbreaks vary from person to person.
2. Genital herpes is caused by a virus.
3. Genital herpes was discovered five years ago.
4. Genital herpes recurrences can be triggered by menstruation (in females) or sexual intercourse.
5. Every person who has a primary (first) outbreak of genital herpes will have recurrence within the next year.
6. Genital herpes makes males infertile (sterile).
7. Between recurrences, the genital herpes virus lies dormant (inactive) in the nerve cells.
8. Herpes Type 1 cannot occur on the genitals.
9. A person having recurrences of genital herpes often experiences prodromal (early warning) sensations.
10. Years may pass between genital herpes recurrences.
11. Every sore on the genitals is herpes.
12. Once a genital herpes sore has healed, the person will never develop another herpes sore.
13. A person who gets cold sores on the mouth is immune to genital herpes.
14. Genital herpes usually looks like blisters on the genitals.
15. Prodromal (early warning) sensations of genital herpes recurrences include tingling or itching in the area where the genital herpes sores usually appear.
16. If a person has sexual intercourse with someone who has genital herpes, s/he will definitely get genital herpes too.
17. Several hundred people are expected to catch genital herpes from toilet seats this year.
18. A woman who has genital herpes will become sterile because of the herpes infection.
19. People who wear contact lenses and have oral (mouth) herpes should avoid putting the lenses in their mouths because the herpes infection could spread to their eyes.
20. A person with genital herpes is instructed to keep the sore area clean and dry.
21. Genital herpes leads to death.
22. There is a cure for genital herpes at present.
23. Genital herpes recurrences do not typically become less frequent over time.
24. A person who has genital herpes often has more psychological complications than physical complications.
25. When a person has an active outbreak of genital herpes, it is advisable not to have sexual intercourse.
26. People who have genital herpes can sometimes predict when they will have a recurrence.
27. A woman who has genital herpes should have a Pap smear at least once a year.
28. Genital herpes can be contagious even if the herpes sore has a scab on it.
29. First episodes of genital herpes infection are usually more severe than the recurrences.
30. A person who has genital herpes is immune to oral (mouth) herpes.
31. Between recurrences, the genital herpes virus lies dormant (inactive) near the spinal cord.
32. Stress can often trigger a genital herpes recurrence.
33. Herpes can be fatal to a newborn if s/he contracts the infection.
34. Genital herpes can often be detected by the use of a Pap smear.
35. After a person is exposed to genital herpes, s/he will often show symptoms in 2-20 days.
36. Anxiety can trigger a genital herpes recurrence.
37. Condoms offer 100% protection from catching genital herpes.
38. A genital herpes infection usually leads to syphilis.
39. A woman who had genital herpes must have a Caesarean section if she has a baby.
40. Most people have been exposed to oral herpes at one time or another.
41. A woman with genital herpes can deliver a baby through her vagina if she doesn't have an active herpes infection at the time of delivery.
42. If both parents have genital herpes, their children will be born with herpes.
43. A woman who has genital herpes can never have a baby.
44. Genital herpes is not contagious.
45. L-lysine is a cure for genital herpes.
46. Genital herpes may be associated with cancer of the cervix.
47. Contraceptive foam has been proven to kill genital herpes in humans.
48. In a primary (first) case of genital herpes, the person may feel like s/he has the flu.
49. Oral herpes is contagious.
50. The best way to treat genital herpes sores is to keep them moist.
51. Acyclovir (also called Zovirax), an anti-viral drug, can cure genital herpes.
52. A person with genital herpes is not contagious during the prodromal (early warning) stage.
53. Genital herpes is not prevalent (common) on college campuses.
54. Oral herpes cannot be transferred to the genitals during oral-genital sex.

Genital Herpes Perceived Severity Scales

Jerrold Mirotznik,[1] *Brooklyn College, City University of New York*

The Genital Herpes Perceived Severity Scales (GHPSS; Mirotznik, 1991) measure attitudes about contracting this sexually transmitted disease. The scales were developed to test the speculations, frequently reported as facts in the media, that (a) single, sexually active, and consequently at-risk young adults had become highly anxious about infection with the herpes virus; and (b) as a result of this heightened concern, those at risk had dramatically altered their dating behaviors. Although several researchers had addressed these issues (Aral, Cates, & Jenkins, 1985; Simkins & Eberhage, 1984; Simkins & Kushner, 1986), they used measures that suffered from important limitations, including vague conceptualizations and operationalizations in terms of a single questionnaire item. Single-item measures tend to be less reliable and, as such, have the untoward effect of attenuating associations with other measures. Another limitation concerned the use of dichotomous response options. Dichotomous response options fail to capture the variability of reactions to genital herpes. Finally, little evidence was presented regarding these measures' psychometric properties. (See Mirotznik, 1991, for a detailed discussion of these limitations.)

The primary theoretical orientation guiding the conceptualization of the GHPSS was the health belief model (HBM; Janz & Becker, 1984). In the HBM, it is hypothesized that people are likely to take steps to avoid a particular disease if they perceive that disease as personally threatening. A major component of perceived threat is the degree to which a disease is thought to be severe. Perceived severity, in turn, has been defined not just in terms of a disease's medical/clinical consequences but also its social and psychological effects. Accordingly, the GHPSS were constructed to measure the degree to which people believe that contracting genital herpes would lead to the latter type of consequences.

Description

Three scales were developed de novo. Each scale was hypothesized to measure a particular social or psychological consequence of infection. To enhance content and face validity, all items were constructed with the help of two clinicians, a sex therapist and a psychologist, both with expertise in treating people with genital herpes.

The Fear Scale measures whether respondents are frightened about contracting this disease by determining the degree to which they embrace seven items that characterize herpes and those who contract it in highly negative, stigmatizing terms. Each item has a 6-point Likert-type re-

sponse format ranging from (1) *strongly disagree* to (6) *strongly agree.*

The Family Impediment Scale measures the degree to which respondents believe that contracting genital herpes would be a hindrance in establishing a family. It consists of one overall question asking respondents to rate how difficult it would be for a single person with genital herpes to experience each of five family life-course events. Each item has a 6-point Likert-type response format ranging from (1) *not difficult at all* to (6) *very difficult.*

The Emotional Response Scale assesses possible emotional reactions to infection with genital herpes. The scale lists seven emotions. For each emotion, respondents indicate on a 4-point Likert-type format whether they would (1) *not react* with the emotion or (4) *strongly experience* the emotion.

Response Mode and Timing

For the items for each scale, respondents can circle on the questionnaire the number of the response option that best corresponds to their attitude or they can mark the number on separate machine-scorable answer sheets. The three scales take approximately 5 minutes to complete.

Scoring

Items within each scale and between scales are keyed in the same direction with higher scores indicating that respondents perceive herpes to be more severe. For each scale, a total score is calculated by first summing the response number for all answered items and then dividing by the number of answered items. The resulting mean score has the beneficial properties of having the same range as the individual items and also of adjusting for any missing items.

Reliability

To assess the psychometric properties of the GHPSS and the consistency of those properties across varied populations, the scales were initially administered to two convenience samples: 998 college and graduate students and 178 residents of a therapeutic community for alcohol and drug rehabilitation (Mirotznik, 1991). Subsequently, the questionnaire was administered to an additional sample of 439 college students. Each sample was subdivided into those who were single and sexually active and therefore at risk of infection and those not at risk. For each of the resulting six subsamples, internal consistency reliability was then calculated using Cronbach's alpha. For the Fear Scale the mean alpha across the six subsamples was .80 with a range of .73 to .83. The mean alpha for the Family Impediment Scale was .77 with a range of .73 to .81, and for the Emotional Response Scale it was .77 with a range of .75 to .82.

[1]Address correspondence to Jerrold Mirotznik, Department of Health and Nutrition Sciences, Brooklyn College, 2900 Bedford Avenue, Brooklyn, NY 11210.

Generally, the scales exhibited somewhat better reliability for the student subsamples than for the therapeutic community subsamples.

Validity

Two tests were conducted to assess validity (Mirotznik, 1991). Given that these three scales were hypothesized to measure the same overarching construct, perceived severity of genital herpes, they should be more highly correlated with each other than with measures of other constructs. As Nunnally (1978) pointed out, an indication that variables cluster as theoretically predicted is important evidence of construct validity. A principal components factor analysis with varimax rotation conducted on the initial subsample of at-risk students indicated that the GHPSS generally factored as expected. Specifically, all three scales loaded highly on one factor (i.e., Fear Scale, .76; Family Impediment Scale, .75; Emotional Reaction Scale, .68), whereas measures of knowledge about genital herpes and preventive behaviors loaded on other factors. When the factor analysis was rerun on the remaining five subsamples, generally the same factor structure appeared.

A second important test of construct validity involves determining if a measure of a construct fits predictions from a well-accepted theory (Nunnally, 1978). According to the HBM, the greater people's perceived severity of disease, the more likely they are to engage in preventive health behaviors. To assess this, a measure of preventive behavior (i.e., change in dating behaviors in light of knowledge about genital herpes) was correlated with the three perceived severity scales separately for the at-risk respondents from each of the three convenience samples. Each scale was significantly associated in the theoretically predicted direction, albeit modestly so, with the measure of preventive behavior in the two subsamples of at-risk students. The mean correlations for these two subsamples were .25 for the Fear Scale, .17 for the Family Impediment Scale, and .18 for the Emotional Response Scale. It is conceivable that the magnitude of these correlations may have been attenuated by the single-item used to operationalize preventive behavior.

References

Aral, S. O., Cates, W., & Jenkins, W. C. (1985). Genital herpes: Does knowledge lead to action? *American Journal of Public Health, 75,* 69-71.

Janz, N. K., & Becker, M. H. (1984). The health belief model: A decade later. *Health Education Quarterly, 11,* 1-47.

Mirotznik, J. (1991). Genital herpes: A survey of the attitudes, knowledge, and reported behaviors of college students at-risk for infection. *Journal of Psychology and Human Sexuality, 4,* 73-99.

Nunnally, J. C. (1978). *Psychometric theory.* New York: McGraw-Hill.

Simkins, L., & Eberhage, M. G. (1984). Attitudes toward AIDS, herpes II, and toxic shock syndrome. *Psychological Reports, 55,* 779-786.

Simkins, L., & Kushner, A. (1986). Attitudes toward AIDS, herpes II, and toxic shock syndrome: Two years later. *Psychological Reports, 59,* 883-891.

Exhibit

Genital Herpes Perceived Severity Scales

Instructions: The following items measure your beliefs about genital herpes. Some of the questions concern your views about others who have contracted the virus and the general consequences of infection. Other questions concern how you would personally react if you contracted the virus. For each item, please circle the response option that best corresponds to your feelings.

Fear Scale

For the following statements please select a number from 1 to 6, 1 meaning that you strongly disagree and 6 that you strongly agree.

1. Genital herpes will ruin your sex life.
2. Having genital herpes is as bad as having cancer.
3. No one will want me if I had genital herpes.
4. Genital herpes is a dirty disease.
5. I would not trust anybody who has genital herpes.
6. My opinion of a person would change if I found out he/she had genital herpes.
7. Even though I would be very understanding of people I knew had genital herpes, I would be tempted to stay away from them.

Family Impediment Scale

How difficult to deal with would each of the following things be for a single person who has genital herpes? Choose a number from 1 to 6, 1 indicating not difficult at all and 6 very difficult.

1. Meeting a boyfriend/girlfriend.
2. Telling a boyfriend or girlfriend that you have genital herpes.

3. Having sex.
4. Getting married.
5. Having children.

Emotional Reaction Scale

People may have different reactions to contracting genital herpes. How would you react? For each emotion listed below indicate if you would: 1. not react with the emotion, 2. mildly feel the emotion, 3. moderately feel the emotion, or 4. strongly experience the emotion.

1. Angry.
2. Punished.
3. Fearful.
4. Numbed.
5. Damaged.
6. That it was expected.
7. Guilty.

Source. These scales are reprinted with permission of the author.

Inventory of Dyadic Heterosexual Preferences and Inventory of Dyadic Heterosexual Preferences–Other

Daniel M. Purnine, Michael P. Carey,[1] and Randall S. Jorgensen,
Syracuse University

The Inventory of Dyadic Heterosexual Preferences (IDHP) was developed to measure men's and women's affinity for a broad range of fairly conventional sexual behavior preferences within the context of a dyadic heterosexual relationship. Six scales, reflecting different domains of behavioral preference, are derived. The IDHP allows researchers to explore relationships between specific preferences or profiles of preference and various behavioral, personality, or dyadic correlates. Sex therapists may be interested in comparing the profile of one's sexual preferences with that of one's partner. An other-focused version of the inventory (IDHP-O) asks the respondent to indicate how he or she believes the partner would respond to the IDHP.

Description

A complete description of the IDHP and its development may be found elsewhere (Purnine, Carey, & Jorgensen, 1996). The IDHP is a 27-item self-report inventory that measures the following six areas of sexual preference: Erotophilia, Use of Contraception, Conventionality, Use of Erotica, Use of Drugs/Alcohol, and Romantic Foreplay.

Seventy-four statements, applicable to both men and women, were generated to elicit responses to specific behaviors or elements of a sexual scene. Each item was followed by a 6-point Likert-type scale, ranging from *strongly agree* to *strongly disagree*. Items regarding fantasy, opinion,

[1]Address correspondence to Michael P. Carey, Department of Psychology, 430 Huntington Hall, Syracuse University, Syracuse, NY 13244-2340; email: mpcarey@psych.syr.edu.

or motivation were generally excluded. The perfect tense ("I would enjoy") rather than the present tense ("I enjoy") was employed so that items outside one's habitual range of experience may be applicable. This use of the hypothetical allows the IDHP to be applicable to those not currently involved in a sexually intimate relationship.

The 74 items were administered to 258 undergraduate and graduate university students (Sample 1), 18 to 59 years of age (M = 23). After eliminating items that failed to elicit a broad range of responses or that were unreliable during a 1- to 2-week period, 46 items remained. Factor analyses suggested a six-factor, 27-item solution. This solution was based on a covariance matrix in which the variance attributable to gender had been removed. A gender-neutral factor structure was considered necessary to allow meaningful comparisons between the profiles of male and female partners.

These results were cross-validated using new data (Sample 2) from 228 students, aged 17 to 53 (M = 21). Six items were reworded to improve their clarity. Three new items were introduced to enlarge certain factors. A six-factor maximum likelihood solution, with promax rotation, incorporated the new items and suggested the elimination of three others. The final 27-item factor structure accounted for 51% of the variance among the 27 items.

Response Mode and Timing

Using a paper-and-pencil format, respondents circle the number indicating their personal level of agreement or disagreement with each statement of preference. It takes approximately 5 minutes to complete the IDHP and, if administered, an additional 5 minutes to complete the IDHP-O.

Scoring

IDHP scale scores (individual preferences). Higher scores on each of the six IDHP scales indicate stronger preference for the behaviors in that scale. First, Items 3, 24, and 26 must be reverse scored by subtracting the number circled from 7. Each scale is then derived by adding across the items; Erotophilia: 1, 7, 8, 11, 16, 17, 18; Use of Contraception: 3, 6, 13, 26; Conventionality: 5, 10, 22, 23; Use of Erotica: 4, 9, 24, 27; Use of Drugs/Alcohol: 12, 14, 15, 20; and Romantic Foreplay: 2, 19, 21, 25. To standardize the scales, each ranging from 1 to 6, sums may be divided by the number of items added.

Exploratory scores. Several dyadic variables are currently under investigation: Agreement, or similarity between two partners' preferences, may be observed by comparing the IDHP of each partner; Female Understanding (of the male) is reflected by comparing the male's IDHP with the IDHP-O of the female; and Male Understanding (of the female) is reflected by comparing the female's IDHP with the male's IDHP-O. An individual variable, Perceived Agreement, is reflected in the difference between one's own IDHP and IDHP-O. These variables may be generated through correlational procedures or as difference scores (by adding the absolute value of point differences across

the 27 items). Because these variables are exploratory, the following sections pertain only to the IDHP scale scores.

Reliability

Listed in Table 1 are alpha coefficients, test-retest reliability correlations, means, and standard deviations across the six IDHP scales, based on data from Sample 2. The scales are internally consistent (M alpha coefficient = .72) and stable over time (M test-retest r = .84). Item analysis

Table 1 Psychometric Properties of the Inventory of Dyadic Heterosexual Preferences Scale

Scale	Alpha coefficients	Test-retest correlations[a]	Means (SD) Male	Female
1. Erotophilia	.73	.84	4.77 (0.56)	4.27 (0.73)
2. Use of Contraception	.65	.80	4.36 (0.93)	4.59 (0.84)
3. Conventionality	.59	.83	2.89 (0.83)	3.20 (0.91)
4. Use of Erotica	.83	.92	4.04 (0.97)	3.22 (1.12)
5. Use of Drugs/ Alcohol	.87	.91	3.15 (1.34)	2.43 (1.18)
6. Romantic Foreplay	.62	.73	4.43 (0.71)	4.91 (0.71)

a. Test-retest interval was 2 weeks, including 45 women and 20 men (N = 65).

from Sample 1 required a test-retest reliability of .70 for each item.

Validity

In a subgroup of 45 women and 20 men from Sample 2, seven additional scales were administered for purposes of establishing concurrent and discriminant validity with the six IDHP scales. Of 42 predictions in this 6 × 7 matrix of correlations, 36 were supported. Absence of any relationship between each IDHP scale and the Crowne and Marlowe (1960) Social Desirability Scale provides discriminant evidence that the IDHP is not confounded by a bias toward presenting oneself in a socially desirable light. The Sexual Opinion Survey (SOS; Fisher, White, Byrne, & Kelley, 1988), a 21-item measure of erotophilia, correlated with the IDHP scale, Erotophilia (r = .54). However, discriminant validity for this scale is currently lacking, because the SOS also was related to Use of Erotica, Use of Drugs/ Alcohol, and Conventionality. It should be noted, however, that similar relationships exist among the IDHP factors themselves. This is an allowance of oblique factor rotation. In fact, it would be surprising if erotophilia were *not* related to other, possibly more specific, domains of preference.

Both concurrent and discriminant validity were evidenced for the following IDHP scales: Use of Contraception, Conventionality, and Use of Drugs/Alcohol. The Use of Contraception scale positively correlated only with the measure Affective Response Toward Contraceptive Topics and Behavior (Kelley, 1979). Conventionality was related to the Sexual Irrationality Questionnaire (Jordan & McCormick, 1988), a measure with factors such as "conformity" and "cautious control." Both the global and sexual subscales of the Alcohol Expectancy Questionnaire (Brown, Christiansen, & Goldman, 1987) were positively related to the IDHP Use of Drugs/Alcohol only. Validity of Romantic Foreplay and Use of Erotica remain without support, as the former was uncorrelated with its criterion measure and no relevant measure was available to test the latter.

Other Information

Further research regarding reliability, validity, and factor structure across diverse populations is encouraged for clinicians and researchers using the IDHP and IDHP-O.

References

Brown, S. A., Christiansen, B. A., & Goldman, M. S. (1987). The Alcohol Expectancy Questionnaire: An instrument for the assessment of adolescent and adult alcohol expectancies. *Journal of Studies on Alcohol, 48*, 483-491.

Crowne, D. P., & Marlowe, D. (1960). A new scale of social desirability independent of psychopathology. *Journal of Consulting Psychology, 24*, 349-354.

Fisher, W. A., White, L. A., Byrne, D., & Kelley, K. (1988). Erotophilia-erotophobia as a dimension of personality. *The Journal of Sex Research, 25*, 123-151.

Jordan, T. J., & McCormick, N. B. (1988). Sexual Irrationality Questionnaire. In C. M. Davis, W. L. Yarber, & S. L. Davis (Eds.), *Sexually-related measures: A compendium* (pp. 46-49). Lake Mills, IA: Davis, Yarber, & Davis.

Kelley, K. (1979). Socialization factors in contraceptive attitudes: Roles of affective responses, parental attitudes, and sexual experience. *The Journal of Sex Research, 15*, 6-20.

Purnine, D. M., Carey, M. P., & Jorgensen, R. S. (1996). The Inventory of Dyadic Heterosexual Preferences: Development and psychometric evaluation. *Behaviour Research and Therapy, 34*, 375-387.

Exhibit

Inventory of Dyadic Heterosexual Preferences

Instructions:[a] Please read the following statements carefully and indicate how much you agree or disagree that the statement is true for you. Respond to each item as you would actually like things to be in relations with your partner. Feel free to ask the investigator about any statement that is not clear to you. Please respond to all items.

There are no right or wrong answers; respond as truthfully as possible.

1. I would like to initiate sex.

Strongly agree	Agree	Somewhat agree	Somewhat disagree	Disagree	Strongly[b] disagree
6	5	4	3	2	1

2. An intimate, romantic dinner together would be a real turn on to me.
3. Using spermicide would spoil sex for me.
4. I would like to use a vibrator or other sexual toy (or aid) during sex.
5. I would prefer to have sex under the bedcovers and with the lights off.
6. Having myself or my partner use a condom would not spoil sex for me.
7. Having sex in rooms other than the bedroom would turn me on.
8. I would prefer to have sex everyday.
9. Looking at sexually explicit books and movies would turn me on.
10. I would not enjoy looking at my partner's genitals.
11. I would like to have sex after a day at the beach.
12. I would like to mix alcohol and sex.
13. Using a contraceptive would not affect my sexual satisfaction or pleasure.
14. I would enjoy having sex after smoking marijuana.
15. I would prefer to have sex while using drugs that make me feel aroused.
16. I would enjoy having sex outdoors.
17. My preferred time for having sex is in the morning.
18. Swimming in the nude with my partner would be a turn-on.
19. I would enjoy dressing in sexy/revealing clothes to arouse my partner.
20. I would like to mix drugs and sex.
21. I would get turned on if my partner touched my chest and nipples.
22. I would prefer to avoid having sex during my (partner's) period.
23. I would not enjoy having my partner look at my genitals.
24. Sexually explicit books and movies are disgusting to me.

25. I would find deep kissing with the tongue quite arousing to me.
26. Using a vaginal lubricant (KY jelly) would spoil sex for me.
27. Watching erotic movies with my partner would turn me on.

Source. This inventory is reprinted with permission of the author.

a. Instructions for the IDHP-O: Please read the following statements carefully and indicate how much you believe that *your partner* would agree or disagree that the statement is true for him/her. That is, respond to each item *as you think your partner would respond*—how he or she would actually like things to be in relations with you.

b. This scale is repeated after each item.

Assessing AIDS-Related Concern, Beliefs, and Communication Behavior

William J. Brown[1] and Mihai C. Bocarnea, *Regent University*

The AIDS-Related Concern, Beliefs, and Communication Behavior Inventory (AIDS CBCI) was developed in 1991 to assess audience responses to an AIDS prevention campaign designed to increase concern about AIDS, knowledge of the disease, and communication behavior regarding AIDS and HIV transmission. The AIDS prevention campaign used the entertainment-education communication strategy in which entertainment media are used to promote educational messages (Brown & Singhal, in press). In this case an entertainment video hosted by Ronald Reagan, Jr. was distributed to educators to promote AIDS education among young adults with a high risk for HIV infection (Brown, 1991). The AIDS CBCI is designed to be especially useful to researchers studying the effects of AIDS educational programs on target audiences' concern about AIDS, beliefs about the disease, and interpersonal communication with others about the disease.

Description

The AIDS CBCI consists of three scales: 5 items measure concern about AIDS, 14 items measure beliefs about AIDS, and 4 items measure AIDS-related communication behavior. The concern scale and communication behavior scale are both interval scales that use a 7-point Likert-type format

[1]Address correspondence to William J. Brown, Dean, College of Communication and the Arts, Regent University, 1000 Regent University Drive, Virginia Beach, VA 23464-5041; email: willbro@beacon.regent.edu.

(response options ranging from *none at all* or *not at all* (1) to *a lot* (7). The AIDS belief scale is a nominal scale that provides three options to respondents: *true, false,* and *don't know.* Multivariate and correlation analyses were conducted with data from 257 completed questionnaires to develop the inventory (Brown, 1992). Each scale is designed to measure a distinct dependent variable often targeted by AIDS prevention messages.

Response Mode and Timing

Two methods of scoring responses can be used for completing the AIDS CBCI. Respondents can either record their responses on the inventory questionnaire to the left of each question, or they can record their responses on a separate scantron form. Scantron forms allow for electronic input of respondents' answers and thus reduce the error of transferring data from questionnaires to computer files. The 23-item AIDS CBCI takes about 5-7 minutes to complete.

Scoring

The 11 Likert-type items in the inventory are keyed in the same direction, with 1 indicating the lowest level of concern and communication behavior and 7 indicating the highest levels of each variable. The concern scale ranges from a low score of 5 to a high score of 35, and the communication behavior scale ranges from 4 to 28. The 14-item nominal scale is coded on a range of 0 to 14, indicating the total number of correct answers (Items 7, 9,

10, 11, 16, 19, and 20 are coded true; Items 8, 12, 13, 14, 15, 17, and 18 are coded false).

Reliability

Separate reliability analyses were conducted for each scale. Based on a data set of 257 completed inventories, the two interval scales were assessed using Cronbach's coefficient alpha. The concern scale yielded a reliability coefficient of .65, and the communication behavior scale yielded a reliability coefficient of .84 (Brown, 1992). The reliability of the 14-item nominal belief scale was assessed by using the Spearman-Brown formula and computing the split-half correlation of the first seven scale items with the second seven scale items (see Pedhazur & Schmelkin, 1991, p. 90). Results yielded a reliability coefficient of .98 for the belief scale.

Validity

Attention was given to the content validity of the three scales by using previously published research designed to measure concern about AIDS and AIDS-related knowledge and communication behavior. The questionnaire items assessing AIDS-related concern and communication behavior were based on the work of Bowen and Michal-Johnson (1989); Cline, Freeman, and Johnson (1990); Cline, Johnson, and Freeman (1992); Goodwin and Roscoe (1988); and Probart (1989). The belief scale was first developed as an instrument to assess the effects of Britain's national AIDS prevention television campaign, reported by Wober (1987) and Worchester (1988). Many of the belief items are also contained in scales developed by DiClemente, Boyer, and Morales (1988); DiClemente, Zorn, and Temoshok (1986); and Goodwin and Roscoe (1988).

Construct validity of the AIDS CBCI was also evaluated by testing hypothesized relationships between the measured variables and several related variables and by examining correlations among related variables. Regression analyses indicate concern about AIDS is a significant predictor of discussing AIDS with others, including open discussions with sexual partners or potential sexual partners ($\beta = .22$, $p < .05$). Accurate beliefs about AIDS is also a significant predictor of interpersonal communication about the disease ($\beta = .67$, $p < .01$). Concern about AIDS is highly correlated with having an accurate knowledge of the disease ($r = .67$, $p < .001$) and with taking precautions to protect oneself against the disease ($r = .63$, $p < .001$). Openly talking with actual or potential sexual partners about AIDS is also highly correlated with taking precautions to protect oneself against the disease ($r = .48$, $p < .001$). Accurate knowledge of AIDS is correlated highly with taking precautions to prevent exposure to HIV infection ($r = .48$, $p < .001$). These regression and correlation analyses all support the predictive validity of the AIDS CBCI.

References

Bowen, S. P., & Michal-Johnson, P. (1989). The crisis of communication relationships: Confronting the threat of AIDS. *AIDS and Public Policy, 4,* 10-19.

Brown, W. J. (1991). An AIDS prevention campaign: Effects on attitudes, beliefs, and communication behavior. *American Behavioral Scientist, 34,* 666-678.

Brown, W. J. (1992). Culture and AIDS education: Reaching high-risk heterosexuals in Asian-American communities. *Journal of Applied Communication Research, 20,* 275-291.

Brown, W. J., & Singhal, A. (in press). Entertainment-education strategies for social change. In D. P. Demers & K. Viswanath (Eds.), *Mass media, social control and social change.*

Cline, R. J. W., Freeman, K. E., & Johnson, S. J. (1990). Talk among sexual partners about AIDS: Factors differentiating those who talk from those who do not. *Communication Research, 17,* 792-808.

Cline, R. J. W., Johnson, S. J., & Freeman, K. E. (1992). Talk among sexual partners about AIDS: Interpersonal communication for risk reduction or risk enhancement? *Health Communication, 4,* 39-56.

DiClemente, R. J., Boyer, C. B., & Morales, E. S. (1988). Minorities and AIDS: Knowledge, attitudes, and misconceptions among Black and Latino adolescents. *American Journal of Public Health, 78,* 55-57.

DiClemente, R. J., Zorn, J., & Temoshok, L. (1986). Adolescents and AIDS: A survey of knowledge, beliefs, and attitudes about AIDS in San Francisco. *American Journal of Public Health, 76,* 1443-1445.

Goodwin, M. P., & Roscoe, B. (1988). AIDS: Students' knowledge and attitudes at a midwestern university. *Journal of American College Health, 36,* 214-222.

Pedhazur, E. J., & Schmelkin, L. P. (1991). *Measurement, design, and analysis: An integrated approach.* Hillsdale, NJ: Lawrence Erlbaum.

Probart, C. K. (1989). A preliminary investigation using drama in community AIDS education. *AIDS Education and Prevention, 1,* 268-276.

Wober, J. M. (1987). *Informing the public about AIDS: Measurement of knowledge, attitudes, and behaviour.* London: Independent Broadcasting Authority.

Worchester, R. M. (1988, August/September). *British attitudes to AIDS and the effect of the government's TV advertising campaign.* Paper presented at the 14th World Congress of the International Political Science Association, Washington, DC.

Exhibit

AIDS Concern, Beliefs, and Communication Behavior Inventory

Instructions: The following questions are intended to gain an understanding of (1) the degree to which you are concerned about AIDS, (2) what you believe about AIDS, and (3) how much you discuss AIDS with others. Several questions use a 1 to 7 scale, with 1 indicating the lowest level of concern and communication about AIDS and 7 indicating the highest level of concern and communication about AIDS. Record your answers either on the blank line to the left of each question or on the scantron form if provided. Your answers are anonymous; therefore please answer each question as honestly as you can.

_____ 1. How important is the AIDS issue to you?[a]
_____ 2. How much do you feel you know about AIDS?
_____ 3. How much do you know about those who have suffered from AIDS?
_____ 4. If you are sexually active, what precautions do you take to protect yourself from AIDS? or If you are not sexually active, what precautions will you take in the future to protect yourself from AIDS?
_____ 5. How much do you seek out more information about AIDS?
_____ 6. If you are sexually active, how much do you openly talk to your sexual partner(s) about AIDS? or If you are not sexually active, how much would you openly talk to a future sexual partner about AIDS?
_____ 7. How much have you discussed the AIDS issue with others during the last month?
_____ 8. How much do you talk to those of the opposite sex about AIDS?
_____ 9. How much do you talk to those of the same sex about AIDS?

For the next set of questions, please indicate whether you think the statement is true or false. Mark "don't know" if you are not able to judge whether the statement is true or false.

                    1. True   2. False   3. Don't Know

_____ 10. You can get AIDS if you are infected with a needle which has been used by someone who has the AIDS virus.
_____ 11. You can get AIDS by breathing air infected by the coughs and sneezes of someone who has the AIDS virus.
_____ 12. A person who has the AIDS virus may appear healthy.
_____ 13. Everyone who develops AIDS will eventually die as a result of it (if no other tragedy takes that person's life).
_____ 14. Everyone who has the AIDS virus will develop AIDS.
_____ 15. The symptoms of people dying from AIDS are always the same.
_____ 16. You can get AIDS if you swallow the saliva of someone who has the AIDS virus.
_____ 17. You can get AIDS if you are bitten by an insect which has drawn blood from someone who has the AIDS virus.
_____ 18. Just as there is a test which shows that a woman is *not* pregnant, there is also a test that shows a person definitely does *not* have the AIDS virus.
_____ 19. The AIDS virus can enter the body through any open cut or graze from contact with the body fluids of an infected person.
_____ 20. A woman who has the AIDS virus can *not* pass it on to a man with whom she has had sexual intercourse.
_____ 21. You can *not* get the AIDS virus through oral sex.
_____ 22. A spermicidal gel or product is effective in killing any AIDS virus that may be present from either partner during sexual intercourse.
_____ 23. You can *not* get AIDS by using a toilet seat that has recently been used by someone who has the AIDS virus.

a. A 7-point scale anchored by *not very important* to *very important, not very much* to *a lot,* or *none* to *a lot,* as appropriate to the item, follows each item.

The HIV-Knowledge Questionnaire

Michael P. Carey,[1] *Syracuse University*
Dianne Morrison-Beedy, *Niagara University*
Blair T. Johnson, *Syracuse University*

The HIV-Knowledge Questionnaire (HIV-K-Q) was developed to measure knowledge about the transmission, prevention, and consequences of HIV infection. We sought to develop a measure that was reliable and valid; understandable to those with an eighth-grade education or less; and appropriate for use regardless of respondent age, gender, race/ethnicity, and sexual orientation. Our aim was to develop a measure that was brief but sensitive because we needed a measure to use in community-based studies of risk reduction interventions. We also believe that this measure will be helpful in theoretical model building and testing; assessment and evaluation of focused HIV education, prevention, testing, and counseling programs; and in more general educational and primary care settings.

Description

A complete description of the HIV-K-Q, its development and psychometric evaluation, may be found elsewhere (Carey, Morrison-Beedy, & Johnson, 1997). The HIV-K-Q is a 45-item self-administered questionnaire designed to measure knowledge about the following HIV-related domains: *transmission* (e.g., vaginal, anal, and oral sexual intercourse; blood products; needle sharing; and perinatal) and *nontransmission* (e.g., saliva, insect bites, touching, sharing food); effective (male and female condom, abstinence, monogamy following antibody testing) and ineffective (e.g., douching, birth control pills, vaccine) *prevention methods* (e.g., condom use, needle sterilization); and *consequences of infection* (e.g., treatment, disease course). The HIV-K-Q emphasizes sexual transmission over needle sharing and other modes of transmission.

Development of the HIV-K-Q began with a formative research phase in which we held eight focus groups with 45 economically disadvantaged urban women to learn what information and myths were widely held in the community. Based on this formative work, as well as consultation with leading researchers and other HIV experts, we developed a 62-item version of the HIV-K-Q. This version was administered to 669 adults, including economically disadvantaged men and women ($n = 350$), university students ($n = 279$), and HIV experts ($n = 40$). We employed item analyses to eliminate 17 items that were too easy or not associated with the total score. Principal factor analysis on the remaining 45 items resulted in a single factor labeled *HIV Knowledge*. This one-factor solution was cross-validated with data

from two community-based samples that included 285 women and 76 men.

Response Mode and Timing

Using a paper-and-pencil format, respondents circle *True, False,* or *I Don't Know* for each of the 45 items. Using a computer-administered form of the HIV-K-Q, and an undergraduate sample, we learned that completing the HIV-K-Q takes an average of 4.12 minutes ($SD = 0.77$; range = 1.37 to 5.85 min). The time to complete the HIV-K-Q was unrelated to the score attained on it, $r(48) = .02$. The mean time to respond to any given item ranged from a low of 2.73 s (for Item 2) to a high of 10.28 s (for Item 41). Our experience with community-based samples suggests that the paper-and-pencil format takes low-literacy adults longer to complete, but nearly everyone has completed the measure within 10 minutes.

We have also completed reading-level analyses on the HIV-K-Q. Analysis with the Flesch formula indicated that the material was at the primary-grade level, with most passages in the "fairly easy" to "very easy" range. Analysis using the Spache formula revealed that most of the material was below fourth-grade level. However, several words increased the level to approximately the seventh-grade level; these "foreign" words include vaccine, antibiotics, genitals, Pap smears, that is, words that are either medical or sexual in nature. Although these words increase the reading level, they are likely to be understood by low-literacy readers due to their common use in the popular culture.

Scoring

Based on the results of the principal factor analysis, we advise the use of a single summary score, which is obtained by summing the number of items correctly answered. Items scored *I Don't Know* are scored incorrect. The range of possible scores is 0–45; transformation of the raw score into a percentage correct score (i.e., number correct/45) facilitates interpretation. Higher scores on the HIV-K-Q indicate greater knowledge.

Reliability

Internal consistency was determined with Cronbach's alpha. Using data obtained from five separate samples—urban primary care patients ($n = 350$), university students ($n = 279$), community-based couples ($n = 152$), community-based urban women ($n = 212$), and HIV experts ($n = 40$)—alpha for the total sample ($N = 1,033$) was .91. Alpha

[1]Address correspondence to Michael P. Carey, Department of Psychology, 430 Huntington Hall, Syracuse University, Syracuse, NY 13244-2340; email: mpcarey@psych.syr.edu.

was also calculated separately for each subsample and ranged from .83 to .93 across the subsamples.

To determine the test-retest stability of the HIV-K-Q, a Pearson product-moment correlation coefficient was calculated for the urban women who took the HIV-K-Q on three occasions, with 2-week and 3-month retest intervals ($ns =$ 33 and 25, respectively). These calculations indicated high test-retest reliability ($rs = .91$ and $.90$ at 2 and 12 weeks, respectively; both $ps < .0001$). The test-retest correlations for the university students who retook the HIV-K-Q was $r(130) = .83$, $p < .0001$.

Validity

To provide known-groups evidence for the validity of the HIV-K-Q, we compared HIV-K-Q scores among groups expected to differ in their knowledge as a function of prior training or experience related to HIV and AIDS. Pairwise comparisons revealed that the experts (91%) were significantly better informed than the other four groups; the university students (82%) were more knowledgeable than were the primary care patients (69%), urban women (72%), and community couples (52%); and the primary care and urban women, who did not differ from each other, were more knowledgeable than the community couples. All groups exceeded the score that would be achieved by chance (i.e., 33%).

Additional evidence of the validity of the HIV-K-Q came from a subsample of the urban women who participated in an HIV risk reduction program (Carey et al., 1995). This intervention program was designed to enhance HIV-related knowledge as well as motivation and skills needed to reduce risk. Scores on the HIV-K-Q indicated that women assigned to the intervention condition significantly improved their scores from pre- ($M = 75\%$) to postintervention ($M = 87\%$) assessments, $t(42) = 6.08$, $p = .0001$. In contrast, women in the control condition of this study did not improve their scores, $Ms = 71\%$ and 72%, respectively, $t(31) = 0.79$, $p > .10$.

Discriminant evidence was provided by the absence of significant correlations between the HIV-K-Q and (a) the Social Desirability Scale (Crowne & Marlowe, 1960), $r(271) = -0.09$; (b) positive or negative mood subscales from the Positive and Negative Affect Scale (Watson, Clark, & Tellegen, 1988), $rs(277) = .00$ and -0.05, respectively; (c) the Rosenberg Self-Esteem Scale (Wylie, 1977), $r(268)$

$= -0.05$; (d) any of the five subscales from the Multidimensional Condom Attitudes Scale (Helweg-Larson & Collins, 1994), rs ranging from -0.05 to $.11$; (e) the Center for Epidemiological Studies Depressed Mood scale (Radloff, 1977), $r(148) = -0.11$; (f) the Dyadic Adjustment Scale (Spanier, 1976), $r(148) = .16$; or (g) the Index of Sexual Satisfaction (Hudson, Harrison, & Crosscup, 1981), $r(148) = -0.05$.

Other Information

Further research regarding reliability, validity, and factor structure across diverse populations is encouraged. This research was supported by grants from the National Institute of Mental Health to Michael P. Carey and Blair T. Johnson, and a grant from the National Institute of Nursing Research to Dianne Morrison-Beedy.

References

Carey, M. P., Maisto, S. A., Kalichman, S. C., Forsyth, A. D., Wright, E., & Johnson, B. T. (1995). *Enhancement, behavioral skills training, and education reduces the risk of HIV infection for ethnically diverse urban women.* Manuscript submitted for publication.

Carey, M. P., Morrison-Beedy, D., & Johnson, B. T. (1997). The HIV-Knowledge Questionnaire. *AIDS & Behavior, 1*(1), 61-74.

Crowne, D. P., & Marlowe, D. (1960). A new scale of social desirability independent of psychopathology. *Journal of Consulting Psychology, 24,* 349-354.

Helweg-Larson, M., & Collins, B. E. (1994). The UCLA Multidimensional Condom Attitudes Scale: Documenting the complex determinants of condom use in college students. *Health Psychology, 13,* 224-237.

Hudson, W. W., Harrison, D. F., & Crosscup, P. C. (1981). A short-form scale to measure sexual discord in dyadic relationships. *The Journal of Sex Research, 17,* 157-174.

Radloff, L. S. (1977). The CES-D scale: A self-report depression scale for research in the general population. *Applied Psychological Measurement, 1,* 385-401.

Spanier, G. B. (1976). Measuring dyadic adjustment: New scales for assessing the quality of marriage and similar dyads. *Journal of Marriage and the Family, 38,* 15-28.

Watson, D., Clark, L. A., & Tellegen, A. (1988). Development and validation of brief measures of positive and negative affect: The PANAS scales. *Journal of Personality and Social Psychology, 54,* 1063-1070.

Wylie, R. C. (1977). *The self-concept: A review of methodological considerations and measuring instruments.* Lincoln: University of Nebraska Press.

Exhibit

HIV-Knowledge Questionnaire

For each statement, please circle true (T), *false* (F), *or I don't know* (DK). If you do not know, please do not guess; instead, please circle *DK*.

	True	False	I don't know
1. HIV and AIDS are the same thing.	T	F	DK
2. There is a cure for AIDS.	T	F	DK

		True	False	I don't know
3.	A person can get HIV from a toilet seat.	T	F	DK
4.	Coughing and sneezing DO NOT spread HIV.	T	F	DK
5.	HIV can be spread by mosquitoes.	T	F	DK
6.	AIDS is the cause of HIV.	T	F	DK
7.	A person can get HIV by sharing a glass of water with someone who has HIV.	T	F	DK
8.	HIV is killed by bleach.	T	F	DK
9.	It is possible to get HIV when a person gets a tattoo.	T	F	DK
10.	A pregnant woman with HIV can give the virus to her unborn baby.	T	F	DK
11.	Pulling out the penis before a man climaxes or cums keeps a woman from getting HIV during sex.	T	F	DK
12.	A woman can get HIV if she has anal sex with a man.	T	F	DK
13.	Showering, or washing one's genitals or private parts, after sex keeps a person from getting HIV.	T	F	DK
14.	Eating healthy foods can keep a person from getting HIV.	T	F	DK
15.	All pregnant women infected with HIV will have babies born with AIDS.	T	F	DK
16.	Using a latex condom or rubber can lower a person's chance of getting HIV.	T	F	DK
17.	A person with HIV can look and feel healthy.	T	F	DK
18.	People who have been infected with HIV quickly show serious signs of being infected.	T	F	DK
19.	A person can be infected with HIV for 5 years or more without getting AIDS.	T	F	DK
20.	There is a vaccine that can stop adults from getting HIV.	T	F	DK
21.	Some drugs have been made for the treatment of AIDS.	T	F	DK
22.	Women are always tested for HIV during their Pap smears.	T	F	DK
23.	A person *cannot* get HIV by having oral sex, mouth-to-penis, with a man who has HIV.	T	F	DK
24.	A person can get HIV even if she or he has sex with another person only one time.	T	F	DK
25.	Using a lambskin condom or rubber is the best protection against HIV.	T	F	DK
26.	People are likely to get HIV by deep kissing, putting their tongue in their partner's mouth, if their partner has HIV.	T	F	DK
27.	A person can get HIV by giving blood.	T	F	DK
28.	A woman cannot get HIV if she has sex during her period.	T	F	DK
29.	You can usually tell if someone has HIV by looking at them.	T	F	DK
30.	There is a female condom that can help decrease a woman's chance of getting HIV.	T	F	DK
31.	A natural skin condom works better against HIV than does a latex condom.	T	F	DK
32.	A person will NOT get HIV if she or he is taking antibiotics.	T	F	DK
33.	Having sex with more than one partner can increase a person's chance of being infected with HIV.	T	F	DK
34.	Taking a test for HIV one week after having sex will tell a person if she or he has HIV.	T	F	DK
35.	A person can get HIV by sitting in a hot tub or a swimming pool with a person who has HIV.	T	F	DK
36.	A person can get HIV through contact with saliva, tears, sweat, or urine.	T	F	DK
37.	A person can get HIV from the wetness from a woman's vagina.	T	F	DK
38.	A person can get HIV if having oral sex, mouth on vagina, with a woman.	T	F	DK
39.	If a person tests positive for HIV, then the test site will have to tell all of his or her partners.	T	F	DK
40.	Using Vaseline or baby oil with condoms lowers the chance of getting HIV.	T	F	DK
41.	Washing drug use equipment with cold water kills HIV.	T	F	DK
42.	A woman can get HIV if she has vaginal sex with a man who has HIV.	T	F	DK
43.	Athletes who share needles when using steroids can get HIV from the needles.	T	F	DK
44.	Douching after sex will keep a woman from getting HIV.	T	F	DK
45.	Taking vitamins keeps a person from getting HIV.	T	F	DK

Source. This questionnaire was originally published in "The HIV-Knowledge Questionnaire," by M. P. Carey, D. Morrison-Beedy, and B. T. Johnson, 1997, *AIDS & Behavior, 1*(1), 61-74. Reprinted with permission.

The Meharry Questionnaire: The Measurement of Attitudes Toward AIDS-Related Issues

Frederick A. Ernst,[1] Rupert A. Francis, Joyce Perkins, Quintessa Britton-Williams, and Ajaipal S. Kang, *Meharry Medical College*

The Meharry Questionnaire was developed to measure the attitudes and behaviors of workers in health care facilities concerning AIDS-related issues. We were particularly concerned about attitudes that would be expected to compromise quality of care. Furthermore, we wished to identify differences in attitudes related to specific differences in demographics, specifically race, gender, education, and religious preference. In 1989, we used a convenience sample of 2,006 employees in the mental health and retardation residential facilities throughout the state of Tennessee. A follow-up questionnaire was administered in 1994 for the same population, using Items 4, 5, 6, and 8 from the original survey. The 1994 sample consisted of 857 respondents. Each administration of the survey achieved a fairly representative cross-section of socioeconomic strata by including respondents from all occupational categories at each of the facilities.

The combined 1989 and 1994 populations had a racial composition of 38% Blacks and 55% Whites; 68% of the sample were females. The highest levels of education completed by the respondents were as follows: 45% with high school or less, 33% with bachelor's degree or some college, and 8% with master's or doctorate degrees. The respondents who chose not to answer any of the demographics were not included in the statistics above.

Previous analyses from this data set revealed that Blacks were significantly more likely than Whites to affirm personal habit changes to prevent HIV infection and significantly more likely to reject the notion that AIDS is not a threat to rural areas of the United States (Ernst, Francis, Nevels, Collipp, & Lewis, 1991). Findings from the same questionnaire demonstrated that condemnation of homosexuality is stronger in the Black community deriving primarily from relatively less tolerant attitudes of Black females (Ernst, Francis, Nevels, & Lemeh, 1991).

Description

The Meharry Questionnaire consists of 13 statements to which respondents answer on a 6-point Likert-type scale of 0 (*strongly disagree*) to 5 (*strongly agree*). It was originally designed to assess attitudes of physicians and was later modified for general public comprehension.

Response Mode and Timing

The questionnaire requires approximately 5 to 10 minutes to complete, including the time in which respondents are providing cursory demographic information.

Scoring

Each of the 13 items was analyzed independently to compare differences in responses that might have been related to specific demographic characteristics. In unpublished work, a moral conservatism score was derived from responses to Items 2, 4, 6 (scored in reverse), 9, 10, 11, and 13. The mean score on this measure of moral conservatism was 6.11, $SD = .18$ (range: -5 to 30).

Reliability

Reliability analyses yielded a Cronbach alpha of 0.696 with an average interitem correlation of 0.16. Split-half reliability was 0.74. Test-retest correlation coefficients ranged from 0.24·to 0.72 for the 13 items.

Validity

Although no validity studies have been published to date, we have data supporting the validity of the questionnaire. For example, we have found that moral conservatism is strongly and inversely related to educational level ($p < .000001$). Religious preference is also predictable from scores on moral conservatism but this relationship is more complex because the more conservative religions (e.g., Church of God) tend to be overrepresented by respondents with less formal education.

References

Ernst, F. A., Francis, R. A., Nevels, H., Collipp, D., & Lewis, A. (1991). Racial differences in affirmation of personal habit change to prevent HIV infection. *Preventive Medicine, 20*, 529-533.

Ernst, F. A., Francis, R. A., Nevels, H., & Lemeh, C. A. (1991). Condemnation of homosexuality in the Black community: A gender-specific phenomenon? *Archives of Sexual Behavior, 20*, 579-585.

---

[1]Address correspondence to Frederick A. Ernst, Department of Family and Preventive Medicine, Meharry Medical College, 1005 D. B. Todd Jr. Boulevard, Nashville, TN 37208.

Exhibit

The Meharry Questionnaire: The Measurement of Attitudes Toward AIDS-Related Issues

Age _____ Sex _____ Race _____ Occupation _____

Education _____ Religious preference _____

Marital status _____

Please *circle the number* which reflects the amount of your agreement or disagreement with each statement.

1. AIDS will never be a threat to the rural areas of the U.S.A.

0	1	2	3	4	5[a]
Strongly disagree				Strongly agree	

2. AIDS is the result of God's punishment ("Divine Retribution").
3. Most of the AIDS patients in the 1990s will have to be treated by family doctors.
4. AIDS will help the society by decreasing the number of homosexuals (gay people).
5. I have made changes in my personal habits to prevent being infected by the AIDS virus.
6. Sterilized needles should be made available to needle-using drug abusers to prevent the spread of AIDS.
7. All pregnant women should be required to have their blood tested for the AIDS virus.
8. It is easier to catch the AIDS virus than the experts are leading us to believe.
9. The AIDS epidemic is a fulfillment of biblical prophecy.
10. AIDS will help the society by decreasing the number of drug abusers.
11. People with AIDS have gotten what they deserve.
12. In the 1990s, a large increase in health care manpower will be required because of AIDS.
13. Needle-using drug abusers who get AIDS are not worthy of extensive medical attention.

Source. This questionnaire is reprinted with permission of the authors.
a. This scale follows each of the statements.

HIV/AIDS Knowledge and Attitudes Scales for Teachers

Patricia Barthalow Koch[1] and Maureen D. Singer,
Pennsylvania State University

HIV is rapidly increasing among children and adolescents in the United States (Centers for Disease Control, 1992,

[1]Address all correspondence to Patricia Barthalow Koch, Department of Biobehavioral Health, Pennsylvania State University, University Park, PA 16802; email: p3k@psu.edu.

1993). Education about prevention and how best to live with HIV-infected family members, friends, and co-workers, as well as how to deal with the disease if one is personally infected, is the key to disarming the horrible effects of this disease. Education at each school level (elementary, intermediate, and high school) has been recommended so that children can grow up knowing how to protect themselves. Yet researchers have indicated that children and adolescents continue to have many fears and questions about HIV/AIDS arising from a lack of education and from misunderstanding (Anderson & Christenson, 1991; Brown & Fritz, 1988). Although the majority of states have kindergarten through 12th grade HIV/AIDS education mandates, the implementation of these is questionable (di Mauro, 1989-1990). Researchers have shown that teachers at various levels lack basic factual knowledge of the cause, transmission, and prevalence of HIV/AIDS (Ballard, White, & Glascoff, 1990; Bowd, 1987; Price, Desmond, & Kukulka, 1985).

Thus, the HIV/AIDS Knowledge and Attitudes Scales for Teachers were developed to serve as measurement instruments in determining teachers' level of knowledge and attitudes toward HIV disease, in general, and specific educational issues. These scales can be used with preservice education students; the data can be useful in designing college programs to better prepare our future teachers. The scales can also be used with practicing educators with the data guiding the design of in-service workshops to prepare more effective AIDS educators.

Description

The HIV/AIDS Knowledge Scale for Teachers consists of two parts. The first part, General Knowledge, includes 14 true-false items regarding the HIV-disease process (e.g., cause, symptoms, diagnosis, effects, treatment) and 4 true-false items specific to classroom issues. The second part, Likelihood of Transmission, contains 17 possible modes of HIV transmission. Thus, the entire knowledge scale contains 35 items.

The HIV/AIDS Attitudes Scale for Teachers contains 25 items regarding HIV/AIDS, persons with HIV/AIDS, and educational issues. The respondent indicates her or his attitudes using a 5-point Likert-type scale.

Response Mode and Timing

For the General Knowledge part of the HIV/AIDS Knowledge Scale for Teachers, respondents identify the statements as either (1) true, (2) false, or (3) not sure. For the Likelihood of Transmission part of the knowledge scale, respondents are given 17 possible modes of HIV transmission and asked if transmission through each mode is (1) very likely, (2) somewhat likely, (3) somewhat unlikely, (4) very unlikely, (5) definitely not possible, or (6) don't know. The entire scale takes approximately 20 minutes to complete.

For the HIV/AIDS Attitudes Scale for Teachers, respondents indicate, using a Likert-type scale, if they (1) strongly agree, (2) agree, (3) are uncertain, (4) disagree, or (5) strongly disagree with each of the 25 statements. This scale takes approximately 10-15 minutes to complete.

Scoring

The highest possible score on the HIV/AIDS Knowledge Scale for Teachers is 35. One point is given for every correct

answer on the General Knowledge part of the knowledge scale, with the highest possible score being 18. Correct answers are as follows: definitely true (1) for Items 3, 4, 6, 7, 9, 11, 14, 15, 17, 18; definitely false (2) for Items 1, 2, 5, 8, 10, 12, 13, 16. All unsure responses are considered incorrect.

The highest possible score for the Likelihood of Transmission part of the knowledge scale is 17 with one point given for each correct answer. The correct answers are as follows: very likely (1) for Items 27, 30, 32; very likely or somewhat likely (1 or 2) for Items 20, 29, 34; very unlikely for Items 21, 23, 31, 33, 35; definitely not possible for Items 19, 22, 24, 25, 26, 28.

Scores on the HIV/AIDS Attitudes Scale for Teachers can range from 25 (most unsupportive attitudes) to 125 (most supportive attitudes). A mean score can be calculated, with a mean of 1.00 representing the most unsupportive attitudes and 5.00 indicating the most supportive attitudes toward dealing with HIV disease inside and outside of the classroom. The following items on the scale are reverse scored: 1, 5, 7, 9, 10, 13, 15, 17, 20, 21, 22, 25.

Research using these instruments involving 128 elementary education students completing their student teaching experiences indicated that they had very poor knowledge about HIV disease, ($M = 18.9$) representing a 54% correct response level (Singer, 1991). These student teachers possessed uncertain to slightly positive attitudes toward dealing with HIV disease, with an average score of 87.6 ($M = 3.46$).

Reliability

Reliability for the knowledge and attitudes scales was established using two different methods (Singer, 1991). First, a test-retest of the instruments was conducted with 59 elementary education majors. Pearson product-moment correlations were established for the knowledge scale at .87 and for the attitudes scale at .89. Internal reliability for the knowledge scale, using Kuder-Richardson's statistic, was established using a sample of 128 elementary education student teachers. The reliability for the General Knowledge section was .78 and for the Likelihood of Transmission section was .88, yielding an overall reliability for the entire scale of .89. Cronbach's alpha coefficient was used to establish reliability for the attitude scale at .89. It is recommended that reliability be further tested with groups of education majors, student teachers, and teachers of differing content areas and levels of school (elementary, intermediate, and high school).

Validity

The HIV/AIDS Knowledge and Attitude Scales for Teachers were constructed adapting items and/or format from the National Health Interview Survey (Hardy, 1989), the Nurses' Attitudes About AIDS Scale (Preston, Young, Koch, & Forti, 1995), and an instrument previously used in a study of preservice elementary education teachers (Ballard et al., 1990). A panel of three experts in the area of HIV/AIDS disease and education reviewed the items and answers for relevancy and accuracy. A pilot test for content validity was then conducted with 10 elementary education majors. It is recommended that construct validity be further tested with groups of education majors, student teachers, and teachers of differing content areas and levels of school.

References

Anderson, D. & Christenson, G. (1991). Ethnic breakdown of AIDS related knowledge and attitudes from the National Adolescent Student Health Survey. *Health Education, 22*, 30-34.

Ballard, D., White, D., & Glascoff, M. (1990). HIV/AIDS education for preservice elementary teachers. *Journal of School Health, 60*, 262-269.

Bowd, A. (1987). Knowledge and opinions about AIDS and related educational issues among student teachers and experienced teachers. *Canadian Journal of Public Health, 78*, 84-87.

Brown, L., & Fritz, G. (1988). Children's knowledge and attitudes about AIDS. *Journal of the American Academy of Child and Adolescent Psychiatry, 27*, 504-508.

Centers for Disease Control. (1992). Sexual behaviors among high school students—United States 1990. *Morbidity and Mortality Weekly Report, 41*, 885-888.

Centers for Disease Control. (1993, December). *HIV/AIDS surveillance report*. Atlanta, GA: Author.

di Mauro, D. (1989-1990, December/January). Sexuality education 1990: A review of state sexuality and AIDS education curricula. *SIECUS Report, 18*(2), 1-9.

Hardy, A. M. (1989). *AIDS knowledge and attitudes for April-June 1989*. Provisional data from the National Health Interview Survey. (Advance Data from Vital and Health Statistics, No. 179) (DHHS Publication No. PHS 90-1250). Hyattsville, MD: National Center for Health Statistics.

Preston, D. B., Young, E. W., Koch, P. B., & Forti, E. M. (1995). The Nurses' Attitudes About AIDS Scale (NAAS): Development and psychometric analysis. *AIDS Education and Prevention, 7*, 443-454.

Price, J., Desmond, S., & Kukulka, G. (1985). High school students' perceptions and misperceptions of AIDS. *Journal of School Health, 55*, 107-109.

Singer, M. D. (1991). *Elementary student teachers' knowledge and attitudes of HIV/AIDS and HIV/AIDS education*. Unpublished thesis, Pennsylvania State University, University Park, PA.

Exhibit

HIV/AIDS Knowledge Scale for Teachers

Please indicate, to the best of your knowledge, if the following statements are true (1) or false (2) by circling a number from the scale for your answer. If you are not sure of the correct answer, circle 3.

1 = True   2 = False   3 = Not sure[a]

1. AIDS is an infectious disease caused by a bacteria.
2. AIDS breaks down the body's immunity by destroying the B cells in the endocrine system.
3. AIDS can damage the brain.
4. It may be more than 5 years before an HIV-infected person develops AIDS.
5. HIV lives and functions in warm, moist environments for days outside of the body.
6. Early symptoms of HIV infection include fatigue, fever, weight loss, and swelling of the lymph nodes.
7. A person who has tested negatively on one HIV antibody blood test could still transmit HIV to a sexual partner.
8. The number of HIV-infected persons will be decreasing during the next two years.
9. Two common disorders found in persons with AIDS are pneumocystis carinii pneumonia and Kaposi's sarcoma.
10. Latex condoms are not as effective as "lambskin" or natural membrane condoms in preventing the spread of HIV.
11. Drugs can be used to slow down the rate of reproduction of HIV and lengthen the life of an infected person.
12. It is possible to detect HIV antibodies in the bloodstream immediately after becoming infected.
13. There is a vaccine available in Europe that can protect a person from getting AIDS.
14. There have been no cases of AIDS spread by students to their teachers or classmates through usual daily contact.
15. In recent years, adolescents are among the groups with the largest increase of HIV infection.
16. Less than one-half of the states have mandated that AIDS education be included in their schools' curricula.
17. There is a federal law that protects children with HIV or AIDS from educational discrimination.
18. There is no cure for AIDS at the present time.

To what degree do you think the following are likely to transmit HIV. Please use the numbers from the scale for your answers.

1 = Very likely   2 = Somewhat likely   3 = Somewhat unlikely
4 = Very unlikely   5 = Definitely not possible   6 = Don't know

19. Working near someone with AIDS
20. HIV-infected mother to baby during pregnancy/birth
21. Kissing someone who has AIDS

22. Eating in a restaurant where the cook has AIDS
23. Receiving a blood transfusion
24. Sharing plates, forks, or glasses with someone who has AIDS
25. Living with a person who has AIDS (without sexual involvement)
26. Donating blood
27. Sharing needles for drug use with someone who has AIDS

How likely do you think the following situations are in transmitting HIV? Please use the numbers from the scale for your answers.

> 1 = Very likely   2 = Somewhat likely   3 = Somewhat unlikely
> 4 = Very unlikely   5 = Definitely not possible   6 = Don't know

28. Mosquito bites
29. HIV-infected mother to baby through nursing
30. Receiving anal intercourse from an HIV-infected person without using a condom
31. Receiving anal intercourse from an HIV-infected person with using a condom
32. Having sexual intercourse with an HIV-infected person without using a condom
33. Having sexual intercourse with an HIV-infected person with using a condom
34. Performing oral sex on an HIV-infected man without using a condom
35. Performing oral sex on an HIV-infected woman using a dental dam

HIV/AIDS Attitudes Scale for Teachers

The following statements reflect attitudes about HIV and AIDS. Circle the number that best describes your reactions to each statement.

> 1 = Strongly agree   2 = Agree   3 = Uncertain   4 = Disagree   5 = Strongly disagree

1. I believe I have enough information about HIV/AIDS to protect myself in my social life.
2. I worry about possible casual contact with a person with AIDS.
3. Activities that spread HIV, such as some forms of sexual behavior, should be illegal.
4. I feel uncomfortable when coming in contact with gay men because of the risk that they may have AIDS.
5. I believe I have enough information about HIV/AIDS to protect myself in my future work setting.
6. Persons with AIDS are responsible for getting their illness.
7. Civil rights laws should be enacted/enforced to protect people with AIDS from job and housing discrimination.
8. Male homosexuality is obscene and vulgar.
9. HIV antibody blood test results should be confidential to avoid discrimination against people with positive results.
10. I feel that more time should be spent teaching future teachers about HIV/AIDS in their college courses.
11. I feel disgusted when I consider the state of sinfulness of male homosexuality.
12. I would quit my job before I would work with someone who has AIDS.
13. People should not blame the homosexual community for the spread of AIDS in the U.S.
14. AIDS is a punishment for immoral behavior.
15. I feel secure that I have reduced all risks of personally contracting HIV.
16. I think all children should be tested for HIV before entering school.
17. I believe it is the regular elementary classroom teacher's responsibility to teach AIDS education.
18. In my opinion, parents of all students in the class should be notified if there is a student with HIV or AIDS in the class.
19. I feel that all school personnel who have direct contact with a student with HIV or AIDS should be notified.
20. I think that students with HIV or AIDS should be allowed to fully participate in the day-to-day activities of the regular classroom.
21. I would support including AIDS education in the curriculum in a school where I was teaching.
22. A teacher with HIV or AIDS should be allowed to continue teaching.
23. It scares me to think that I may have a student with HIV or AIDS in my classroom.
24. I believe that teachers should have the right to refuse to have students with HIV or AIDS in their classroom.
25. I feel that I could comfortably answer students' questions about HIV/AIDS.

---

a. The appropriate scale of numbers follows each item in the scale.

Assessment of Knowledge and Beliefs About HIV/AIDS Among Adolescents

Cheryl Koopman,[1] *Stanford University*
Helen Reid, *University of California, Los Angeles*

Assessment is essential to the evaluation of interventions designed to increase knowledge and encourage the adoption of safer beliefs about preventing HIV/AIDS. We developed two measures for adolescents, a particularly high-risk population for HIV/AIDS due to their sexual risk behaviors and high prevalence of sexually transmitted diseases (Hein, 1992).

Description

Two measures were developed, one to assess knowledge and the other to assess beliefs about preventing HIV/AIDS. After a review of the literature on HIV/AIDS prevention for adolescents, we generated a list of items to assess knowledge and beliefs in this area, items that would apply specifically to high-risk youths as well as ones that applied to everyone.

Knowledge items tapped seven domains: definitions, risk behavior, transmission of the virus, outcomes of HIV infection, HIV testing, prevention, and distinguishing safer from less safe behavior. Beliefs items were generated to tap five domains: perceived threat, peer support for safe acts, self-efficacy, self-control in high-risk sexual situations, and expectation to prevent pregnancy.

Two advisory councils were created, composed of experts on content and reading level. They evaluated the items on the basis of content, accuracy, reading level, and clarity. After revising the items based on this feedback, we developed measures of knowledge and beliefs, which were then revised on the basis of pilot testing with adolescents. After pilot testing, the measures included 52 items for the AIDS Knowledge Test, 8 items for the Safer Alternatives Test, and 39 items for the Beliefs About Preventing AIDS Test. Upon review of the knowledge measure, and prior to analysis, three items were excluded due to inconsistencies across states in laws governing adolescent HIV testing.

From June 1988 to February 1991, a consecutive series of 450 youths aged 11 to 19 years ($M = 15.98, SD = 1.72$) were recruited at four homeless shelters and one agency providing social and recreational services to gay-identified youths in New York City. Youths of African American (49%), Hispanic/Latino (35%), White (10%), and other ethnicities (6%) voluntarily participated. Of those participating, 153 were homeless females, 158 were homeless males, and 139

[1]Address correspondence to Cheryl Koopman, Department of Psychiatry and Behavioral Sciences, Stanford University School of Medicine, Stanford, CA 94305-5544; email: hf. cko@forsythe.stanford.edu.

were gay or bisexual males. Lesbian youths at the agency participated in the comprehensive intervention program but were not assessed.

Response Mode and Timing

The response format is true-false for the knowledge items. For the safer-alternative items, the respondent is asked to identify the safer action of two alternatives. The response format for the beliefs about prevention items is a 4-point Likert-type scale for each item (1 = *agree strongly* to 4 = *disagree strongly*). Each instrument takes fewer than 10 minutes to complete.

Scoring

Total-score subscales are computed by summing items if a minimum of 75% of the items for each subscale are present. The mean value of an item on the scale is substituted for missing items. Nineteen items are reverse scored in the computation of the beliefs about prevention scale score.

Reliability and Validity

Using baseline data collected at each youth's entry into the study, we conducted principal components analyses of (a) 49 knowledge items, (b) 8 safer-alternative items, and (c) 39 beliefs items. Internal consistency coefficients (Cronbach's alpha) were estimated for each of the factors that emerged in the rotated factor (varimax) solutions.

Forty-five of the original 49 AIDS knowledge items loaded on three factors: medical/scientific knowledge (23 items, $M = 17.7$, $SD = 3.4$, range = 7 to 23, alpha = .71), myths of HIV transmission (9 items, $M = 6.9$, $SD = 2.0$, range = 0 to 9, alpha = .72), and knowledge of high-risk and prevention behaviors (13 items, $M = 10.4$, $SD = 2.3$, range = 3 to 13, alpha = .68).

In the examination of the safer-alternative items, seven of the eight items were retained ($M = 5.6$, $SD = 1.6$, range = 0 to 7, alpha = .69).

The best factor structure for representing the items comprising the measure of beliefs about preventing AIDS was a five-factor solution after varimax rotation. Three items were dropped from the original measure due to their failure to load on any of these five factors. The resulting measure includes 36 items, comprising five scales based on these factors: perceived threat, self-control, self-efficacy, peer support for safe acts, and expectation to prevent pregnancy. Internal consistency was calculated on scales based on these five factors, using Cronbach's alpha: peer support for safe acts, alpha = .61; expectation to prevent pregnancy, alpha = .72; perceived threat, alpha = .81, self-control, alpha = .82, and self-efficacy, alpha = .90. The mean overall score on this measure was 109.0, with a standard deviation of 22.6 (range from 39 to 142).

Within the measures, all subscales are significantly correlated. Correlations among the Knowledge/Safer Alternatives subscales range from .26 to .61 ($p < .0001$); among the Beliefs subscales the range is .37 to .74 ($p < .0001$ for all pairs). However, the correlations between Knowledge and Beliefs subscales range from .00 to .19. Subscales are significantly correlated with age ($r = .12$ to $r = .34$) with the exception of expectation to prevent pregnancy ($r = .07$, $p = .18$).

Homeless females scored significantly lower than gay/ bisexual males on the scale measuring expectation to prevent pregnancy. There were no significant differences between male homeless, female homeless, and gay/bisexual male youths on the Beliefs scales measuring peer norms, perceived HIV risk, self-efficacy, or self-control. Gay/ bisexual males scored highest on every subscale of the Knowledge and Safer Alternative measures. Overall, gay/ bisexual males answered 85% of the items correctly (44 of 52), whereas homeless youths answered correctly 75% of the time, significantly lower.

Other Information

This research was funded by Grant 1P50 MH 43520 to the HIV Center for Clinical and Behavioral Studies from the National Institute of Mental Health and the National Institute on Drug Abuse (Mary Jane Rotheram-Borus, principal investigator), and Grant 1R01 MH 54930 from the National Institute of Mental Health (David Spiegel, principal investigator).

References

Hein, K. (1992). Adolescents at risk for HIV infection. In R. J. DiClemente (Ed.), *Adolescents and AIDS: A generation in jeopardy* (pp. 3-16). Newbury Park, CA: Sage.

Koopman, C., Rotheram-Borus, M. J., Henderson, R., Bradley, J. S., & Hunter, J. (1990). Assessment of knowledge of AIDS and beliefs about AIDS prevention among adolescents. *AIDS Education and Prevention, 2*(1), 58-70.

Rotheram-Borus, M. J., Koopman, C., Haignere, C., & Davies, M. (1991). Reducing HIV sexual risk behaviors among runaway adolescents. *Journal of the American Medical Association, 266,* 1237-1245.

Rotheram-Borus, M. J., Rosario, M., Reid, H., & Koopman, C. (1995). Predicting patterns of sexual acts among homosexual and bisexual youths. *American Journal of Psychiatry, 152,* 588-595.

Exhibit 1

AIDS Knowledge Test

Directions: Read each of the following statements and decide whether you think the statement is true or false. If you think the statement is true, mark "T." If you think the statement is false, mark "F."

1. AIDS means Acquired Immune Deficiency Syndrome.
2. Most scientists today believe that AIDS is caused by a virus, called HIV (Human Immunodeficiency Virus).
3. Most people who develop AIDS eventually recover.
4. A baby born to a mother with HIV infection can get AIDS.
5. HIV is carried in the blood.
6. Most people who have HIV infection are sick with AIDS.
7. Prostitutes in New York City have a low chance of getting HIV (which can lead to AIDS).
8. HIV (which can lead to AIDS) is carried in men's cum (semen).
9. The number of men and women infected with HIV will probably be less in the next several years than it is now.
10. AIDS weakens the body's ability to fight off disease.
11. People have been known to get HIV and develop AIDS from toilet seats.
12. A negative HIV antibody test means that a person probably has AIDS.
13. You can't get HIV (which can lead to AIDS) if you only have intercourse with one person for the rest of your life.
14. It is a good idea to ask someone about his/her past sexual activities before having sex with them, even though some partners may lie to you.
15. If the HIV test comes out negative, it means that the person has AIDS.
16. People get other diseases because of AIDS.
17. You can die from AIDS.
18. Men have a higher chance of getting AIDS from having sex with a woman than from having sex with a man.
19. Using a condom will lessen the chance of getting AIDS.

20. People who have AIDS get pneumonia more often than the average person.
21. Women are more likely to get AIDS from having sex with a straight (heterosexual) man than with a bisexual man.
22. It is safe to have intercourse without a condom with a person who shoots drugs as long as you don't shoot drugs.
23. People have been known to get HIV and develop AIDS from a swimming pool used by someone with AIDS.
24. People of any race can get HIV and develop AIDS.
25. People have been known to get HIV and develop AIDS by tongue kissing a person who is infected.
26. Lambskin condoms are better than latex condoms for preventing HIV infection.
27. People usually become very sick with AIDS a few days after being infected with HIV.
28. Getting AIDS depends on whether or not you practice safe sex, not on the group you hang out with.
29. People have been known to get HIV and develop AIDS from insect bites.
30. It is safer not to have sexual intercourse at all than to have sexual intercourse using a condom.
31. You only need one HIV test to come out positive to be sure that you are infected.
32. Pregnant women are safe from getting HIV infection.
33. A vaccine has recently been developed that prevents people from getting HIV infection (which can lead to AIDS).
34. The virus that can lead to AIDS can be passed by an infected person even though that person isn't sick.
35. If you are really healthy, then exercising daily can prevent getting HIV (which can lead to AIDS).
36. If the person you are now having sex with has been tested and does not have HIV infection, it means that you are not infected.
37. People have been known to get HIV and develop AIDS by eating at a restaurant where a worker has AIDS.
38. When using condoms, it is better to use one with a spermicide like Nonoxynol-9.
39. You can get HIV and eventually AIDS through an open cut or wound.
40. You are safe from AIDS if you have oral sex (with mouth to penis or mouth to vagina) without a condom.
41. If you get a "false positive" result on your HIV antibody test, it means you are infected.
42. Anal (rear end) sex without a condom is one of the safer sexual practices.
43. You can get HIV and eventually AIDS by donating blood.
44. Using drugs like marijuana, alcohol, cocaine and crack makes it more likely that you may have unsafe sex.
45. You can get HIV (which can lead to AIDS) by getting tested for it.

Safer Alternatives

Directions: For each pair of choices below, show which you think is safer by marking your choice (either A or B) on your answer sheet. If you do not know, take a guess.

Which is safer?

1. A) Giving blood
   B) Getting a blood transfusion
2. A) Working in the same office with someone who has AIDS or HIV
   B) Contact with HIV or the AIDS virus through an open cut or sore.
3. A) Heterosexual vaginal intercourse with a woman who has AIDS
   B) Anal intercourse with a man who has AIDS
4. A) Using a needle just used by a person with HIV
   B) A man having unprotected vaginal intercourse with a woman who has AIDS
5. A) Having sexual intercourse with a person who shoots drugs
   B) Spending time in the same house or room with a person who has AIDS
6. A) Homosexual anal intercourse with someone who has AIDS
   B) Receiving a blood transfusion
7. A) Unprotected sexual intercourse with a lesbian
   B) Unprotected sexual intercourse with a bisexual man

Note. True-false answer key: 1-T, 2-T, 3-F, 4-T, 5-T, 6-F, 7-F, 8-T, 9-F, 10-T, 11-F, 12-F,13-F, 14-T, 15-F, 16-F, 17-T, 18-F, 19-T, 20-T, 21-F, 22-F, 23-F, 24-T, 25-F, 26-F, 27-F, 28-T, 29-F, 30-T, 31-F, 32-F, 33-F, 34-T, 35-F, 36-F, 37-F, 38-T, 39-T, 40-F, 41-F, 42-F, 43-F, 44-T, 45-F. Scales: Medical/Scientific Knowledge (1, 2, 3, 4, 5, 6, 8, 9, 10, 12, 15, 16, 17, 20, 26, 31, 33, 34, 35, 36, 38, 39, 41); Myths of HIV Transmission (11, 23, 25, 27, 29, 32, 37, 43, 45); Knowledge of High Risk/Prevention Behaviors (7, 13, 14, 18, 19, 21, 22, 24, 28, 30, 40, 42, 44). Safer Alternatives answer key: 1-A, 2-A, 3-A, 4-B, 5-B, 6-B, 7-A.

Beliefs About Preventing AIDS

Directions: Read each statement carefully. Then show your agreement or disagreement by marking A, B, C, or D.

Mark: "1" if you agree strongly
          "2" if you agree somewhat
          "3" if you disagree somewhat
          "4" if you disagree strongly

1.   I would feel uncomfortable buying condoms.
2.   I would be too embarrassed to carry a condom around with me, even if I kept it hidden.
3.   It doesn't bother me if others make fun of me because I believe in having safe sex.
4.   If my partner won't use (or let me use) a condom, I won't have sex.
5.   My friends have changed the way they have sex because of the AIDS epidemic.
6.   I will have safe sex even if people make fun of me for it.
7.   AIDS is a health scare that I take very seriously.
8.   There is a good chance I will get AIDS during the next five years.
9.   If I ask to use condoms, it might make my partner not want to have sex with me.
10. A person who gets AIDS has a good chance of being cured.
11. I plan on being very careful about who I have sex with.
12. My friends practice safe sex.
13. I have no control over my sexual urges.
14. My friends feel that it is too much trouble to use condoms.
15. I have a high chance of getting AIDS because of my past history.
16. My partner will know I really care about him/her if I ask to use condoms.
17. I don't know how to use a condom.
18. AIDS is the scariest disease I know.
19. If I was going to have sex with someone and they made fun of me for wanting to have safe sex, I would probably give in.
20. There is still time for me to protect myself against AIDS.
21. Trying to have safe sex gets in the way of having fun.
22. I feel almost sure that I will get AIDS.
23. I know how to have safe sex.
24. Using condoms would be a sexual "turn off" for me.
25. I am not doing anything now that is sexually unsafe.
26. In the future I will always be able to practice safe sex.
27. Before I decide to have intercourse, I will make sure we have a condom.
28. Once I get sexually excited, I lose all control over what happens.
29. Most of my friends think that practicing safe sex can lower the spread of AIDS.
30. If I ask to use a condom, it will look like I don't trust my partner.
31. Carrying condoms with me every day is a habit I can keep.
32. I am too young to take care of a baby right now.
33. Not getting pregnant (or not getting a girl pregnant) is very important to me.
34. I will not bother with birth control when I have intercourse with a member of the opposite sex.
35. In the future, whenever I have sexual intercourse with a member of the opposite sex, I plan to make sure we are using birth control.
36. If I wanted to have sex with a member of the opposite sex, and did not have protection, I would go ahead and have intercourse anyway.

Source. These scales were originally published in "Assessment of Knowledge of AIDS and Beliefs About AIDS Prevention Among Adolescents," by C. Koopman, M. J. Rotheram-Borus, R. Henderson, J. S. Bradley, and J. Hunter, 1990, *AIDS Education and Prevention, 2*(1), 58-70. Reprinted with permission.

Note. Reverse scored: 3, 4, 5, 6, 7, 11, 12, 16, 18, 20, 23, 25, 26, 27, 29, 31, 32, 33, 35. Scales: Perceived Threat (7, 8, 10, 15, 18, 22); Self-Control (9, 13, 19, 21, 24, 28, 30, 36); Self-Efficacy (1, 2, 3, 4, 6, 11, 16, 17, 20, 23, 25, 26, 27, 31); Peer Support for Safe Acts (5, 12, 14, 29); Expectation to Prevent Pregnancy (32, 33, 34, 35, 36).

HIV/AIDS Knowledge and Attitudes Scales for Hispanics

Raffy R. Luquis,[1] *University of Arkansas*
Patricia Barthalow Koch, *Pennsylvania State University*

The HIV/AIDS Knowledge and Attitudes Scales for Hispanics were developed to fill a void for assessing knowledge and attitudes among people, particularly college students, with Hispanic (Latino) ethnic backgrounds. Although a number of scales had previously been developed to measure HIV/AIDS knowledge and attitudes, none emphasized issues of primary cultural importance to Hispanic populations, such as "virginity" and "promiscuity," highly structured gender roles, appropriateness of sexual discussions, barriers toward condom use, and culturally specific attitudes toward homosexuality (Carballo-Dieguez, 1989; Lifshitz, 1990-1991; Maldonado, 1990-1991; Marin, 1989; Medina, 1987). In addition, few of the existing scales have been translated appropriately into Spanish. Yet Hispanics are the fastest growing racial/ethnic group in the United States being affected by HIV disease, with persons with Hispanic backgrounds representing approximately 7% of the U.S. population but 17% of AIDS cases in the United States (Centers for Disease Control, 1993).

Description

The HIV/AIDS Knowledge Scale for Hispanics, consisting of two parts, was adapted from a survey used by the Centers for Disease Control (Dawson, 1990). The first part, General Knowledge, contains 21 statements about the prevalence, risk factors, course of the disease, diagnosis, and prevention of HIV/AIDS. The second part of the knowledge scale, Likelihood of Transmission, concentrates on HIV transmission modes and contains 16 statements about possible ways to transmit HIV.

The HIV/AIDS Attitudes Scale for Hispanics was adapted from the attitudes survey used by the Centers for Disease Control (Dawson, 1990) and the Nurses' Attitudes About AIDS Scale (NAAS; Preston, Young, Koch, & Forti, 1995). Relevant parts of these previous scales were used and supplemented with statements more specific to Hispanic college students to create a scale of 26 items. These items include attitudes about the HIV and people who may be infected, sexual behavior and safer-sex practices, and discussions and learning about HIV/AIDS.

The knowledge and attitudes scales are available in both English and Spanish versions.

---
[1]Address correspondence to Raffy R. Luquis, Department of Health Sciences, HPER 306, University of Arkansas, Fayetteville, AR 72701.

Response Mode and Timing

For the General Knowledge part of the HIV/AIDS Knowledge Scale for Hispanics, respondents identify the first 20 statements as either *(1) definitely true*, (2) *probably true*, (3) *probably false*, (4) *definitely false*, or (5) *don't know*. Question 21 is a multiple-choice question from which the respondent chooses the correct answer. For the Likelihood of Transmission part of the knowledge scale, respondents are given 15 ways that HIV might be transmitted and asked if transmission through this mode is (1) *very likely*, (2) *somewhat likely*, (3) *somewhat unlikely*, (4) *very unlikely*, (5) *definitely not possible*, or (6) *don't know*. The final question asks the respondent to circle all of the fluids through which HIV has been transmitted. It takes approximately 15 minutes to complete the entire knowledge scale.

For the HIV/AIDS Attitudes Scale for Hispanics, respondents indicate, using a Likert-type scale, if they *(1) strongly agree*, (2) *agree*, (3) are *uncertain*, (4) *disagree*, or (5) *strongly disagree* with each of the 26 statements. This scale takes about 10 minutes to complete.

Scoring

One point is given for every correct answer on the General Knowledge part of the knowledge scale, with the highest possible score being 21. Correct answers are as follows: *definitely true* (1) for Items 1, 3, 5, 8, 10, 11, 12, 14, 15, 18, 19, 20; *definitely true* (1) or *probably true* for Item 7; and *definitely false* (4) for Items 2, 4, 6, 9, 13, 16, 17. The correct multiple-choice answer to Item 21 is 4.

The highest possible score for the Likelihood of Transmission part of the knowledge scale is 23. One point is given for each correct answer for Items 22-36. The correct answers are *very likely* (1) for Items 28, 35, 36; *very unlikely* (4) for Items 24, 29; and *definitely not possible* for Items 22-23, 25-27, 30-34. For Item 37, one point each is given for circling b, c, f, h and not circling a, d, e, g.

A mean score is calculated for the HIV/AIDS Attitudes Scale for Hispanics. This score can range from 1, representing the most unsupportive attitudes toward HIV/AIDS and safer sex, to 5, representing the most supportive attitudes. The following items are reversed scored: 1, 5, 8, 9, 10, 12, 13, 15, 16, 20, 21, 23, 25, 26.

In a comparison study of 144 Hispanic and 232 non-Hispanic college students, no significant difference was found in their General Knowledge of HIV/AIDS ($M = 12.94$ and $M = 12.70$, respectively), representing about a 60% level of correct responses (Luquis, 1991). Additionally, no significant difference was found in their Likelihood of Transmission knowledge ($M = 15.17$ and $M = 15.19$, respectively), indicating about a 65% level of correct responses. However, significant differences in attitudes were found based on gender and ethnicity, with mean scores as follows: Hispanic male ($M = 3.76$), Hispanic female ($M = 3.89$), non-Hispanic male ($M = 3.61$), and non-Hispanic female ($M = 3.94$). These attitude scores ranged from slightly positive/liberal to somewhat positive/liberal.

Reliability

Internal reliability for the knowledge and attitudes scales, using Cronbach's alpha coefficient, was established using a sample of 144 Hispanic and 232 non-Hispanic college students (Luquis, 1991). The item analyses produced an alpha of .61 for the HIV/AIDS Knowledge Scale for Hispanics and an alpha of .85 for the HIV/AIDS Attitudes Scale for Hispanics.

Validity

Initial versions of the scales were subjected to focus group analysis and discussion with separate groups of Hispanic male and female university students. This process was extremely helpful in determining the culturally relevant issues to be included. The revised instruments were then pilot tested with Hispanic and non-Hispanic students for feedback concerning content, format, and vocabulary. The English versions of the instruments were then translated into Spanish by the primary researcher. They were back-translated into English by another bilingual professional to ensure the validity of the Spanish versions of the scales.

References

Carballo-Dieguez, A. (1989, September/October). Hispanic culture, gay male culture, and AIDS: Counseling implications. *Journal of Counseling & Development, 68*, 26-30.

Centers for Disease Control. (1993, December). *HIV/AIDS surveillance report*. Atlanta, GA: Author.

Dawson, D. A. (1990). *AIDS knowledge and attitudes for July-September*. Provisional data from the National Health Interview Survey. (Advance Data From Vital and Health Statistics No. 183). Hyattsville, MD: Department of Health and Human Services, Public Health Services, Centers for Disease Control, National Center for Health Statistics.

Lifshitz, A. (1990-1991, December/January). Critical cultural barriers that bar meeting the needs of Latinas. *SIECUS Report, 19*(2) 16-17.

Luquis, R. (1991). *Knowledge of and attitudes about HIV/AIDS among Hispanic college students at the Pennsylvania State University*. Unpublished master's thesis, Pennsylvania State University, University Park, PA.

Maldonado, M. (1990-1991, December/January). Latinas and HIV/AIDS: Implications for the 90s. *SIECUS Report, 19*(2), 11-17.

Marin, G. (1989). AIDS prevention among Hispanics: Needs, risk behavior, and cultural values. *Public Health Report, 104*, 411-414.

Medina, C. (1987). Latino culture and sex education. *SIECUS Report, 15*(3), 1-4.

Preston, D. B., Young, E. W., Koch, P. B., & Forti, E. M. (1995). The Nurses' Attitudes About AIDS Scale (NAAS): Development and psychometric analysis. *AIDS Education and Prevention, 7*, 443-454.

Exhibit

HIV/AIDS Knowledge Scale for Hispanics[a]

Please indicate, to the best of your knowledge, if the following statements are *definitely true* (1), *probably true* (2), *probably false* (3), or *definitely false* (4). If you are not sure of the correct answer, circle 5.

Scale: 1 = Definitely true   2 = Probably true   3 = Probably false
          4 = Definitely false   5 = Don't know

1. AIDS can reduce the body's natural protection against diseases.[b]
2. AIDS is especially common in older people.
3. AIDS can damage the brain.
4. AIDS usually leads to heart disease.
5. AIDS results from an infectious disease caused by a virus.
6. College students are not at risk of contracting AIDS.
7. AIDS leads to death.
8. A person can be infected with HIV and not have the disease AIDS.
9. Looking at a person is enough to tell if he or she has HIV.
10. Any person with AIDS can pass it on to someone else during unprotected sexual intercourse.
11. A person who has HIV can look and feel healthy and well.
12. A pregnant woman who has HIV can give the virus to her baby.
13. There is a vaccine available to the public that protects a person from getting HIV.
14. There is no cure for AIDS at the present time.
15. It may be more than five years before a person infected by HIV develops AIDS.
16. A person can be diagnosed with AIDS by taking one special blood test.
17. Using any type of condom can help protect you from AIDS.
18. Minorities, like Blacks and Hispanics, are at greater risk of getting AIDS than the rest of the population.

19. The number of HIV-infected persons will be decreasing in the U.S. during the next two years.
20. In the United States, every 2 minutes a Hispanic/Latino is infected with HIV.
21. Hispanics represent what percentage of AIDS cases in the U.S.?
    1. 2%
    2. 5%
    3. 10%
    4. 17%
    5. 25%

How likely do you think it is that a person will get AIDS or HIV infection from each of the following? Please circle the number from the scale for your answer.

Scale: 1 = Very likely   2 = Somewhat likely   3 = Somewhat unlikely
         4 = Very unlikely   5 = Definitely not possible   6 = Don't know

22. Living near a hospital or home for AIDS patients.
23. Working near someone with HIV.
24. Kissing with exchange of saliva someone who has HIV.
25. Eating in a restaurant where the cook has HIV.
26. Shaking hands, touching, or kissing on the cheek someone who has HIV.
27. Using public toilets.
28. Sharing needles for drug use with someone who has AIDS.
29. Receiving a blood transfusion from a hospital blood bank.
30. Mosquito or other insect bites.
31. Donating blood.
32. Being coughed or sneezed on by someone who has HIV.
33. Attending class with a student who has HIV.
34. Sharing a dorm room with a student who has HIV.
35. Unprotected (without a condom) sexual intercourse with an HIV-infected person.
36. Unprotected (without a condom) anal intercourse with an HIV-infected person.
37. Circle all the fluids through which HIV has been transmitted:
    1. saliva   5. urine
    2. semen   6. blood
    3. vaginal secretions 7. tears
    4. perspiration   8. mother's milk

HIV/AIDS Attitudes Scale for Hispanics

The following statements reflect attitudes about HIV and AIDS. Circle the number that best describes your reactions to each statement.

Scale: 1 = Strongly agree   2 = Agree   3 = Uncertain   4 = Disagree   5 = Uncertain

1. I believe I have enough information about AIDS to protect myself.
2. I believe women should not have sexual intercourse before marriage.
3. Activities that spread AIDS, such as some forms of sexual behavior, should be illegal.
4. I feel uncomfortable when coming in contact with gay men because of the risk that they may have for AIDS.
5. Civil rights laws should be enacted/enforced to protect people with AIDS from job and housing discrimination.
6. Male homosexuality is obscene and vulgar.
7. I believe men should not have sexual intercourse before marriage.
8. AIDS antibody blood test results should be confidential to avoid discrimination against people with positive results.
9. I feel that more time should be spent teaching students about AIDS.
10. People should not blame the homosexual community for the spread of AIDS in the U.S.
11. AIDS is a punishment for immoral behavior.
12. I feel secure that I have reduced all risk of personally contracting AIDS.
13. It would not bother me to attend class with a person with AIDS.
14. Anyone who has had more than one sexual partner is promiscuous.
15. I could comfortably discuss AIDS with a friend.
16. I would not avoid a friend if she/he had AIDS.
17. If I discovered that my roommate had AIDS, I would move out.
18. I do not believe in using condoms.

19. I could not discuss AIDS with my parents.
20. I would date a person with HIV.
21. I would feel comfortable discussing AIDS in a classroom situation.
22. I would not engage in sexual intercourse before marriage.
23. I would feel comfortable asking a new partner about his/her sexual history.
24. I would use AIDS as an excuse to avoid any sexual relationships.
25. I would limit myself to one sexual partner.
26. I would use a condom every time I had sex.

a. The Spanish translation of the scales are available from Raffy R. Luquis.
b. The appropriate scale follows each item.

A Measure of AIDS Prevention Information, Motivation, Behavioral Skills, and Behavior

Steven J. Misovich, *University of Connecticut*
William A. Fisher,[1] *University of Western Ontario*
Jeffrey D. Fisher, *University of Connecticut*

The information, motivation, and behavioral skills (IMB) model of AIDS risk behavior change (J. Fisher & Fisher, 1992; W. Fisher & Fisher, 1993) has been developed and validated to serve as general conceptualization for understanding and promoting AIDS risk reduction behavior change. The IMB model proposes that *information* that is directly relevant to AIDS preventive behavior, *motivation* to act on this information, and *behavioral skills* for acting on it effectively are fundamental determinants of AIDS preventive behavior. According to the IMB model, AIDS prevention information and AIDS prevention motivation work through AIDS prevention behavioral skills to affect the initiation and maintenance of AIDS preventive behavior. The IMB model proposes that AIDS prevention information and AIDS prevention motivation may also have direct effects on AIDS preventive behavior, when such preventive behavior does not require the performance of complicated or novel behavioral acts. The propositions of the IMB model concerning the relationship of AIDS prevention information, motivation, behavioral

skills, and behavior have been consistently and strongly confirmed in research conducted with samples of gay men and heterosexual university students (J. Fisher, Fisher, Williams, & Malloy, 1994) and ethnically diverse heterosexual high school students (W. Fisher, Williams, Fisher, & Malloy, 1998).

In addition to specifying the determinants of AIDS preventive behavior, the IMB model provides a highly generalizable approach to the design, implementation, and evaluation of AIDS risk reduction interventions that are empirically targeted at the needs of specific populations at risk. Three phases of activity are involved in the application of the IMB model for the design, deployment, and evaluation of AIDS risk reduction interventions. First, *elicitation research* is conducted using open- and closed-ended assessment strategies to empirically determine strengths and weaknesses in a target population's existing levels of AIDS prevention information, motivation, behavioral skills, and behavior. Second, *targeted interventions* are constructed to address deficits and to capitalize on strengths that have been identified in elicitation research in the target population's AIDS prevention information, motivation, behavioral skills, and behavior, and to create changes in these factors to facilitate AIDS risk behavior change. Third, methodologically rigorous *evaluation research* is conducted to

[1]Address correspondence to William A. Fisher, Department of Psychology, University of Western Ontario, London, Ontario N6A 5C2, Canada; email: fisher@sscl.uwo.ca.

determine the extent to which the IMB model-based targeted intervention has resulted in short- and long-term changes in AIDS prevention information, motivation, behavioral skills, and behavior per se. The IMB model has been successfully used as the basis for elicitation, intervention, and evaluation research in a sample of heterosexual university students, and findings have demonstrated that the IMB model-based intervention resulted in significant changes in AIDS risk reduction information, motivation, and behavioral skills, and in significant, sustained improvement in AIDS preventive behaviors such as condom use during sexual intercourse (J. Fisher, Fisher, Misovich, Kimble, & Malloy, 1996).

The questionnaire presented herein was constructed to serve as an IMB model-based instrument for assessing AIDS prevention information, motivation, behavioral skills, and behavior. This questionnaire was used as a premeasure and postmeasure of these factors in the multisession AIDS risk reduction intervention with university students referred to earlier (J. Fisher et al., 1996), and versions of these measures have been used in correlational studies of the determinants of AIDS preventive behavior among gay men, heterosexual university students, and ethnically diverse heterosexual high school students (J. Fisher et al., 1994; W. Fisher et al., 1998).

Description, Scoring, Reliability, and Validity

The questionnaire is designed to be used with heterosexual college students and heterosexual post-college-age adults. With modifications based on appropriate elicitation research, this questionnaire could be adapted for use with other populations, and variations of this questionnaire that have been used with gay men, and with ethnically diverse heterosexual high school students, are available from the first author. The questionnaire presented in the exhibit and the data and means reported here, however, are based on a questionnaire version designed for use with heterosexual college students and completed by the subset of the experimental and control respondents (J. Fisher et al., 1996) who reported engaging in sexual intercourse during the month prior to administration of the questionnaire.

Demographic Measures:
Questionnaire Page 1

This section includes measures of respondent's sex, ethnic background, and age.

AIDS Prevention Information Measures:
Questionnaire Pages 2-4

The "Health and Relationships Survey" assesses respondents' levels of AIDS prevention information in categories that have relevance to the practice of preventive behavior and that elicitation research in heterosexual university student and adult populations (Misovich, Pittman, Fisher, & Fisher, 1993) indicates may be deficient. Items 1 through 33 measure areas of AIDS prevention information that are relevant to preventive behavior, and they focus on issues, such as knowledge about the effectiveness of condoms in preventing AIDS, and knowledge about likely and unlikely

vectors of HIV transmission. Items 34 through 37 tap information that is specifically relevant to university students, covering rates of HIV infection in the student population, knowledge about where to purchase condoms on campus, and the fact that members of that college-age population may be HIV-positive without showing any overt symptoms. These four items may be replaced with information items that cover the same three topics but that are specifically relevant to different populations under study. Items 38 through 46 measure respondents' endorsement of incorrect "AIDS information heuristics": simple but invalid decision rules that individuals invoke to make rapid but incorrect judgments about whether to practice safer sex and that have been found to be directly related to levels of AIDS risk behavior (Misovich, Fisher, & Fisher, 1996, 1997).

Scoring the AIDS information scale is accomplished by dichotomizing each item into a value of 1 (correct) or 0 (incorrect) and then summing the item values. To do this, with true items, responses of 1 (*strongly agree*) or 2 (*agree somewhat*) should be recoded as 1, and all other responses (including missing values) should be recoded as 0. For false items, responses of 4 (*disagree somewhat*) or 5 (*strongly disagree*) should be recoded as 1, and all other responses should be coded as 0. The items should then be summed to form an AIDS prevention information scale score. Cronbach's alpha for this scale when used with a university student population was .75, and the mean for the sample was 33.5. Evidence of validity is provided by results that show that AIDS prevention information scores improved significantly in response to an intervention that stressed relevant AIDS prevention information, but not in the control condition of this intervention (J. Fisher et al., 1996), and by findings confirming the role of AIDS prevention information as specified by the IMB model using a variety of similar items in diverse populations at risk (J. Fisher et al., 1994; W. Fisher et al., 1998).

Measures of Motivation to Perform AIDS Preventive Behavior: Questionnaire Pages 5-9

Questionnaire measures of motivation to perform AIDS preventive behavior were based on the concepts and operations of the theory of reasoned action (e.g., Ajzen & Fishbein, 1980; Fishbein & Ajzen, 1975; Fishbein & Middlestadt, 1989). For each of eight critical AIDS preventive behaviors (e.g., not having sexual intercourse at all, talking with my partner about safer sex, always using latex condoms during intercourse), the first three items measure the respondent's attitude toward the AIDS-preventive act in question using bipolar evaluative scales. The next questionnaire item measures the respondent's subjective norms, or perceptions of whether significant others wish them to perform the preventive behavior in question. The final questionnaire item measures the respondent's behavioral intention to perform the preventive practice in question.

Attitudes toward AIDS preventive acts. To determine respondents' attitudes toward performing specific AIDS preventive behaviors, respondents rate their performance of eight preventive acts on three 5-point semantic differential scales (*good-bad, nice-awful,* and *pleasant-unpleasant*).

These ratings should be reversed such that each item is scored from 1 (positive evaluation) to 5 (negative evaluation) and summed to produce an attitudes toward AIDS preventive behaviors scale score (Ajzen & Fishbein, 1980; Fishbein & Ajzen, 1975). Cronbach's alpha for this scale with university students was .86, and the mean score was 65.9. Validity evidence for the scale is provided by the fact that an AIDS prevention intervention that sought to improve attitudes toward preventive behaviors resulted in more favorable attitudes toward AIDS preventive acts scale scores, whereas control conditions had no impact on these scores (J. Fisher et al., 1996), and by evidence concerning the ability of very similar attitude items to predict AIDS prevention behavioral intentions to practice AIDS prevention across diverse samples at risk (W. Fisher, Fisher, & Rye, 1995).

Subjective norms regarding AIDS preventive acts. This scale assesses respondents' subjective norms (Ajzen & Fishbein, 1980; Fishbein & Ajzen, 1975) or generalized perceptions of social support for their practice of AIDS preventive behaviors. To assess respondents' social norms for AIDS preventive behavior, they are asked to complete items measuring the extent to which they believe that "most people who are important to them" think they should perform each of the eight critical AIDS preventive behaviors at focus. These items should be scored (1 = *very true*, 5 = *very untrue*, that "Most people who are important to me think I should . . . ") and summed to create an overall measure of social norms concerning the practice of AIDS preventive behaviors (Ajzen & Fishbein, 1980; Fishbein & Ajzen, 1975). Cronbach's alpha for this scale with university students was .87, and the mean was 20.4. Validity evidence for the scale includes the ability of very similar social norm items to predict AIDS prevention behavioral intentions across diverse samples at risk (W. Fisher et al., 1995).

Behavioral intentions for AIDS prevention. Respondents' behavioral intentions (Ajzen & Fishbein, 1980; Fishbein & Ajzen, 1975) to perform each of the AIDS preventive behaviors under study are measured by asking them to rate, on a 5-point scale ranging from *very likely* (1) to *very unlikely* (5), how probable it is that they will perform each of the eight AIDS preventive acts sampled over a specified time period (e.g., over the next month). Respondents' scores (1 = *very likely*, 5 = *very unlikely*) should be summed to form a measure of AIDS prevention behavioral intentions. Cronbach's alpha for this scale with university students was .80, and the mean was 18.7. Validity evidence for the scale includes the fact that an AIDS prevention intervention produced changes in these AIDS prevention behavioral intentions, whereas a control condition did not (J. Fisher et al., 1996), and evidence of the ability of very similar behavioral intention items to predict AIDS preventive behavior across time and across diverse samples at risk (W. Fisher et al., 1995).

Behavioral Skills Measures:
Questionnaire Pages 9-13

AIDS prevention behavioral skills are assessed with the subscales tapping perceived difficulty of AIDS preventive

behaviors (all items with the response format *very easy to do* to *very hard to do*) and perceived effectiveness at AIDS preventive behavior (all items with the response format *very effectively* to *very ineffectively*).

The Perceived Difficulty of AIDS Preventive Behavior subscale asks respondents to rate, on 5-point scales, how hard or easy it would be for them to perform 12 critical AIDS preventive behaviors. These items should be summed (1 = *very hard*, 5 = *very easy*) to form an overall Perceived Difficulty of AIDS Preventive Behavior score. Cronbach's alpha for this scale when used with university students was .74, and the mean of the scale was 44.8. Validity evidence is provided by findings that show that perceived difficulty of AIDS preventive behavior scores changed as expected in response to an AIDS prevention intervention experimental condition, but not in a control condition (J. Fisher et al., 1996), and by evidence that shows that responses to similar items are significantly correlated with trained raters' evaluations of the effectiveness of respondents' written and videotaped role plays of AIDS preventive behaviors (Williams et al., in press).

The Perceived Effectiveness at AIDS Preventive Behavior Scale asks respondents to rate, on 5-point scales, how effectively they believe they could engage in a range of 24 AIDS preventive behaviors. These items should be scored (1 = *very effectively*, 5 = *very ineffectively*) and summed to form an overall perceived effectiveness of AIDS preventive behavior score. Cronbach's alpha for this scale within a university student sample was .88, and the scale mean was 90. Validity evidence is again provided by findings that show that perceived effectiveness scores changed in response to an AIDS prevention intervention experimental condition, but did not change in a control condition (J. Fisher et al., 1996), and by evidence that shows that responses to similar items are significantly correlated with trained raters' evaluations of the effectiveness of respondents' written and videotaped role plays of AIDS preventive behaviors (Williams et al., in press).

AIDS Preventive Behaviors:
Questionnaire Pages 13-16

AIDS preventive behaviors are assessed with four subscales measuring discussion of safer sex, condom accessibility, condom use, and HIV testing, and with a number of single items that may be employed alone or in combination to reflecting a variety of safer versus riskier sexual practices. *Safer-sex discussion* is measured with two items (6 and 19) that ask if the respondent has discussed AIDS prevention with a sexual partner and if he or she has tried to persuade a sexual partner to practice only safer sex using a condom. These two items, which correlate .42 with one another ($N = 263, p < .001$), may be summed to create an indicator of discussion of AIDS preventive behavior. *Condom accessibility* is assessed with two items (7 and 8) that asking respondents how often they have purchased condoms and the extent to which they have kept condoms easily available. These two items, which correlate .51 with one another ($N = 325, p < .001$), may be summed to create a behavioral indicator of condom accessibility. *Condom use during sexual intercourse* is assessed with three items (9, 13, and 14) that ask respondents about their frequency of condom use during intercourse. These items should be standardized (because of their varying response formats) and summed to produce an indicator of condom use; within a university student sample, Cronbach's alpha for these items was .98. Finally, *HIV testing behavior* is assessed by asking respondents to report whether or not they have made an appointment for an HIV test (Item 22), and whether or not they have actually had an HIV test (Item 21). These two items, which correlate .49 with one another, may be summed to form an indicator of HIV testing behavior.

Several additional items measuring AIDS risk and AIDS preventive behaviors are included in the AIDS preventive behavior portion of the questionnaire. Items 1 through 5 and 10 through 12 may be used to classify respondents into risk categories (e.g., never had intercourse, have had intercourse but in a monogamous relationship with no previous partners). Items 15 through 18 of this section of the questionnaire involve anal intercourse, and Item 20 assesses the sex of the respondent's sexual partners. Items 23 and 24 assess the respondent's HIV testing behavior prior to the time interval of the questionnaire and ask about the type of site (e.g., an anonymous or a confidential site) they may have used for an HIV test.

Response Mode and Timing

This questionnaire is a self-administered questionnaire and takes approximately 45 minutes to complete when used in a university student population. Additional time and additional instructions, as well as other modifications, may be required if using this questionnaire in other populations.

References

Ajzen, I., & Fishbein, M. (1980). *Understanding attitudes and predicting social behavior.* Englewood Cliffs, NJ: Prentice Hall.

Fishbein, M., & Ajzen, I. (1975). *Belief, attitude, intention, and behavior: An introduction to theory and research.* Reading, MA: Addison-Wesley.

Fishbein, M., & Middlestadt, S. E. (1989). Using the theory of reasoned action as a framework for understanding and changing AIDS-related behaviors. In V. M. Mays, G. W. Albee, & S. F. Schneider (Eds.), *Primary prevention of AIDS: Psychological approaches* (pp. 93-110). London: Sage.

Fisher, J. D., & Fisher, W. A. (1992). Changing AIDS risk behavior. *Psychological Bulletin, 111*, 455-474.

Fisher, J. D., Fisher, W. A., Misovich, S. J., Kimble, D. L., & Malloy, T. E. (1996). Changing AIDS risk behavior: Effects of an intervention emphasizing AIDS risk reduction information, motivation, and behavioral skills in a college student population. *Health Psychology, 15*, 114-123.

Fisher, J. D., Fisher, W. A., Williams, S. S., & Malloy, T. E. (1994). Empirical tests of an information-motivation-behavioral skills model of AIDS preventive behavior. *Health Psychology, 14*, 238-250.

Fisher, W. A., Fisher, J. D. (1993). A general social psychological model for changing AIDS risk behavior. In J. Pryor & G. Reeder (Eds.), *The social psychology of HIV infection.* Hillsdale, NJ: Lawrence Erlbaum.

Fisher, W. A., Fisher, J. D., & Rye, B. J. (1995). Understanding and promoting AIDS preventive behavior: Insights from the theory of reasoned action. *Health Psychology, 14*, 255-264.

Fisher, W. A., Williams, S. S., Fisher, J. D., & Malloy, T. E. (1998). *Predicting AIDS risk behavior among urban adolescents: An empirical test of the information-motivation-behavioral skills model.* Manuscript submitted for publication.

Misovich, S. J., Fisher, J. D., & Fisher, W. A. (1996). The perceived AIDS-preventive utility of knowing one's partner well: A public health dictum and individuals' risky sexual behavior. *Canadian Journal of Human Sexuality, 5*, 83-90.

Misovich, S. J., Fisher, J. D., & Fisher, W. A. (1997). Close relationships and elevated HIV risk behavior: Evidence and possible underlying psychological processes. *General Psychology Review, 1*, 72-107.

Misovich, S. J., Pittman, L., Fisher, J. D., & Fisher, W. A. (1993). *New measures of AIDS knowledge: Scale development, validation, and relationship with behavior.* Unpublished manuscript, University of Connecticut, Storrs.

Williams, S. S., Doyle, T. M., Pittman, L. D., Weiss, L. H., Fisher, J. D., & Fisher, W. A. (in press). Roleplayed safer sex skills of heterosexual college students influenced by both personal and partner factors. *AIDS and Behavior.*

Exhibit

The Health and Relationships Survey

Please answer each question below by circling a number to its right, according to this scale: 1 = Strongly Agree, 2 = Agree Somewhat, 3 = Neither Agree nor Disagree 4 = Disagree Somewhat, 5 = Strongly Disagree

1. More of the virus that causes AIDS is found in blood and semen than in other body fluids.[a]
2. It is estimated that more than one million Americans are currently infected with the virus that causes AIDS.
3. If you do not use condoms, withdrawal of the penis immediately before orgasm reduces the risk of getting the virus that causes AIDS to the point where it is highly unlikely that a person will get it.
4. A person is not very likely to get AIDS by sharing IV-drug needles with someone who has the virus.
5. These days, it is very unlikely that a blood transfusion would give a person the virus that causes AIDS.
6. Unprotected oral sex is less risky for transmitting the virus that causes AIDS than unprotected vaginal sex.
7. Most people who have been exposed to the virus that causes AIDS show clearly visible symptoms of serious illness.
8. The virus that causes AIDS is not spread by sneezing or coughing.
9. There are no cases of people getting the virus that causes AIDS from contact with saliva.
10. A person can be infected with the virus that causes AIDS for five or more years without developing AIDS.

11. Several people have gotten the virus that causes AIDS by donating blood.
12. It is unsafe to use drinking fountains or public toilets that might have been used by somebody who has the virus that causes AIDS.
13. Some people have gotten the virus that causes AIDS from infected people's sweat in gymnasiums or health clubs.
14. If you kiss someone who has the virus that causes AIDS, you will probably get the disease.
15. A woman who is infected with the virus that causes AIDS cannot pass the disease to her infant.
16. The virus that causes AIDS is not spread by mosquitoes.
17. Through sexual intercourse, men can transmit the virus that causes AIDS somewhat more easily to women than women can transmit it to men.

(page 3)[b]

18. Oil-based lubricants such as Vaseline should be used to lubricate condoms.
19. Condoms may be safely stored in one's wallet for up to two months.
20. In order for a condom to effectively reduce one's risk for the virus that causes AIDS, it must be put on before any sexual intercourse takes place.
21. Natural condoms made of animal products are as effective as latex condoms in preventing the virus that causes AIDS.
22. Medical experts believe that most people infected with the virus that causes AIDS will eventually develop AIDS.
23. In order for the virus that causes AIDS to be transmitted from one person to another, there must be direct contact between one person's blood, vaginal secretions or semen, and the other person's blood.
24. Condoms have an "expiration date" like food does, and you should not buy condoms whose expiration date has passed.
25. Nonoxynol-9 (found in some spermicides and foams) has been shown to kill the virus that causes AIDS.
26. If you have a "confidential" HIV blood test, you have to give your name to the testing site.
27. People can get the virus that causes AIDS by eating food that has been prepared by someone who has the disease.
28. Children who have the virus that causes AIDS can easily spread the disease to other children.
29. It is unsafe to share drinking glasses and eating utensils with people who have the virus that causes AIDS.
30. Many health-care workers have become infected as a result of treating AIDS patients.
31. Household pets can spread the virus that causes AIDS to people.
32. If a person has unsafe sex and an HIV blood test two weeks later indicates that they do not have the virus that causes AIDS, they can be fairly certain that they were not exposed to the AIDS virus.
33. When properly used, latex condoms greatly reduce the chance that the virus that causes AIDS will be transmitted through sexual intercourse.

(page 4)

34. According to a recent study, about 1 in 500 college students have been exposed to the virus that causes AIDS.
35. There are several locations on campus where condoms can be purchased at any hour of the night.
36. Most college students who get infected with the virus that causes AIDS during college will feel fine and show no symptoms of AIDS throughout their college career.
37. At UConn, condoms may be purchased at the Student Infirmary, and charged to your next semester's fee bill.
38. If you know a person's sexual history and lifestyle before you have sex with them, it is unnecessary to use condoms.
39. The way a person behaves around you when you first meet them is probably a good indicator of whether or not they are the type of person who may have been exposed to the virus that causes AIDS.
40. You really only need to use condoms during "one night stands."
41. You can tell whether a potential sex partner is at risk for AIDS by how they dress and how they look.
42. When you feel you have gotten to know someone very well, you no longer need to practice safer sex with them.
43. Asking your partner about their sexual history is a good way to find out whether or not to practice safer sex with them.
44. As long as a person doesn't belong to a "high risk" group such as gays or drug users, you really don't need to worry about getting the virus that causes AIDS from them.
45. If two people have sex only with each other, they really don't have to practice safer sex.
46. Individuals in urban areas should definitely follow safer-sex guidelines, but individuals in rural areas really don't need to.

(page 5)

Each question below is asked in the context of what you would think or do *in the next month*. Although many of the situations discussed might be relevant for a much longer period of time, for research purposes, we need to have a standard time frame.

Answer each of the questions below by putting an X on the part of the line that best represents your feelings. Be sure to put your mark *within one of the five intervals on each line.*

For example, if your answer to a question below was "very good," "somewhat nice," and "neither pleasant nor unpleasant" your response would look like this:

My getting a new car during the next month would be:

very good		__X__	_____	_____	_____	_____		very bad
very awful		_____	_____	_____	___X___	_____		very nice
very pleasant		_____	_____	___X___	_____	_____		very unpleasant

The questions below deal with not having sexual intercourse at all.

Note: When we say "sexual intercourse," we mean sex where the penis is put into the vagina or sex where the penis is put into the rectum (the behind).

1. My *not* having sexual intercourse at all during the next month would be:[c]
2. Most people who are important to me think I should not have sexual intercourse at all during the next month.

     very true |_____|_____|_____|_____|_____| very untrue

3. I intend to not have sexual intercourse at all during the next month.

     very likely |_____|_____|_____|_____|_____| very unlikely

(page 7)

Please Note:

Many of the questions in this section ask you to describe your feelings about a specific behavior that involves a sexual partner. If you do not currently have a sexual partner, please answer those questions *as if you had a sexual partner.*

The questions below deal with discussing safer sex with sexual partners.

4. My talking about safer sex (how to keep from getting the virus that causes AIDS) with my sexual partner(s) before having sex with them during the next month would be:[c]
5. Most people who are important to me think I should talk about safer sex with my partner(s) before having sex with them during the next month.

     very true |_____|_____|_____|_____|_____| very untrue

6. If I have sex during the next month, I intend to talk about safer sex with my partner(s) before having sex with them.

     very likely |_____|_____|_____|_____|_____| very unlikely

The questions below deal with trying to persuade your partner(s) to practice only safer sex.

7. Trying to persuade my partner(s) to practice only safer sex (for example, to use latex condoms) during the next month would be:[c]
8. Most people who are important to me think I should try to persuade my partner(s) to practice only safer sex during the next month.

     very true |_____|_____|_____|_____|_____| very untrue

9. If I have sex during the next month, I intend to try to persuade my partner(s) to practice only safer sex.

     very likely |_____|_____|_____|_____|_____| very unlikely

The questions below deal with buying latex condoms.

10. My buying latex condoms during the next month would be:[c]
11. Most people who are important to me think I should buy latex condoms during the next month.

     very true |_____|_____|_____|_____|_____| very untrue

12. I intend to buy latex condoms during the next month.

     very likely |_____|_____|_____|_____|_____| very unlikely

The next questions deal with always making sure you have latex condoms handy.

13. Always having latex condoms handy during the next month would be:[c]

14. Most people who are important to me think I should always have latex condoms handy during the next month.

very true |_____|_____|_____|_____|_____| very untrue

15. I intend to always have latex condoms handy during the next month.

very likely |_____|_____|_____|_____|_____| very unlikely

(page 11)

The questions below deal with always using latex condoms during sexual intercourse.

16. In the next month, my partner(s) and I always using latex condoms during sexual intercourse would be:[c]

17. Most people who are important to me think my partner(s) and I should always use latex condoms during sexual intercourse in the next month.

very true |_____|_____|_____|_____|_____| very untrue

18. If I have sexual intercourse during the next month, I intend to have my partner(s) and I always use latex condoms.

very likely |_____|_____|_____|_____|_____| very unlikely

The questions below are about getting a blood test for the virus that causes AIDS.

19. Getting a blood test during the next month to check whether I have the virus that causes AIDS would be:[c]

20. Most people who are important to me think I should get a blood test during the next month to check whether I have the virus that causes AIDS.

very true |_____|_____|_____|_____|_____| very untrue

21. I intend to get a blood test during the next month to check whether I have the virus that causes AIDS.

very likely |_____|_____|_____|_____|_____| very unlikely

The questions below deal with asking your partner to get a blood test for the virus that causes AIDS.

22. Asking my partner(s) to get a blood test during the next month to check whether they have the virus that causes AIDS would be:[c]

23. Most people who are important to me think I should ask my partner(s) to get a blood test during the next month to check whether they have the virus that causes AIDS.

very true |_____|_____|_____|_____|_____| very untrue

24. I intend to ask my partner(s) to get a blood test during the next month to check whether they have the virus that causes AIDS.

very likely |_____|_____|_____|_____|_____| very unlikely

For the following questions, please circle the answer you feel best applies to you. We realize that some of these questions may seem a bit repetitive or awkward, but for scientific reasons, the questions have to be phrased in a particular way. Each of the questions is different, and each is important to the outcome of this study. Please be patient and answer as best you can.

Please circle how *hard* or *easy* it would be for you to do each of the following things.

1. How hard would it be for you to buy condoms?[d]
2. How hard would it be for you to be supportive if your sexual partner brought up the topic of using condoms to reduce the risk of getting the virus that causes AIDS?
3. How hard would it be for you to make safer sex with a latex condom sexually exciting for your partner?
4. How hard would it be for you to discuss safer sex (for example, always using latex condoms) with your partner in a nonsexual setting, such as while riding in your car?
5. How hard would it be for you to consistently use condoms with a partner *every time* you have a one-night stand?
6. How hard would it be for you to use a condom with your partner while under the influence of alcohol or drugs?
7. How hard would it be for you to avoid using alcohol or drugs if you think you might be having sex later?

Please circle how *effectively* or *ineffectively* you feel you could do each of the following things.

8. How effectively could you discuss safer sex (such as using latex condoms) with your partner before having sex with them?[e]

9. How effectively could you refuse to have unsafe sexual intercourse? (Note: unsafe sexual intercourse means (1) penis-in-vagina intercourse, no condom; or (2) penis-in-rectum intercourse, no condom).
10. If you were about to have sex, how effectively could you show your partner nonverbally (for example, through body movements) that you want to practice only safer sex?
11. How effectively could you tell your partner through a joke or a "one-liner" that you want to practice only safer sex?
12. How effectively could you convince your partner to practice only safer sex?
13. How effectively could you convince your partner to use a condom for *vaginal sex*?
14. How effectively could you convince your partner to use a condom (or other latex barrier) for *oral sex*?
15. How effectively could you plan ahead to be sure you always have condoms on hand whenever you have sex?
16. How effectively could you make safer sex (using a latex condom) enjoyable for your partner?
17. How effectively could you make your partner feel good about using condoms during *vaginal intercourse*?
18. How effectively could you make your partner feel good about using condoms (or another latex barrier) during *oral sex*?
19. How effectively could you refuse to have *oral sex* without a condom or other latex barrier?

> For the items below, we want you to answer as if you were *currently in a long-term relationship,* in which you have been having sexual intercourse *without* using condoms (e.g., if you or your partner are using birth control pills).

20. How effectively could you discuss initiating safer sexual practices (e.g., using a latex condom) with your partner?
21. How effectively could you persuade your partner to begin practicing only safer sex (sex with a latex condom) with you?
22. If you were able to persuade your partner to begin using latex condoms with you, how hard would it be for you to continue using condoms *every time* you have sexual intercourse until both of you get an HIV blood test?[d]
23. How effectively could you persuade your partner to get an HIV blood test with you?

> For the items below, we want you to answer as if you were *currently in a long-term relationship,* in which you have been having sexual intercourse *with* a condom.

24. How effectively could you persuade your partner to continue to use condoms with you *every time* you have sexual intercourse?
25. How hard would it be for you to continue using condoms with your partner *every time* you have sexual intercourse until both of you get an HIV blood test?[d]

> Imagine that you are in your room with an attractive person whom you have recently met and you like very much. It is clear from their behavior that they want to have sexual intercourse with you, and you also want to have sex with them. However, when you have sex you want you and your partner to use a condom to reduce both of your risk of becoming infected with the virus that causes AIDS.

26. How effectively could you discuss safer sexual practices with this new partner before having sex with them?
27. How effectively could you persuade them to practice only safer sex (sex with a condom) with you?
28. If you were about to have sex, how effectively could you show them nonverbally (for example, through body movements) that you want to practice only safer sex?
29. How effectively could you tell them through a joke or a "one-liner" that you want to practice only safer sex?
30. How effectively do you think you could use a condom without discussing it at all with them, by just putting it on before sex?
31. Overall, how effectively could you make sure that a condom is used?
32. If no condom is available, instead of having intercourse, how hard would it be for you to engage in another pleasurable activity (such as mutual masturbation) where a condom isn't needed?[d]
33. If no condom is available, how hard would it be for you to stop sexual activity while you or your partner go to get a condom?[d]

> Now imagine that your attractive partner who you've recently met says that using a condom is unnecessary, because one of you is on the pill. You still want to use a condom because of your concerns about getting the virus that causes AIDS.

34. How effectively do you think you could convince this partner that the two of you should use a condom, without making them refuse to have sex with you?

35. How effectively do you think you could negotiate a safer sexual alternative with them? For instance, if they refused to use a condom, how effectively could you convince them to engage in another sexual activity, such as mutual masturbation?

36. How hard would it be for you to refuse to have sex with them if they refused to use a condom with you?[d]

We would like you to tell us whether you have done each of the following things during the time interval which is indicated.

---

1. Have you had *sexual intercourse* (sex in which the penis is put into the vagina, or sex where the penis is put into the rectum) at all during the past *month*?

   Circle one:

   Yes: I have had sexual intercourse   **No:** I have not had sexual intercourse
   during the past *month*.   during the past *month*.

2. Have you ever had sexual intercourse during your lifetime?

   Circle one: Yes   No

3. Please circle *any* of the alternatives below that apply to both you and your sexual partner(s) during the past *month*.
   A. Both I and all my sexual partners have tested HIV negative.
   B. Both I and my sexual partner have never had any other sexual partners.
   C. Neither of the above are true for me and my partner(s) during the past month.
   D. I have not had any sexual partners during the past month.

4. Are you in a close relationship involving sexual intercourse?

   Circle one: Yes   No

5. If you answered "Yes" to number 4 (above), is your relationship with your partner monogamous (neither of you has sexual intercourse with other people)?

   Circle one:
   Yes   No   Uncertain   Not applicable: I was not in a close sexual relationship.

6. I have discussed safer sex with a sexual partner (or sexual partners) before having sex with them during the past *month*.

   Circle one:
   Yes   No   Not applicable: I have not had sexual intercourse during the past month.

7. I have bought latex condoms during the past *month*.

   Circle one:
   Often   A few times   Once   Never

8. I kept latex condoms some place nearby where they were easily available during the past *month*.

   Circle one:
   Always   Often   Sometimes   Rarely   Never

9. My partner(s) and I have used latex condoms when having *sexual intercourse* (sex in which the penis is put into the vagina, or sex where the penis is put into the rectum) during the past *month*.

   Circle one:
   Never   Rarely   Sometimes   Often   Always   Not applicable: I have not had sexual
                                                        intercourse during the past month.

Fill in Number Below

10. How many different people have you had vaginal intercourse (penis-in-vagina) with during the last month?	
11. With how many of these partners were condoms used *all the time*?	
12. How many of these partners had an AIDS blood test and you knew they had not been exposed to the virus that causes AIDS?	

13. When you had *vaginal intercourse* during the past *month*, how often were condoms used?

   Circle one:
   Never   Rarely   Sometimes   Often   Always   Not applicable: I have not had vaginal
                                                        intercourse during the past month.

14. When you had *vaginal intercourse* during the past *month*, what percentage of the time were condoms used?

   _____ %   Not applicable: I have not had vaginal intercourse during the past month.

Fill in Number Below

15. How many different people have you had *anal intercourse* (penis-in-rectum) with during the last month?	
16. With how many of these partners were condoms used *all the time*?	
17. How many of these partners had an AIDS blood test and you knew they had not been exposed to the virus that causes AIDS?	

18. When you had *anal intercourse* during the past *month*, how often were condoms used?
    Circle one:
    Never   Rarely   Sometimes   Often   Always   Not applicable: I have not had anal intercourse
    during the past month.

19. I have tried to convince or persuade my sex partner(s) to practice only safer sex (always using condoms) during the past *month*.
    Circle one:
    Always   Sometimes   Never   Not applicable: I have not had sex   Does not apply: My partner has
    during the past month.   wanted to have only safer sex
    (always using a latex condom)
    during the past month.

20. *Circle the letter which applies to you:*
    A.   I have sex only with men.
    B.   I have sex with both men and women.
    C.   I have sex only with women.
    D.   I don't have sexual intercourse.

The following questions concern having a blood test to find out if you have been exposed to the virus that causes AIDS.

21. I have had a blood test to check whether I have been exposed to the virus that causes AIDS during the past *month*.
    Circle one:
    Yes   No   Not applicable: I have never had sexual intercourse or used injection drugs.

22. I have made an appointment to get a blood test to check whether I have been exposed to the virus that causes AIDS during the past *month*.
    Circle one:
    Yes   No   Not applicable: I have never had sexual intercourse or used injection drugs.

23. At *some time in the past*, I have had a blood test to determine whether I have been exposed to the virus that causes AIDS.
    Circle one: Yes   No

24. If you had a blood test for the virus that causes AIDS, where did you have this blood test?
    Circle the letter which applies to you:
    A.   Anonymous test site (you don't give your name)
    B.   Confidential test site (you give your name, but it is kept confidential)
    C.   Doctor's office
    D.   Through the military or ROTC
    E.   Blood donation
    F.   Other

a. Each item is followed by 1 2 3 4 5.

b. See the text for an explanation.

c. This item is followed by the good-bad, awful-nice, and pleasant-unpleasant scales.

d. Each item is followed by the following five options: *very hard to do, fairly hard to do, neither hard nor easy to do, fairly easy to do,* and *very easy to do.*

e. Each item is followed by the following five options: *very effectively, somewhat effectively, neither effectively nor ineffectively, somewhat effectively,* and *very effectively.*

Beliefs About AIDS Questionnaire

Philip R. Nader,[1] *University of California, San Diego*

The Beliefs About AIDS Questionnaire (Nader, Wexler, Patterson, McKusick, & Coates, 1989) was developed to assess adolescents' beliefs and attitudes about AIDS. The scale specifically examines perceptions of personal susceptibility and peer norms related to risky sexual behavior, in addition to knowledge about AIDS transmission. The questionnaire was developed for the American Social Health Association to assist in development of an AIDS education project.

Description

The Beliefs About AIDS Questionnaire consists of 14 items, with responses indicated on a 6-point Likert-type scale. The items were theoretically derived to reflect four constructs: (a) knowledge of and agreement with health guidelines concerning AIDS transmission (5 items), (b) perceived personal threat of contracting AIDS (4 items), (c) personal efficacy for preventing infection of self or others (2 items), and (d) perceived peer norms regarding risky sexual behaviors (3 items). A group of AIDS educators developed the items.

Response Mode and Timing

Respondents answer each item on a 6-point Likert-type scale ranging from *strongly disagree* to *strongly agree*. No time limit for completion is indicated. With only 14 items, most respondents should be able to complete the questionnaire in less than 5 minutes.

[1] Address correspondence to Philip R. Nader, Child and Family Health Studies, Department of Pediatrics, M-031F, University of California, San Diego, La Jolla, CA 92093-0631; email: pnader@ucsd.edu. This chapter was prepared by Robert Bauserman.

Scoring

Separate scores are calculated for each of the four theoretically derived scales. All items are scored in the same direction, except for two items on the Perceived Threat scale (belief that AIDS does not affect high school students and belief that AIDS affects only gay men and IV drug users).

Reliability and Validity

The authors report that the questionnaire has acceptable test-retest reliability. The items were tested in two administrations with more than 2,000 high school students.

The Beliefs About AIDS Questionnaire has face validity. Other evidence for validity comes from a large-scale survey conducted for a pilot AIDS education project (Nader et al., 1989), including 1,341 urban high school students and three additional opportunistic samples of adolescents: 131 students from affluent, suburban private high schools; 74 youths incarcerated in a detention facility; and 26 members of a gay youth group. Incarcerated youths scored lower than the other groups on all four scales, indicating less knowledge of transmission and health guidelines, less perceived personal threat, lower personal efficacy to avoid infection, and lower levels (norms) of safe sex practices among their peers. In contrast, gay youths perceived significantly higher levels of safe sex norms among peers than did urban high school youths, and scored higher than the other groups as well. Both urban and suburban youths fell between the other two groups on all scales, although the differences were not statistically significant.

Reference

Nader, P. R., Wexler, D. B., Patterson, T. L., McKusick, L., & Coates, T. (1989). Comparison of beliefs about AIDS among urban, suburban, incarcerated, and gay adolescents. *Journal of Adolescent Health Care, 10,* 413-418.

Exhibit

Beliefs About AIDS Questionnaire (sample items)

For this section, we are interested in your opinions: thus please do not be concerned whether your answers are right or wrong. This is not a test. Circle the number next to each statement that best describes your agreement or disagreement with that statement.

I.   Agreement with health guidelines
     The risk of getting AIDS increases as the number of partners increases.[a]
II. Perceived threat
     I am fearful of getting AIDS.
III. Personal efficacy
     I can do the things necessary to prevent my getting the AIDS virus.
IV. Perceived norms
     My friends support the idea of avoiding risky sexual activity.

a. Each item is followed by a 6-point (*strongly disagree* to *strongly agree*) scale.

AIDS-Contact Scale

Joseph H. Pleck,[1] *University of Illinois at Urbana-Champaign*

Persons with AIDS now require care in many health institutions. Within any specific institution, however, individual staff will vary in the extent and the nature of contact. These differences may be due to the structure of their jobs or to personal preferences. The AIDS-Contact Scale (O'Donnell, O'Donnell, Pleck, Snarey, & Rose, 1987; Pleck, O'Donnell, O'Donnell, & Snarey, 1988), designed for health care workers, assesses the degree of contact with persons with AIDS. This measure could be useful to survey levels of contact among different staff groups and to assess staff self-selection into groups of varying contact.

Description

The AIDS-Contact Scale is a 15-item, self-administered questionnaire concerning the number of different AIDS patients seen, time spent with AIDS patients, the number of contacts with family and friends of patients, and the

frequency of a variety of specific physical contact (touching, handling bedclothes, handling blood and other fluids, and handling equipment contaminated by such fluids) and social contact (general conversation with patients, discussion of physical and emotional problems related to the disease). Items 1-4 require respondents to estimate their amount of contact with AIDS patients, their friends, and their relatives on several different dimensions (e.g., amount of time per week spent with AIDS patients). For Items 5-15, participants use a 4-point Likert-type scale (1 = *never* to 4 = *often*) to indicate frequency of contact with AIDS and AIDS patients in a variety of settings.

Response Mode and Timing

The AIDS-Contact Scale is a self-administered instrument. For Items 1-4, participants report numbers to indicate the number of AIDS patients seen, hours per week spent with AIDS patients, percentage of time spent with AIDS patients, and number of interactions with families or friends of AIDS patients. For Items 5-15, participants can circle a number from 1 to 4 to indicate the extent of contact with AIDS, AIDS patients, and their families. The scale requires approximately 5 minutes to complete.

[1]Address correspondence to Joseph H. Pleck, Division of Human Development and Family Studies, University of Illinois at Urbana-Champaign, Bevier Hall 155, MC-180, 905 S. Goodwin, Urbana, IL 61801; email: jhpleck@uiuc.edu.

Scoring

A higher score indicates greater AIDS contact. Items 1-4 are standardized so they have a standard deviation of 1. In the validation test sample, the remaining items had standard deviations that varied around the value of 1. Therefore, with Items 1-4 standardized, the items contribute equally to the scale score. The mean of all 15 items represents the score for the scale.

Reliability

The AIDS-Contact Scale was derived empirically from a larger pool of items. Starting with the conceptually core items from the pool, further items from the pool were added until no meaningful increment in internal reliability (as assessed by coefficient alpha) resulted. In a sample of 237 hospital workers at a hospital caring for AIDS patients, Cronbach's alpha for the 8-item scale was .83.

Validity

Pleck et al. (1988) found that the mean score of the AIDS-Contact Scale is significantly negatively correlated with the AIDS-Phobia Scale score ($r = -.23$, $p < .01$) and the AIDS-Stress Scale score ($r = -.25$, $p < .01$) (described elsewhere in this volume). In multivariate analyses, AIDS contact is associated with being in a job other than social services ($b = -.48$, $p = .01$) and holding negative attitudes toward AIDS ($b = -.31$, $p = .01$). AIDS contact is a significant predictor of both AIDS phobia ($b = -.13$, $p = .05$) and AIDS stress ($b = -.22$, $p = .01$).

References

O'Donnell, L., O'Donnell, C., Pleck, J. H., Snarey, J., & Rose, R. (1987). Psychological responses of hospital workers to acquired immune deficiency syndrome (AIDS). *Journal of Applied Sociology, 17*, 269-285.

Pleck, J. H., O'Donnell, L., O'Donnell, C., & Snarey, J. (1988). AIDS-phobia, contact with AIDS, and AIDS-related job stress in hospital workers. *Journal of Homosexuality, 15*, 41-54.

Exhibit

AIDS-Contact Scale

Instructions: Listed below you will find a list of questions regarding your amount of contact with AIDS, people with AIDS, and with family and friends of people with AIDS. In the space provided, please provide the response that best represents your experience.[a]

1. Over the past year, approximately how many AIDS patients have you seen?
2. Over the past month, on the average, about how much time per week have you spent with AIDS patients?
3. Over the past year, what percentage of your time would you say you've spent with AIDS patients?
4. Over the past year, approximately how many interactions have you had with the families or friends of AIDS patients?
5. Overall, how frequent would you say you interact with AIDS patients?
6. Regarding AIDS patients themselves, how often do you work in the same room?
7. Regarding AIDS patients themselves, how often do you come into direct physical contact (e.g., touch)?
8. Regarding AIDS patients themselves, how often do you handle bedclothes?
9. Regarding AIDS patients themselves, how often do you obtain and/or handle blood?
10. Regarding AIDS patients themselves, how often do you handle sputum, urine, or feces?
11. Regarding AIDS patients themselves, how often do you handle equipment which has come into contact with body fluids?
12. In terms of more social contact, how often do you have general conversations with AIDS patients?
13. How often do you talk about physical problems or diseases with AIDS patients?
14. How often do you talk about emotional problems related to the disease with AIDS patients?
15. How often do you talk with family/friends of AIDS patients?

a. For Items 1-4 respondents fill in a number. For the remaining items, respondents use a 4-point Likert-type scale, where 1 = *never*, 2 = *rarely*, 3 = *sometimes*, and 4 = *often*.

AIDS-Phobia Scale

Joseph H. Pleck,[1] *University of Illinois at Urbana-Champaign*

The AIDS-Phobia Scale (O'Donnell, O'Donnell, Pleck, Snarey, & Rose, 1987; Pleck, O'Donnell, O'Donnell, & Snarey, 1988) was developed to assess attitudes toward AIDS and persons with AIDS. Persons with AIDS have become a socially stigmatized group. As a result, many individuals have negative attitudes toward AIDS and actively avoid persons with AIDS. If individuals are in occupational roles that require contact with persons with AIDS, holding such negative attitudes could lead to increased stress and avoidance.

Description

The AIDS-Phobia Scale is a 16-item, self-administered questionnaire concerning perceptions of AIDS and persons with AIDS in general, as well as attitudes about the exclusion of persons with AIDS from certain jobs, and issues about AIDS directly relevant to health care workers. Using a 7-point Likert-type scale, respondents indicate the extent to which they agree (1 = *strongly agree*, 4 = *no opinion*, 7 = *strongly disagree*) with each of 12 statements. Respondents then answer three further questions regarding these issues, choosing from *yes*, *no*, or *don't know*. A final question asks, given the growing number of AIDS cases, how the participant's level of tolerance concerning homosexuality has changed with response options from *more tolerant*, *no change*, and *less tolerant*.

Response Mode and Timing

The AIDS-Phobia Scale is a self-administered instrument. For Items 1-12, respondents can circle the number from 1 to 7 corresponding to their degree of agreement. They can circle *yes*, *no*, or *don't know* for Items 13-15 and *more tolerant*, *no change*, or *less tolerant* for Item 16. The scale requires approximately 5 minutes to complete.

Scoring

So that a higher score indicates a greater degree of AIDS phobia, responses to Items 1, 3, 4, 5, 6, 7, 8, and 10 are reversed so that 1 = *strongly disagree* and 7 = *strongly agree*. For Items 13-16, which have three response catego-

ries each, the coding is adjusted so these item responses have the same range (7 points) as Items 1-12 and therefore contribute equally to the overall scale score. For Items 13-15, *yes* is coded 1, *no* is coded 7, and *don't know* is assigned the midpoint value of 4. For Item 16, *more tolerant* is coded 1, *no change* is coded 4, and *less tolerant* is coded 7. The mean of all 16 items represents the score for the scale.

Reliability

The AIDS-Phobia Scale was derived empirically from a larger pool of items. Starting with the conceptually core items from the pool, further items from the pool were added until no meaningful increment in internal reliability (as assessed by coefficient alpha) resulted. In a sample of 237 hospital workers at a hospital caring for AIDS patients, the Cronbach alpha for the 16-item scale was .76.

Validity

Pleck et al. (1988) found that the mean score of the AIDS-Phobia Scale was significantly negatively correlated with the AIDS-Contact Scale score ($r = -.23, p < .01$), and significantly positively correlated with the AIDS-Stress Scale score ($r = .54, p < .01$) (described elsewhere in this volume). Hierarchical multiple regression analyses showed homophobia to be the single strongest predictor of AIDS phobia ($b = .54, p < .01$). Additionally, AIDS phobia was found to be a statistically significant predictor of AIDS contact ($b = -.31, p < .01$) and AIDS stress ($b = .48, p < .01$). With AIDS phobia in the model, homophobia accounts for no additional variance in these outcomes.

References

O'Donnell, L., O'Donnell, C., Pleck, J. H., Snarey, J., & Rose, R. (1987). Psychological responses of hospital workers to acquired immune deficiency syndrome (AIDS). *Journal of Applied Social Psychology, 17*, 269-285.

Pleck, J. H., O'Donnell, L., O'Donnell, C., & Snarey, J. (1988). AIDS-phobia, contact with AIDS, and AIDS-related job stress in hospital workers. *Journal of Homosexuality, 15*, 41-54.

[1]Address correspondence to Joseph H. Pleck, Division of Human Development and Family Studies, University of Illinois at Urbana-Champaign, Bevier Hall 155, MC-180, 905 S. Goodwin, Urbana, IL 61801; email: jhpleck@uiuc.edu.

Exhibit

AIDS-Phobia Scale

Instructions: Listed below you will find a list of statements and questions regarding AIDS and people with AIDS. For numbers 1-12, please indicate the degree to which you agree or disagree with the statement. For numbers 13-16, please circle the response that best represents your opinion.[a]

1. A hospital worker should not be required to work with AIDS patients.
2. AIDS patients have as much right to quality medical care as anyone else.
3. AIDS makes my job a high risk occupation.
4. AIDS is God's punishment for immorality.
5. Dealing with AIDS patients is different than dealing with other types of patients.
6. The high cost of treating AIDS patients is unfair to other people in need of care.
7. AIDS patients offend me morally.
8. If I learned someone I knew had AIDS, it would be hard for me to continue my relationship with him or her.
9. Having a co-worker who had AIDS would not bother me.
10. If I got AIDS, I would worry that other people would think I was a homosexual.
11. Working with AIDS patients can be a rewarding experience.
12. It's important to go out of your way to be helpful to a patient with AIDS.
13. Do you think people with AIDS should be allowed to work in public schools?
14. Do you think people with AIDS should be allowed to handle food in restaurants?
15. Do you think people with AIDS should be allowed to work with patients in hospitals?
16. Has the growing number of AIDS cases made you more tolerant, less tolerant, or not changed your attitude at all about homosexuality?

a. For Items 1-12, respondents use a Likert-type scale where 1 = *strongly agree*, 2 = *somewhat agree*, 3 = *slightly agree*, 4 = *no opinion*, 5 = *slightly disagree*, 6 = *somewhat disagree*, and 7 = *strongly disagree*. For Items 13-15, respondents choose between *yes, no,* and *don't know*. For Item 16, respondents choose between *more tolerant, no change,* and *less tolerant*.

AIDS-Stress Scale

Joseph H. Pleck,[1] *University of Illinois at Urbana-Champaign*

The AIDS-Stress Scale (O'Donnell, O'Donnell, Pleck, Snarey, & Rose, 1987; Pleck, O'Donnell, O'Donnell, & Snarey, 1988) was developed to assess the challenges posed to health care workers as a result of working with AIDS and persons with AIDS. Health care workers may find themselves treating individuals with AIDS who have lifestyles and values quite different from their own. Differences such as these between patient and health care provider have been shown to be stressful for both parties (Graham & Reeder, 1972). Additionally, the increasing

[1]Address correspondence to Joseph H. Pleck, Division of Human Development and Family Studies, University of Illinois at Urbana-Champaign, Bevier Hall 155, MC-180, 905 S. Goodwin, Urbana, IL 61801; email: jhpleck@uiuc.edu.

disability and eventual death of persons with AIDS, so many of whom are relatively young, can have a demoralizing effect on medical personnel, causing them to withdraw from such patients or to suffer from feelings of frustration and helplessness. Also, the high mortality rate associated with AIDS and the potential transmissibility of the disease via body fluids creates a situation in which staff perceive themselves to be at risk for developing AIDS by virtue of direct contact with patients or clinical specimens. This can lead to fear when caring for persons with AIDS and anger at having to do so.

Description

The AIDS-Stress Scale is an 8-item, self-administered questionnaire concerning the experience, by health care workers, of stress related to contact with AIDS patients. Using a 4-point Likert-type scale, respondents indicate their degree of comfort with AIDS patients and with friends and family of persons with AIDS, as well as the degree of risk they perceive as a result of their jobs. Respondents also answer 5 *yes-no* questions regarding stress of working with AIDS patients and whether they feel their knowledge is sufficient to deal with the physical and emotional needs of AIDS patients and with the family and friends of patients.

Response Mode and Timing

The AIDS-Stress Scale is a self-administered instrument. For Items 1, 2, 6, 7, and 8, respondents can circle *yes* or *no*. For Items 3 and 4, respondents can circle a number from 1 to 4 to indicate the degree to which they feel comfortable in a given situation and, for Item 5, to indicate the amount of risk they perceive in their jobs. The scale requires approximately 5 minutes to complete.

Scoring

For Items 1-2 and 6-8, which have two response categories each, the answers are coded 1 = *yes* to 4 = *no* so these item responses have the same range (4 points) as Items 3-5 and therefore contribute equally to the overall scale score. So that high score indicates a greater degree of AIDS stress, Items 1, 2, 3, and 4 are reverse scored. The mean of all eight items represents the score for the scale.

Reliability

The AIDS-Stress Scale was derived empirically from a larger pool of items. Starting with the conceptually core items from the pool, further items from the pool were added until no meaningful increment in internal reliability (as assessed by coefficient alpha) resulted. In a sample of 237 hospital workers at a hospital caring for AIDS patients, Cronbach's alpha for the 8-item scale was .668.

Validity

Pleck et al. (1988) found that the mean score of the AIDS-Stress Scale was significantly negatively correlated with AIDS-Contact Scale score ($r = -.25$, $p < .01$) and significantly positively correlated with the AIDS-Phobia Scale score ($r = .54$, $p < .01$) (described elsewhere in this volume). In multivariate analyses, AIDS stress is associated with being an LPN/aide or technical service worker ($b = .18$, $p = .01$ and $b = .18$, $p = .01$, respectively), having low contact with AIDS ($b = -.13$, $p = .01$), and being AIDS phobic ($b = .48$, $p = .01$).

References

Graham, S., & Reeder, L. G. (1972). Social factors in chronic illness. In H. E. Freeman, S. Levine, & L. G. Reeder (Eds.), *Handbook of medical sociology* (pp. 63-107). Englewood Cliffs, NJ: Prentice Hall.

O'Donnell, L., O'Donnell, C., Pleck, J. H., Snarey, J., & Rose, R. (1987). Psychological responses of hospital workers to acquired immune deficiency syndrome (AIDS). *Journal of Applied Social Psychology, 17,* 269-285.

Pleck, J. H., O'Donnell, L., O'Donnell, C., & Snarey, J. (1988). AIDS-phobia, contact with AIDS, and AIDS-related job stress in hospital workers. *Journal of Homosexuality, 15,* 41-54.

Exhibit

AIDS-Stress Scale

Instructions: Listed below you will find a list of questions regarding AIDS and people with AIDS. Please circle the response that best represents your answer.[a]

1. Do you feel that working with AIDS patients is one of the more stressful parts of your job?
2. Do you think it will be hard for you to deal with a larger number of AIDS patients in the future?
3. On a scale of 1 to 4, where 1 is *not comfortable at all* and 4 is *very comfortable,* how comfortable would you say you are with AIDS patients?
4. How comfortable would you say you are with friends and families of AIDS patients?
5. On a scale of 1 to 4, where 1 is *no risk at all* and 4 is *high risk,* how much risk to do you think *you* have of getting AIDS because of your job?
6. Do you feel the knowledge you have is sufficient to deal with the physical needs of AIDS patients?
7. Do you feel the knowledge you have is sufficient to deal with the emotional needs of AIDS patients?
8. Do you feel the knowledge you have is sufficient to deal with the families and friends of AIDS patients?

a. For Items 1-2 and 6-8, respondents choose between *yes* and *no.* For the remaining items, respondents use a Likert-type scale ranging from 1 to 4. For Items 3 and 4, 1 = *not comfortable at all,* 2 = *somewhat uncomfortable,* 3 = *somewhat comfortable,* and 4 = *very comfortable.* For Item 5, 1 = *no risk at all,* 2 = *very little risk,* 3 = *some risk,* and 4 = *high risk.*

The Nurses' Attitudes About AIDS Scale

Deborah Bray Preston,[1] *Pennsylvania State University*
Elaine Wilson Young, *Massachusetts General Hospital Institute
    of Health Professions*
Patricia Barthalow Koch, *Pennsylvania State University*

Caring for HIV-positive individuals and AIDS patients and providing AIDS education and counseling are central to the nursing profession. Nurses' attitudes may affect their caregiving (Koch, Preston, Young, & Wang, 1991). Therefore, crucial to research about nursing practice regarding AIDS is the development of a sound, theoretically based, empirically tested instrument to measure nurses' attitudes about AIDS and persons with AIDS (PWAs). The Nurses' Attitudes About AIDS Scale (NAAS) was developed to meet this need (Preston, Young, Koch, & Forti, 1995). Suggested applications of the NAAS are (a) as a descriptive tool to investigate AIDS-related attitudes in a variety of nursing populations; (b) as a means of describing models of nursing practice behavior related to PWAs; (c) as a means of predicting practice outcomes related to care of PWAs in varying nursing populations, specifically the use of universal precautions; (d) as a needs assessment for educational programming related to AIDS; and (e) as an evaluative tool to assess attitude change as the result of educational programming.

Description

The NAAS contains 53 attitudinal statements to which the respondent can reply on a Likert-type scale from 1 = *strongly agree* to 5 = *strongly disagree*. Principal axis factor analysis, using a varimax rotation, has established two subject areas and three subscales with a purposive sample of 731 working RNs. Part One of the NAAS is composed of two subscales. The first consists of 12 questions related to attitudes concerning AIDS and society in general (Societal Concerns), and the other subscale consists of 13 questions related to attitudes concerning AIDS and nursing practice (Nursing Care Concerns). These two factors accounted for 32% of the explained variance. Part Two contains 28 questions related to attitudes toward homosexuality, accounting for 45% of the explained variance. Further development of the scale is under way involving the testing of items that represent attitudes toward intravenous drug users and women with AIDS (Preston & Romeo, 1993).

Response Mode and Timing

Respondents choose the response (1 = *strongly agree*, 2 = *agree*, 3 = *neither agree nor disagree*, 4 = *disagree*, and 5 = *strongly disagree*) that best reflects their attitude toward each statement. The scale requires approximately 20 minutes to complete.

Scoring

A score of 53 indicates low tolerance or unfavorable attitudes concerning AIDS issues and homosexuality, and a score of 165 indicates high tolerance or favorable attitudes. Many items need to be reverse scored.

Reliability

A purposive sample of 731 working RNs established the Cronbach alpha coefficient for the Societal Concerns subscale at .72, the Nursing Care Concerns subscale at .83, and the Homosexuality subscale at .96 (Preston et al., 1995).

Validity

Establishing content validity was begun by developing 273 attitudinal statements, using the Ajzen and Fishbein (1980) model, representing opinions, feelings, and judgments about AIDS and PWAs. These items were evaluated by a panel of 10 nurses practicing in several nursing settings and 7 experts in the areas of AIDS education and attitude measurement. Thirty-three practicing nurses then reviewed the shortened and revised instrument for clarity and readability. Construct validity was established using the principal components factor analysis, described above, on the responses of 731 nurses. Criterion validity of the NAAS was evaluated by relating scores on all three subscales to respondents' willingness to care for PWAs, which had been found to be a criterion variable for positive attitudes in previous research (Barrick, 1988). Examining the responses from the sample of 731 nurses, those who stated they were willing to care for PWAs held significantly more favorable attitudes on all three subscales than those who stated they were not willing.

Other Information

Requests for permission to use the NAAS should be sent to Deborah B. Preston, School of Nursing, Pennsylvania State University, University Park, PA 16802.

---

[1]Address correspondence to Deborah B. Preston, School of Nursing, Pennsylvania State University, University Park, PA 16802.

References

Ajzen, I., & Fishbein, M. (1980). *Understanding attitudes and predicting social behavior.* Englewood Cliffs, NJ: Prentice Hall.

Barrick, B. (1988). The willingness of nursing personnel to care for patients with acquired immune deficiency syndrome: A survey and recommendations. *Journal of Professional Nursing, 4,* 366-372.

Koch, P. B., Preston, D. B., Young, E. W., & Wang, M. Q. (1991). Factors associated with AIDS-related attitudes among rural nurses. *Health Values, 15*(6), 32-40.

Preston, D. B., & Romeo, K. (1993). *Nurses and AIDS: A comparison of urban and rural practice in acute-care settings.* Proposal to the Northeast Regional Center for Rural Development, University Park, PA.

Preston, D. B., Young, E. W., Koch, P. B., & Forti, E. M. (1995). The Nurses' Attitudes About AIDS Scale (NAAS): Development and psychometric analysis. *AIDS Education and Prevention, 7,* 443-454.

Exhibit

The Nurses' Attitudes About AIDS Scale (sample items)

Following are examples of the 53 questions from the three subscales. Respondents indicate whether they strongly agree or strongly disagree with the statements.

Societal Concerns Subscale

Civil rights laws should be enacted to protect people with AIDS from job and housing discrimination.

Public school officials should not be required to accept an AIDS child into classes.

Nursing Care Concerns Subscale

I feel worried about the possibility of acquiring AIDS from patients.

Homosexuality Subscale

Male homosexuality should be considered immoral.

Homosexual men are mistreated in our society.

AIDS Attitude Scale

Jacque Shrum, Norma Turner, and Katherine Bruce,[1]
University of North Carolina at Wilmington

The purpose of the AIDS Attitude Scale (AAS) is to measure attitudes about AIDS and people who have AIDS or HIV infection. The scale can be used to discriminate people who are more empathetic or tolerant toward people who have HIV infection from those who are less tolerant or empathetic. Subject areas on the AAS include fears related to contagion and casual contact, moral issues, and topics related to legal and social welfare issues.

Description

This scale is a 54-item Likert-type scale (5 points) with response options labeled *strongly agree, agree, neither agree nor disagree, disagree,* and *strongly disagree.* The items on the scale were selected from an initial pool of 94 items written by undergraduate students in health education and nursing classes, or derived from literature review and interviews with experts knowledgeable about AIDS. They were reviewed for readability by five different undergraduate and graduate students and for acceptability for inclusion in the scale by a panel of four expert judges. The judges agreed on 67 of the original items for inclusion in the scale. The scale was administered to 164 undergraduate students in health education courses, and an item analysis was conducted to identify the statements that could best discriminate high and low scorers. Fifty-four items had statistically significant item-total correlations ($p < .001$). These items were arranged in random order, and the scale was tested for reliability. This scale was designed to measure students' attitudes about AIDS, but could be used for other populations.

Response Mode and Timing

Respondents circle or blacken one response option for each item on a separate answer sheet. Most respondents complete the scale within 15 minutes.

Scoring

The 25 tolerant items (2, 3, 5, 6, 9, 12, 14, 15, 19, 21, 22, 23, 24, 26, 28, 31, 32, 34, 36, 38, 41, 46, 51, 52, and 53) are scored such that *strongly agree* has a value of 5, *agree* a value of 4, and so forth. For the intolerant items (1, 4, 7, 8, 10, 11, 13, 16, 17, 18, 20, 25, 27, 29, 30, 33, 35, 37, 39, 40, 42, 43, 44, 45, 47, 48, 49, 50, and 54), reverse scoring is used. The total attitude score is obtained by the following formula: AAS score = $(X - N)\ (100)/(N)\ (4)$,

where X is the total of the scored responses and N is the number of items properly complete. Scores may range from 0 to 100; higher scores indicate more empathy or tolerance related to AIDS and people who have AIDS.

Reliability

To measure internal consistency (split-half reliability), 135 undergraduates completed the scale. Reliability was high (Cronbach's alpha = .96; Shrum, Turner, & Bruce, 1989).

Validity

Content and face validity were evaluated by a panel of four expert judges: a social worker, a university health educator, a health education faculty member, and an experimental psychologist. Experts were chosen because of their expertise related to AIDS, either in education, counseling, or support services, or related to attitude scale development. The panel assessed the relevance of each item, as well as the content of the entire scale (Shrum et al., 1989). Evidence for construct validity through factor analysis shows three consistent factors related to contagion concerns, moral issues, and legal/social welfare issues. These account for over 40% of the variance (Bruce, Shrum, Trefethen, & Slovik, 1990; Shrum et al., 1989). Evidence for known-groups, convergent, and discriminant validity of the AAS has been documented by Bruce and Reid (1995).

Other Information

The scale is published in its entirety in Shrum et al. (1989). In the original scale, *AIDS* was used throughout the scale. Now half of the references to AIDS have been changed to *HIV infection* as more appropriate.

References

Bruce, K., & Moineau, S. (1991). A comparison of sexually transmitted disease clinic patients and undergraduates: Implications for AIDS prevention and education. *Health Values, 15,* 5-12.

Bruce, K., Pilgrim, C., & Spivey, R. (1994). Assessing the impact of Magic Johnson's HIV positive announcement on a university campus. *Journal of Sex Education and Therapy, 20,* 264-276.

Bruce, K., & Reid, B. (1995, March). *The AIDS Attitude Scale: Validity assessment.* Paper presented at the 41st annual meeting of the Southeastern Psychological Association, Savannah, GA.

Bruce, K., Shrum, J., Trefethen, C., & Slovik, L. (1990). Students' attitudes about AIDS, homosexuality, and condoms. *AIDS Education and Prevention, 2,* 220-234.

Shrum, J., Turner, N., & Bruce, K. (1989). Development of an instrument to measure attitudes towards AIDS. *AIDS Education and Prevention, 1,* 222-230.

[1]Address correspondence to Katherine Bruce, Department of Psychology, UNC-Wilmington, 601 South College Road, Wilmington, NC 28403-3297; email: bruce@uncwil.edu.

Exhibit

AIDS Attitude Scale

Instructions: For each of the following statements, please note whether you agree or disagree with the statement. There are no correct answers, only your opinions. Use the following scale:

SA: Strongly agree with the statement
A: Agree with the statement
N: Neither agree nor disagree with the statement
D: Disagree with the statement
SD: Strongly disagree with the statement

1.   Limiting the spread of AIDS is more important than trying to protect the rights of people with AIDS.
2.   Support groups for people with HIV (Human Immunodeficiency Virus) infection would be very helpful to them.
3.   I would consider marrying someone with HIV infection.
4.   I would quit my job before I would work with someone who has AIDS.
5.   People should not be afraid of catching HIV from casual contact, like hugging or shaking hands.
6.   I would like to feel at ease around people with AIDS.
7.   People who receive positive results from the HIV blood test should not be allowed to get married.
8.   I would prefer not to be around homosexuals for fear of catching AIDS.
9.   Being around someone with AIDS would not put my health in danger.
10. Only disgusting people get HIV infection.
11. I think that people with HIV infection got what they deserved.
12. People with AIDS should not avoid being around other people.
13. People should avoid going to the dentist because they might catch HIV from dental instruments.
14. The thought of being around someone with AIDS does not bother me.
15. People with HIV infection should not be prohibited from working in public places.
16. I would not want to be in the same room with someone who I knew had AIDS.
17. The "gay plague" is an appropriate way to describe AIDS.
18. People who give HIV to others should face criminal charges.
19. People should not be afraid to donate blood because of AIDS.
20. A list of people who have HIV infection should be available to anyone.
21. I would date a person with AIDS.
22. People should not blame the homosexual community for the spread of HIV infection in the United States.
23. No one deserves to have a disease like HIV infection.
24. It would not bother me to attend class with someone who has AIDS.
25. An employer should have the right to fire an employee with HIV infection regardless of the type of work s/he does.
26. I would allow my children to play with the children of someone known to have AIDS.
27. People get AIDS by performing unnatural sex acts.
28. People with HIV should not be looked down upon by others.
29. I could tell by looking at someone if s/he had AIDS.
30. It is embarrassing to have so many people with HIV infection in our society.
31. Health care workers should not refuse to care for people with HIV infection regardless of their personal feelings about the disease.
32. Children who have AIDS should not be prohibited from going to schools or day care centers.
33. Children who have AIDS probably have a homosexual parent.
34. HIV blood test results should be confidential to avoid discrimination against people with positive results.
35. HIV infection is a punishment for immoral behavior.
36. I would not be afraid to take care of a family member with AIDS.
37. If I discovered that my roommate had AIDS, I would move out.
38. I would contribute money to an HIV infection research project if I were making a charitable contribution.
39. The best way to get rid of HIV infection is to get rid of homosexuality.
40. Churches should take a strong stand against drug abuse and homosexuality to prevent the spread of AIDS.
41. Insurance companies should not be allowed to cancel insurance policies for AIDS-related reasons.
42. Money being spent on HIV infection research should be spent instead on diseases that affect innocent people.
43. A person who gives HIV to someone else should be legally liable for any medical expenses.
44. The spread of AIDS in the United States is proof that homosexual behavior should be illegal.
45. A list of people who have HIV infection should be kept by the government.
46. I could comfortably discuss AIDS with others.

47. People with AIDS are not worth getting to know.
48. I have no sympathy for homosexuals who get HIV infection.
49. Parents who transmit HIV to their children should be prosecuted as child abusers.
50. People with AIDS should be sent to sanitariums to protect others from AIDS.
51. People would not be so afraid of AIDS if they knew more about the disease.
52. Hospitals and nursing homes should not refuse to admit patients with HIV infection.
53. I would not avoid a friend if s/he had AIDS.
54. The spread of HIV in our society illustrates how immoral the United States has become.

Source. This scale was originally published in "Development of an Instrument to Measure Attitudes Towards AIDS," by J. Shrum, N. Turner, and K. Bruce, 1989, *AIDS Education and Prevention, 1,* 222-230. Reprinted with permission.

The AIDS Discussion Strategy Scale

William E. Snell, Jr.,[1] *Southeast Missouri State University*

To gain insight into the nature of how people discuss sexual topics, such as AIDS, with a potential sex partner, Snell and Finney (1990) developed the AIDS Discussion Strategy Scale (ADSS), an objective self-report instrument designed to measure the types of interpersonal discussion strategies that women and men use if they want to discuss AIDS with an intimate partner. The ADSS was found to have subscales involving the use of six specific types of discussion tactics: *rational strategies,* defined as straightforward, reasonable attempts to discuss AIDS in a forthright manner with an intimate partner; *manipulative strategies,* defined as deceptive and indirect efforts to persuade an intimate partner to engage in conversation about AIDS; *withdrawal strategies,* defined as attempts to actually avoid any extended interpersonal contact with an intimate partner until this individual agrees to a discussion about AIDS; *charm strategies,* defined as acting in pleasant and charming ways toward an intimate partner to promote a discussion about AIDS; *subtlety strategies,* defined as involving the use of hinting and subtle suggestions to elicit a conversation about AIDS; and *persistence strategies,* defined as persistent and continuous attempts to try to influence an intimate partner to discuss AIDS.

Description

The ADSS consists of 72 items. Respondents answer the items using a 5-point Likert-type scale: −2 = *definitely would not do this,* −1 = *might not do this,* 0 = *not sure whether I would do this,* 1 = *might do this,* and 2 = *would definitely do this.* To determine whether the 72 items on the ADSS would form independent clusters of items, a principal components factor analysis with varimax rotation was conducted. Six factors with eigenvalues greater than 1 were extracted. Those items that loaded on unique factors (coefficients greater than .30) were used to construct six subscales for the ADSS. The number of items on the respective subscales were as follows: rational (26 items), manipulation (20 items), withdrawal (4 items), charm (5 items), subtlety (3 items), and persistence (4 items).

Response Mode and Timing

Respondents indicate their response on a computer scan sheet by darkening in a response from A to E for each item. The questionnaire usually requires about 45 minutes to complete.

Scoring

The labels and items for the ADSS subscales are Rational (Items 2, 4, 8, 9, 11, 12, 14, 16, 17, 18, 21, 23, 25, 28, 29, 31, 32, 35, 37, 43, 49, 53, 55, 61, 65, 67); Manipulation (Items 5, 6, 13, 20, 22, 24, 27, 38, 40, 42, 44, 45, 48, 52, 54, 57, 58, 69, 70, 72); Withdrawal (Items 39, 51, 56, 63);

[1]Address correspondence to William E. Snell, Jr., Department of Psychology, Southeast Missouri State University, One University Plaza, Cape Girardeau, MO 63701; email: wesnell@semovm.semo.edu.

Charm (Items 9, 36, 60, 64, 66); Subtlety (Items 3, 10, 50); and Persistence (Items (7, 41, 46, 47). The ADSS items are coded so that A = –2, B = –1, C = 0, D = +1, and E = +2 (no items are reverse coded). Then, the items on each subscale are averaged so that higher scores indicate a greater likelihood of using this type of AIDS-related discussion strategy.

Reliability

Reliability analyses were conducted on each subscale using Cronbach's alpha measure of interitem consistency. In two investigations reported by Snell and Finney (1990), all six subscales were found to have more than adequate internal consistency: rational (.96, .96), manipulation (.93, .92), withdrawal (.83, .85), charm (.81, .82), subtlety (.74, .66), and persistence (.81, .80).

Validity

Gender comparisons on the ADSS (Snell & Finney, 1990) indicate that females reported they would be more likely than males to use rational approaches to discuss AIDS with an intimate partner; that females were less likely than males to report that they would use manipulative tactics to persuade an intimate partner to discuss the topic of AIDS; and that females reported that they would be less likely than males to use charm to persuade an intimate partner to talk about AIDS. Although no other gender effects were found, it is informative to note that both males and females reported that they would use subtlety in trying to discuss AIDS with an intimate partner. By contrast, both males and females indicated that they would be less likely to use withdrawal tactics to elicit a discussion on AIDS with a close partner.

Correlations between the ADSS and the Stereotypes About AIDS Scale (Snell & Finney, 1990) indicated that people's use of AIDS-related discussion strategies were associated with their privately held stereotypes about AIDS. Also, people's willingness to use a variety of strategies to discuss the topics of AIDS with an intimate partner was associated with their own personal sexual dispositions, sexual attitudes, and sexual behaviors. Moreover, the pattern of findings indicated both some similar and some unique gender-related findings. For both males and females, the use of manipulative AIDS-related discussion strategies was directly related to their sexual traits (i.e., sexual depression and sexual preoccupation), their sexual attitudes (i.e., manipulative and casual sexual attitudes), and their sexual behaviors (i.e., an exchange orientation to sexual relations). Other gender similarities showed that both men and women who held sexually manipulative attitudes endorsed the use of charm as a tactic for discussing AIDS with a potential sexual partner, and both men and women whose orientation toward their sexual relations was based on mutual caring and concern reported that they would use persistence as a strategy for discussing AIDS with a potential sex partner. Although there was considerable similarity in the way that men's and women's sexual dispositions, attitudes, and behaviors affected their use of AIDS-related discussion strategies, other findings were more gender specific. For example, women with greater sexual esteem were more likely to report that they would use rational and less likely to use manipulation and charm as avenues for discussing AIDS. Among males, by contrast, sexual esteem was associated with less willingness to use charm to elicit a conversation about AIDS with a partner.

Reference

Snell, W. E., Jr., & Finney, P. D. (1990). Interpersonal strategies associated with the discussion of AIDS. *Annals of Sex Research, 3*, 425-451.

Exhibit

The AIDS Discussion Strategy Scale

Instructions: Suppose you wanted to talk to a potential or current sexual partner about AIDS. The following statements concern the types of things you might do if you wanted to discuss the topic of AIDS (Acquired Immune Deficiency Syndrome) with a sexual partner (either a current sexual partner or a future sexual partner). More specifically, we are interested in whether you would use each of the behaviors listed below. To provide your responses, use the following scale:

A	=	Definitely would not do this.
B	=	Might not do this.
C	=	Not sure whether I would do this.
D	=	Might do this.
E	=	Would definitely do this.

Remember: Be sure to respond to each and every statement; leave no blanks.

1. My partner and I would compromise about the aspects of the topic of AIDS we'd discuss.
2. I would try to reason with my partner to influence him/her to discuss AIDS.
3. I would drop hints about wanting to discuss the topic of AIDS.
4. I would simply tell my partner that I wanted to discuss AIDS with him/her.
5. I would put on a sweet face to induce my partner to discuss AIDS-related issues.

 6. I would try to get my partner to discuss AIDS by doing some fast talking.
 7. I would continually attempt to discuss the issue of AIDS.
 8. I would try to discuss AIDS with my partner.
 9. I would explain the reason that it's important for us to discuss AIDS.
10. I would subtly bring up the topic of AIDS.
11. I would state in a matter-of-fact way that I wanted to talk about AIDS.
12. I would try to look sincere to make the person more willing to talk about AIDS.
13. I would persuade my partner to discuss AIDS by telling some small white lies.
14. I would try to discuss the topic of AIDS, despite any obstacles from my partner.
15. I would try to negotiate what AIDS-related topics we'd be willing to discuss.
16. I would argue in a logical way that it's important for us to discuss AIDS.
17. I would make suggestions that we discuss AIDS.
18. I would simply ask to discuss AIDS with my partner.
19. I would try to put my partner in a good mood before trying to talk about AIDS.
20. I would use deception to get my partner to talk about AIDS.
21. I would talk with my partner about AIDS even if s/he didn't want to.
22. I would tell my sexual partner that I'd do something special if s/he'd discuss AIDS with me.
23. I would explain the reason why I want to discuss AIDS.
24. I would try to make my partner think that s/he wanted to talk about AIDS.
25. I would tell my partner it's in his/her best interest to discuss the issue of AIDS.
26. I would get mad if my partner didn't want to discuss the topic of AIDS.
27. I would make my partner believe that s/he would be doing me a favor by discussing AIDS.
28. I would try to persuade my partner to discuss AIDS-related issues.
29. I would try to discuss the topic by convincing my partner that it's really important.
30. I would make my partner realize that I have a legitimate right to demand we talk about AIDS.
31. I would try to make my partner feel like discussing topics related to AIDS.
32. I would demand to discuss aspects of our relationship that deal with AIDS.
33. I would try to make my partner feel bad or guilty if s/he didn't discuss AIDS with me.
34. I would moralize about the topic of AIDS.
35. I would talk my partner into discussing issues dealing with AIDS.
36. I would give my partner a big hug to put her/him in a good mood to discuss AIDS.
37. I would tell my partner that it's important for us to discuss AIDS.
38. I would con my partner into discussing things about AIDS.
39. I would tell my partner that we couldn't have sex until we discussed AIDS.
40. I would try to manipulate my partner into a discussion on AIDS.
41. I would keep bugging my partner to discuss the topic of AIDS.
42. I would use flattery to persuade my partner to discuss AIDS.
43. I would tell my partner I want to talk about AIDS.
44. I would pout or threaten to cry if I didn't get my way in discussing AIDS.
45. I would promise sexual rewards if we first discussed AIDS.
46. I would repeatedly remind my partner that I want to discuss AIDS.
47. I would keep trying to discuss AIDS issues with my partner.
48. I would become especially affectionate so my partner would agree to discuss AIDS issues.
49. I would insist that my partner and I discuss AIDS.
50. I would drop subtle hints that I want to talk about AIDS.
51. I would refrain from sexual contact until we discussed AIDS.
52. I would try to use coercion or blackmail to make my partner discuss AIDS.
53. I would try my hardest to make my partner discuss AIDS.
54. I would blow up in anger if s/he would not discuss the issue of AIDS.
55. I would state my need to discuss AIDS with my partner.
56. I would withhold affection and act cold until s/he discusses the topic of AIDS with me.
57. I would tell my partner that unless we discussed AIDS, I would never talk with him/her again.
58. I would get angry and demand that s/he talk about AIDS with me.
59. I would give up if my partner refused to discuss any AIDS-related issues.
60. I would appeal to my partner's love/affection for me as a basis for our discussing AIDS.
61. I would ask my partner if s/he wanted to discuss AIDS.
62. I would argue until my partner agreed to discuss the topic of AIDS with me.
63. I would refuse to interact further with my partner unless we first discussed AIDS.
64. I would act nice so that my partner could not refuse to discuss AIDS with me.
65. I would convince my partner that we need to discuss AIDS.

66. I would be especially sweet, charming, and pleasant before bringing up the subject of AIDS.
67. I would tell my partner we are close enough to discuss AIDS.
68. I would loudly voice my desire to discuss the topic of AIDS.
69. I would pretend to be an expert about AIDS.
70. I would plead or beg my partner to talk about the disease AIDS.
71. I would get someone else to help persuade my partner to discuss AIDS.
72. I would tell my partner I have a lot of knowledge about the topic of AIDS.

Source. This scale is reprinted with permission of the authors.

The Multidimensional AIDS Anxiety Questionnaire

William E. Snell, Jr.[1] and Phillip D. Finney, *Southeast Missouri State University*

Although considerable medical attention has been recently focused on AIDS, relatively little is known about the amount and nature of anxiety that this disease may be fostering in segments of society. To better understand the public's reaction to AIDS, a multidimensional self-report measure of anxiety experienced about AIDS was developed, the Multidimensional AIDS Anxiety Questionnaire (MAAQ; Finney & Snell, 1989; Snell & Finney, 1996). Factor analysis indicated that the MAAQ items correspond to five concepts concerned with AIDS anxiety: (a) AIDS-related anxiety manifested as physiological arousal, (b) AIDS-related anxiety manifested as fear, (c) AIDS-related anxiety manifested as cognitive worry, (d) AIDS-related anxiety manifested as sexual inhibition, and (e) AIDS-anxiety manifested as discussion inhibition.

Description

The MAAQ consists of 50 items. In responding to the MAAQ, individuals are asked to indicate how characteristic each statement is of them. A 5-point Likert-type scale is used to collect data on the responses, with each item being scored from 0 to 4: *not at all characteristic of me* (A), *slightly characteristic of me* (B), *somewhat characteristic of me* (C), *moderately characteristic of me* (D), and *very characteristic of me* (E). To create subscale scores, the items on each subscale are averaged. Higher scores thus correspond to greater amounts of each respective type of AIDS-related anxiety.

Response Mode and Timing

Individuals are asked to record their responses to the MAAQ on a computer scan sheet by darkening in a response from A to E for each MAAQ item. Alternatively, one could prepare the MAAQ so that respondents write directly on the instrument itself. The questionnaire usually takes between 20 and 25 minutes to complete.

Scoring

The MAAQ consists of five subscales designed to measure several aspects of anxiety about AIDS. (The items on the sixth subscale are indicated here also, although the eigenvalue from the factor analysis for this subscale was less than 1. Although this sixth subscale appears to be psychometrically weak, we anticipate that it will gain more prominence in future research.) The labels for these subscales are (with a listing of the items on each subscale): Physiological Arousal (Items 13, 14, 23, 27, 28, 29, 31, 33, 34, 38, 39, 43, 44, 46, 47, 48); Fear of AIDS (Items 5, 6, 10, 15, 16, and 21); Sexual Inhibition (Items 18, 30, 35, 37, 40, 42); Cognitive Worry (Items 1, 3, 4, 8, and 9); Discussion Inhibition (Items 2, 7, 12, 19, and 24); and Anxiety About AIDS Exposure (Items 20, 49, 50). The MAAQ items are scored so that A = 0, B = 1, C = 2, D = 3, and E = 4. Next, they are averaged for each subscale so that higher scores correspond to greater amounts of anxiety about AIDS (score range for each subscale = 0 to 4).

[1]Address correspondence to William E. Snell, Jr., Department of Psychology, Southeast Missouri State University, One University Plaza, Cape Girardeau, MO 63701; email: wesnell@semovm.semo.edu.

Reliability

Internal consistency coefficients for the MAAQ were reported by Finney and Snell (1989). All five scales had high internal consistency, with Cronbach alphas ranging from a low of .85 to a high of .94. Test-retest reliability coefficients for the Physiological Arousal (.65), Fear of AIDS (.78), and Sexual Inhibition (.63) subscales of the MAAQ were quite high; the coefficients for the Cognitive Worry (.40) and Discussion Inhibition (.40) subscales were somewhat lower.

Validity

To determine whether the 50 MAAQ items would cluster into unique groups, a principal components factor analysis with varimax rotation was conducted. There were five factors with eigenvalues greater than 1. Factor 1 had an eigenvalue of 17.00 (accounting for 34% of the variance) and consisted of 16 items concerned with signs of general physiological arousal about AIDS. Factor 2 had an eigenvalue of 4.43 (accounting for 9% of the variance) and consisted of six items reflecting a stronger fear of AIDS. Factor 3 consisted of six statements concerned specifically with sexual inhibition resulting from AIDS (eigenvalue = 2.24; 4% of the variance). The five items that characterized Factor 4 concerned cognitive worry about AIDS (eigenvalue = 1.23; 2% of the variance). Factor 5 consisted of five items concerned with discussion inhibition about AIDS (eigenvalue = 1.16; 2% of the variance). As anticipated, physiological (the arousal and fear factors), cognitive (the worry factor), and behavioral (the sexual inhibition and discussion inhibition factors) manifestations of AIDS anxiety were apparent in these data.

Researchers (Finney & Snell, 1989; Snell & Finney, 1996) have indicated that physiological arousal about AIDS and discussion inhibition about AIDS are associated with more positive personal approaches to AIDS. Additional research findings indicate that the MAAQ is related to the Stereotypes About AIDS Scale and the AIDS Discussion Strategy Scale. Still other results demonstrate convergent validity for the MAAQ with other measures of general anxiety and discriminant validity from social desirability and other personality characteristics. Also, AIDS anxiety was also found to be broadly related to individuals' underlying general anxiety level but unrelated to other specific forms of anxiety (e.g., relationship anxiety). Furthermore, scores on the MAAQ have been shown to be related to the contraceptive behavior of university students: More specifically, the physiological arousal type of AIDS anxiety was positively correlated with reliable contraceptive behaviors among males. Males who reported AIDS anxiety, manifested as physiological arousal, were also more likely to report a change in sexual practices due to the possibility of contracting AIDS. In addition, there was a trend for physiological arousal to be positively related to self-reported use of condoms or spermicides to protect against AIDS among males.

References

Finney, P., & Snell, W. E., Jr. (1989, April). *The AIDS Anxiety Scale: Components and correlates.* Paper presented at the annual meeting of the Southwestern Psychological Association, Houston, TX.

Snell, W. E., Jr., & Finney, P. (1996). *The Multidimensional AIDS Anxiety Questionnaire.* Unpublished manuscript.

Exhibit

The Multidimensional AIDS Anxiety Questionnaire

Instructions: The items listed below refer to feelings and reactions that people may experience about the disease AIDS (Acquired Immune Deficiency Syndrome). As such, there are no right or wrong answers, only the individual reactions that people have. We are interested in how typical these feelings and behaviors are of you. To provide your responses, use the following scale to indicate how characteristic the following statements are of you:

A = *Not at all* characteristic of me.
B = *Slightly* characteristic of me.
C = *Somewhat* characteristic of me.
D = *Moderately* characteristic of me.
E = *Very* characteristic of me.

NOTE: Remember to respond to all items, even if you are not completely sure. Also, please be honest in responding to these statements.

1. Thinking about AIDS makes me feel anxious.
2. I sometimes find it hard to discuss issues dealing with AIDS.
3. I feel tense when I think about the threat of AIDS.
4. I feel quite anxious about the epidemic of AIDS.
5. I feel scared about AIDS when I think about sexual relationships.
6. I'm afraid of getting AIDS.
7. I have trouble talking about AIDS with an intimate partner.

8. I feel flustered when I realize the threat of AIDS.
9. The disease AIDS makes me feel nervous and anxious.
10. I feel scared when I think about catching AIDS from a sexual partner.
11. I'm not worried about getting AIDS.
12. I would feel shy discussing AIDS with an intimate partner.
13. My heart beats fast with anxiety when I think about AIDS.
14. I feel anxious when I talk about AIDS with people.
15. Because of AIDS, I feel nervous about initiating sexual relations.
16. All these discussions of AIDS leave me feeling a bit alarmed.
17. I would not find it hard to discuss AIDS with an intimate partner.
18. AIDS makes me feel jittery about having sex with someone.
19. I feel uncomfortable when discussing AIDS.
20. I sometimes worry that one of my past sexual partners may have had AIDS.
21. Thinking about catching AIDS leaves me feeling concerned.
22. I would not hesitate to ask a former sex partner about AIDS-related concerns.
23. The issue of AIDS is a very stressful experience for me.
24. I feel nervous when I discuss AIDS with another person.
25. The threat of getting AIDS makes me feel uneasy about sex.
26. I worry about what I should do about AIDS.
27. Anxiety about AIDS is beginning to affect my personal relationships.
28. In general, the media attention on AIDS makes me feel restless.
29. I have feelings of worry when I think about AIDS.
30. Were I to have sexual relations, I would worry about getting AIDS.
31. All this recent media attention about AIDS leaves me feeling on edge.
32. AIDS does not influence my willingness to engage in sexual relationships.
33. When I think about AIDS, I feel tense.
34. I am more anxious than most people are about the disease AIDS.
35. If I were to have sex with someone, I would worry about AIDS.
36. I'm pretty indifferent to the idea of catching AIDS.
37. I would hesitate to involve myself in a sexual relationship because of AIDS.
38. When talking about AIDS with someone, I feel jumpy and high-strung.
39. I become really frightened when I think about the threat of AIDS.
40. The fear of AIDS makes me feel nervous about engaging in sex.
41. The increased chances of being infected with AIDS leaves me feeling troubled.
42. Because of AIDS, I feel too nervous to start a new sexual relationship.
43. The spread of AIDS is causing me to feel quite a bit of stress.
44. I worry that AIDS may directly influence my life.
45. I had a better attitude towards sex before the AIDS epidemic.
46. I get pretty upset when I think about the possibility of catching AIDS.
47. The discussion of AIDS makes me feel uncomfortable.
48. All this talk about AIDS has left me feeling strained and tense.
49. I'm concerned that I might be carrying the AIDS virus.
50. I feel nervous when I think that a past sexual partner could have given me AIDS.

The Stereotypes About AIDS Scale

William E. Snell, Jr.,[1] Phillip D. Finney, and Lisa J. Godwin,
Southeast Missouri State University

The spread of AIDS poses such a severe threat to society that a variety of stereotypes have proliferated about this disease. Snell, Finney, and Godwin (1991) conducted an investigation to examine several stereotypes about AIDS. More specifically, they developed and provided preliminary validation of the psychometric properties of the Stereotypes About AIDS Scale (SAAS), a multidimensional measure of stereotypes about AIDS. The selection of the particular stereotypes about AIDS measured by the SAAS was based on a literature review about AIDS stereotypes. Four categories of AIDS-related stereotypes (with multiple subscales in each category) are measured by the SAAS: (a) global stereotypic beliefs about AIDS, (b) personal attitudes about AIDS, (c) medical issues about AIDS, and (d) sexual issues about AIDS. The items in Section A of the SAAS (Global Stereotypes About AIDS) form four separate subscales concerned with stereotypes about the need for AIDS-related education, AIDS-related confidentiality, the transmission of AIDS, and AIDS is caused by homosexuality. The items in Section B of the SAAS (Personal Attitudes About AIDS) form five separate subscales concerned with stereotypes about the desire to avoid those afflicted with AIDS, AIDS is not perceived as self-relevant, a closed-minded approach to AIDS, the issue of AIDS is being exaggerated, and the notion that AIDS is a moral punishment. The items in Section C of the SAAS (Medical Issues About AIDS) form four separate subscales concerned with stereotypes about the belief that AIDS is a threat to medical staff, protecting the U.S. blood supply system from AIDS, a cure for AIDS, and AIDS testing should be conducted. The items in Section D of the SAAS (Sexual Issues About AIDS) form two separate subscales concerned with stereotypes about the relationship between AIDS and sexual activity and the prevention of AIDS through the use of condoms.

Description

The SAAS consists of four sections. Section A has 30 items, Section B has 35 items, Section C has 30 items, and Section D has 20 items. In responding to the SAAS, individuals are asked to indicate how much they agree or disagree with each statement, using a 5-point Likert-type format: *agree* (+2), *slightly agree* (+1), *neither agree nor disagree* (0), *slightly disagree* (−1), and *disagree* (−2). To create subscale scores, the items on each subscale are aver-

aged. Higher positive (negative) scores correspond to greater agreement (disagreement) with the stereotypes measured by the SAAS.

Response Mode and Timing

People respond to the SAAS by using a computer scan sheet to darken a response (either A, B, C, D, or E) for each item. The entire questionnaire (i.e., all four sections) usually takes about 35-45 minutes to complete.

Scoring

The SAAS consists of 15 separate subscales. Several SAAS items are reversed scored (A8, A20, A21, C2, C12, AND D4) before the subscales are computed. The four subscales for Section A are the need for AIDS-related education (A4, A6, A12, A18, A20, A22, A24, A28, A30), AIDS-related confidentiality (A2, A3, A8, A9, A14, A21, A26, A27), the transmission of AIDS (A5, A11, A15, A17, A23, A29), and AIDS is caused by homosexuality (A1, A7, A13, A19, A25). The five subscales for Section B are the desire to avoid those afflicted with AIDS (B1, B22, B23, B24, B34, B35), AIDS was not perceived as self-relevant (B5, B6, B7, B8), a closed-minded approach to AIDS (B13, B16, B17), the issue of AIDS is being exaggerated (B3, B10, B25, B29), and the notion that AIDS is a moral punishment (B9, B32, B33). The four subscales for Section C are the belief that AIDS is a threat to medical staff (C3, C4, C6, C11, C12, C18), protecting the U.S. blood supply system from AIDS (C2, C5, C7, C17, C25, C27), cure for AIDS (C9, C10, C23), and AIDS testing should be conducted (C13, C14). The two subscales for Section D are the relationship between AIDS and sexual activity (D1, D2, D4 TO D12, D13) and the prevention of AIDS through the use of condoms (D3, D10, D17, D18, D19).

Reliability

Snell et al. (1991) found that for Section A of the SAAS, the reliabilities ranged from a low of .75 to a high of .85, for Section B of the SAAS, the reliabilities ranged from a low of .72 to a high of .87, for Section C of the SAAS, the reliabilities ranged from a low of .64 to a high of .83, and for Section D of the SAAS, the Cronbach alphas were .86 and .78, respectively.

Validity

Snell et al. (1991) reported that those individuals who endorsed a wide range of negative, inaccurate stereotypes about AIDS, as measured by their responses to SAAS, reported greater AIDS-related anxiety. In particular, people

[1]Address correspondence to William E. Snell, Jr., Department of Psychology, Southeast Missouri State University, One University Plaza, Cape Girardeau, MO 63701; email: wesnell@semovm.semo.edu.

who believed that AIDS was not relevant to them, who were closed-minded about AIDS, and who believed that the media was exaggerating the issue of AIDS indicated that they felt sufficient AIDS anxiety to inhibit their sexual activity. Additionally, it was found that those who believed in the importance of AIDS education reported that they would be more likely to use direct, rational strategies to start a conversation about AIDS with a potential sexual partner. One other set of findings reported by Snell et al. dealt with the issue of men's and women's stereotypic reactions to AIDS. It was found that both males and females were supportive of greater educational efforts about AIDS, although, interestingly enough, they also were somewhat supportive of widespread mandatory testing for AIDS. In addition, other evidence indicated a consistent pattern of gender differences in men's and women's stereotypic beliefs about AIDS, with the findings generally suggesting that women ex-

pressed more positive and less prejudicial AIDS-related attitudes than did males. Snell et al. also found that females' endorsement of several socially undesirable stereotypes about women was predictive of their agreement (and disagreement) with a number of prejudicial (and nonprejudicial) stereotypes about AIDS and AIDS-afflicted individuals, as measured by the SAAS. Females who held a set of disparaging beliefs about women (e.g., that women are more passive, vulnerable, and moral than men; that women are sexually passive and sexual teases) reported adhering to a variety of stigmatizing beliefs and attitudes about AIDS, as measured by the SAAS.

Reference

Snell, W. E., Jr., Finney, P. D., & Godwin, L. J. (1991). Stereotypes about AIDS. *Contemporary Social Psychology, 15*, 18-38.

Exhibit

The Stereotypes About AIDS Scale

AIDS–Section A

Instructions: The items listed below refer to people's beliefs about the topic of AIDS (Acquired Immune Deficiency Syndrome). We are interested in whether you agree or disagree with these statements. As such, there are no right or wrong answers, only your own individual opinions. To indicate your reactions to these statements, use the following scale:

A	=	Agree
B	=	Slightly agree
C	=	Neither agree nor disagree
D	=	Slightly disagree
E	=	Disagree

Remember: There are no right or wrong responses; only your opinions. Be sure to respond to each and every statement; leave no blanks.

1. Homosexuality is the cause of AIDS.
2. People with AIDS don't really have a right to confidentiality about their disease.
3. People ought to notify their employees if they contract AIDS.
4. Not enough money is being spent on AIDS-related research.
5. AIDS can be transmitted by being in the same room with an AIDS patient.
6. People need education to learn how to avoid getting the virus AIDS.
7. If it weren't for homosexuals, we wouldn't have the disease AIDS.
8. AIDS victims have a right to privacy about their lives and lifestyles.
9. Businesses should have the right to fire people if they have AIDS.
10. The cost of medical care for AIDS patients should be paid by the government.
11. AIDS can be transmitted by shaking hands with an AIDS patient.
12. AIDS education is an appropriate task for schools to perform.
13. The sexual promiscuity of homosexuals is the reason why AIDS exists.
14. The government should be able to test anyone for AIDS.
15. A person can get AIDS from fellow workers at a job.
16. The government is not doing enough to fight AIDS.
17. AIDS can be transmitted by sharing eating utensils with an AIDS patient.
18. Sexual education about AIDS is necessary at school.
19. AIDS is really a punishment sent from God for the sinful acts of homosexuality.
20. AIDS-infected children should be kept out of public school.
21. Having a co-worker with AIDS would not bother me.
22. AIDS is a serious national problem that deserves government attention.

23. AIDS can be transmitted by kissing an individual with AIDS.
24. It is important that students learn about AIDS in their classes.
25. AIDS is God's way of getting rid of homosexuals.
26. Identifying those people with AIDS should be a high priority.
27. Employees have a right to know if any of their co-workers have AIDS.
28. The federal government ought to fund education on AIDS.
29. People can catch AIDS by giving CPR to an individual with AIDS.
30. Children need instruction about AIDS in their school curriculum.

AIDS–Section B

Instructions: The items listed below refer to people's beliefs about the topic of AIDS (Acquired Immune Deficiency Syndrome). We are interested in whether you agree or disagree with these statements. As such, there are no right or wrong answers, only your own individual opinions. To indicate your reactions to these statements, use the following scale:

A	=	Agree
B	=	Slightly agree
C	=	Neither agree nor disagree
D	=	Slightly disagree
E	=	Disagree

Remember: There are no right or wrong responses; only your opinions. Be sure to respond to each and every statement; leave no blanks.

1. I don't want to talk or interact with anyone with AIDS.
2. We have a social obligation to help those with AIDS.
3. People who describe AIDS as an epidemic are exaggerating its true nature.
4. As always, science will eventually find a cure for AIDS.
5. AIDS is really not my problem; it's somebody else's.
6. AIDS is not my problem.
7. AIDS is not a threat to me.
8. The AIDS crisis is really removed from me.
9. People who die from AIDS are being punished for their past wrongs.
10. People are blowing the issue of AIDS way out of proportion.
11. People should test themselves for AIDS.
12. People who get AIDS can blame only themselves.
13. Only people from California have been affected by AIDS.
14. Part of the problem with AIDS is that people don't talk about it.
15. The AIDS epidemic will soon be a financial burden on the U.S. economy.
16. You can't teach young children about AIDS.
17. Men and women don't really need to discuss AIDS with each other.
18. AIDS has become a significant problem in prison populations.
19. A cure for AIDS is inevitable.
20. AIDS is easy to get.
21. AIDS may eventually bankrupt the U.S. health care system.
22. People with AIDS should not be allowed to work in public schools.
23. People with AIDS should not be allowed to handle food in restaurants.
24. People with AIDS should not be allowed to work with patients in hospitals.
25. AIDS is not as big a problem as the media suggests.
26. I am not the kind of person who is likely to get AIDS.
27. I am less likely than most people to get AIDS.
28. I'd rather get any other disease than AIDS.
29. I've heard enough about AIDS, and I don't want to hear any more about it.
30. Living in San Francisco would increase anyone's chances of getting AIDS.
31. If a free blood test were available to see if you have the AIDS virus, I would take it.
32. AIDS is God's punishment for immorality.
33. AIDS patients offend me morally.
34. If I knew someone with AIDS, it would be hard for me to continue that relationship.
35. Children with AIDS should not be allowed to attend public schools.

AIDS–Section C

Instructions: The items listed below refer to people's beliefs about the topic of AIDS (Acquired Immune Deficiency Syndrome). We are interested in whether you agree or disagree with these statements. As such, there are no right or wrong answers, only your own individual opinions. To indicate your reactions to these statements, use the following scale:

A	=	Agree
B	=	Slightly agree
C	=	Neither agree nor disagree
D	=	Slightly disagree
E	=	Disagree

Remember: There are no right or wrong responses; only your opinions. Be sure to respond to each and every statement; leave no blanks.

1. The family of AIDS victims ought to have the right to participate in medical decisions.
2. People with AIDS should not be admitted to medical hospitals.
3. Doctors can catch AIDS if they treat patients with this disease.
4. AIDS patients will contaminate medical staff and other hospital patients.
5. It's important to maintain a safe blood banking system, because of AIDS.
6. Health care workers can catch AIDS in medical situations.
7. Medicine has a test to identify whether a person has AIDS.
8. The medical test for AIDS will not always identify a recently infected person.
9. There's a vaccine that prevents the spread of AIDS.
10. There are effective medical treatments for those with AIDS.
11. Doctors and nurses are at risk for catching AIDS from infected patients.
12. No medical assistance person has ever caught AIDS from a patient.
13. AIDS blood tests should be administered to everyone in hospitals.
14. Hospitals should have the right to test all patients for AIDS.
15. A doctor with AIDS should not be allowed to treat patients.
16. A hospital worker should not be required to work with AIDS patients.
17. AIDS patients have as much right to quality medical care as anyone else.
18. AIDS makes a medical job a high-risk occupation.
19. Dealing with AIDS patients is different from dealing with other types of patients.
20. The high cost of treating AIDS patients is unfair to other people in need of care.
21. Working with AIDS patients can be a rewarding experience for medical personnel.
22. Hospital personnel should go out of their way to be helpful to a patient with AIDS.
23. People with AIDS can be cured if they seek medical attention.
24. To get AIDS, a person must have intimate sexual or blood contact with an AIDS carrier.
25. The disease AIDS can be transmitted by the exchange of blood (or blood products).
26. AIDS has been identified in hemophiliacs (people who bleed easily).
27. AIDS has been linked to blood transfusion.
28. AIDS is probably in most of the nation's blood supply.
29. A blood test can identify testing for AIDS.
30. People get AIDS from blood transfusion.

AIDS–Section D

Instructions: The items listed below refer to people's beliefs about the topic of AIDS (Acquired Immune Deficiency Syndrome). We are interested in whether you agree or disagree with these statements. As such, there are no right or wrong answers, only your own individual opinions. To indicate your reactions to these statements, use the following scale:

A	=	Agree
B	=	Slightly agree
C	=	Neither agree nor disagree
D	=	Slightly disagree
E	=	Disagree

Remember: There are no right or wrong responses; only your opinions. Be sure to respond to each and every statement; leave no blanks.

1. AIDS is a serious challenge to the notion of recreational sex.
2. Because of AIDS, everyone has a responsibility to practice healthful sexual behaviors.
3. Condoms offer protection against the spread of AIDS.
4. AIDS cannot be transmitted by heterosexual (male-female) sexual activity.
5. People catch AIDS from their sexual partners.
6. The more sexual partners people have, the greater their chance of acquiring AIDS.
7. AIDS is associated with multiple anonymous sexual contacts.
8. AIDS is transmitted by intimate sexual contact.
9. People can contact AIDS even though they have had sex with only one person.
10. Condoms are a safe shield against AIDS.
11. AIDS is essentially a sexually transmitted disease.
12. People can contract AIDS from sexual contact with a single infected person.
13. Any sexually active people can get AIDS.
14. People get AIDS from sex.
15. People don't engage in sex very much nowadays because of AIDS.
16. AIDS is transmitted primarily through sexual relations.
17. Proper use of condoms can reduce the risk of catching AIDS.
18. The use of condoms can prevent the spread of AIDS.
19. Heterosexuals who use condoms can lessen their risk for getting AIDS.
20. People who have "one-night stands" will probably catch AIDS.

Alternate Forms of HIV Prevention Attitude Scales for Teenagers

Mohammad R. Torabi and William L. Yarber,[1] *Indiana University*

The lack of valid devices for measuring attitudes toward HIV prevention for adolescents has remained an obstacle to HIV/AIDS education evaluation. Many national authority groups, such as the National Research Council (Coyle, Boruch, & Turner, 1989), have recognized the importance of constructing reliable survey questionnaires in evaluating HIV prevention programs. In addition to knowledge and behavioral outcomes, it is imperative to determine attitude status and how it changes in health education settings.

Research indicates that attitudes are best described as multidimensional, having the three components of cognitive (belief), affective (feeling), and conative (intention to act) (Ajzen & Fishbein, 1980; Kothandapani, 1971; Ostrom, 1969). This model has been successfully applied in

measurement of attitudes toward alcohol among teenagers (Torabi & Veenker, 1986), prevention of cancer for college students (Torabi & Seffrin, 1986), and sexually transmitted diseases (Yarber, Torabi, & Veenker, 1989).

In testing situations, especially for test-retest design, there is a need for parallel, equivalent, or alternate forms of tests. Tests are considered to be parallel whenever their information functions are identical (Timminga, 1990). For most educational evaluation using pretest-posttest design, the use of alternate forms is preferred over single forms. Our purpose was to develop alternate, attitude-scale forms, using the three-component model, to measure adolescents' attitudes toward HIV and prevention of HIV infection.

Description

A large pool of Likert-type items was generated, guided by a table of specifications using a three-component attitude theory and conceptual areas related to HIV and HIV pre-

[1]Address correspondence to William L. Yarber, Department of Applied Health Science, Indiana University, HPER Building, Bloomington, IN 47405; email: yarber@ucs.indiana.edu.

vention. A preliminary scale with 50 items was prepared and reviewed by a jury of experts. The jurors provided feedback regarding clarity and content validity. Following revision, the preliminary scale was administered to 210 midwestern high school students. After extensive item analyses, two comparable forms with 15 maximally discriminatory items were identified. These alternate forms were simultaneously administered to a representative sample of 600 teenagers in a midwestern high school. Data were subjected to various techniques of item analyses, factor analysis, and reliability estimation.

The item analyses results provided strong evidence of internal consistency and comparability. The item correlation coefficients were positive and statistically significant for both forms. Additionally, the normative data regarding means, the standard deviations of item scores, and the total scale scores for the two forms were comparable.

Response Mode and Timing

Respondents indicate whether they *strongly agree, agree, undecided, disagree,* or *strongly disagree* to each statement. It takes about 10 minutes to complete the scale.

Scoring

The minimum and maximum possible points for each form are 15 and 75 points, the higher score indicating the more positive attitudes toward HIV and HIV prevention.

Scoring for Form A. For Items 7, 8, 11, 13, and 15, *strongly agree* = 5 points, *agree* = 4, *undecided* = 3, *disagree* = 2, and *strongly disagree* = 1. For the remaining items, *strongly agree* = 1, *agree* = 2, *undecided* = 3, *disagree* = 4, and *strongly disagree* = 5.

Scoring for Form B. For Items 1, 3, 8, 9, 10, 11, 12, 13, 14, and 15, *strongly agree* = 5, *agree* = 4, *undecided* = 3, *disagree* = 2, and *strongly disagree* = 1. For the remaining items, *strongly agree* = 1, *agree* = 2, *undecided* = 3, *disagree* = 4, and *strongly disagree* = 5.

Reliability

Alternate reliability across the form was .82. The alpha reliability for Forms A and B was .78 and .77, and split-half method was .76 and .69, respectively (Torabi & Yarber, 1992).

Validity

Evidence of content validity was provided by using a jury of experts, table of specifications, and factor analysis procedures. The factor analyses of both forms identified reasonably comparable factor structures for each form, indicating further evidence of content validity and comparability. It would have been ideal to provide evidence of criterion-related validity by surveying actual behaviors or practices. However, due to serious resistance to assessing minors' sexual and injecting drug behaviors, no such data were obtained.

Because the evidence of validity and reliability of the alternate forms was obtained from a sample of predominantly White, in-school students, the forms may not be very appropriate for minority or out-of-school youths.

Other Information

The scales may be used for needs assessment and evaluation of HIV/AIDS education measuring teenagers attitudes toward prevention of HIV infection. The alternate forms are probably more suitable to pretest-posttest HIV education evaluation design.

References

Ajzen, I., & Fishbein, M. (1980). *Understanding attitudes and predicting social behavior.* Englewood Cliffs, NJ: Prentice Hall.

Coyle, S., Boruch, R. F., & Turner, C. F. (1989). *Evaluating AIDS prevention programs.* Washington, DC: National Academy Press.

Kothandapani, V. (1971). *A psychological approach to the prediction of contraceptive behavior.* Chapel Hill: University of North Carolina, Carolina Population Center.

Ostrom, T. M. (1969). The relationship between the affective, behavioral, and cognitive components of attitude. *Journal of Experimental Psychology, 5,* 12-30.

Timminga, E. B. (1990). The construction of parallel test from IRT-based item banks. *Journal of Educational Statistics, 15*(2), 129-145.

Torabi, M. R., & Seffrin, J. R. (1989). A three component cancer attitude scale. *Journal of School Health, 56*(5), 170-174.

Torabi, M. R., & Veenker, C. H. (1986). An alcohol attitude scale for teenagers. *Journal of School Health, 6*(3), 96-100.

Torabi, M. R., & Yarber, W. L. (1992). Alternate forms of the HIV prevention attitude scales for teenagers. *AIDS Education and Prevention, 4,* 172-182.

Yarber, W. L., Torabi, M. R., & Veenker, C. H. (1989). Development of a three component sexually transmitted diseases attitude scale for young adults. *Journal of Sex Education and Therapy, 15,* 36-49.

Exhibit

Alternate Forms of HIV Prevention Attitude Scales for Teenagers

Form A

Directions: Please read each statement carefully. *Record your immediate reaction to the statement by blackening the proper oval on the answer sheet.* There is no right or wrong answer for each statement, so mark your own response. Use the below key:

Key: A = Strongly agree
      B = Agree
      C = Undecided
      D = Disagree
      E = Strongly disagree

Example: Doing something to prevent getting HIV is the responsibility of each person.

                A   B   C   D   E

1. I would feel very uncomfortable being around someone with HIV.
2. I feel that HIV is a punishment for immoral behavior.
3. If I were having sex, it would be insulting if my partner insisted we use a condom.
4. I dislike the idea of limiting sex to just one partner to avoid HIV infection.
5. I would dislike asking a possible sex partner to get the HIV antibody test.
6. It would be dangerous to permit a student with HIV to attend school.
7. It is easy to use the prevention methods that reduce one's chance of getting HIV.
8. It is important to talk to a sex partner about HIV prevention before having sex.
9. I believe that sharing IV drug needles has nothing to do with HIV.
10. HIV education in schools is a waste of time.
11. I would be supportive of a person with HIV.
12. Even if a sex partner insisted, I would not use a condom.
13. I intend to talk about HIV prevention with a partner if we were to have sex.
14. I intend not to use drugs so I can avoid HIV.
15. I will use condoms when having sex if I'm not sure if my partner has HIV.

Form B

Directions: Please read each statement carefully. *Record your immediate reaction to the statement by blackening the proper oval on the answer sheet.* There is no right or wrong answer for each statement, so mark your own response. Use the below key:

Key: A = Strongly agree
      B = Agree
      C = Undecided
      D = Disagree
      E = Strongly disagree

Example: Doing something to prevent getting HIV is the responsibility of each person.

                A   B   C   D   E

1. I am certain that I could be supportive of a friend with HIV.
2. I feel that people with HIV got what they deserve.
3. I am comfortable with the idea of using condoms for sex.
4. I would dislike the idea of limiting sex to just one partner to avoid HIV infection.
5. It would be embarrassing to get the HIV antibody test.
6. It is meant for some people to get HIV.
7. Using condoms to avoid HIV is too much trouble.
8. I believe that AIDS is a preventable disease.
9. The chance of getting HIV makes using IV drugs stupid.
10. People can influence their friends to practice safe behavior.
11. I would shake hands with a person having HIV.
12. I will avoid sex if there is a slight chance that the partner might have HIV.
13. If I were to have sex I would insist that a condom be used.
14. If I used IV drugs, I would not share the needles.
15. I intend to share HIV facts with my friends.

Source. These scales are reprinted with permission of the authors.

HIV Prevention Knowledge Test for Teenagers

William L. Yarber[1] and Mohammad R. Torabi, *Indiana University*

Several surveys of teenagers' knowledge about HIV infection and AIDS reveal cognitive deficiencies, especially concerning the prevention of HIV infection (DiClemente, Zorn, & Temoshok, 1989; Koopman, Rotheram-Borus, Henderson, Bradley, & Hunter, 1990). This is problematic, because misconceptions and incomplete information may lead to unintended high-risk HIV behaviors. Given the philosophy that proper HIV education emphasizes preventive behaviors, the cognitive component of such programs should likewise provide accurate concepts concerning prevention (Yarber, 1989b). A measure designed specifically to assess knowledge of HIV preventive behaviors can assist in the formative and summative evaluations of educational programs. The HIV Prevention Knowledge Test for Teenagers was developed to measure teenagers' knowledge of HIV, with emphasis focused on HIV preventive behaviors.

Description

In developing this knowledge test, the multiple-choice approach was used, with items generated that represent both the knowledge level (HIV concepts) and application level (HIV situations) of the cognitive domain (Bloom, 1956). A pool of items based on literature (Haffner, 1988; National Coalition of Advocates for Students, 1987; Yarber, 1989a, 1989b) was developed according to a table of specifications containing four conceptual areas, each with specific categories, the HIV/AIDS problem: social impact of HIV/AIDS, HIV infection, and AIDS; HIV transmission: sexual contact, blood transmission, mother to child, fears, and fallacies; individual HIV prevention: knowing of infection, sexual, drug use, and mother to child; and HIV/-AIDS control efforts: testing/medical, education/research, individual activism, help sources.

A panel of experts, including federal government HIV officials, health educators, and teenagers, reviewed the items, which resulted in the elimination of some questions. Attempts were made to make the reading level of the items at the junior high school level. A preliminary test consisting of 50 items (44 knowledge domain, 6 application) and 5 demographic questions was developed. This form was reviewed by a small group of eighth-grade students, which resulted in further verbal clarification of some items. Subsequently, the form was administered to high school students.

The sample consisted of 246 students who were enrolled in an urban high school located in a large midwestern city. Their ages ranged from 13 to 20 years or older; the majority

were between 16 and 19 years old. There was a nearly equal proportion of females and males, with about 72% and 17% of the sample being White and Black students, respectively. The students were sampled in 1990.

The collected data were analyzed to provide evidence of reliability and validity of the test using correlation techniques, difficulty index, and factor analysis. From the item analysis, a pool of the 30 most functional items (25 knowledge domain, 5 application domain) were selected for the final test. The data were then reanalyzed using only the 30 items. The items of the final test had the highest item correlation and were within the average item difficulty range. The mean score of the final test is 17 with a standard deviation of 6.6.

Response Mode and Timing

The test is multiple choice; respondents select the one best answer to each question. The test takes about 15 minutes to complete.

Scoring

Possible scores range from 0 to 30. Correct answers are identified in the exhibit by an asterisk.

Reliability

The reliability coefficient of the final test was .85 (alpha) and .86 (Kuder-Richardson).

Validity

The use of a jury of experts and a table of specifications provided evidence of content validity.

Other Information

Because the test largely assesses knowledge of HIV/AIDS prevention behaviors, it has application for curriculum development and for the evaluation of educational programs designed for teenagers that emphasize HIV/AIDS prevention.

References

Bloom, B. S. (Ed.). (1956). *Handbook of educational objectives: Handbook I. Cognitive domain.* New York: McKay.

DiClemente, R. J., Zorn, J., & Temoshok, T. (1989). Adolescents and AIDS: A survey of knowledge, beliefs and attitudes about AIDS in San Francisco. *American Journal of Public Health, 76,* 1443-1445.

Haffner, D. (1988). The AIDS epidemic: Implications for the sexuality education of youth. *SIECUS Report, 16*(6), 1-5.

Koopman C., Rotheram-Borus, M. J. Henderson, R., Bradley, J. S., & Hunter, J. (1990). Assessment of knowledge of AIDS and beliefs about AIDS prevention among adolescents. *AIDS Education and Prevention, 2*(1), 58-69.

[1]Address correspondence to William L. Yarber, Department of Applied Health Science, Indiana University, HPER Building, Bloomington, IN 47405; email: yarber@ucs.indiana.edu.

National Coalition of Advocates for Students. (1987). *Criteria for evaluating an AIDS curriculum.* Boston: Author.

Yarber, W. L. (1989a). *AIDS: What young adults should know.* Reston, VA: Association for the Advancement of Health Education.

Yarber, W. L. (1989b). Performance standards for the evaluation and development of school HIV/AIDS education curricula for adolescents. *SIECUS Report, 17*(6), 18-26.

Exhibit

HIV Prevention Behaviors Knowledge Test for Teenagers

Note: HIV means the virus that causes AIDS, which is also called the AIDS virus. STD means sexually transmitted diseases, such as syphilis, gonorrhea, or herpes. IV drugs means intravenous drugs.

Part I. Directions: Choose the best answer for each question.

1. The *most* common way HIV has been transmitted is
   *a. by sexual contact.
   b. by IV drug use.
   c. by blood transfusions.
   d. from mother to child.
2. How long does it take for the symptoms of HIV infection to develop after a person becomes infected?
   a. 2 to 6 weeks.
   b. 1 to 2 weeks.
   c. few weeks to 3 years.
   *d. few months to 10 years or more.
3. The *surest* way to avoid HIV and other STD is by
   a. having only one sex partner.
   b. using condoms during sex.
   c. carefully selecting sex partners.
   *d. not having sex or injecting drugs.
4. Sexual fidelity is *100 percent* effective in avoiding HIV or other STD only if
   a. a condom is used for every sexual contact.
   b. anal intercourse is avoided.
   *c. neither partner was infected when sex started, and both avoid IV drugs and sex with others.
   d. each partner states that he/she has not had sex with high-risk persons.
5. Which statement concerning having an HIV infection and AIDS is *true?*
   *a. One can be infected with HIV without having symptoms.
   b. Many persons with an HIV infection have recovered.
   c. All persons with an HIV infection have developed AIDS.
   d. Nearly all persons diagnosed with AIDS have already died.
6. Which statement concerning HIV infection is *true?*
   a. An HIV infection causes sterility.
   *b. HIV can be transmitted to others, even if symptoms of infection are absent.
   c. The exact percentage of HIV-infected persons who will develop AIDS is known.
   d. The outcome of having AIDS is *not* very severe.
7. Which statement concerning HIV transmission is *true?*
   a. HIV is transmitted like the flu or common cold.
   b. HIV can be spread by casual contact.
   c. HIV can be spread by mosquitoes.
   *d. Family members living with HIV-infected persons have not acquired HIV just by being near the person.
8. Which statement concerning the HIV-antibody test is *true?*
   a. A positive HIV-antibody test result means that the person will develop AIDS.
   *b. A positive HIV-antibody test result means that the person has been infected with HIV.
   c. The HIV-antibody test can be purchased at a drugstore by anyone.
   d. The HIV-antibody test will be positive very soon after a person becomes infected.
9. Which statement concerning teenagers and AIDS is *false?*
   a. AIDS among teenagers is increasing.
   *b. Teenagers are safe from HIV infection.
   c. Teenagers can get HIV from sex and IV drug use.
   d. Some HIV-infected people in the 20-29 age group acquired HIV when they were teenagers.

10. Which statement concerning AIDS and the HIV infection problem is *false*?
    a. There are many more persons infected with HIV than those actually having AIDS.
    *b. HIV infection has been limited to a few large cities.
    c. Both sexes and children have been infected with HIV.
    d. The number of AIDS cases is increasing in the United States.

11. Which statement concerning symptoms of HIV infection is *false*?
    a. Sometimes it takes a long time for symptoms to appear.
    b. Early symptoms of HIV infection are like some common illnesses.
    c. Most persons with HIV have periods of both health and illness.
    *d. A person can usually guess who is infected.

12. Which statement about having an HIV infection is *false*?
    a. Many HIV-infected persons do not know they are infected until symptoms appear.
    b. HIV itself usually does not kill the person.
    *c. Only a small percentage of HIV-infected persons will develop AIDS.
    d. Persons with HIV may get severe illnesses healthy persons do not get.

13. Which statement concerning HIV transmission is *false*?
    a. There have been very few female-to-female sexual transmissions of HIV.
    *b. HIV is transmitted only if the infected person has been diagnosed as having AIDS.
    c. A person with an STD has a greater chance of getting HIV if he/she has sex with an HIV-infected person.
    d. HIV probably can be transmitted by oral sex.

14. Which statement concerning blood donation and transfusion is *false*?
    *a. One can get HIV from *donating* blood.
    b. It is very unlikely to get HIV from blood transfusions.
    c. All donated blood is tested for HIV antibodies.
    d. Persons who might have HIV should not donate blood.

15. Which statement concerning multiple sex partners is *false*?
    a. Condoms reduce the risk of acquiring HIV or other STD if a person has multiple sex partners.
    b. The more sex partners a person has, the greater the chance of getting HIV.
    *c. There is little chance of getting HIV or other STD from multiple partners if all are heterosexual.
    d. There is a risk of getting HIV or other STD from having multiple sex partners even if you know each partner.

16. Which statement concerning HIV-infected women and pregnancy is *false*?
    *a. All children of HIV-infected women are born with HIV.
    b. It is risky for an HIV-infected women to breast-feed.
    c. The HIV-infected woman should delay pregnancy.
    d. Babies born with HIV usually die within two years.

17. Which statement concerning the fear of getting HIV or other STD is *false*?
    a. Some people should fear getting HIV or other STD.
    b. Myths about the transmission of HIV and other STD have increased people's fears.
    *c. For most people, fear of getting HIV or other STD is justified.
    d. There is nothing to fear about acquiring HIV or other STD from just being around others.

18. Which statement concerning HIV-infected persons is *false*?
    a. HIV-infected persons should practice sexual abstinence or low-risk behavior.
    *b. HIV-infected persons should avoid donating blood, but they can donate body organs and semen.
    c. HIV can be transmitted soon after a person becomes infected.
    d. HIV-infected persons should never share IV drug needles.

19. Which statement concerning the prevention of HIV and other STD is *false*?
    a. The precautions for avoiding HIV infection also prevent other STD.
    b. Some behaviors that prevent HIV and other STD also prevent unwanted pregnancy.
    *c. Scientists are unsure about how a person can avoid HIV and other STD.
    d. Individual prevention is the most important solution to stopping HIV and other STD.

20. Which statement about preventing HIV and other STD by sexual fidelity is *false*?
    *a. Sexual fidelity works only if it is practiced in marriage.
    b. Uninfected partners who practice sexual fidelity will avoid HIV or other STD from sex.
    c. Sexual fidelity works unless one's partner uses IV drugs or was infected when the relationship started.
    d. It is sometimes impossible to know if a partner is sexually faithful.

21. Which statement concerning the selection of new sex partners is *false*?
    *a. Insisting that new sex partners get tested for HIV and other STD *eliminates* the risk of becoming infected.
    b. It is difficult to know for sure if a partner is infected.
    c. It is impossible to determine who is uninfected just by looking at the person.
    d. A person thinking of having sex should consider that anyone could be infected.

22. Which statement about using condoms for preventing HIV and other STD is *false*?
    *a.   Intercourse is the only sexual activity for which condoms are needed.
    b.   Each condom should be used only once.
    c.   An empty space should be left at the end of the condom when it is used.
    d.   A condom should be used even if one carefully selects sex partners.
23. Which statement concerning the HIV-antibody test is *false*?
    *a.   All persons with positive test results have AIDS.
    b.   Persons having a positive test result can transmit HIV.
    c.   Test results may be negative shortly after a person has become infected with HIV.
    d.   The test results are very accurate, but not perfect.
24. Which statement concerning calling the National AIDS Information Line is *false*?
    a.   The hot line is available 24 hours daily.
    b.   The caller will not be asked his/her age or phone number.
    c.   The person answering will not ask for the caller's name.
    *d.   The call will be charged as a long distance call on the telephone bill.
25. Which statement concerning the medical treatment of AIDS patients and persons with HIV is *false*?
    a.   Some drugs improve the health of persons with AIDS.
    *b.   An HIV infection can be cured.
    c.   There is no vaccine to prevent an HIV infection.
    d.   Drugs that help restore the immune system are being tested.

Part II. Directions: Read the HIV life situations below and answer the questions concerning them.

26. Margarita and Carlos have decided to have sex with each other. But they want to avoid getting HIV or other STD. Both have had sex with other people. What would be their *wisest* choice to avoid HIV or other STD?
    a.   Both would urinate and wash their genitals after sex.
    b.   Margarita would take the birth control pill.
    *c.   Carlos would wear a condom during all sexual activity.
    d.   Both would not have sex with other people.
27. Naoko thinks she might be infected with HIV or another STD. But, she does not have symptoms. She wants to do something about her concern. Which behavior would be the *wisest*?
    *a.   She could immediately talk to a health counselor.
    b.   She could ask her sex partners if they have symptoms.
    c.   She could wait to see if she develops symptoms.
    d.   She could take some medicine she got from a friend.
28. Stacey and Daryl are high school students who are dating each other. They are considering having sex, and have decided to talk about HIV and other STD. Some of their statements are correct and others are incorrect. Which statement is *incorrect*?
    *a.   It would be safe for us to have sex, since neither one of us looks like we are infected.
    b.   If we have sex, Daryl should use a condom.
    c.   Even though neither one of us is homosexual, there is still a chance of getting HIV or another STD.
    d.   It is impossible to know for sure if there is no risk of HIV or other STD, since we cannot be perfectly sure of each other's past.
29. Chris and Paul sometimes shoot IV drugs together and with their friends. Often they share the drug needles. However, they do not have sex with each other. They have certain beliefs about their lifestyle and HIV infection. Which belief listed below is *incorrect*?
    *a.   We have no chance of getting HIV, since we are shooting drugs only with friends.
    b.   We should get counseling about whether we should take the HIV-antibody test.
    c.   It would be wise to stop sharing needles, even if we shared them before.
    d.   We could be infected with HIV, even though we do not have sex.
30. Jamal and Cantrise are students in the same high school and have dated each other for a long time. Jamal uses IV drugs, but Cantrise does not. They had too much to drink at a recent party, and afterwards had sex for the first time. Cantrise had some beliefs about their relationship and HIV infection. Which of Cantrise's beliefs is *incorrect*?
    a.   Women have acquired HIV from men who use IV drugs.
    b.   If we continue to have sex, I should insist that Jamal use a condom.
    *c.   I have no chance of getting HIV if we have more sex as long as I do not use IV drugs.
    d.   I have a chance of getting HIV.

Source. This test was originally published in "HIV Prevention Knowledge Test for Teenagers," by W. Yarber and M. Torabi, 1990-1991, December/January, *SIECUS Report,* 19(2), 28-32. Reprinted with permission of SIECUS, 130 W. 42nd Street, Suite 350, New York, NY 10036-7802.

Adolescent AIDS Knowledge Scale

Gregory D. Zimet,[1] *Indiana University School of Medicine*

The Adolescent AIDS Knowledge Scale was developed as part of a comprehensive questionnaire to evaluate adolescents' knowledge, beliefs, and attitudes about AIDS (Zimet et al., 1989). The knowledge scale was developed with two principal issues in mind. First of all, we wanted to ensure that the scale covered relevant material. To accomplish this goal, item content was derived from a 1988 informational brochure distributed to every household by the U.S. government (Centers for Disease Control, 1988). As a result, the scale addresses multiple AIDS-related domains, including modes of transmission, high-risk behaviors, mortality, the existence of a cure, prevention of transmission, and the appearance of persons with AIDS (PWAs).

A second issue considered during scale development was that most existing AIDS knowledge scales confounded knowledge (i.e., awareness of scientific facts about AIDS) with beliefs. It seemed likely that a person might "know" the facts according to experts, but not believe them. In considering the design of AIDS education interventions, it appeared particularly important to assess AIDS awareness/knowledge separately from AIDS beliefs. To address this issue, each item on the Adolescent AIDS Knowledge Scale was constructed to begin with the phrase "Do most experts say . . . ?" A separate but parallel AIDS Beliefs scale was developed to evaluate the extent to which adolescents believed what experts were saying.

Description

The Adolescent AIDS Knowledge Scale has 22 items. Each item takes the form of a question (e.g., "Do most experts say you can get AIDS by giving blood?"). Transmission-related items cover true modes of transmission (e.g., sharing needles), low- or no-risk behaviors (e.g., sharing a glass of water), behaviors that increase risk of transmission (e.g., prostitution), and transmission of HIV without clinical AIDS. Two protection items address effective (i.e., condom use) and ineffective (i.e., eating healthy foods) protective behaviors. Finally, single items cover such topics as the mortality associated with AIDS, whether there is a cure for AIDS, and whether it is possible to determine if someone has AIDS by looking at him or her.

Response Mode and Timing

To each question, respondents are asked to circle *yes, no,* or *don't know.* Response times vary, but typically the scale requires less than 5 minutes to complete.

---
[1]Address correspondence to Gregory D. Zimet, Division of Adolescent Medicine, Riley Children's Hospital, Room 1740N, 702 Barnhill Drive, Indianapolis, IN 46202; email: gzimet@indyvax.iupui.edu.

Scoring

A correct response receives a score of 1. An incorrect answer or a *don't know* response each receives a score of 0. For the following items, *no* is the correct response: 1, 3, 4, 5, 9, 11, 13, 15, 17, and 19. For the following items, *yes* is the correct response: 2, 6, 7, 8, 10, 12, 14, 16, 18, 20, 21, and 22. The total score for the scale, which is calculated by summing across items, can range from 0 to 22.

Reliability

An AIDS knowledge scale such as this one represents multiple content areas, not a single construct. Therefore, standard measures of internal reliability that assess overall internal consistency (e.g., Cronbach's coefficient alpha or Kuder-Richardson formula 20) are inappropriate (Anastasi, 1982; Zimet, 1992b). A more useful approach involves a specialized form of Spearman-Brown split-half reliability in which items from one half are matched for content with items from the other half (Zimet, 1992b). Given that the Adolescent AIDS Knowledge Scale was not designed with this approach to reliability in mind, it is not possible to match all items perfectly (e.g., only one item addresses mortality associated with AIDS). Nonetheless, in a sample of 721 junior and senior high school students, the Spearman-Brown matched-item split-half method resulted in a coefficient of .82, indicating good internal reliability (Zimet, 1992b).

Validity

The content validity of the scale was established through the use of the U.S. government brochure on AIDS to guide item selection (Centers for Disease Control, 1988). Furthermore, in addressing major AIDS-related domains (HIV transmission, protection, mortality, appearance, etc.), the scale demonstrates good face validity.

Support for the construct validity of the Adolescent AIDS Knowledge Scale is demonstrated by expected relationships with other variables. For example, it may be expected that older students have more accurate knowledge about AIDS than younger students. For the Adolescent AIDS Knowledge Scale, analysis of variance indicated a linear increase in scores across grade level among 617 7th to 12th graders: $F(5, 611) = 8.8, p < .0001$ (Zimet, DiClemente, et al., 1993).

Another expectation is that greater AIDS knowledge is likely to be negatively correlated to inaccurate beliefs about AIDS. Among 438 junior and senior high school students, increases in scores on the Adolescent AIDS Knowledge Scale, in fact, were associated significantly with decreases in inaccurate beliefs about AIDS: $r = -.65, p < .001$ (Zimet et al., 1991).

Finally, it is reasonable to expect that more accurate knowledge about AIDS will be negatively related to fears about interacting with PWAs. Among the same 438 students, Adolescent AIDS Knowledge Scale scores correlated significantly and negatively with anxiety about interacting with PWAs: $r = -.28$, $p < .001$ (Zimet et al., 1991).

References

Anastasi, A. (1982). *Psychological testing* (5th ed.). New York: Macmillan.

Centers for Disease Control. (1988). Understanding AIDS [An information brochure mailed to all U.S. households]. *Morbidity and Mortality Weekly Report, 37,* 261-269.

Zimet, G. D. (1992a). Attitudes of teenagers who know someone with AIDS. *Psychological Reports, 70,* 1169-1170.

Zimet, G. D. (1992b). Reliability of AIDS knowledge scales: Conceptual issues. *AIDS Education and Prevention, 4,* 338-344.

Zimet, G. D., Anglin, T. M., Lazebnik, R., Bunch, D., Williams, P., & Krowchuk, D. P. (1989). Adolescents' knowledge and beliefs about AIDS: Did the government brochure help? *American Journal of Diseases of Children, 143,* 518-519.

Zimet, G. D., Bunch, D. L., Anglin, T. M., Lazebnik, R., Williams, P., & Krowchuk, D. P. (1992). Relationship of AIDS-related attitudes to sexual behavior changes in adolescents. *Journal of Adolescent Health, 13,* 493-498.

Zimet, G. D., DiClemente, R. J., Lazebnik, R., Anglin, T. M., Ellick, E. M., & Williams, P. (1993). Changes in adolescents' knowledge and attitudes about AIDS over the course of the AIDS epidemic. *Journal of Adolescent Health, 14,* 85-90.

Zimet, G. D., Hillier, S. A., Anglin, T. M., Ellick, E. M., Krowchuk, D. P., & Williams, P. (1991). Knowing someone with AIDS: The impact on adolescents. *Journal of Pediatric Psychology, 16,* 287-294.

Zimet, G. D., Lazebnik, R., DiClemente, R. J., Anglin, T. M., Williams, P., & Ellick, E. M. (1993). The relationship of Magic Johnson's announcement of HIV infection to the AIDS attitudes of junior high school students. *The Journal of Sex Research, 30,* 129-134.

Exhibit

Adolescent AIDS Knowledge Scale

Instructions: Experts on AIDS have talked about the spread and prevention of AIDS. Please circle your answer for each question.

1. Do most experts say there's a high chance of getting AIDS by kissing someone on the mouth who has AIDS?   Yes No Don't Know
2. Do most experts say AIDS can be spread by sharing a needle with a drug user who has AIDS?   Yes No Don't Know
3. Do most experts say you can get AIDS by giving blood?   Yes No Don't Know
4. Do most experts say there's a high chance that AIDS can be spread by sharing a glass of water with someone who has AIDS?   Yes No Don't Know
5. Do most experts say there's a high chance you can get AIDS from a toilet seat?   Yes No Don't Know
6. Do most experts say AIDS can be spread if a man has sex with a woman who has AIDS?   Yes No Don't Know
7. Do most experts say AIDS can be spread if a man has sex with another man who has AIDS?   Yes No Don't Know
8. Do most experts say a pregnant woman with AIDS can give AIDS to her unborn baby?   Yes No Don't Know
9. Do most experts say you can get AIDS by shaking hands with someone who has AIDS?   Yes No Don't Know
10. Do most experts say a woman can get AIDS by having sex with a man who has AIDS?   Yes No Don't Know
11. Do most experts say you can get AIDS when you masturbate by yourself?   Yes No Don't Know
12. Do most experts say using a condom (rubber) can lower your chance of getting AIDS?   Yes No Don't Know
13. Do most experts say that there's a high chance of getting AIDS if you get a blood transfusion?   Yes No Don't Know
14. Do most experts say that prostitutes have a higher chance of getting AIDS?   Yes No Don't Know
15. Do most experts say that eating healthy foods can keep you from getting AIDS?   Yes No Don't Know
16. Do most experts say that having sex with more than one partner can raise your chance of getting AIDS?   Yes No Don't Know
17. Do most experts say that you can always tell if someone has AIDS by looking at them?   Yes No Don't Know
18. Do most experts say that people with AIDS will die from it?   Yes No Don't Know
19. Do most experts say there is a cure for AIDS?   Yes No Don't Know
20. Do most experts say that you can have the AIDS virus without being sick from AIDS?   Yes No Don't Know
21. Do most experts say that you can have the AIDS virus and spread it without being sick from AIDS?   Yes No Don't Know
22. Do most experts say that if a man or woman has sex with someone who shoots up drugs, they raise their chance of getting AIDS?   Yes No Don't Know

Index of Homophobia
(Index of Attitudes Toward Homosexuals)

Wendell A. Ricketts
Walter W. Hudson,[1] *WALMYR Publishing Co.*

The Index of Homophobia (IHP) is a short-form scale designed to measure homophobic versus nonhomophobic attitudes (the fear of being in close quarters with homosexuals).

Description

The IHP contains 25 category-partition (Likert-type) items, some of which are worded negatively to partially offset the potential for response set bias. Each item is scored on a relative frequency scale as shown in the scoring key of the instrument. Obtained scores range from 0 to 100 where higher scores indicate greater degrees of homophobia. The IHP has a cutting score of 50, such that scores above that value indicate the presence of an increasingly homophobic attitude toward human sexual expression and scores below that value indicate the presence of an increasing nonhomophobic orientation. A score of 0 represents the most nonhomophobic position, and a score of 100 represents the most homophobic position. The IHP can be used with all English-speaking populations aged 12 or older.

The readability statistics for the IHP are as follows: Flesch Reading Ease: 68, Gunning's Fog Index: 10, and Flesch-Kincaid Grade Level: 7.

Response Mode and Timing

The IHP is normally completed in 5-7 minutes.

Scoring

Items noted below the copyright notation on the scale must first be reverse scored by subtracting the item response from $K + 1$ where K is the number of response categories in the scoring key. After making all appropriate item reversals, compute the total score as $S = (\Sigma X_i - N)(100) / [(K - 1)N]$ where X is an item response, i is item, K is the number of response categories, and N is the number of properly completed items. Total scores remain valid in the face of missing values (omitted items) provided the respondent completes at least 80% of the items. The effect of the scoring formula is to replace missing values with the mean item response value so that scores range from 0 to 100 regardless of the value of N.

Reliability

Cronbach's alpha = .90, and *SEM* = 4.43. Test-retest reliability is not available.

Validity

Known-groups validity is not available for the IHP. Detailed information about content, factorial, and construct validity is reported in the *WALMYR Assessment Scale Scoring Manual,* which is available from the publisher.

Other Information

The IHP is a copyrighted commercial assessment scale and may not be copied, reproduced, altered, or translated into other languages. It may be obtained in tear-off pads of 50 copies per pad at $0.30 per copy ($15.00 per pad) by writing the WALMYR Publishing Co., P.O. Box 6229, Tallahassee, FL 32314-6229; phone and fax: (850) 656-2787; email: walmyr@syspak.com.

References

Hudson, W. W., & Ricketts, W. A. (1980). A strategy for the measurement of homophobia. *Journal of Homosexuality, 5,* 357-372.

Nurius, P. S., & Hudson, W. W. (1993), *Human services practice, evaluation & computers.* Pacific Grove, CA: Brooks/Cole.

[1]Address correspondence to Walter W. Hudson, WALMYR Publishing Co., P.O. Box 6229, Tallahassee, FL 32314-6229; email: walmyr@syspak.com.

Exhibit

 INDEX OF ATTITUDES TOWARD HOMOSEXUALS (IAH)

Name: _____ Today's Date: _____

This questionnaire is designed to measure the way you feel about working or associating with homosexuals. It is not a test, so there are no right or wrong answers. Answer each item as carefully and as accurately as you can by placing a number beside each one as follows.

1 = Strongly agree
2 = Agree
3 = Neither agree nor disagree
4 = Disagree
5 = Strongly disagree

1. _____ I would feel comfortable working closely with a male homosexual.
2. _____ I would enjoy attending social functions at which homosexuals were present.
3. _____ I would feel uncomfortable if I learned that my neighbor was homosexual.
4. _____ If a member of my sex made a sexual advance toward me I would feel angry.
5. _____ I would feel comfortable knowing that I was attractive to members of my sex.
6. _____ I would feel uncomfortable being seen in a gay bar.
7. _____ I would feel comfortable if a member of my sex made an advance toward me.
8. _____ I would be comfortable if I found myself attracted to a member of my sex.
9. _____ I would feel disappointed if I learned that my child was homosexual.
10. _____ I would feel nervous being in a group of homosexuals.
11. _____ I would feel comfortable knowing that my clergyman was homosexual.
12. _____ I would be upset if I learned that my brother or sister was homosexual.
13. _____ I would feel that I had failed as a parent if I learned that my child was gay.
14. _____ If I saw two men holding hands in public I would feel disgusted.
15. _____ If a member of my sex made an advance toward me I would be offended.
16. _____ I would feel comfortable if I learned that my daughter's teacher was a lesbian.
17. _____ I would feel uncomfortable if I learned that my spouse or partner was attracted to members of his or her sex.
18. _____ I would feel at ease talking with a homosexual person at a party.
19. _____ I would feel uncomfortable if I learned that my boss was homosexual.
20. _____ It would not bother me to walk through a predominantly gay section of town.
21. _____ It would disturb me to find out that my doctor was homosexual.
22. _____ I would feel comfortable if I learned that my best friend of my sex was homosexual.
23. _____ If a member of my sex made an advance toward me I would feel flattered.
24. _____ I would feel uncomfortable knowing that my son's male teacher was homosexual.
25. _____ I would feel comfortable working closely with a female homosexual.

3, 4, 6, 9, 10, 12, 13, 14, 15, 17, 19, 21, 24.

Source. This scale is reprinted with permission of WALMYR Publishing Co.

Homophobic Behavior of Students Scale

Paul Van de Ven,[1] Laurel Bornholt, and Michael Bailey, *University of Sydney*

The Homophobic Behavior of Students Scale (HBSS; Van de Ven, Bornholt, & Bailey, 1993, 1996) was developed to measure students' behavioral intentions toward gay males and lesbians, in the context of teaching about homosexuality. The HBSS complements existing cognitive and affective measures of homophobia, thereby giving researchers of antigay and antilesbian prejudice an efficient strategy to measure the much neglected, though highly important, behavioral dimension of homophobic responses (Van de Ven, 1994a). Previous assessments of homophobic behavior have relied on highly contrived experimental manipulations that are unsuitable for everyday classroom use and, with their reliance on naive participants, cannot be used in the repeated measures designs of behavior change studies. The HBSS has the advantages of being practical and plausible, and of being a measure of personal commitment to action that can be assessed on multiple occasions. The HBSS can be treated as an individual differences measure of homophobic behavioral intentions or as a dependent variable when evaluating the impact on behavioral intentions of homophobia reduction strategies (see Van de Ven, 1994b, 1995a, 1995b).

Description

The HBSS consists of 10 items arranged in a 5-point Likert-type format to rate strength of intention from 1 (*definitely false*) to 5 (*definitely true*). The first six items were designed to measure, across classroom and social situations, the extent to which students associated willingly or avoided contact with gay males and lesbians. These items were construed as a measure of social distance aspects of behavior. The remaining items were selected to measure additional and related aspects of behavior expressed as willingness to act in support of gay and lesbian rights. Separate analyses of the responses of 97 undergraduate students (26 males, 71 females) and 40 high school students (24 males, 16 females) suggested that the items contributed to a single factor of behavioral intentions. The HBSS is appropriate to use with both high school and college populations. A posttest version of the HBSS is created by changing the instructions minimally as specified in the accompanying exhibit.

Response Mode and Timing

Students circle the number from 1 to 5 that corresponds with their willingness to participate in each activity. The HBSS takes approximately 3 minutes to complete.

Scoring

A combination of positive and negative items is used to control for potential response set bias. The positively phrased items (Items 1, 2, 4, 6, 7, 9, and 10) have their scoring reversed in the analysis so that higher scores, following convention, indicate more negative behavioral intentions toward homosexuals. Computed HBSS scores, which can range from 0 (least homophobic) to 100 (most homophobic), are determined by using the equation: HBSS computed score = (HBSS summed raw score − 10) × 2.5.

Reliability

For the sample of 97 undergraduate students, Cronbach's alpha was .81, $M = 37.65$, $SD = 19.94$. For the sample of 40 high school students, Cronbach's alpha was .86, $M = 65.25$, $SD = 24.29$ (Van de Ven et al., 1993, 1996).

Validity

As expected, Van de Ven et al. (1993, 1996) found that the computed score of the HBSS was significantly correlated with Homophobic Cognition, $r = .78$, as measured by the Modified Attitudes Toward Homosexuality Scale (Price, 1982). Also in line with expectations, homophobic behavioral intentions were significantly correlated with both Homophobic Anger, $r = .66$, and Homophobic Guilt, $r = .38$, and significantly negatively correlated with Warmth Toward Homosexuals, $r = −.56$, as measured by the Affective Reactions to Homosexuality Scale (Van de Ven, 1994a; Van de Ven et al., 1993, 1996; after Ernulf & Innala, 1987).

To assess the predictive validity of the HBSS, the 40 high school students were given the opportunity to participate in each of the 10 activities of the HBSS (Van de Ven et al., 1993, 1996). As expected, the group of participants for each activity had a lower HBSS mean than the corresponding group that abstained from participation. Group means were significantly different at the .005 alpha level (for a family-wise error rate of .05) for six of the HBSS activities.

Other Information

If the HBSS is used by researchers, notification to the first author of the use and the results obtained would be appreciated.

This scale was developed while the authors were at the School of Educational Psychology, Measurement and Technology, University of Sydney. Laurel Bornholt is now in the Psychology Department at the University of Sydney.

[1]Address correspondence to Paul Van de Ven, National Centre in HIV Social Research, School of Behavioral Sciences, Macquarie University, Sydney NSW 2109, Australia.

References

Ernulf, K. E., & Innala, S. M. (1987). The relationship between affective and cognition components of homophobic reaction. *Archives of Sexual Behavior, 16,* 501-509.

Price, J. H. (1982). High school students' attitudes toward homosexuality. *Journal of School Health, 52,* 469-474.

Van de Ven, P. (1994a). *Challenging homophobia in schools.* Unpublished doctoral thesis, University of Sydney.

Van de Ven, P. (1994b). Comparisons among homophobic reactions of undergraduates, high school students, and young offenders. *The Journal of Sex Research, 31,* 117-124.

Van de Ven, P. (1995a). Effects on high school students of a teaching module for reducing homophobia. *Basic and Applied Social Psychology, 17,* 153-172.

Van de Ven, P. (1995b). Effects on young offenders of two teaching modules for reducing homophobia. *Journal of Applied Social Psychology, 25,* 632-649.

Van de Ven, P., Bornholt, L., & Bailey, M. (1993, November). *Homophobic attitudes and behaviours: Telling which teaching strategies make a difference.* Paper presented at the annual conference of the Australian Association for Research in Education, Fremantle, Western Australia.

Van de Ven, P., Bornholt, L., & Bailey, M. (1996). Measuring cognitive, affective, and behavioral components of homophobic reaction. *Archives of Sexual Behavior, 25,* 155-179.

Exhibit

Homophobic Behavior of Students Scale

Instructions: As part of the unit of work (Posttest version: As part of the follow-up to the unit of work) on lesbian and gay issues, it may be possible to organize some additional activities and guest speakers. So that these can be planned, please indicate in which of the following activities, if any, you would participate. Circle the number that comes closest to representing your willingness to participate. Please do not leave any statements unanswered.

1. I would speak in a small class group with a gay person or lesbian about homosexual issues.

    Definitely false   1   2   3   4   5   Definitely true[a]

2. I would speak individually, in class, with a gay person or lesbian about homosexual issues.
3. I would NOT like to have a gay person or lesbian address the class about homosexual issues.
4. I would take the opportunity to talk in an informal lunch-time meeting with a group of four lesbians or gay males.
5. I would NOT attend a lunch-time barbecue at which four gay males or lesbians were present.
6. I would watch a video in class in which a lesbian or gay person is featured.
7. I would sign my name to a petition asking the government to do more to stop violence against gay men and lesbians.
8. I would NOT sign my name to a petition asking the government to make sure gays and lesbians have equal rights with everybody else.
9. I would sign my name to a petition asking the government to allow lesbian and gay couples to officially register their marriage or partnership.
10. I would sign my name to a petition asking the government to allow lesbian and gay couples to adopt children.

a. The scale is repeated after each item.

Internalized Homophobia Scale

Glenn J. Wagner,[1] *New York State Psychiatric Institute*

The Internalized Homophobia Scale (IHS) was developed for use with gay men and is intended to measure the extent to which negative attitudes and beliefs about homosexuality are internalized and integrated into one's self-image and identity as gay. The significance of measuring internalized homophobia is its negative impact on the mental health of gay and lesbian individuals as it is often associated with guilt, shame, depression, and feelings of worthlessness. Several clinical reports documenting the effects and dynamics of internalized homophobia have been published, but research studies in which internalized homophobia has been systematically measured have been confined (by and large) to studies of gay men with HIV. In research conducted by our group, and others, we have found that internalized homophobia is associated with demoralization, depression, and general psychological distress, as well as low self-esteem and avoidant coping.

Description

The IHS consists of 20 items, 9 of which are from the Nungesser Homosexual Attitudes Inventory (Nungesser, 1983), with the other 11 items developed by the HIV Center for Clinical and Behavioral Studies at the New York State Psychiatric Institute. A principal components factor analysis with a varimax rotation was performed on a sample of 142 gay men who completed the IHS and a 22-item scale of demoralization (Dohrenwend, Shrout, Egri, & Mendelsohn, 1987), and the 7-item depression subscale of the Brief Symptom Inventory (Derogatis & Melisaratos, 1983). Using all items, a two-factor solution resulted, with all but one (Item 4) of the IHS items loading on Factor 1. All of the items from the depression scale loaded on Factor 2, as did 17 of the items from the demoralization scale. None of the items from the three factors loaded on discrepant factors (Wagner, Brondolo, & Rabkin, in press).

Response Mode and Timing

Each item is scored on a 5-point Likert-type scale where 1 = *strongly disagree* and 5 = *strongly agree*, and each response represents the degree to which the respondent endorses the statement or item. The scale requires approximately 5 minutes to complete.

Scoring

Ten items are positively keyed, and 10 are negatively keyed. The range for the total score is 20 to 100, with higher scores representing greater internalized homophobia.

Reliability

The scale was tested for internal consistency reliability in a sample of 142 gay men, yielding a Cronbach alpha of .92 for the total score (Wagner, Serafini, Rabkin, Remien, & Williams, 1994). Based on this statistic and the previously described factor analysis, it is recommended that the total summed score of the 20 items be regarded as a homogeneous measure of internalized homophobia.

Validity

Research using the IHS has revealed the construct to be positively correlated with mental health measures including demoralization ($r = .49$), global psychological distress ($r = .37$), and depression ($r = .36$) (Wagner et al., in press; Wagner et al., 1994). Other correlates include age at which one first accepted being gay ($r = .46$) and degree of integration into the gay community ($r = -.54$) (Wagner et al., 1994). In a study of HIV+ gay men in which the scale was completed twice, with a 2-year interval, results indicated that greater internalized homophobia, specifically among those who had not yet experienced any HIV-related physical symptoms, predicted higher levels of distress over time; within this subgroup, internalized homophobia at the first assessment was correlated .61 with distress 2 years later.

These research findings indicate that internalized homophobia may have a negative impact on mood, self-esteem, and quality of life. Mental health professionals working with gay men, regardless of HIV status, may be more effective in targeting resources and interventions aimed at improving mental health and overall quality of life if they address issues related to internalized homophobia.

References

Derogatis, L. R., & Melisaratos, N. (1983) The Brief Symptom Inventory: An introductory report. *Psychological Medicine, 13,* 595-605.

Dohrenwend, B. P., Shrout, P. E., Egri, G., & Mendelsohn, F. S. (1987). Nonspecific psychological distress and other dimensions of psychopathology. *Archives in General Psychiatry, 9,* 114-122.

Nungesser, L. G. (1983). *Homosexual acts, actors and identities.* New York: Praeger.

Wagner, G., Brondolo, E., & Rabkin, J. G. (in press). Internalized homophobia in a sample of HIV+ gay men, and its relationship to psychological distress, coping, and illness progression. *Journal of Homosexuality, 32*(2).

Wagner, G., Serafini, J., Rabkin, J., Remien, R., & Williams, J. (1994). Integration of one's religion and homosexuality: A weapon against internalized homophobia? *Journal of Homosexuality, 26*(4), 91-109.

[1]Address correspondence to Glenn J. Wagner, New York State Psychiatric Institute, 722 W. 168th Street, Unit #335, New York, NY 10032.

Exhibit

Internalized Homophobia Scale

Instructions: The following are some statements that individuals can make about being gay. Please read each one carefully and decide the extent to which you agree with the statement, then circle the number which best reflects how much you agree or disagree with the statement.

Response format: 1 Strongly Disagree
2 Disagree
3 Neutral
4 Agree
5 Strongly Agree

1. Male homosexuality is a natural expression of sexuality in human males.
2. I wish I were heterosexual.
3. When I am sexually attracted to another gay man, I do not mind if someone else knows how I feel.
4. Most problems that homosexuals have come from their status as an oppressed minority, not from their homosexuality per se.
5. Life as a homosexual is not as fulfilling as life as a heterosexual.
6. I am glad to be gay.
7. Whenever I think a lot about being gay, I feel critical about myself.
8. I am confident that my homosexuality does not make me inferior.
9. Whenever I think a lot about being gay, I feel depressed.
10. If it were possible, I would accept the opportunity to be completely heterosexual.
11. I wish I could become more sexually attracted to women.
12. If there were a pill that could change my sexual orientation, I would take it.
13. I would not give up being gay even if I could.
14. Homosexuality is deviant.
15. It would not bother me if I had children who were gay.
16. Being gay is a satisfactory and acceptable way of life for me.
17. If I were heterosexual, I would probably be happier.
18. Most gay people end up lonely and isolated.
19. For the most part, I do not care who knows I am gay.
20. I have no regrets about being gay.

Source. This scale is reprinted with permission of the author.

Gay Identity Questionnaire

Stephen Brady,[1] *Boston University School of Medicine*

The Gay Identity Questionnaire (GIQ) can be used by clinicians and researchers to identify gay men in the developmental stages of "coming out" proposed by Cass (1979) in the homosexual identity formation (HIF) model. These stages include confusion, comparison, tolerance, acceptance, pride, and synthesis. Test construction procedures included the selection of questionnaire items based on the constructs of the HIF model and the establishment of reliability and validity for the GIQ through two pilot tests and one final administration of the instrument (Brady, 1983; Brady & Busse, 1994).

Description

The GIQ is composed of 45 true-false items and can easily be scored for the purpose of identifying the respondent's stage of HIF. Findings suggest that the GIQ is a reliable and valid measure that can be used by clinicians and researchers to examine the coming-out process. Two-hundred twenty-five male respondents were administered the final version of the GIQ and a Psychosocial/Background Questionnaire. Efforts were made to recruit a developmentally heterogeneous sample of men with same-sex thoughts, feelings, and/or behavior. The majority of the respondents (179) were young (*M* age = 28.8 years), non-Hispanic White men residing in southern California in 1983. All respondents indicated they had homosexual thoughts, feelings, or engaged in homosexual behavior. In addition to the author's use, the instrument has been used in a number of doctoral dissertations and master's theses over the past 10 years.

Response Mode and Timing

The GIQ consists of 45 randomly ordered, true-false statements to which subjects respond by circling either the letter T or F depending upon whether they agree or disagree with the statement. The instrument takes approximately 15-20 minutes to complete.

Scoring

The scoring of the GIQ includes the following. Three items (Items 4, 22, and 40) are used as validity checks and identify that an individual has thoughts, feelings, or engages in behavior that can be labeled as homosexual. Respondents must mark at least one of these three items as true for the instrument to be considered appropriate for use in classifying the stage of HIF.

The other 42 items are used to determine respondents' stage designation. Each of the six stages of HIF is represented by seven items that are characteristic of individuals at that stage. For each item, a respondent marks as true, he accrues 1 point in the HIF stage represented by that item. For every item a respondent marks false, he receives a 0. The subset of items in which a respondent accrues the most points is his given stage designation. If a respondent accrues the same number of points in two or more stages, he is given a dual-stage designation.

Reliability

Interitem consistency scores for the GIQ were obtained using the Kuder-Richardson formula (Hays, 1973). Too few respondents were identified in the first two stages of HIF for data analytic procedures to be used. The reliabilities for the other four stages were as follows: Stage 3 (Identity Tolerance), $r = .76$; Stage 4 (Identity Acceptance), $r = .71$; Stage 5 (Identity Pride), $r = .44$; and Stage 6 (Identity Synthesis), $r = .78$.

Validity

No statistically significant relationships were found between respondent age, education, income, religiosity, political values, and HIF stages. Findings that most demographic variables did not confound the HIF process supports the validity of the HIF model for predicting stages of coming out independent of those variables.

Findings also support a central construct of the HIF model that describes the importance of psychological factors in the evolution of a homosexual identity. Statistical tests revealed a significant positive relationship between respondent stage of HIF and a composite measure of nine self-report items assessing psychological well-being, $F(3, 189) = 8.67$, $p < .01$. Subsequent post hoc analysis of ANOVA results using Tukey's HSD test (Hays, 1973) revealed that respondents in Stage 3, Identity Tolerance, reported having less psychological well-being compared to their counterparts in Stages 4, 5, and 6.

Significant relationships were also found between respondents' stage of HIF and five indexes assessing homosexual adjustment. More specifically, respondents in Stage 3, Identity Tolerance, compared with respondents in the later stages of HIF, reported homosexuality as being a less viable identity, $F(3, 190) = 9.86$, $p < .01$; they were less exclusively homosexual, $F(3, 188) = 14.34$, $p < .01$; they were less likely to have come out to significant others, $F(3, 190) = 25.04$, $p < .01$; they were less sexually active, $F(3, 191) = 4.52$, $p < .01$); and they had fewer involvements in intimate homosexual relationships, $\chi^2 (3, N = 194) = 9.68$, $p < .01$.

[1]Address correspondence to Stephen Brady, Division of Psychiatry, Boston University School of Medicine, Dr. Solomon Carter Fuller Mental Health Center, 85 East Newton Street, Boston, MA 02118.

Respondents in the latter three stages of HIF did not differ appreciably from one another on measures of psychological well-being or homosexual adjustment. These latter findings suggest that HIF may be a two-stage process rather than the six stages proposed by Cass (1979) in the HIF model. In the first stage (Identity Confusion/Comparison/Tolerance) respondents remain unclear about or do not like their homosexual identity, whereas in the second stage (Identity Acceptance/Pride/Synthesis) respondents know and approve of their identity while maintaining different public identities.

Findings support the use of the GIQ as a brief measure for identifying young, middle-class, White men at one of the stages of HIF proposed by Cass (1979). To increase the generalizability of the instrument, future researchers should recruit a sample that includes women and people of color. In addition, a refinement of the instrument so that homosexual identity is treated as a continuous variable with a summed scale score, rather than a categorical variable with a stage designation, would be an improvement in the measurement of HIF.

References

Brady, S. M. (1983). The relationship between differences in stages of homosexual identity formation and background characteristics, psychological well-being and homosexual adjustment. *Dissertation Abstracts International, 45,* 3328(10B).

Brady, S. M., & Busse, W. J. (1994). The Gay Identity Questionnaire: A brief measure of homosexual identity formation. *Journal of Homosexuality, 26*(4), 1-22.

Cass, V. C. (1979). Homosexual identity formation: A theoretical model. *Journal of Homosexuality, 4,* 219-235.

Cass, V. C. (1984). Testing a theoretical model. *The Journal of Sex Research, 20,* 143-167.

Hays, W. L. (1973). *Statistics for the social sciences.* New York: Holt, Rinehart & Winston.

Exhibit

Gay Identity Questionnaire

Directions: Please read each of the following statements carefully and then circle whether you feel the statements are true (T) or false (F) for you at this point in time. A statement is circled as true if the entire statement is true, otherwise it is circled as false.

		True	False
1.	I probably am sexually attracted equally to men and women. (Stage 2)	T	F
2.	I live a homosexual lifestyle at home, while at work/school I do not want others to know about my lifestyle. (Stage 4)	T	F
3.	My homosexuality is a valid private identity, that I do not want made public. (Stage 4)	T	F
4.	I have feelings I would label as homosexual. (validity check item)	T	F
5.	I have little desire to be around most heterosexuals. (Stage 5)	T	F
6.	I doubt that I am homosexual, but still am confused about who I am sexually. (Stage 1)	T	F
7.	I do not want most heterosexuals to know that I am definitely homosexual. (Stage 4)	T	F
8.	I am very proud to be gay and make it known to everyone around me. (Stage 5)	T	F
9.	I don't have much contact with heterosexuals and can't say that I miss it. (Stage 5)	T	F
10.	I generally feel comfortable being the only gay person in a group of heterosexuals. (Stage 6)	T	F
11.	I'm probably homosexual, even though I maintain a heterosexual image in both my personal and public life. (Stage 3)	T	F
12.	I have disclosed to 1 or 2 people (very few) that I have homosexual feelings, although I'm not sure I'm homosexual. (Stage 2)	T	F
13.	I am not as angry about treatment of gays because even though I've told everyone about my gayness, they have responded well. (Stage 6)	T	F
14.	I am definitely homosexual but I do not share that knowledge with most people. (Stage 4)	T	F
15.	I don't mind if homosexuals know that I have homosexual thoughts and feelings, but I don't want others to know. (Stage 3)	T	F
16.	More than likely I'm homosexual, although I'm not positive about it yet. (Stage 3)	T	F
17.	I don't act like most homosexuals do, so I doubt that I'm homosexual. (Stage 1)	T	F
18.	I'm probably homosexual, but I'm not sure yet. (Stage 3)	T	F
19.	I am openly gay and fully integrated into heterosexual society. (Stage 6)	T	F
20.	I don't think that I'm homosexual. (Stage 1)	T	F
21.	I don't feel as if I'm heterosexual or homosexual. (Stage 2)	T	F
22.	I have thoughts I would label as homosexual. (validity check item)	T	F
23.	I don't want people to know that I may be homosexual, although I'm not sure if I am homosexual or not. (Stage 2)	T	F
24.	I may be homosexual and I am upset at the thought of it. (Stage 2)	T	F
25.	The topic of homosexuality does not relate to me personally. (Stage 1)	T	F

26. I frequently confront people about their irrational, homophobic (fear of homosexuality) feelings. (Stage 5)   T   F
27. Getting in touch with homosexuals is something I feel I need to do, even though I'm not sure I want to. (Stage 3)   T   F
28. I have homosexual thoughts and feelings but I doubt that I'm homosexual. (Stage 1)   T   F
29. I dread having to deal with the fact that I may be homosexual. (Stage 2)   T   F
30. I am proud and open with everyone about being gay, but it isn't the major focus of my life. (Stage 6)   T   F
31. I probably am heterosexual or non-sexual. (Stage 1)   T   F
32. I am experimenting with my same sex, because I don't know what my sexual preference is. (Stage 2)   T   F
33. I feel accepted by homosexual friends and acquaintances, even though I'm not sure I'm homosexual. (Stage 3)   T   F
34. I frequently express to others, anger over heterosexuals' oppression of me and other gays. (Stage 5)   T   F
35. I have not told most of the people at work that I am definitely homosexual. (Stage 4)   T   F
36. I accept but would not say I am proud of the fact that I am definitely homosexual. (Stage 4)   T   F
37. I cannot imagine sharing my homosexual feelings with anyone. (Stage 1)   T   F
38. Most heterosexuals are not credible sources of help for me. (Stage 5)   T   F
39. I am openly gay around heterosexuals. (Stage 6)   T   F
40. I engage in sexual behavior I would label as homosexual. (validity check item)   T   F
41. I am not about to stay hidden as gay for anyone. (Stage 5)   T   F
42. I tolerate rather than accept my homosexual thoughts and feelings. (Stage 3)   T   F
43. My heterosexual friends, family, and associates think of me as a person who happens to be gay, rather than as a gay person. (Stage 6)   T   F
44. Even though I am definitely homosexual, I have not told my family. (Stage 4)   T   F
45. I am openly gay with everyone, but it doesn't make me feel all that different from heterosexuals. (Stage 6)   T   F

Source. This questionnaire is reprinted with permission of the author.

Homosexual Identity Questionnaire

The Editors

The Homosexual Identity Questionnaire (HIQ) was developed by Cass (1979, 1986) to measure varying levels of development in the process of adopting or acquiring a homosexual identity. It was derived from Cass's theory of gay identity formation and was designed, in part, to assess the validity of aspects of this theory (Cass, 1984). There are six stages of identity formation described in this theory and measured by the HIQ.

The HIQ contains 210 items in 17 subscales: Commitment, Disclosure, Generality, Identity, Evaluation, Group Identification, Social Interaction, Alienation, Inconsistency, Sexual Orientation Activity, Acculturation, Deference to Others, Dichotomization, Personal Control, Strategies, Per-

sonal Satisfaction, and Professional Contact. It takes an average of 45 minutes to complete the HIQ.

Additional information and the instrument can be obtained from Vivienne Cass, Darley House, 4 Darley Street, South Perth, Western Australia, 6151.

References

Cass, V. C. (1979). Homosexual identity formation: A theoretical model. *Journal of Homosexuality, 4,* 219-235.

Cass, V. C. (1984). Homosexual identity formation: Testing a theoretical model. *The Journal of Sex Research, 20,* 143-176.

Cass, V. C. (1986). *Homosexual identity formation: The presentation and testing of a socio-cognitive model.* Unpublished manuscript, Murdoch University, Murdoch, Western Australia.

Lesbian Degree of Involvement and Overtness Scale

K. D. Ferguson[1] and Deana C. Finkler, *Utica College*

The Lesbian Degree of Involvement and Overtness (DIOS) scale was developed to measure (a) the degree of interpersonal lesbian involvement and (b) the overtness of lesbianism.

Description

The scale is a 37-item summated rating scale (10-point) with response options labeled from *very comfortable* to *very uncomfortable*. Respondents also indicate which behaviors they have performed and at what age the behavior first occurred. An original list of 39 items was subjected to two Q sorts, one for the degree of interpersonal homosexual involvement and the other for the degree of overtness of one's lesbianism. Twenty-six items reflecting involvement and 15 items reflecting overtness were retained.

Response Mode and Timing

Respondents circle the number indicating their comfortableness with each statement, circle the item number for each statement that is true for them (that they have done), and indicate the age at which that behavior first occurred. The scale requires an average of 20 minutes for completion.

Scoring

Items, 1, 4, 6, 9, 11, 13, 14, 16, 17, 19, 24, 26, 29, 32, and 36 comprise the Involvement scale. Items 2, 3, 5, 7, 8, 10, 11, 12, 15, 17, 18, 19, 20, 21, 22, 23, 24, 25, 27, 28,

30, 31, 33, 34, 35, and 37 comprise the Overtness scale. (Note that Items 11, 17, 19, and 24 appear on both scales.) Higher scores indicate greater involvement and overtness.

Reliability

Scale homogeneity was demonstrated for both the Involvement scale ($KR_{21} = .78$, $p < .01$) and the Overtness scale ($KR_{21} = .70$, $p < .01$). In scale testing, odd-even, split-half reliability, corrected with the Spearman-Brown formula, also showed high internal consistency for both the Involvement scale, $r = .95$, $p < .001$, and the Overtness scale, $r = .92$, $p < .001$ (Ferguson & Finkler, 1978). A second sample also revealed high internal consistency for both the Involvement scale, $r = .86$, $p < .01$, and the Overtness scale, $r = .84$, $p < .01$, using the Spearman-Brown split-half step-up technique with an odd-even split.

Validity

The scale discriminated, in the expected direction, between lesbians, feminists, and introductory psychology students, with lesbians scoring higher than feminists, who scored higher than students (Ferguson & Finkler, 1978).

Reference

Ferguson, K. D., & Finkler, D. C. (1978). An involvement and overtness measure for lesbians: Its development and relation to anxiety and social zeitgeist. *Archives of Sexual Behavior, 7,* 211-227.

[1]Address correspondence to K. D. Ferguson, Division of Behavioral Sciences, Utica College, Burrstone Road, Utica, NY 13502.

Sexual Correlates of Female Homosexual Experience

Erich Goode,[1] *State University of New York at Stony Brook*

Description

Goode and Haber (1977) investigated whether and to what extent there were differences in prior sexual experiences and behavior between college women who have had

[1]Address correspondence to Erich Goode, Department of Sociology, State University of New York at Stony Brook, Stony Brook, NY 11794-4356; email: egood@sbccvm.edu.

homosexual experiences and those with no such experiences. The instrument is a questionnaire consisting of 60 questions dealing with a wide variety of sexual experiences and behaviors. These include age at first intercourse, total number of partners with whom the respondent has engaged in sexual intercourse, number of sexual partners the respondent was not in love with, experiences with fellatio and cunnilingus, types of sexual experiences with another woman, age of the respondent when she first engaged in homosexual experience, experience with masturbation, and experience with orgasm.

Response Mode and Timing

The questions are framed either in the form of a forced-choice checklist or a question requesting the respondent write out a specific answer, often a number. Most respondents require between 30 and 60 minutes to complete the questionnaire.

Scoring

No scoring is required (see below).

Reliability and Validity

Because the study for which the instrument was developed (Goode & Haber, 1977) was descriptive and exploratory, and not explanatory and definitive, tests of reliability and validity were not undertaken. Simple percentage differences—as determined by magnitude—were used to determine the differences between the two groups of women.

Reference

Goode, E., & Haber, L. (1977). Sexual correlates of homosexual experience: An exploratory study of college women. *The Journal of Sex Research, 13,* 12-21.

Exhibit

Sexual Experience Questionnaire

The intent of this study is to find out what and how women feel about their own sexuality. The questions are designed as a means of understanding what women experience in their sexual relationships and activities.

It is my belief that we, as women, have been letting one another down by allowing men to define our sexuality for us. The time has come for us to speak candidly and frankly about our sexual lives. Only in this way can we know the nature of our collective experiences.

It will not be easy to shed the beliefs we were taught and expect to accept pertaining to our sexuality, but it is something we must do for ourselves, and for each other.

Several hundred questionnaires will be distributed to a sample of women on the Stony Brook campus. *All returned questionnaires will remain confidential.* There is no need to write your name on this questionnaire.

Please answer all questions honestly, completely, and seriously. Your cooperation is very much appreciated. Thank you![a]

1. Have you ever engaged in sexual intercourse with a man or a boy? (*Please check one*) Yes _____ No _____
   (If *no*, skip to Question 2; if *yes*, proceed to Question 1a)
   1a. Please write in your age when you first engaged in sexual intercourse with a man or boy _____
   1b. Please write in the total number of men that you have engaged in sexual intercourse with _____
   1c. Have you ever engaged in sexual intercourse with a man that you were not in love with? Yes _____ No _____
   1d. If yes to Question 1c, with how many men have you engaged in sexual intercourse that you were not in love with? (Please write in the number) _____
   1e. If yes to Question 1c, how did you usually feel right after engaging in intercourse with a man that you were not in love with? (Please check the alternative that comes closest to your feelings)
   Negative (sad, depressed, guilty, etc.) _____
   Positive (it was what I wanted to do at the time) _____
   Neutral (it didn't both me) _____
   It depended on the man; I felt different with different men _____
   It depended on my mood at the time _____
   Other (Please explain) _____
   1f. About what proportion of the time do you generally achieve orgasm during intercourse with a man? (Please check the appropriate category)
   Never _____
   Rarely (less than 10 percent of the time) _____
   Occasionally (less than a quarter of the time, but more than 10 percent of the time) _____
   About half the time, more or less _____
   Usually _____
   Always or almost always _____
   1g. Do you think that you could estimate the total number of *times* that you have had intercourse, with any man?

About how many times would you say that you had sexual intercourse with a man? (Please write in the number) _____

2. Have you ever engaged in fellatio with a man (oral stimulation of a man's penis) *whether or not it led to his orgasm*? Yes _____ No _____

(If *no*, please skip to Question 3; if *yes*, proceed with Question 2a)

2a. Could you estimate about the total number of times that you have engaged in fellatio, with any man? _____

2b. About what proportion of this number of times did your oral stimulation of a man's penis lead to his orgasm? (Please write in about what percentage of the time this happened) _____

2c. With how many men have you engaged in fellatio when it did not lead to his orgasm? _____

2d. With how many men have you engaged in fellatio when it did lead to his orgasm? _____

2e. How old were you when you first engaged in fellatio with a man? _____

2f. How old were you when you first engaged in fellatio with a man when it led to his orgasm? _____

2g. Do you usually enjoy fellating a man? Yes _____ No _____

About half and half—sometimes yes, sometimes no _____

It depends _____

If it depends, what does it depend on? _____

2h. Do you usually fellate a man spontaneously, or does the man usually request you to do it?

Usually spontaneously _____

At first I was asked; later it's usually been spontaneously _____

It depends on how much I like the man _____

I usually have to be asked to do it _____

There's no particular pattern to it _____

It's some other way (Please explain) _____

3. Has a man ever engaged in cunnilingus (oral stimulation of a woman's genitals) with you? Yes _____ No _____

If *no*, have your ever wanted a man to engage in cunnilingus with you? Yes _____ No _____

If *yes*, could you please estimate the total number of times that a man has engaged in cunnilingus with you? _____

(If a man has not engaged in cunnilingus with you, please skip to Question 4; if one has, please continue with Question 3a)

3a. About what proportion of the time would you say that you have achieved orgasm during cunnilingus with a man? (Please check the appropriate category)

Never _____

Rarely (less than 10 percent of the time) _____

Occasionally (less than a quarter of the time, but more than 10 percent of the time) _____

About half the time, more or less _____

Usually _____

Always or almost always _____

3b. If you achieve orgasm during cunnilingus with a man less than half the time, why do you think this is so? (Please explain) _____

3c. If a man has engaged in cunnilingus with you, do you usually have to ask him to do it, or does he usually do it without your asking him?

I always have to ask _____

I usually have to ask _____

It depends on the man _____

It happens both ways about half the time _____

The man usually does it without my asking _____

The man always does it without my asking _____

3d. How many men have performed cunnilingus with you? _____

3e. How old were you when a man first performed cunnilingus with you? _____

3f. How old were you when a man first performed cunnilingus with you, and it led to your orgasm? _____

3g. Have you ever been afraid to ask a man to perform cunnilingus with you because you thought he wouldn't like it? Yes _____ No _____

3h. If yes, about how many times have you been afraid to ask a man to perform cunnilingus with you because you thought he wouldn't like it? _____

3i. If yes, with how many men have you been afraid to ask to perform cunnilingus with you because you thought they wouldn't like it? _____

4. Have you ever engaged in any of the following sexual experiences with another woman?

Nude hugging and kissing and caressing, without genital contact: Yes _____ No _____

Cunnilingus: Yes _____ No _____

Mutual pubic rubbing: Yes _____ No _____

Manual genital contact: Yes _____ No _____

(If you have not engaged in any of these activities, please skip to Question 5; if you have, please proceed with Question 4a)
If you have engaged in any other sexual experiences with another woman, what were they? (Please explain) ____

4a. About what is the total number of times that you have engaged in the sexual experiences with another woman asked about in question 4—caressing, cunnilingus, pubic rubbing, and manual genital contact? (Please write in the total number) ____

4b. About what proportion of the time have you engaged in each of the following activities when you have a sexual experience with another woman? (Please write in the percentage)
Nude hugging, kissing, and caressing, without genital contact ____%
Cunnilingus ____%
Mutual pubic rubbing ____%
Manual genital contact ____%
Other (Please explain) ____

4c. How old were you when you first had any of these sexual experiences with another woman? ____

4d. With how many women have you engaged in any of these sexual experiences? ____

4e. Have you ever engaged in any of these sexual experiences with another woman, with a man present?
Yes ____ No ____

4f. If so, how often has this happened? ____

4g. About what proportion of the time that you have had a sexual experience with another woman did you achieve orgasm?
Never ____
Rarely ____
Occasionally ____
About half the time ____
Usually ____
Always or almost always ____

5. Have you ever masturbated yourself? Yes ____ No ____
(If no, skip to Question 6; if yes, proceed with Question 5a)

5a. How old were you when you first masturbated yourself? ____

5b. How old were you when you first masturbated yourself to orgasm? ____

5c. About how frequently would you say that you have masturbated yourself per month in the past year? ____

5d. About what proportion would you say that you achieve orgasm when you masturbate yourself?
Never ____
Rarely ____
Occasionally ____
About half the time ____
Usually ____
Always or almost always ____

5e. Do you feel that masturbation is a substitute for having orgasms during regular intercourse, or do you think it is an enjoyable activity in itself?
A substitute ____
Enjoyable in itself ____
Something else (Please explain) ____

6. Are some of your orgasms significantly more enjoyable than others, or are they about equally enjoyable?
Yes, some are far more enjoyable than others ____
They are about equally enjoyable ____
I have never had an orgasm ____

6a. If some of your orgasms are far more pleasurable than others, what do you think it is that makes it this way? (Please explain) ____

6b. Which of the following activities gives you the most pleasurable orgasm? Which one the least? Please *rank* all of the following activities in terms of how pleasurable your orgasms have been when you have engaged in each one:
Intercourse with a man ____
Cunnilingus with a man ____
Masturbating myself ____
A man masturbating me ____
Sexual experience with another woman ____
My orgasms are about equally enjoyable ____
I have had orgasms only one way ____
I have never had an orgasm ____
Something else (Please explain) ____

7. If you fail to achieve an orgasm during intercourse with a man, are you usually:
   Extremely disappointed and frustrated _____
   Somewhat disappointed and frustrated _____
   Indifferent; if it happens, it happens, if it doesn't, it doesn't, that's all _____
   I usually feel some other way (Please explain) _____

8. How do you know when you are having an orgasm? What are the signs, what happens to your body or mind that tells you you are having an orgasm? (Please explain) ____

9. Are there any sexual activities in general that you have not participated in, but you would like to try?
   Yes _____   No _____
   If yes, what are they? ____

10. When you have been in bed with another person have there been times when you would have liked to engage in a certain activity, but didn't because you were afraid to ask your partner? Yes _____   No _____
    If yes, what were they? (Please describe) _____

11. When you have been in bed with someone for the first time, have you ever felt reluctant to take your clothes off because you were afraid that the other person might not like your body? Yes _____   No _____
    If yes, about how many times has this happened? _____

12. About how many orgasms per week do you feel is ideal for yourself? _____

13. If you had things your way, how often would you want to have sex each week? _____

14. Do you fantasize during sex—any form of sex? Yes _____   No _____

15. When you have sex, any form of sex, and have an orgasm, do you feel that one orgasm is satisfying for the next few hours, or do you usually feel that you would like to have more than one?
    One is usually satisfying _____
    I usually would like to have more than one _____
    It depends _____
    (If it depends, what does it depend on?) _____
    Something else (Please explain) ____
    I rarely or never have orgasms _____

16. If you could have things more or less exactly the way you wanted them sexually, what would they be like? How would you change your life? What would your sex life be like? ____

17. Age _____

18. What is your grandparent's religion? ____

19. How religious would you say you are?
    Very religious _____
    Somewhat religious _____
    Not very religious _____
    I'm not religious at all _____

20. Father's education _____

21. Mother's education _____

22. Race: Black _____   White _____   Oriental _____   Puerto Rican _____   Other (Please write in your race) _____

23. How influential do you feel your parents are now on your life?
    Very influential now _____
    Somewhat influential now _____
    Not very influential now _____
    Not at all influential now _____

24. Have you ever smoked marijuana? Yes _____   No _____

25. How frequently would you estimate that you have smoked marijuana in the past six months or so?
    Not at all _____
    Less than monthly _____
    More than monthly, but less than weekly _____
    About once a week _____
    Several times a week _____
    Daily or so _____
    More than once a day _____

26. What are your impressions of this questionnaire? _____

27. Are there any questions that should have been asked, but were not? _____

a. The introduction to the questionnaire was written by Goode's collaborator, Lynn Haber.

Evaluation Thermometer Measure for Assessing Attitudes Toward Gay Men

Geoffrey Haddock,[1] *University of Michigan*
Mark P. Zanna, *University of Waterloo*

The framework from which the use of the "evaluation thermometer" is derived comes from contemporary theorizing in the general area of attitudes. Drawing on recent theoretical perspectives on the attitude concept presented by Zanna and Rempel (1988) and Eagly and Chaiken (1993), attitude is defined as an overall or summary evaluation of an attitude object along a dimension of favorability (e.g., positive-negative). Both Zanna and Rempel and Eagly and Chaiken perceive such evaluations as having multiple antecedents. According to this perspective, the attitude concept is viewed as being based on three general sources of information: (a) cognitive information (e.g., beliefs about the attitude object), (b) affective information (e.g., feelings or emotions associated with the attitude object), and (c) information concerning past behaviors or behavioral intentions toward the attitude object.

Defining attitude as an overall evaluation implies that measures of the construct should not be restrictive in their content. For instance, using responses to items such as "I would feel comfortable being in a gay bar" and "Homosexuality is sinful" may not accurately reflect an individual's attitude toward gay men because, for many individuals, these questions are not important in determining their overall evaluation of the group. Thus, the unrestrictive nature of the evaluation thermometer is beneficial in conforming to the Zanna and Rempel (1988) definition of attitude in the sense that it allows respondents to make a judgment based on the information most relevant to themselves.

Description

The evaluation thermometer is adapted from the "feeling thermometer" used in past survey research (e.g., Campbell, 1971), but modified so as to remove its affective nature and make it more purely evaluative. In assessing attitudes toward gay men, respondents are asked to "provide a number between 0/deg and 100/deg to indicate your overall evaluation of gay men." The extreme ends of the scale, 0/deg and 100/deg, are labeled *extremely unfavorable* and *extremely favorable*, with the adjectives *very, quite, fairly,* and *slightly unfavorable/favorable* marked at 10/deg increments. The midpoint of the scale, 50/deg, is labeled *neither favorable nor unfavorable*.

The evaluation thermometer measure can be easily used with diverse populations. Previous research suggests that college and adult samples are able to respond effortlessly to the evaluation thermometer.

Response Mode and Timing

Respondents are asked to simply indicate a number between 0/deg and 100/deg. This is a very simple task that requires very little time. Indeed, one major advantage of the evaluation thermometer is its simplicity. Attitudes toward numerous social groups can be assessed quickly in a single setting. Because attitudes toward several groups are being obtained simultaneously, respondents naturally provide differentially favorable evaluations, allowing the researcher to compare the favorability of respondents' evaluations.

Scoring

Given that the measure is a single item, no computations are required to create an attitude score. In past research in the intergroup context, mean scores on the measure have ranged from approximately 80 (for the target group "English Canadians") to 35 (for the group "feminists"). Generally, in assessing attitudes toward gay men, the evaluation thermometer results in mean scores between 40 and 50. In studies assessing attitudes toward multiple social groups, gay men are typically evaluated less favorably than most groups (Esses, Haddock, & Zanna, 1993).

Reliability

It has been suggested that a single-item attitude measure might be less reliable than multi-item measures. However, research by Jaccard, Weber, and Lundmark (1975) has revealed that single-item attitude measures that are purely evaluative are as reliable as multi-item measures and yield the same results as multiple-item assessment devices. Consistent with this opinion, Haddock, Zanna, and Esses (1993) revealed that the test-retest reliability of the evaluation thermometer, over a 2-week period, was .77.

Validity

Numerous studies have been conducted assessing the validity of the evaluation thermometer. For instance, Haddock (1994) established that scores on the evaluation thermometer were correlated .91 with a multiple-item semantic differential measure. Furthermore, in assessing attitudes

[1]Address correspondence to Geoffrey Haddock, Research Center for Group Dynamics, Institute for Social Research, P.O. Box 1248, University of Michigan, Ann Arbor, MI 48109; email: ghaddock@umich.edu.

toward the target group "Jews," Stangor, Sullivan, and Ford (1991) found a correlation of −.73 between thermometer scores and scores on a 10-item anti-Semitism scale.

Other Information

In a recent study, Haddock et al. (1993, Study 1) assessed the extent to which attitudes toward gay men, as assessed by the evaluation thermometer, were predicted by the favorability of respondents' stereotypes, symbolic beliefs, and affective responses about the group. Stereotypes refer to the attributes or characteristics associated with the group (e.g., the belief that gay men are "intelligent"). Symbolic beliefs refer to the values believed to be hindered or promoted by the group (e.g., the belief that gay men "promote freedom of expression"). Affective responses refer to the feelings or emotions elicited by the group (e.g., gay men may make an individual feel "proud"). The results of this research revealed that symbolic beliefs, affective responses, and behavioral information were all uniquely predictive of attitudes, but that their relative importance was moderated by individual differences in authoritarianism. The attitudes of high authoritarians were derived primarily from symbolic beliefs, whereas the attitudes of low authoritarians were derived primarily from affective responses and stereotypic beliefs. In addition, high authoritarians reported more negative stereotypes, symbolic beliefs, and affective responses about gay men.

References

Campbell, D. T. (1971). *White attitudes toward Black people.* Ann Arbor, MI: Institute for Social Research.

Eagly, A. H., & Chaiken, S. (1993). *The psychology of attitudes.* Fort Worth, TX: Harcourt Brace Jovanovich.

Esses, V. M., Haddock, G., & Zanna, M. P. (1993). Values, stereotypes, and emotions as determinants of intergroup attitudes. In D. M. Mackie & D. L. Hamilton (Eds.), *Affect, cognition and stereotyping: Interactive processes in group perception* (pp. 137-166). New York: Academic Press.

Haddock, G. (1994). *Feeling versus believing: Investigating the existence of individual differences in attitude structure.* Unpublished doctoral dissertation, University of Waterloo, Canada.

Haddock, G., Zanna, M. P., & Esses, V. M. (1993). Assessing the structure of prejudicial attitudes: The case of attitudes toward homosexuals. *Journal of Personality and Social Psychology, 65,* 1105-1118.

Jaccard, J., Weber, J., & Lundmark, J. (1975). A multitrait-multimethod analysis of four attitude assessment procedures. *Journal of Experimental Social Psychology, 11,* 149-154.

Stangor, C., Sullivan, L. A., & Ford, T. E. (1991). Affective and cognitive determinants of prejudice. *Social Cognition, 9,* 359-391.

Zanna, M. P., & Rempel, J. K. (1988). Attitudes: A new look at an old concept. In D. Bar-Tal & A. W. Kruglanski (Eds.), *The social psychology of knowledge* (pp. 315-334). Cambridge, UK: Cambridge University Press.

Exhibit

Evaluation Thermometer Measure for Assessing Attitudes Toward Gay Men

Please provide a number between 0/deg and 100/deg to indicate your overall evaluation of:

GAY MEN _____

POSITIVE	100/deg	Extremely favorable
	90/deg	Very favorable
	80/deg	Quite favorable
	70/deg	Fairly favorable
	60/deg	Slightly favorable
	50/deg	Neither favorable nor unfavorable
	40/deg	Slightly unfavorable
	30/deg	Fairly unfavorable
	20/deg	Quite unfavorable
	10/deg	Very unfavorable
NEGATIVE	0/deg	Extremely unfavorable

Knowledge About Homosexuality Questionnaire

Mary B. Harris,[1] *University of New Mexico*

The Knowledge About Homosexuality Questionnaire was developed by Harris, Nightengale, and Owen (1995) to measure the accuracy of nurses', psychologists', and social workers' knowledge about homosexuality and about issues related to sexual orientation. It has also been used to measure information possessed by college and high school students (Harris & Vanderhoof, 1995). The intent of the instrument is to measure factual knowledge, rather than evaluative opinions.

Description

The Knowledge About Homosexuality Questionnaire is a 20-item, true-false factual test. The first 14 items were based on the work of Sears (1992), and the other questions were developed by the authors, based partially on material in Crooks and Baur (1990).

Response Mode and Timing

This instrument has thus far been given only as part of a longer survey. It has been scored by having respondents write T or F after each item or by having them circle the correct answer (T or F). Alternatively, they could mark the correct answer on a machine-scorable answer sheet. The instrument takes approximately 5 minutes to complete.

Scoring

The correct responses are indicated on the instrument. The total number of correct responses is counted, with omissions scored as incorrect. This procedure produces possible scores ranging from 0 to 20, with a 10 representing chance. Mean scores were 16.3 or 82% correct for a sample of 97 health care professionals (Harris et al., 1995), 14.4 or 72% correct for a sample of 210 college students, and 12.7 or 63% correct for a sample of 31 high school students (Harris & Vanderhoof, 1995).

[1]Address correspondence to Mary B. Harris, College of Education, University of New Mexico, Albuquerque, NM 87131; email: mharris@unm.edu.

Reliability

Cronbach's alpha was .70 for the sample of health care professionals, .74 for the college students, and .28 for the high school students.

Validity

Construct validity, suggesting that people who have more relevant education score higher on the instrument, comes from several sources. An expert in sexuality, who teaches a human sexuality course, took the test and got all of the items correct. Scores on the knowledge test were significantly higher for psychologists and social workers than for nurses and significantly higher for people with more advanced degrees than for those with less education (Harris et al., 1995). The mean score was higher for health care professionals than for college students and was higher for college students than for high school students.

People with higher scores were significantly less prejudiced against gays and lesbians in all three studies, with correlations on various measures ranging from –.41 to –.61. They also held less politically and socially conservative opinions on a number of issues (Harris & Vanderhoof, 1995).

The instrument is currently being administered to a sample of teachers as part of a questionnaire concerning their interactions with gay and lesbian parents.

References

Crooks, R., & Baur, K. (1990). *Our sexuality* (4th ed.). Redwood, CA: Benjamin Cummings.

Harris, M. B., Nightengale, J., & Owen, N. (1995). Health care professionals' experience, knowledge, and attitudes concerning homosexuality. *Journal of Gay and Lesbian Social Services, 2*(2), 91-107.

Harris, M. B., & Vanderhoof, J. (1995). Attitudes toward gays and lesbians serving in the military. *Journal of Gay and Lesbian Social Services, 3*(4), 23-51.

Sears, J. T. (1992). Educators, homosexuality, and homosexual students: Are personal feelings related to professional beliefs? *Journal of Homosexuality, 22*(3/4), 29-79.

Exhibit

Knowledge About Homosexuality Questionnaire

Please respond to each of the following statements by circling T if you think that it is true and F if you think that it is false.

Item	Scoring
1. Homosexuality is a phase which children outgrow.	F
2. There is a good chance of changing homosexual persons into heterosexual men and women.	F

3. Most homosexuals want to be members of the opposite sex.	F
4. Some church denominations have condemned legal and social discrimination against homosexuals.	T
5. Sexual orientation is established at an early age.	T
6. According to the American Psychological Association, homosexuality is an illness.	F
7. Homosexual males are more likely to seduce young boys than heterosexual males are to seduce young girls.	F
8. Gay men are more likely to be victims of violent crime than the general public.	T
9. A majority of homosexuals were seduced in adolescence by a person of the same sex, usually several years older.	F
10. A person becomes a homosexual (develops a homosexual orientation) because he/she chooses to do so.	F
11. Homosexual activity occurs in many animals.	T
12. Kinsey and many other researchers consider sexual behavior as a continuum from exclusively homosexual to exclusively heterosexual.	T
13. A homosexual person's gender identity does not agree with his/her biological sex.	F
14. Historically, almost every culture has evidenced widespread intolerance toward homosexuals, viewing them as "sick" or as "sinners."	F
15. Heterosexual men tend to express more hostile attitudes toward homosexuals than do heterosexual women.	T
16. "Coming out" is a term that homosexuals use for publicly acknowledging their homosexuality.	T
17. One difference between homosexual men and women is that lesbians tend to have more partners over their lifetime.	F
18. The National Gay and Lesbian Task Force is an agency founded to work with homosexual men and women to help achieve legal rights.	T
19. Bisexuality can be characterized by overt behaviors and/or erotic responses to both males and females.	T
20. Recent research has shown that homosexuality is caused by a chromosomal abnormality.	F

Source. This questionnaire is reprinted with permission of the author.

Gay and Lesbian Parents Questionnaire

Mary B. Harris[1] and Pauline H. Turner, *University of New Mexico*

The Gay and Lesbian Parents Questionnaire is designed to gather descriptive information about the relationships between gay and lesbian parents and their children. In particular, it is intended to permit comparisons of children with gay and lesbian parents to children of heterosexual single parents and to identify particular problems or issues that these children might be facing.

Description

The Gay and Lesbian Parents Questionnaire consists of two sections. Section A contains questions that could also be answered by heterosexual single parents. These questions include (a) demographic data on age, sex, ethnicity, education, religion, occupation and income; (b) information on current and past marital status; age, sex, and custody of children; others living in household; and time spent with children; (c) questions about problems commonly found in single-parent families and blended families; (d) questions about gender roles; (e) for each child, up to a maximum of four, five questions about interaction with the child; (f) a question regarding the respondent's willingness to be inter-

[1]Address correspondence to Mary B. Harris, College of Education, University of New Mexico, Albuquerque, NM 87131; email: mharris@unm.edu.

viewed; and (g) an open-ended question asking for any other information the respondent might care to share.

Section B includes additional questions specifically concerned with sexual orientation: (a) personal and family history relevant to sexual orientation; (b) respondent's children's and (ex-) spouse's knowledge of and reactions to his or her homosexuality; (c) problems and benefits the respondents' homosexuality causes for their children and themselves as parents; (d) the relationship between the respondent's partner and children (if applicable); and (e) another open-ended question asking for additional comments.

Response Mode and Timing

The items are primarily answered by checking appropriate alternatives, but some require short answers, and the open-ended questions permit longer responses. An interview protocol that involves extended probing of the responses also is available (Turner, Scadden, & Harris, 1990). The questionnaire requires 10 to 30 minutes to complete, depending on the number of children and the details the respondent provides.

Scoring

There is no formal scoring or scaling of the questionnaire, because it is not intended to provide either a single measure or a number of factors.

Reliability

Because the measure is not a unitary scale, a measure of internal consistency is not appropriate. There has been no formal assessment of test-retest reliability, although extended interviews conducted several months later with 21 of the original respondents did not reveal any obvious discrepancies in their responses over time.

Validity

Little information is available on the criterion-referenced validity of the instrument, although its face validity appears high. The responses of the original participants were very similar to those of a sample of heterosexual single parents (Harris & Turner, 1986), suggesting that sexual orientation is not a major factor affecting the relationships single parents have with their children.

References

Harris, M. B., & Turner, P. H. (1986). Gay and lesbian parents. *Journal of Homosexuality, 12*(2), 101-113.

Turner, P. H., Scadden, L., & Harris, M. B. (1990). Parenting in gay and lesbian families. *Journal of Gay and Lesbian Psychotherapy, 1*(3), 55-66.

Exhibit

Gay and Lesbian Parents Questionnaire

Dear Parent:

We are conducting a research study concerning gay and lesbian parents and their children. Specifically, we are interested in identifying specific problems or benefits these parents and their children may have, examining relationships between parents and children, and comparing attitudes of these parents and their children to attitudes of heterosexual parents and children.

Should you decide to participate, we will ask you to complete a questionnaire which should take 20-30 minutes. We will also ask if you would be willing to participate in a more in-depth interview, which would last approximately 45 minutes to one hour. Finally, we will ask permission to administer a questionnaire or some verbal measure to your child(ren) which will take approximately 30 minutes. Even if you do not wish to be interviewed or to have your child(ren) participate in the study, we would like to have you fill out the questionnaire if you are willing to do so. Naturally, the responses you and your child(ren) make will remain completely confidential. No one except the researchers will see your questionnaires or hear or read your comments or those of your children. No names will be used in the study; results will be reported statistically. In fact, if you only fill out the questionnaire and are not interviewed, we will never learn your name.

We realize that truthfully answering some of the questions may cause you some discomfort. We wish to emphasize that your participation is strictly voluntary and that you may choose to withdraw from the study at any point. Refusal by you or your child(ren) to participate will not result in any penalty or discrimination.

Since very little research exists concerning the specific problems of gay and lesbian parents and their children and how these problems might be unique, we hope to obtain results that would contribute to the well-being of these parents and their children. Should you desire a summary of the results of this study, please send a stamped, self-addressed envelope to one of the researchers. Results probably will not be available for at least six months, but we will send you the summary as soon as we can.

If you have any questions concerning this project, please feel free to contact one of us (address and phone below). If you have any concerns, problems, or complaints about the study, you may call . . .

Your return of the completed questionnaire constitutes your permission to participate in this study. Please note that attached to the questionnaire is a consent form for your child(ren) to be asked to participate. Your signed return of the consent form constitutes your permission for us to ask your child(ren) to participate. You will be contacted about a convenient time and place.

Thank you for your cooperation.

Sincerely,

Your completion of this questionnaire constitutes your consent to participate in this project. Do not put your name or any identifying marks on this questionnaire. Please answer every question as accurately as possible.

Section A

General information

1. Year of birth _____ 2. Sex _____ Male _____ Female
3. Ethnic background _____
4. Circle the highest year of school that you have completed.
    Elem/HS   1 2 3 4 5 6 7 8 9 10 11 12
    College   1 2 3 4
    Post Grad.   1 2 3 4 5
5. What is your religious preference? _____
6. What is your work or occupation? _____
7. Your total household income for the past year was: (check closest one)
    _____ Below $6,000   _____ $12,000-$15,000   _____ $22,000-$27,000
    _____ $6,000-$9,000   _____ $15,000-$18,000   _____ $27,000-$30,000
    _____ $9,000-$12,000   _____ $18,000-$22,000   _____ Above $30,000
8. At what age were you first married? _____
9. How many times have you been married? _____
10. How many children age 18 and under do you have that either live with you or that you see and are responsible for on a regular basis? _____
11. List the *age* and *sex* of each child. _____
12. Estimate the total number of days per year that you spend with your children under age 18. _____
13. Who else lives with you?
    _____ Spouse   _____ Female friend
    _____ Male lover   _____ No one
    _____ Female lover   _____ Other (specify) _____
    _____ Male friend
14. Are you: _____ Heterosexual _____ Homosexual _____ Bisexual
15. Are you: (check one)
    _____ A single parent
    _____ A stepparent with children of your own
    _____ Other (specify) _____
16. If you are currently single, indicate in the blank beside A how long you have been single. If you have remarried, indicate in the blank beside B how long you have been remarried.
    Single A. _____ Years _____ Months Remarried B. _____ Years _____ Months
17. How long were you married before you became a single parent?
    _____ Years _____ Months _____ Never married
18. How much time per week do you spend away from your child(ren), not counting the time spent at work and/or school? (check one)
    _____ More than 10 hours
    _____ 6-10 hours
    _____ 3-6 hours
    _____ Less than 3 hours

19. Below are listed some common problems of single parents. Using the scale below, rate each problem as to its degree of difficulty to you now (if you are single) or formerly (when you were single).

    1 = Not a problem at all   2 = A slight problem   3 = A moderate problem   4 = A significant problem

    _____ Managing household tasks
    _____ Finances
    _____ Lack of emotional support (someone to help with decision making, problem solving)
    _____ Lack of physical support (someone to help with repairs, chauffeuring, etc.)
    _____ Lack of adult companionship
    _____ Development and maintenance of yourself
    _____ Child care
    _____ Visitation with other parent
    _____ Loss of friends
    _____ Dating
    _____ Other (explain) _____

20. Below are listed some common problems of parents in blended families (stepparents). Using the scale below, rate each problem as to its degree of difficulty for your family. Respond to this question *only* if you are a member of a blended family *or* if you are living with a lover who acts as a stepparent to your children.

    1 = Not a problem at all   2 = A slight problem   3 = A moderate problem   4 = A significant problem

    _____ Finances, including disagreements with spouse/lover about financial arrangements for children
    _____ Lack of emotional support from spouse/lover (decision making, problem solving)
    _____ Lack of physical support from spouse/lover (help with children, household tasks, etc.)
    _____ Development and maintenance of self
    _____ Child care
    _____ Visitation with us of children living with other biological parent
    _____ Visitation of children living with us to other biological parent
    _____ Disagreements with spouse/lover on discipline techniques
    _____ Other (explain) _____

21. If you have custody or joint custody of your children, how difficult was it to obtain?
    _____ Not very   _____ Considerably
    _____ Slightly   _____ N/A—I do not have custody or joint custody
    _____ Average

22. If you *do not* have or share custody, but see your children regularly, how difficult was that arrangement to obtain and implement, both legally and practically?
    _____ Not very   _____ Considerably
    _____ Slightly   _____ N/A—I have shared or full custody
    _____ Average

23. To what extent do you identify with the feminist movement?
    _____ None   _____ Moderately
    _____ Somewhat   _____ Strongly

24. To what extent did each of your parents encourage sex-typed toys and activities? Answer for *each* parent.
    Mother: Father:
    _____ None   _____ None
    _____ Somewhat _____ Somewhat
    _____ Moderately _____ Moderately
    _____ Strongly _____ Strongly
    _____ N/A   _____ N/A

25. To what extent did your parents encourage you to play with same-sex, rather than opposite-sex, friends?
    Mother: Father:
    _____ None   _____ None
    _____ Somewhat _____ Somewhat
    _____ Moderately _____ Moderately
    _____ Strongly _____ Strongly

26. To what extent do you now encourage sex-type toys and activities with your children, i.e., giving dolls to girls and cars/trucks to boys?
    _____ None   _____ Moderately
    _____ Somewhat   _____ Strongly

27. To what extent do you attempt to provide a role model who is the opposite sex of you for your children?
    _____ None   _____ Moderately
    _____ Somewhat   _____ Strongly

28. For each of the household chores listed below, indicate whether your children perform them. Mark M if only your male children perform them, F if only your female children perform them, and B if children of both sexes perform them. Leave blank if *no* child performs them. Mark N/A if all children are too young to perform these tasks.
_____ Cooking, or assisting with meal preparation, including setting table
_____ After-meal clean-up
_____ Making beds, dusting, vacuuming
_____ Mowing lawn
_____ Washing car
_____ Doing laundry
_____ Repairing car
_____ Doing household repairs/maintenance
29. Are you willing to participate in a more in-depth interview?
_____ Yes   _____ No
30. Are you willing for any or all of your children to participate in this study?
_____ Yes   _____ No
31. If the answer to either Question 29 or 30 was yes, please provide your name and a phone number where you can be reached. _____

Please answer the following questions for *each* of your children separately. There are four identical sets of questions allowing for four children. If you have more than four children, answer for the two oldest and the two youngest only. Identify the age and sex of each child at the beginning of each set of five questions.

Age _____   Sex _____

How often do you become angry at your child? (check one)
_____ Very frequently
_____ Quite often
_____ Sometimes
_____ Seldom
_____ Never
How do you get along with your child? (check one)
_____ Very well
_____ Well
_____ Fairly well
_____ Not very well
_____ Poorly
How often does your child get on your nerves? (check one)
_____ Frequently
_____ Quite often
_____ Sometimes
_____ Seldom
_____ Never
How much satisfaction do you get from your child? (check one)
_____ Very much
_____ Considerable
_____ Some
_____ Very little
_____ None
Using the following scale, indicate the kind of relationship you have with your child in each of the areas listed.
1 = Poor   2 = Fair   3 = Average   4 = Good   5 = Excellent
_____ Communication
_____ Cooperation
_____ Discipline
_____ Togetherness (feeling of closeness)
_____ Mutual enjoyment

If there is any area in regard to your child(ren) which you think is important that has not been covered, please explain.
_____

Age _____   Sex _____

How often do you become angry at your child? (check one)
_____ Very frequently
_____ Quite often
_____ Sometimes
_____ Seldom
_____ Never

How do you get along with your child? (check one)
_____ Very well
_____ Well
_____ Fairly well
_____ Not very well
_____ Poorly

How often does your child get on your nerves? (check one)
_____ Frequently
_____ Quite often
_____ Sometimes
_____ Seldom
_____ Never

How much satisfaction do you get from your child? (check one)
_____ Very much
_____ Considerable
_____ Some
_____ Very little
_____ None

Using the following scale, indicate the kind of relationship you have with your child in each of the areas listed.
      1 = Poor   2 = Fair   3 = Average   4 = Good   5 = Excellent
_____ Communication
_____ Cooperation
_____ Discipline
_____ Togetherness (feeling of closeness)
_____ Mutual enjoyment

If there is any area in regard to your child(ren) which you think is important that has not been covered, please explain.

Section B

1. List the age of all your siblings.   Brothers   Sisters
                                 _____   _____
                                 _____   _____
                                 _____   _____
                                 _____   _____

2. Are any of your siblings gay or lesbian? _____ Yes _____ No _____ Don't know _____ N/A
   If yes, how many of each sex? _____ Brother(s) _____ Sister(s)
3. Is/was either of your parents gay/lesbian? _____ Yes _____ No _____ Don't know
   If yes, which one? _____ Mother _____ Father _____ Both
4. At what age did you *suspect* you were gay/lesbian? _____ Years
5. At what age were you *certain* you were gay/lesbian? _____ Years
6. At what age did you begin to tell friends you were gay/lesbian? _____ Years
7. At what age did you begin to tell your parents, siblings, spouse you were gay/lesbian?
   _____ Parent(s) _____ Sibling(s) _____ Spouse _____ Parents do not know
   _____ Siblings do not know _____ spouse does/did not know or never married
8. How old were your children when they knew you were gay/lesbian? (List age of each child.) If any or all of your children do not know, please write in DK.
   _____ (youngest child) _____ _____ _____ _____ oldest child)

9. How long did you remain married after you *knew* you were gay/lesbian?
   _____ Years _____ Months
   How long did you remain married after your spouse/child knew?
   _____ Years _____ Months   N/A (never married) _____

10. How did any or all of your children find out you were gay/lesbian?
    _____ I told them
    _____ My spouse (ex-spouse) told them
    _____ Another relative told them
    _____ An adult friend told them
    _____ Children overheard remarks between spouse and me
    _____ Children's friend(s) told them
    _____ Children discovered me with lover
    _____ Children do not know other (please explain) _____

11. Describe the children's immediate reactions to being told about your homosexuality. Mark all that apply and specify ages and sex of child who demonstrated reaction.

_____ Didn't understand	_____ Age	_____ Sex
_____ Knew it all along	_____ Age	_____ Sex
_____ Confusion	_____ Age	_____ Sex
_____ Sympathy	_____ Age	_____ Sex
_____ Shock	_____ Age	_____ Sex
_____ Pleasure	_____ Age	_____ Sex
_____ Relief	_____ Age	_____ Sex
_____ Disbelief	_____ Age	_____ Sex
_____ Anger	_____ Age	_____ Sex
_____ Disappointment	_____ Age	_____ Sex
_____ Guilt	_____ Age	_____ Sex
_____ Pity	_____ Age	_____ Sex
_____ Worry	_____ Age	_____ Sex
_____ Sadness	_____ Age	_____ Sex
_____ Feelings of closeness	_____ Age	_____ Sex
_____ Shame	_____ Age	_____ Sex
_____ Other (please explain) _____		

12. Describe your spouse's immediate reaction to being told about your homosexuality.

_____ Didn't understand	_____ Guilt
_____ Knew it all along	_____ Pity
_____ Confusion	_____ Worry
_____ Sympathy	_____ Sadness
_____ Shock	_____ Feelings of closeness
_____ Pleasure	_____ Shame
_____ Relief	_____ Was not told
_____ Disbelief	_____ N/A
_____ Anger	_____ Other (please explain) _____
_____ Disappointment	

13. Describe how you think your ex-spouse *now* feels about your homosexuality. Mark all that apply.

_____ Angry, hurt	_____ Ashamed
_____ Hostile	_____ Relieved
_____ Supportive, understanding	_____ Proud
_____ Indifferent	_____ N/A (never married or don't know)
_____ Confused	_____ Other (please explain) _____

14. Describe how you think your children feel *now* about your homosexuality. Mark all that apply and *indicate age and sex of child*.

_____ Angry, hurt	_____ Age	_____ Sex
_____ Hostile	_____ Age	_____ Sex
_____ Supportive, understanding	_____ Age	_____ Sex
_____ Indifferent	_____ Age	_____ Sex
_____ Confused	_____ Age	_____ Sex
_____ Ashamed	_____ Age	_____ Sex
_____ Proud	_____ Age	_____ Sex
_____ N/A—don't know		

15. Using the scale below, indicate to what extent you think your homosexuality has caused any of the following problems for your children.

   1 = None   2 = Slightly   3 = Moderately   4 = Extensively

   _____ Making and keeping friends
   _____ Doubting their sexuality or normality
   _____ Meeting and dating members of the opposite sex
   _____ Being teased or ridiculed by friends
   _____ Poor academic performance
   _____ Discrimination by teachers or other adults
   _____ Obtaining a job
   _____ Tension due to having to keep a secret from others
   _____ Other (please specify) _____

16. Using the scale below, indicate to what extent you think your homosexuality has benefited your children in each of the following areas?

   1 = None   2 = Slightly   3 = Moderately   4 = Extensively

   _____ Facilitating acceptance of their own sexuality
   _____ Facilitating tolerance or empathy for people who are different
   _____ Exposing the child(ren) to new points of view and experiences
   _____ Making friends
   _____ Other (please specify) _____

17. Do you feel that your homosexuality creates different or special problems for your male and female children?
   _____ Yes   _____ No   _____ Don't know
   _____ N/A—I only have children of one sex. If yes, please explain briefly. _____

18. If you knew you were gay/lesbian when you married, what was the *major* reason for your marriage?
   _____ Social pressure to conform
   _____ A desire to have children
   _____ A personal unwillingness to accept my own homosexuality
   _____ To prove my masculinity/femininity
   _____ An escape from a disappointing gay/lesbian relationship
   _____ Genuine affection for spouse
   _____ Other (please explain) _____
   _____ N/A—never married

19. Do you presently have one special lover? _____ Yes _____ No

20. If yes, does s/he live with you? _____ Yes _____ No

21. Does this lover act as a stepparent to your child, i.e., do the child(ren) perceive this person as a member of the family?
   _____ Definitely yes   _____ Definitely no
   _____ To some extent   _____ Don't know

22. How much difficulty do you have reconciling your gay/lesbian role with your role as a parent?
   _____ None   _____ Average
   _____ Some   _____ Considerable

23. How much difficulty does your partner have reconciling your gay/lesbian role with your role as a parent?
   _____ None   _____ Considerable
   _____ Some   _____ N/A—I do not currently have a special partner
   _____ Average

24. To what extent do you feel the gay/lesbian community as a whole accepts your role as parent?
   _____ Not at all   _____ Extensively
   _____ Slightly   _____ Don't know
   _____ Moderately

25. Is your children's jealousy of your lover a problem?
   _____ Yes _____ No _____ Maybe _____ Don't know

26. Are you willing to participate in a more in-depth interview?
   _____ Yes _____ No

27. Are you willing for any or all of your children to participate in this study?
   _____ Yes _____ No

28. If the answer to either question 26 or 27 was yes, please provide your name and a phone number where you can be reached. _____

29. Do you have any other feelings or experiences dealing with being a gay/lesbian parent which you would like to share with us? _____

Attitudes Toward Lesbians and Gay Men Scale

Gregory M. Herek,[1] *University of California, Davis*

The Attitudes Toward Lesbians and Gay Men scale (ATLG) is a brief measure of heterosexuals' attitudes toward gay men and women. The ATLG treats these attitudes as one instance of intergroup attitudes, similar in psychological structure and function to interracial and interethnic attitudes. Borrowing from public discourse surrounding sexual orientation, the scale presents statements that tap heterosexuals' affective responses to homosexuality and to gay men and lesbians.

Description

The ATLG is appropriate for administration to adult heterosexuals in the United States. Scale development included extensive factor analysis, item analysis, and construct validity studies (Herek, 1984, 1987a, 1987b, 1988, 1994). The full ATLG consists of 20 statements, 10 about gay men (ATG subscale) and 10 about lesbians (ATL subscale), to which respondents indicate their level of agreement or disagreement. Because they consist of different items, ATL and ATG subscale scores are not directly comparable. Researchers wishing to compare a subject population's attitudes toward gay men with their attitudes toward lesbians are advised to use parallel forms of one of the subscales (the ATG items have usually been used for this purpose), with each item presented twice, once in reference to gay men and once in reference to lesbians.

When the 20-item ATLG was initially developed, a 10-item short version (ATLG-S) also was formulated. The short version correlated highly with its longer counterpart (ATLG-S with ATLG, $r = .97$), as did the two 5-item subscales (ATG-S5 with ATG, $r = .96$; ATL-S5 with ATL, $r = .95$; Herek, 1988). In the course of several national telephone surveys, even shorter, 3-item subscales were used (the ATG-S3 and ATL-S3), based on three ATG items (Herek & Capitanio, 1995). The short versions have proved sufficiently reliable, valid, and convenient that their use is recommended for most research settings.

Response Mode and Timing

The ATLG can be used as a paper-and-pencil, self-administered questionnaire or can be administered orally (as in a telephone survey). Written versions of the scale typically provide respondents with a 5-, 7-, or 9-point Likert-type scale with anchor points of *strongly disagree* and *strongly agree*. If labeling of each response point is desired, it is recommended that a 4- or 5-point scale be used with the following labels: *strongly disagree, disagree somewhat, neither agree nor disagree* (for 5-point scales only), *agree some-*

what, and *strongly agree.* For oral administration, a 4-point response scale is recommended. Completion time varies depending on whether the long or short form of the instrument is used, and whether the administration is written or oral. For college-educated respondents, each item requires roughly 30-60 seconds.

Scoring

Scoring is accomplished by summing numerical values (e.g., 1 = *strongly disagree*, 9 = *strongly agree*) across items for each subscale. Reverse scoring is used for some items as indicated below. The possible range of scores varies depending on the response scale used. With a 9-point response scale, for example, total scale scores can range from 20 (extremely positive attitudes) to 180 (extremely negative attitudes), with ATL and ATG subscale scores each ranging from 10 to 90.

Reliability

The ATLG and its subscales have consistently shown high levels of internal consistency. As would be expected, alpha levels are usually higher when longer versions of the scale are used and when the scale is administered in paper-and-pencil format. With college student samples completing a written version of the ATLG or its short forms, alpha levels are typically greater than .85 for the subscales and .90 for the full scale (Herek, 1987a, 1987b, 1988). With nonstudent adults completing a self-administered questionnaire, alpha values typically exceed .80 (Herek, 1994; Herek & Glunt, 1991). In national telephone surveys with oral administration to adult probability samples, reliability typically has exceeded .80 for the ATG-S5 (Herek, 1994; Herek & Glunt, 1991, 1993), and .70 for the ATG-S3 and ATL-S3 (Herek, 1994; Herek & Capitanio, 1996).

Test-retest reliability was demonstrated with alternate forms (Herek, 1988, 1994). Respondents completed the original ATLG items and then, 3 weeks later, completed the alternate form (i.e., ATG items reworded to refer to lesbians, ATL items reworded to refer to gay men). Correlations were $r = .83$ for the ATG and its alternate, .84 for the ATL and its alternate, and .90 for the entire ATLG and its alternate.

Validity

The ATLG and its subscales are consistently correlated with other theoretically relevant constructs. Higher scores (more negative attitudes) correlate significantly with high religiosity, lack of contact with gay men and lesbians, adherence to traditional sex role attitudes, belief in a traditional family ideology, and high levels of dogmatism (Herek, 1987a, 1987b, 1988, 1994; Herek & Capitanio,

---

[1]Address correspondence to Gregory M. Herek, P.O. Box 11196, Berkeley, CA 94712-1196.

1995, 1996; Herek & Glunt, 1993). In addition, high ATG scores (more negative attitudes toward gay men) are positively correlated with AIDS-related stigma (Herek, 1995; Herek & Glunt, 1991).

The ATLG's discriminant validity also has been established. Members of lesbian and gay organizations scored at the extreme positive end of the range (Herek, 1988), and nonstudent adults who publicly supported a local gay rights initiative scored significantly lower on the ATLG than did community residents who publicly opposed the initiative (Herek, 1994).

Other Information

For a more thorough discussion of the ATLG's development and usage, and item and scale scores for various samples, see Herek (1994). For a comparison of Black and White adults' ATLG scores in a national telephone survey, see Herek and Capitanio (1995). Researchers need not obtain the author's permission to use the ATLG in not-for-profit research that is consistent with the American Psychological Association's *Ethical Principles of Psychologists*.

References

Herek, G. M. (1984). Attitudes toward lesbians and gay men: A factor analytic study. *Journal of Homosexuality, 10*(1/2), 39-51.

Herek, G. M. (1987a). Can functions be measured? A new perspective on the functional approach to attitudes. *Social Psychology Quarterly, 50,* 285-303.

Herek, G. M. (1987b). Religion and prejudice: A comparison of racial and sexual attitudes. *Personality and Social Psychology Bulletin, 13,* 56-65.

Herek, G. M. (1988). Heterosexuals' attitudes toward lesbians and gay men: Correlates and gender differences. *The Journal of Sex Research, 25,* 451-477.

Herek, G. M. (1994). Assessing attitudes toward lesbians and gay men: A review of empirical research with the ATLG scale. In B. Greene & G. M. Herek (Eds.), *Lesbian and gay psychology: Theory, research, and clinical applications* (pp. 206-228). Thousand Oaks, CA: Sage.

Herek, G. M. (1995). The HIV epidemic and public attitudes toward lesbians and gay men. In M. P. Levine, P. Nardi, & J. Gagnon (Eds.), *A plague of our own: The impact of the HIV epidemic on the lesbian and gay community.* Chicago: University of Chicago Press.

Herek, G. M., & Capitanio, J. P. (1995). Black heterosexuals' attitudes toward lesbians and gay men in the United States. *The Journal of Sex Research, 32,* 95-105.

Herek, G. M., & Capitanio, J. P. (1996). "Some of my best friends": Intergroup contact, concealable stigma, and heterosexuals' attitudes toward gay men and lesbians. *Personality and Social Psychology Bulletin, 22,* 412-424.

Herek, G. M., & Glunt, E. K. (1991). AIDS-related attitudes in the United States: A preliminary conceptualization. *The Journal of Sex Research, 28,* 99-123.

Herek, G. M., & Glunt, E. K. (1993). Interpersonal contact and heterosexuals' attitudes toward gay men: Results from a national survey. *The Journal of Sex Research, 30,* 239-244.

Exhibit

Attitudes Toward Lesbians and Gay Men Scale, Revised Version (ATLG-R)

Attitudes Toward Lesbians (ATL-R) Subscale

1. Lesbians just can't fit into our society. (ATL-R-S5 item)*
2. A woman's homosexuality should not be a cause for job discrimination in any situation. (Reverse scored)
3. Female homosexuality is bad for society because it breaks down the natural divisions between the sexes.*
4. State laws against private sexual behavior between consenting adult women should be abolished. (Reverse scored) (ATL-R-S5 item)*
5. Female homosexuality is a sin. (ATL-R-S5 item)
6. The growing number of lesbians indicates a decline in American morals.
7. Female homosexuality in itself is no problem unless society makes it a problem. (Reverse scored) (ATL-R-S5 item)
8. Female homosexuality is a threat to many of our basic social institutions.
9. Female homosexuality is an inferior form of sexuality.
10. Lesbians are sick. (ATL-R-S5 item)

Attitudes Toward Gay Men (ATG-R) Subscale

11. Male homosexual couples should be allowed to adopt children the same as heterosexual couples. (Reverse scored)
12. I think male homosexuals are disgusting. (ATG-R-S5 item) (ATG-R-S3 item)
13. Male homosexuals should not be allowed to teach school.
14. Male homosexuality is a perversion. (ATG-R-S5 item)
15. Male homosexuality is a natural expression of sexuality in men. (Reverse scored) (ATG-R-S5 item) (ATG-R-S3 item)*
16. If a man has homosexual feelings, he should do everything he can to overcome them.
17. I would not be too upset if I learned that my son were a homosexual. (Reverse scored)
18. Sex between two men is just plain wrong. (ATG-R-S5 item) (ATG-R-S3 item)*
19. The idea of male homosexual marriages seems ridiculous to me.

20. Male homosexuality is merely a different kind of lifestyle that should not be condemned. (Reverse scored)
(ATG-R-S5 item)

Source. This scale was originally published in B. Greene and G. M. Herek (Eds.), *Lesbian and Gay Psychology: Theory, Research, and Clinical Applications.* Thousand Oaks, CA: Sage, 1994.

Note. In the course of empirical research, the items marked with an asterisk have been reworded slightly from the original version of the scale to update their content or clarify their meaning. To avoid confusion with the original version (Herek, 1987b, 1988), the item set presented here is designated the ATLG-R.

Heterosexual Attitudes Toward Homosexuality Scale

Knud S. Larsen,[1] *Oregon State University*

Description

The Heterosexual Attitudes Toward Homosexuality (HATH) scale is a 20-item Likert-type scale (5-point) with response categories labeled *strongly disagree, disagree, uncertain, agree,* and *strongly agree.* The scale was developed on college populations. However, adherence to Edwards's (1957) a priori criteria for attitude scale statements has yielded a scale applicable to a variety of populations.

Three phases were employed in the development of the scale (Larsen, Reed, & Hoffman, 1980). Phase 1, an item analysis, yielded 20 statements with item-total correlations from .57 to .74. Analysis yielded a correct split-half correlation of .92, and the scale was found to discriminate between individuals based on sex, academic major, and church attendance in Phase 2. In Phase 3 (a validation study), the HATH scale was administered with several additional attitude scales and indexes of an exploratory nature. Analysis yielded a corrected split-half correlation of .92. As in Phase 2, a significant effect of sex was found; females appear more tolerant than males. In addition, the HATH scale correlated significantly with peer attitudes, religiosity, and authoritarianism. In a subsequent study (Larsen, Cate, & Reed, 1983), the HATH scale was employed to evaluate three sets of predictors of attitudes toward homosexuality: (a) anti-Black and orthodox religious attitudes, (b) sexual permissiveness, and (c) the effect of an introductory human sexuality course. Results showed significant regression coefficients for anti-Black attitudes and religious orthodoxy, confirming the predictions. Sexual permissiveness did not significantly add to the prediction of attitudes toward homosexuality. The

experimental group showed significantly greater change in attitude toward homosexuality than the control group, $F(1, 291) = 23.70, p < .001$.

Response Mode and Timing

Respondents circle the number corresponding with their agreement or disagreement with each statement. The response categories contain the following weights: *agree strongly* (1), *agree* (2), *uncertain* (3), *disagree* (4), and *disagree strongly* (5). The HATH scale requires approximately 10 minutes for completion.

Scoring

Half of the items are keyed in the negative direction. The following items should have weights reversed: 3, 4, 5, 6, 13, 14, 15, 17, 18, and 20. After weight reversal for negative items, simply sum the 20 items for a total attitude score. A lower score indicates a more positive attitude.

Reliability

Overall internal consistency for Phase 1 was calculated using an alpha coefficient, which yielded a value of .95. In Phase 2, the split-half coefficient of the HATH scale was .86, and, when corrected by the Spearman-Brown prophecy formula (Ghisseli, 1964), the results yielded a coefficient of .92. In Phase 3, the uncorrected split-half coefficient was .85 and corrected, .92.

Validity

The scale has consistently predicted a sex difference with females more positive in attitudes toward homosexuality (Larsen et al., 1983; Larsen et al., 1980). Mean HATH scale

[1]Address correspondence to Knud S. Larsen, Department of Psychology, Oregon State University, Corvallis, OR 97331; email: klarsen@orst.edu.

scores were more positive for upper-class students compared with lower-class students. Liberal arts students are more positive than business students, and less frequent church attenders are more positive than frequent church goers (Larsen et al., 1980).

Furthermore, the HATH scale has also been related to peer attitudes, religiosity, and authoritarianism (Larsen et al., 1980). In a second study (Larsen et al., 1983), the HATH scale predicted anti-Black and orthodox religious attitudes and demonstrated a significant change in attitudes toward homosexuality as a function of a course in human sexuality.

In a later study (1990), the relationship of the HATH scale to attitudes toward persons with AIDS was investigated. Because a disease such as AIDS is at least partially associated with homosexuality, it was predicted that respondents would tend to hold similar attitudes toward persons with AIDS as they hold toward homosexuals. A 20-item attitudes toward AIDS scale (part-whole corrections > .51; alpha = .92) was included with the HATH scale in a survey. One hundred twenty-four undergraduate students at Oregon State University responded to the survey. The Pearson product-moment correlation between the two scales was .84 ($p < .001$). This result adds further construct validity to the HATH scale.

The HATH scale was later employed in a study of 2,364 members of the California San Diego Medical Society (Mathews, Booth, Turner, & Kessler, 1986). Results indicated that the HATH scale differentiated effectively between groups of physicians and contemporary graduates of medical schools (as compared to their predecessors). Thus, the HATH scale would appear to have satisfactory predictive and construct validity.

References

Edwards, A. L. (1975). *Techniques for attitude scale construction*. New York: Appleton-Century-Crofts.

Ghiselli, E. E. (1964). *Theory of psychological measurement*. New York: McGraw-Hill.

Larsen, K. S., Cate, R., & Reed, M. (1983). Anti-Black attitudes, religious orthodoxy, permissiveness, and sexual information: A study of the attitudes of heterosexuals toward homosexuality. *The Journal of Sex Research, 19*, 105-118.

Larsen, K. S., Reed, M., & Hoffman, S. (1980). Attitudes of heterosexuals toward homosexuality: A Likert-type scale and construct validity. *The Journal of Sex Research, 16*, 245-257.

Larsen, K. S., Serra, M., & Long, E. (1990). AIDS victims and heterosexual attitudes. *Journal of Homosexuality, 19*(3), 103-116.

Mathews, W. C., Booth, M. W., Turner, J. D., & Kessler, L. (1986). Physicians' attitudes toward homosexuality—Survey of a California county medical society. *Western Journal of Medicine, 144*, 106-110.

Exhibit

Heterosexual Attitudes Toward Homosexuality Scale

Items	Item-Total Correlations
1. I enjoy the company of homosexuals.	.61
2. It would be beneficial to society to recognize homosexuality as normal.	.67
3. Homosexuals should not be allowed to work with children.	.66
4. Homosexuality is immoral.	.73
5. Homosexuality is a mental disorder.	.64
6. All homosexual bars should be closed down.	.76
7. Homosexuals are mistreated in our society.	.62
8. Homosexuals should be given social equality.	.60
9. Homosexuals are a viable part of our society.	.60
10. Homosexuals should have equal opportunity employment.	.57
11. There is no reason to restrict the places where homosexuals work.	.61
12. Homosexuals should be free to date whomever they want.	.66
13. Homosexuality is a sin.	.66
14. Homosexuals do need psychological treatment.	.57
15. Homosexuality endangers the institution of the family.	.58
16. Homosexuals should be accepted completely into our society.	.65
17. Homosexuals should be barred from the teaching profession.	.74
18. Those in favor of homosexuality tend to be homosexuals themselves.	.72
19. There should be no restrictions on homosexuality.	.64
20. I avoid homosexuals whenever possible.	.67

Source. This scale is reprinted with permission of the author.

Power Sharing in Lesbian Partnerships

Jean M. Lynch,[1] *Miami University*
Mary Ellen Reilly, *University of Rhode Island*

The instrument was developed to determine egalitarianism in lesbian partnerships as a function of similarity in social status variables. Specifically, it investigates whether couples who are similar in age, income, occupation, education, and financial assets tend to characterize their relationships as equal in a variety of areas. Previous researchers have typically investigated one partner's perception of power in the relationship (e.g., Blood & Wolfe, 1960; Peplau, Padesky, & Hamilton, 1982). Our instrument is designed to assess similarities and differences in each partner's assets so that it can be determined whether differences in these demographic variables are related to social status. Additionally, our instrument allows a determination of whether type of couple (i.e., equal, unequal but in agreement about who has more power, and couples with differing perceptions about power sharing) is related to social status variables.

Description

The power sharing instrument consists of demographic items, such as respondent's age as of last birthday, income, educational attainment, occupation and occupational classification, and several items that assess the respondent's assets. A number of items also investigate financial sharing by partners, such as whether the partners are cosignatories on saving and checking accounts, and whether the partner is a sole or partial beneficiary. Respondents also indicate how financial contributions in the household are divided, such as whether the respondent or her partner pays, or whether equal or proportional payments are made for a variety of household needs.

The remainder of the questionnaire measures egalitarianism in a variety of areas. Specifically, these items refer to responsibility for household chores and financial decision making. Three items query respondents regarding sexual equality in terms of initiation, decisions about the frequency of sex, and sexual satisfaction. As above, responses to the items indicate whether respondents are equal or whether the partner or respondent has more control in the relationship.

Finally, single items ask respondents about a number of issues related to equality, for example, self-disclosure, degree of commitment, and yielding in disagreements. Potential responses indicate whether the respondent or her partner or both tend to dominate in these areas. Two items, ideal and actual power (i.e., who has more say and who should have more say) are included from Peplau, Cochran, Rook, and Padesky's (1978) instrument.

Reliability and Validity

No reliability data are available. The instrument evidences face and content validity, covering the areas most significant to power in relationships. Results from studies using the instrument (e.g., Lynch & Reilly, 1986; Peplau et al., 1978; Peplau et al., 1982; Reilly & Lynch, 1990) indicate considerable consistency across diverse samples (college and adult populations in relationships of at least 1 year's duration). For both populations, respondents professed a belief in the importance of power sharing, and there was evidence of a great deal of egalitarianism in lesbian relationships. When inequity was found, power-sharing arrangements did not seem to be explained by social status differences.

References

Blood, R. O., & Wolfe, D. M. (1960). *Husbands and wives.* Glencoe, IL: Free Press.

Lynch, J., & Reilly, M. E. (1985-1986). Role relationships: Lesbian perspectives. *Journal of Homosexuality, 12*(2), 53-69.

Peplau, L., Cochran, S., Rook, K., & Padesky, C. (1978). Loving women: Attachment and autonomy in lesbian relationships. *Journal of Social Issues, 34*(3), 7-27.

Peplau, L., Padesky, C., & Hamilton, M. (1982). Satisfaction in lesbian relationships. *Journal of Social Homosexuality, 8*(2), 23-35.

Reilly, M. E., & Lynch, J. M. (1990). Power-sharing in lesbian partnerships. *Journal of Homosexuality, 19*(3), 1-30.

[1]Address correspondence to Jean M. Lynch, Department of Sociology and Anthropology, Miami University, Oxford, OH 45056; email: lynchjm@casmail.muohio.edu.

Exhibit

Power Sharing in Lesbian Relationships

This questionnaire is the main source of data for a study of lesbian relationships. It should only take a few minutes to complete.

Your replies will be completely anonymous since there are no identifying marks on the questionnaire. *Please do not sign the questionnaire.* It is important that each partner fills out her questionnaire separately and places it in one of the blank envelopes. Both should be returned to me together in the stamped, addressed envelope provided. Since I am studying couples, this is essential. Thank you very much for your time and cooperation.

1. What is your age as of your last birthday? _____ years.
2. What is *your* income (as reported on all W-2 forms)? _____
3. Which of the following best describes your highest level of educational attainment?
   ( ) Completed grammar school   ( ) Master's degree
   ( ) Completed high school   ( ) Ph.D., M.D., Ed.D., J.D.L.
   ( ) Some college or technical school   ( ) Other, please describe _____
   ( ) Completed college
4. What is your occupation? _____
5. Which of the following would you use to describe your occupation?
   ( ) Homemaker   ( ) Farm worker
   ( ) Professional   ( ) Machinist or Transportation Worker
   ( ) Manager or Administrator   ( ) Laborer
   ( ) Sales worker   ( ) Service worker
   ( ) Clerical   ( ) Private household worker
   ( ) Craftsworker   ( ) Other
6. What is the current worth of your *personal* financial assets? (stocks, bonds, property, cars, savings and checking accounts). Please estimate:
   ( ) $0   ( ) $35,000-$49,999
   ( ) $1,001-$9,999   ( ) $50,000-$74,999
   ( ) $10,000-$19,999   ( ) $75,000-$100,000 or more
   ( ) $20,000-$34,999
7. Which of the following are currently held by you? Check all that apply.
   A. ( ) Savings accounts in my name only
   B. ( ) Checking accounts in my name only
   C. ( ) Investments in my name only
   D. ( ) Joint savings accounts
   E. ( ) Joint checking accounts
   F. ( ) Investments in my name and someone else's
8. If you checked A, B, or C in Question 7 above, are the account(s) or investment(s) arranged so that your partner could manage your personal finances in the event that you were unable to do so?
   ( ) Yes
   ( ) No
9. If you checked C, E, or F in Question 7 above, is the other name on the account(s) or investment(s):

	partner	relative	some other person, not related
Checking	( )	( )	( )
Savings	( )	( )	( )
Investments	( )	( )	( )

10. If you have a will, is your partner named as:
    ( ) A beneficiary of all of your estate   ( ) Not mentioned in your will
    ( ) A beneficiary of part of your estate   ( ) I do not have a will
11. If you have life insurance, who is your beneficiary?
    ( ) Partner   ( ) Both partner and relative
    ( ) Relative   ( ) I do not have any insurance
    ( ) Some other person, not related
12. If you are currently renting, and have a lease, whose name is it in?
    ( ) My name   ( ) Someone else's name
    ( ) My partner's name   ( ) No lease
    ( ) Both of our names

13. If you own your own home, whose name is on the mortgage title or title to the house?
    ( ) My name   ( ) My partner and I are tenants in common
    ( ) My partner's name   ( ) My partner and I are joint tenants
14. If you currently own a car, who paid (or is paying) for it?
    ( ) I   ( ) Each has her own car which she owns
    ( ) My partner   ( ) Other. Please explain _____
    ( ) Both own it equally
15. ( ) In our current residence, household furnishings are:
    ( ) Predominantly mine   ( ) Each person owns approximately half of the furnishings
    ( ) Predominantly hers   ( ) Ours jointly
16. In your household, how are contributions to the following arranged:

	I pay	My partner pays	We split bills based on our ability to pay	We split bills equally	Included in the rent	Does not apply
A. Mortgage payments	( )	( )	( )	( )	( )	( )
B. Property taxes	( )	( )	( )	( )	( )	( )
C. Rent payments	( )	( )	( )	( )	( )	( )
D. Insurance (house or apartment)	( )	( )	( )	( )	( )	( )
E. Heating bills	( )	( )	( )	( )	( )	( )
F. Electric bills	( )	( )	( )	( )	( )	( )
G. Telephone bills	( )	( )	( )	( )	( )	( )
H. Groceries	( )	( )	( )	( )	( )	( )
I. Household repairs	( )	( )	( )	( )	( )	( )

17. Reviewing the items in Question 16 above, how would you describe your overall contributions to these household expenses?
    ( ) I contribute more
    ( ) My partner contributes more
    ( ) We contribute according to our ability to pay
    ( ) We contribute equally
18. How long have you and your partner been living together? _____ years
19. When you and your partner first began living together, whose residence did you use?
    ( ) Mine
    ( ) Partner's
    ( ) A new residence chosen by us
20. Our current residence is:
    ( ) Mine, where I lived before meeting my partner
    ( ) Hers, where she lived before meeting me
    ( ) Ours, since we met
21. Do you have children?
    ( ) Yes
    ( ) No (Please skip to Question 25)
22. How many children do you have?
    _____ Girls
    _____ Boys
23. Where are the children presently living? Please describe. _____
24. Who is financially responsible for the support of the children?
    ( ) I am primarily responsible for their support
    ( ) Father is primarily responsible for their support
    ( ) Father and I support them equally
    ( ) Father, partner and I support them
    ( ) Partner and I support them equally
    ( ) Partner is primarily responsible for their support
    ( ) Other. Please describe _____
25. For the following items, please indicate who has the major responsibility for the following chores:

	Always I	Usually I	Partner and I exactly equal	Usually partner	Always partner	Does not apply or done by hired person
A. Cooking	( )	( )	( )	( )	( )	( )
B. Laundry	( )	( )	( )	( )	( )	( )
C. Dishwashing and cleaning up	( )	( )	( )	( )	( )	( )

D. Household repairs	( )	( )	( )	( )	( )	( )
E. Dusting and vacuuming	( )	( )	( )	( )	( )	( )
F. Housecleaning (windows, floors, cleaning drapes)	( )	( )	( )	( )	( )	( )
G. Child care	( )	( )	( )	( )	( )	( )
H. Payment of bills	( )	( )	( )	( )	( )	( )
I. Bathroom cleaning	( )	( )	( )	( )	( )	( )
J. Outdoor maintenance (e.g., washing windows, cleaning gutters, painting)	( )	( )	( )	( )	( )	( )
K. Lawn care	( )	( )	( )	( )	( )	( )
L. Gardening (flowers and vegetables)	( )	( )	( )	( )	( )	( )
M. Car repairs	( )	( )	( )	( )	( )	( )
N. Decorating	( )	( )	( )	( )	( )	( )

26. Who do you think is more involved in your relationship—your partner or you?
_____ Partner is much more involved
_____ Partner is somewhat more involved
_____ We are involved to exactly the same degree
_____ I am somewhat more involved
_____ I am much more involved

27. Who do you think has revealed more about herself to the other—your partner or you?
_____ Partner has revealed much more
_____ Partner has revealed somewhat more
_____ We have revealed exactly the same amount
_____ I have revealed somewhat more
_____ I have revealed much more

28. Who do you think has more of a say about what you and your partner do together—your partner or you?
_____ Partner has much more say
_____ Partner has somewhat more say
_____ We have exactly the same amount of say
_____ I have somewhat more say
_____ I have much more say

29. Who do you think is more satisfied in the relationship—your partner or you?
_____ Partner is much more satisfied
_____ Partner is somewhat more satisfied
_____ We are exactly equally satisfied
_____ I am somewhat more satisfied
_____ I am much more satisfied

30. Who do you think is more committed to the relationship—your partner or you?
_____ Partner is much more committed
_____ Partner is somewhat more committed
_____ We are committed to exactly the same degree
_____ I am somewhat more committed
_____ I am much more committed

31. Who do you think *should* have more of a say about what you and your partner do together—your partner or you?
_____ Partner should have much more say
_____ Partner should have somewhat more say
_____ We should have exactly equal say
_____ I should have somewhat more say
_____ I should have much more say

32. If my partner and I disagreed on political issues or candidates,
_____ Partner would definitely change her opinion
_____ Partner would probably change her opinion
_____ Neither of us would change our opinion
_____ I would probably change my opinion
_____ I would definitely change my opinion

33. When my partner and I argue,
_____ Partner always gives in first
_____ Partner usually gives in first

_____ Sometimes she gives in first, sometimes I give in first
_____ I usually give in first
_____ I always give in first

34. If my partner expressed dislike for a friend of mine,
_____ I would definitely reevaluate my opinion of the friend
_____ I would probably reevaluate my opinion of my friend
_____ Neither of us would change our opinion
_____ I would probably not reevaluate my opinion of the friend
_____ I would definitely not reevaluate my opinion of the friend

35. If my partner were offered an attractive job opportunity in another city, how likely is it that you would move with your partner?
_____ I would definitely move with my partner
_____ I would probably move with my partner
_____ Uncertain if I would move or not
_____ I would probably not move with my partner
_____ I would definitely not move with my partner

36. If I were offered an attractive job opportunity in another city, how likely is it that your partner would move with you?
_____ My partner would definitely move with me
_____ My partner would probably move with me
_____ Uncertain if my partner would move with me
_____ My partner would probably not move with me
_____ My partner would definitely not move with me

37. Who do you think takes more of the initiative in your sexual relationship?
_____ My partner takes much more of the initiative
_____ My partner takes somewhat more of the initiative
_____ We both initiate sex to exactly the same degree
_____ I take somewhat more of the initiative
_____ I take much more of the initiative

38. Who do you think makes more of the decisions about the frequency of sex?
_____ My partner makes much more of the decisions
_____ My partner makes somewhat more of the decisions
_____ We make mutual decisions
_____ I make somewhat more of the decisions
_____ I make much more of the decisions

39. Who do you think is more sexually satisfied in your relationship?
_____ My partner is much more satisfied
_____ My partner is somewhat more satisfied
_____ We are both satisfied to exactly the same degree
_____ I am somewhat more satisfied
_____ I am much more satisfied

40. For the following, please check the appropriate responses:

	Partner always	Partner more than I	Partner and I exactly equal	Usually I	Always I	Does not apply; has never been an issue
A. What car to get	( )	( )	( )	( )	( )	( )
B. Whether or not to buy life insurance	( )	( )	( )	( )	( )	( )
C. How much money to spend per week on food	( )	( )	( )	( )	( )	( )
D. Where to go on vacation	( )	( )	( )	( )	( )	( )
E. What restaurants to frequent	( )	( )	( )	( )	( )	( )
F. How to spend leisure time	( )	( )	( )	( )	( )	( )
G. Which friends to spend time with	( )	( )	( )	( )	( )	( )
H. Where to go on holidays	( )	( )	( )	( )	( )	( )
I. What house or apartment to take	( )	( )	( )	( )	( )	( )

41. Do any of the following know that you are a lesbian?
Your mother _____ our father _____ Brothers _____ Sisters _____ Other relatives _____
Neighbors _____ Friends _____ colleagues at work _____

42. How many friends are aware of your relationship?
   All _____ Most _____ Half _____ A few _____ None _____
43. Do you and your partner participate in any lesbian organizations?
   _____ Yes _____ No
44. How often do you see your family?
   Weekly _____ Monthly _____ Several times a year _____ Never _____

The MacDonald Attitudes Toward Homosexuality Scales

The Editors

The MacDonald Attitudes Toward Homosexuality Scales (ATHS) measure attitudes toward homosexuals and homosexuality. There are three forms: a General Form, a Lesbian Form, and a Gay Male Form. Each form consists of 28 statements about homosexuals in a Likert-type format. The various forms have been administered to a variety of samples (see Falcon, 1976; MacDonald & Games, 1974; MacDonald, Huggins, Young, & Swanson, 1973; White, 1977).

Additional information may be found in MacDonald (1988). A copy of the instrument may be obtained from the first editor (A. P. MacDonald is deceased).

References

Falcon, C. (1976). *The relationship between adherence to sexual role and attitudes toward homosexuals.* Honors thesis, Kent State University.

MacDonald, A. P., Jr. (1974). Instrumental and terminal values: Some new developments. *JSAS Catalogue of Selected Documents in Psychology, 4*(123), Ms. No. 767.

MacDonald, A. P., Jr. (1974-1975). Identification and measurement of multidimensional attitudes toward equality between the sexes. *Journal of Homosexuality, 1,* 165-182.

MacDonald, A. P., Jr. (1988). The MacDonald Attitudes Toward Homosexuality Scales. In C. M. Davis, W. L. Yarber, & S. L. Davis (Eds.), *Sexuality-related measures: A compendium* (pp. 168-170). Lake Mills, IA: Davis, Yarber, and Davis.

MacDonald, A. P., Jr., & Games, R. G. (1974). Some characteristics of those who hold positive and negative attitudes toward homosexuals. *Journal of Homosexuality, 1,* 9-27.

MacDonald, A. P., Jr., Huggins, J., Young, S., & Swanson, R. A. (1973). Attitudes toward homosexuality: Preservation of sex morality or the double standard? *Journal of Consulting and Clinical Psychology, 40,* 161.

White, T. A. (1977). *Attitudes of psychiatric nurses toward lesbianism.* Master's thesis, University of Michigan, Ann Arbor.

Sex-Linked Behaviors Questionnaire

Neil McConaghy,[1] *University of New South Wales*

The questionnaire permits the investigation of the incidence of heterosexual and homosexual feelings, and the relationships of such feelings to sex-linked interests and behaviors and to sexual identity. Using the questionnaire, such data, previously obtained by the difficult and methodologically questionable technique of seeking identified homosexuals and attempting to match them with identified heterosexuals, can be obtained from and reported back to the group being educated.

Description

Respondents anonymously rate the degree of their current and past involvement in outdoor sport, fighting, neatness, music, and performing in public. They also rate their avoidance of being hurt; the frequency they were labeled "sissy" or "tomboy"; their relationships with their father and mother; their use of clothes of the opposite sex for sexual arousal; their wish to be of the opposite sex; their feelings of same and opposite sexual identity and the balance of the degree to which they feel sexually aroused to members of the same, as compared to those of the opposite, sex, currently and until age 15; and the degree to which they are currently aroused to members of the same, as compared to those of the opposite, sex in sexual fantasies and in physical contacts. Items are rated on 4- to 10-point scales.

The questionnaire was developed to help resolve various contradictions in the literature concerning human sexuality. Most surveys, for example, those of Kinsey, Pomeroy, and Martin (1948) and Kinsey, Pomeroy, Martin, and Gebhard (1953), reported that up to half the population have been aware of some homosexual feelings. Yet workers in sexuality research have argued that awareness of bisexual feelings is rare (Freund, 1974) or have based important conclusions on samples that have reported zero incidence of homosexual feelings. For example, Ehrhardt and Baker (1974) concluded that androgenized girls would not develop a higher incidence of lesbianism on the basis that none of the 42 such girls and 26 controls (20 postpubertal) showed homosexual interest.

Considering that many members of representative samples may not be prepared to admit the presence of homosexual feelings openly, I wished to investigate whether they would answer an anonymous questionnaire honestly. If representative samples of various subgroups of the population could be surveyed in this way and reported incidence of heterosexual/homosexual feelings similar to those found in the earlier surveys be obtained, this should establish the earlier finding and force researchers to revise their thinking on this issue.

Despite the wealth of prospective and retrospective studies demonstrating—particularly in males—an association between opposite-sex-linked behaviors and homosexuality (McConaghy, 1982, 1984), this research has been largely ignored or rejected by some workers (e.g., Katchadourian, Lunde, & Trotter, 1979; Pleck, 1981) on the basis that no association has been found between homosexuality and "masculinity-femininity" as measured by such psychological tests as adjective checklists. To determine if the earlier studies could be supported in samples representative of subgroups of the population, items investigating involvement in the behaviors reported in those studies correlating with homosexuality were included in the present questionnaire. Items investigating the respondents' wish to be of the opposite sex and their feelings of opposite-sex identity were also included.

The present questionnaire was developed from that used in an initial study (McConaghy, Armstrong, Birrell, & Buhrich, 1979) by omitting a few items that did not produce significant correlations and adding a few that were considered intuitively to be likely to produce meaningful data.

Researchers have shown the questionnaire to produce reliable and valid data when completed anonymously by second-year medical students who attended a teaching session. It is simply worded and should produce valid data with secondarily educated respondents also. Whether adult patients would answer it honestly if administered nonanonymously would seem worth investigating, but my experience with adolescents with sexual disorders leads me to believe a significant number would not.

Response Mode and Timing

Most items are answered by the respondent putting an X in the appropriate box. Most respondents complete the questionnaire in under 10 minutes.

Scoring

Rated items are converted to numerical scales by numbering each scale item from 1-4 to 1-10, depending on the number of items in each scale. The sex-linked nature of the

[1]Address correspondence to Neil McConaghy, School of Psychiatry, University of New South Wales, P.O. Box 1, Kensington, New South Wales, Australia.

behaviors reported is determined by examining the statistical significance of the difference between their frequency in male and female respondents (McConaghy, 1982). According to the hypotheses being investigated, the appropriate correlations between respondents' scores on the scales are then determined. Spearman rank-order correlations are used, as the scales may not be interval scales. Correlations between respondents' reported degree of current heterosexual to homosexual feeling (on a 15-point scale) and their scores of the degree to which they showed the other behaviors have been investigated (McConaghy, 1982; McConaghy et al., 1979). Other correlations examined have been those between items investigating desire to be of the opposite sex, sex role behaviors, and sexual identity (McConaghy & Armstrong, 1983). Buhrich, Bailey, and Martin (1991) employed the questionnaire to investigate the genetic basis of these behavioral features in male twins.

Reliability

Test-retest reliability on the same respondents has not been investigated. However, over 3 years, samples of 75% to 85% of all second-year medical students of the University of New South Wales reported similar degrees of homosexual to heterosexual feelings and the male students reported similar correlations between degree of homosexual feelings and sex-linked behaviors (McConaghy, 1984, 1987). Over 2 years, similar patterns of relationships between items investigating sexual preference, role, and identity were reported by male medical students with and without a homosexual component (McConaghy & Armstrong, 1983).

Validity

The incidence of homosexual feelings reported in the questionnaire responses of the medical students in the above studies were similar to those of previous surveys of volunteer populations (Davis, 1965; Kinsey et al., 1948; Kinsey et al., 1953). Behaviors were significantly sex linked, as found in previous studies (McConaghy, 1982). Correlations between the presence of homosexual feelings and opposite-sex-linked behaviors consistently reported over the 3 years by the male medical students were similar to those reported in numerous perspective and retrospective studies by self-identified male homosexuals (McConaghy, 1984, 1987). Use of the questionnaire with male Malaysian medical students produced comparable findings to those with New South Wales medical students (Buhrich, Armstrong, & McConaghy, 1982). The presence of these correlations in male but not female medical students was consistent with the finding of the prospective study of Kagan and Moss (1962) that opposite-sex-linked behaviors in male but not female children were associated with avoidance of heterosexual erotic behavior in adulthood.

The validity of the self-ratings of the ratio of homosexual to heterosexual feelings was supported by finding significant correlations between male respondents' reports of these ratios and their penile volume responses to films of male and female nudes (McConaghy & Blaszczynski, 1991). The validity of the assessment of sex-linked behaviors, sex role behaviors, and sexual identity was further supported by findings of significant correlations between the assessments of the behaviors and self-report of the ratio of homosexual to heterosexual interest in male twins, even when respondents reporting bisexual or predominantly homosexual feelings were excluded (McConaghy, Buhrich, & Silove, 1994).

References

Buhrich, N., Armstrong, M. S., & McConaghy, N. (1982). Bisexual feelings and the opposite-sex behavior in male Malaysian medical students. *Archives of Sexual Behavior, 11*, 387-393.

Buhrich, N., Bailey, J. M., & Martin, N. G. (1991). Sexual orientation, sexual identity and sex-dimorphic behaviors in male twins. *Behavior Genetics, 21*, 75-96.

Davis, K. B. (1965). Factors in the sex life of twenty-two hundred women. In A. Krich (Ed.), *The sexual revolution* (pp. 1-86). New York: Dell.

Ehrhardt, A. A., & Baker, S. W. (1974). Fetal androgens, human central nervous system differentiation, and behavior sex differences. In R. C. Friedman & R. M. Richart (Eds.), *Sex differences in behavior* (pp. 31-51). New York: Wiley.

Freund, K. (1974). Male homosexuality: An analysis of the pattern. In J. A. Loraine (Ed.), *Understanding homosexuality: Its biological and psychological bases* (pp. 25-81). St. Leonardgate: Medical and Technical Publishing.

Kagan, J., & Moss, H. A. (1962). *Birth to maturity*. New York: Wiley.

Katchadourian, H. A., Lunde, D. T., & Trotter, R. (1979). *Human sexuality*. New York: Holt, Rinehart & Winston.

Kinsey, A. C., Pomeroy, W. B., & Martin, C. E. (1948). *Sexual behavior in the human male*. Philadelphia: Saunders.

Kinsey, A. C., Pomeroy, W. B., Martin, C. E., & Gebhard, P. H. (1953). *Sexual behavior in the human female*. Philadelphia: Saunders.

McConaghy, N. (1982). Sexual deviation. In A. S. Bellack, M. Hersen, & A. E. Kazdin (Eds.), *International handbook of behavior modification and therapy* (pp. 683-716). New York: Plenum.

McConaghy, N. (1984). Psychosexual disorders. In S. M. Turner & M. Hersen (Eds.), *Adult psychopathology and diagnosis* (pp. 370-405). New York: Wiley.

McConaghy, N. (1987). Heterosexuality/homosexuality: Dimension or dichotomy? *Archives of Sexual Behavior, 16*, 411-424.

McConaghy, N., & Armstrong, M. S. (1983). Sexual orientation and consistency of sexual identity. *Archives of Sexual Behavior, 12*, 317-327.

McConaghy, N., Armstrong, M. S., Birrell, P. C., & Buhrich, N. (1979). The incidence of bisexual feelings and opposite sex behavior in medical students. *Journal of Nervous and Mental Disease, 167*, 685-688.

McConaghy, N., & Blaszczynski, A. (1991). Initial stage of validation by penile volume assessment that sexual orientation is distributed dimensionally. *Comprehensive Psychiatry, 32*, 52-58.

McConaghy, N., Buhrich, N., & Silove, D. (1994). Opposite sex-linked behaviors and homosexual feelings in predominantly heterosexual twins. *Archives of Sexual Behavior, 23*, 565-577.

Pleck, J. H. (1981). *The myth of masculinity*. Cambridge: MIT Press.

Exhibit

Sex-Linked Behaviors Questionnaire

Please answer every question, placing an X in each box where appropriate

Your age: _____ Years
Your sex: Male ( )   Female ( )
Father's (present parent, if mother remarried) occupation (If he is retired, deceased, or not working for any reason give his major past occupation) using two or more words to describe this (e.g., garage mechanic, insurance clerk). _____
Biological father's year of birth (approximate if uncertain) _____
Mother's (present parent, if father remarried) occupation _____
Biological mother's year of birth (approximate if uncertain) _____
All brothers' ages, if any (if none put 0) _____
All sisters' ages, if any (if none put 0) _____
If you were not born in Australia, how many years have you lived here? _____
Until the age of 7 did you prefer
    —to play mainly with boys? ( )
    —to play with boys somewhat more than girls? ( )
    —to play equally with boys and girls?   ( )
    —to play with girls somewhat more than boys? ( )
    —to play mainly with girls? ( )
To what degree did you enjoy outdoor games up until the age of 7 years?

Very much	Moderately	Slightly	Not at all	Disliked	Strongly disliked
( )	( )	( )	( )	( )	( )

If you played outdoor games until the age of 7, to what extent did you prefer rough and tumble (R&T) games (chasing, wrestling) to quiet (Q) games (hop-scotch, dressing up, playing families)?

Markedly preferred R&T	Somewhat R&T	No preference	Somewhat Q	Markedly Q
( )	( )	( )	( )	( )

Between the ages 8-13, to what extent did you enjoy outdoor sports (football, basketball, cricket, tennis, swimming, etc.)?

Very much	Moderately	Slightly	Not at all	Disliked	Strongly disliked
( )	( )	( )	( )	( )	( )

If you played in sports between the ages of 8-13, did you prefer contact (C) (football, basketball, wrestling) to non-contact (N-C) games (tennis, cricket, swimming)?

Markedly preferred C	Somewhat C	No preference	Somewhat N-C	Markedly N-C
( )	( )	( )	( )	( )

Between the ages 14-18, to what extent did you enjoy outdoor sports (football, basketball, cricket, tennis, swimming, etc.)?

Very much	Moderately	Slightly	Not at all	Disliked	Strongly disliked
( )	( )	( )	( )	( )	( )

If you played in sports between the ages of 14-18, did you prefer contact (C) (football, basketball, wrestling) to non-contact (N-C) games (tennis, swimming)?

Markedly preferred C	Somewhat C	No preference	Somewhat N-C	Markedly N-C
( )	( )	( )	( )	( )

To what extent were you involved in physical fighting until the age of 13?

Very often (about weekly for a year or more)	Often (several times a year for a few years)	Regularly (once or twice a year)	Occasionally (Once or twice)	Never
( )	( )	( )	( )	( )

Until the age of 15, did you
    —very often initiate a physical fight?   ( )
    —often initiate a physical fight?   ( )
    —sometimes initiate a physical fight?   ( )
    —rarely initiate a fight but was prepared to fight back?   ( )
    —rarely initiate a fight and tried to avoid fighting back?   ( )
Between the ages 8-15, to what extent did you try to look neat and tidy?

Very much	Moderately	Slightly	Not at all	Looked untidy	Looked very untidy
( )	( )	( )	( )	( )	( )

Since the age of 16, to what extent do you give time and attention to your personal appearance?

| Very much | Moderately | Slightly | Not at all | Regard as waste of time | Strongly regard as waste of time |
| ( ) | ( ) | ( ) | ( ) | ( ) | ( ) |

Between the ages of 8-15, to what extent did you keep your possessions neat and tidy (for example, in your bedroom)?

| Very much | Moderately | Slightly | Not at all | Regard as waste of time | Strongly regard as waste of time |
| ( ) | ( ) | ( ) | ( ) | ( ) | ( ) |

Until the age of 10, to what extent did you try to avoid being physically hurt?

| Very much | Moderately | Slightly | Not at all | Enjoyed activities with risk of being hurt | Strongly enjoyed activities with risk of being hurt |
| ( ) | ( ) | ( ) | ( ) | ( ) | ( ) |

To what extent do you enjoy music?

| Very much | Moderately | Slightly | Not at all | Regard as waste of time | Strongly regard as waste of time |
| ( ) | ( ) | ( ) | ( ) | ( ) | ( ) |

If you do enjoy music, to what extent do you like classical music as opposed to popular music, jazz, etc.?

| Strongly prefer classical | Prefer classical | Both equally | Prefer popular music | Strongly prefer popular music |
| ( ) | ( ) | ( ) | ( ) | ( ) |

Before puberty, to what extent did you like performing (e.g., acting, singing or dancing) before a group?

| Very much | Moderately | Rarely | Not at all | Did not wish to | Strongly did not wish to |
| ( ) | ( ) | ( ) | ( ) | ( ) | ( ) |

Since puberty, to what extent have you performed in public?

| Very much | Moderately | Rarely | Not at all |
| ( ) | ( ) | ( ) | ( ) |

Up to puberty, to what extent did you consider yourself a "loner" as compared with being socially sought after?

| Very much a loner | Moderately a loner | Average | Somewhat socially sought after | Very socially sought after |
| ( ) | ( ) | ( ) | ( ) | ( ) |

Up to puberty, to what extent were you regarded as a leader rather than a follower among your friends?

| Very much a leader | Somewhat of a leader | Average | Somewhat of a follower | Very much a follower |
| ( ) | ( ) | ( ) | ( ) | ( ) |

At any period during your first 15 years were you (if male) every accused of being a sissy or (if female) a tomboy?

| Never | Occasionally (once or twice) | Regularly (once or twice a year) | Often (several times a year) | Very often (about weekly) |
| ( ) | ( ) | ( ) | ( ) | ( ) |

Until the age of puberty, what was the quality of your relationship with your father?

| Very good | Good | Neutral | Rather bad | Very bad | Father absent all or most of the time |
| ( ) | ( ) | ( ) | ( ) | ( ) | ( ) |

Until the age of puberty, what was the quality of your relationship with your mother

| Very good | Good | Neutral | Rather bad | Very bad | Mother absent all or most of the time |
| ( ) | ( ) | ( ) | ( ) | ( ) | ( ) |

At present, what is the quality of your relationship with your father?

| Very good | Good | Neutral | Rather bad | Very bad | Father absent |
| ( ) | ( ) | ( ) | ( ) | ( ) | ( ) |

At present, what is the quality of your relationship with your mother?

| Very good | Good | Neutral | Rather bad | Very bad | Mother absent |
| ( ) | ( ) | ( ) | ( ) | ( ) | ( ) |

Until the age of 16 did you have "crushes" on older members of the same sex as yourself (e.g., teachers)?

| Never | Once | Few times | Often | Very often |
| ( ) | ( ) | ( ) | ( ) | ( ) |

Until the age of 15, did you ever use clothes of the opposite sex to sexually arouse yourself (e.g., in relation to masturbation)?

| Never | Occasionally (once or twice altogether) | Regularly (once or twice a year) | Often (several times a year) | Very often (about weekly) |
| ( ) | ( ) | ( ) | ( ) | ( ) |

After the age of 15, did you ever use clothes of the opposite sex to sexually arouse yourself?

Never	Occasionally (once or twice altogether)	Regularly (once or twice a year)	Often (several times a year)	Very often (about weekly)
( )	( )	( )	( )	( )

Between the ages of 6-12, did you ever wish you were a member of the opposite sex?

Never	Often (about once a week)	Occasionally (about once a month)	Rarely	Never
( )	( )	( )	( )	( )

Since the age of 12, have you ever wished you were a member of the opposite sex?

Never	Often (about once a week)	Occasionally (about once a month)	Rarely	Never
( )	( )	( )	( )	( )

Do you feel you have a component of the opposite sex in your mental make-up (i.e., if male, do you feel you have some degree of femininity in your make-up or, if female, some degree of masculinity)?

Not at all	Slightly	Moderately	Markedly	Extremely
( )	( )	( )	( )	( )

Do you think other people consider you show traits of the opposite sex in your behavior?

Not at all	Slightly	Moderately	Markedly	Extremely
( )	( )	( )	( )	( )

Do you think that you, if male, show effeminate traits or, if female, show the masculine equivalent of effeminate traits (butch)?

Not at all	Slightly	Moderately	Markedly	Extremely
( )	( )	( )	( )	( )

Rate the degree to which, until the age of 15, you felt sexually attracted to members of the same sex as compared to those of the opposite sex on the following scale. (Circle appropriate figure):

To same sex $\underline{0}$ $\underline{10}$ $\underline{20}$ $\underline{30}$ $\underline{40}$ $\underline{50}$ $\underline{60}$ $\underline{70}$ $\underline{80}$ $\underline{90}$ $\underline{100}$ $\underline{0}$
To opposite sex $\overline{100}$ $\overline{90}$ $\overline{80}$ $\overline{70}$ $\overline{60}$ $\overline{50}$ $\overline{40}$ $\overline{30}$ $\overline{20}$ $\overline{10}$ $\overline{0}$ $\overline{0}$

i.e. $\frac{0}{100}$ = Not attracted to same sex / Exclusively attracted to opposite sex

$\frac{100}{0}$ = Exclusively attracted to same sex / Not attracted to opposite sex

and other ratios intermediate between these extremes

Rate the degree to which you *currently* feel sexually attracted to members of the same as compared to those of the opposite sex on the following scale (Circle appropriate figure):

To same sex $\underline{0}$ $\underline{10}$ $\underline{20}$ $\underline{30}$ $\underline{40}$ $\underline{50}$ $\underline{60}$ $\underline{70}$ $\underline{80}$ $\underline{90}$ $\underline{100}$ $\underline{0}$
To opposite sex $\overline{100}$ $\overline{90}$ $\overline{80}$ $\overline{70}$ $\overline{60}$ $\overline{50}$ $\overline{40}$ $\overline{30}$ $\overline{20}$ $\overline{10}$ $\overline{0}$ $\overline{0}$

i.e. $\frac{0}{100}$ = Not attracted to same sex / Exclusively attracted to opposite sex

$\frac{100}{0}$ = Exclusively attracted to same sex / Not attracted to opposite sex

and other ratios intermediate between these extremes

Rate the degree to which in your current sexual fantasies you are aroused by members of the same as compared to those of the opposite sex on the following scale (Circle appropriate figure):

To same sex $\underline{0}$ $\underline{10}$ $\underline{20}$ $\underline{30}$ $\underline{40}$ $\underline{50}$ $\underline{60}$ $\underline{70}$ $\underline{80}$ $\underline{90}$ $\underline{100}$ $\underline{0}$
To opposite sex $\overline{100}$ $\overline{90}$ $\overline{80}$ $\overline{70}$ $\overline{60}$ $\overline{50}$ $\overline{40}$ $\overline{30}$ $\overline{20}$ $\overline{10}$ $\overline{0}$ $\overline{0}$

i.e. $\frac{0}{100}$ = Not attracted to same sex / Exclusively attracted to opposite sex

$\frac{100}{0}$ = Exclusively attracted to same sex / Not attracted to opposite sex

and other ratios intermediate between these extremes

Rate the degree to which in physical contact of any sort you have been conscious of sexual arousal to members of the same as compared to those of the opposite sex on the following scale (Circle appropriate figure):

To same sex $\underline{0}$ $\underline{10}$ $\underline{20}$ $\underline{30}$ $\underline{40}$ $\underline{50}$ $\underline{60}$ $\underline{70}$ $\underline{80}$ $\underline{90}$ $\underline{100}$ $\underline{0}$
To opposite sex $\overline{100}$ $\overline{90}$ $\overline{80}$ $\overline{70}$ $\overline{60}$ $\overline{50}$ $\overline{40}$ $\overline{30}$ $\overline{20}$ $\overline{10}$ $\overline{0}$ $\overline{0}$

i.e. $\frac{0}{100}$ = Not attracted to same sex / Exclusively attracted to opposite sex

$\frac{100}{0}$ = Exclusively attracted to same sex / Not attracted to opposite sex

and other ratios intermediate between these extremes

Do you ever feel uncertain of your identity as a member of your sex, that is, of your identity as a male or as a female?

Never	Very occasionally	Some of the time	Most of the time	All of the time
( )	( )	( )	( )	( )

Rate the strength of your identity as being a member of your sex, rather than as a human being of either sex, on the following scale.

Feel like a member of your sex
—All the time ( )
—Most of the time ( )
—Some of the time ( )
—Very occasionally ( )
—Never ( )

Rate the strength to which you feel like a member of the opposite sex, rather than of the same sex or a human being of either sex, on the following scale:

—All the time ( )
—Most of the time ( )
—Some of the time ( )
—Very occasionally ( )
—Never ( )

Were you ever aware of making a conscious effort to make your behavior more like that you considered typical of your sex?

Very much so	Moderately	To some extent	To a very small extent	Not at all
( )	( )	( )	( )	( )

If so, at what age did you start to make this effort (in years)? _____
At what age did you stop making this effort (in years)? _____
To what extent do you talk with people with whom you are at ease?

A great deal	Moderately	To some extent	To a very small extent
( )	( )	( )	( )

Identification and Involvement With the Gay Community Scale

Peter A. Vanable,[1] David J. McKirnan, and Joseph P. Stokes,
University of Illinois at Chicago

The Identification and Involvement With the Gay Community Scale (IGCS) is designed to measure involvement with and perceived closeness to the gay community among men who have sex with men. Although bisexually and homosexually active men are often considered to be part of the same homogeneous group, there are substantial individual differences in the extent to which these men perceive themselves to be part of a larger gay community and in the degree to which they self-identify as gay (Stokes, McKirnan, & Burzette, 1993; Vanable, McKirnan, Stokes,

[1]Address correspondence Peter A. Vanable at Department of Psychiatry, University of Chicago Hospital, 5841 South Maryland, M/C 3077, Chicago, IL 60637; email: pvanable@uic.edu.

Taywaditep, & Burzette, 1993). The IGCS was developed to characterize these individual differences. The scale was initially developed as part of a larger research program designed to identify both individual- and community-level variables associated with HIV risk behavior among a heterogeneous group of bisexually active men (see McKirnan, Stokes, Doll, & Burzette, 1995, for a description). Thus, although the construct tapped by this scale may be equally relevant to women who have sex with women, reliability and validity data have been gathered only for men.

Description

The scale consists of eight self-report items. Four items require respondents to rate how much their degree of agreement with attitude statements regarding the importance of self-identifying as gay and associating with a gay community. Response options range from *do not agree at all* (1) to *strongly agree* (5). In previous testing of this instrument, these four questions were embedded within a larger set of questions assessing attitudes toward sexuality and AIDS. Three items tap the frequency with which respondents read a gay or lesbian newspaper, attend gay or lesbian organizational activities, and frequent gay bars. The final item assesses the overall number of gay friends in the respondent's social network.

An earlier version of this scale, focussing only on behavioral indexes of involvement in the gay community, was described by Stokes et al. (1993). The present version, which includes subjective ratings of identification with the gay community, was initially tested using a face-to-face interview format in which responses were elicited by trained interviewers. In a more recent study (McKirnan & Vanable, 1995), the scale was administered using a self-report format, yielding similar psychometric properties.

Response Mode and Timing

Respondents are instructed to circle the response that most accurately describes their personal attitudes and experiences. The scale requires 2 to 3 minutes to complete.

Scoring

Prior to computing scale scores, responses to Questions 5 through 8 should be converted to numeric values (A = 1, B = 2, C = 3, D = 4, E = 5). Final scale scores are obtained by computing a mean across the eight items. Item 4 must be reverse coded. Higher scores indicate more identification and involvement with the gay community.

Reliability

Reliability and validity data come from a large, diverse sample of bisexual and gay men living in the metropolitan Chicago area (N = 750). African American (51%) and White (49%) respondents between the ages of 18 and 30 were recruited on the basis of specific sexual behavior criteria. During the first phase of the research, interviews were conducted with men reporting that they had both male and female partners within the past 3 years ($n = 536$). The remaining 214 men were recruited on the basis of having only male sexual partners in the past 3 years. For the complete sample, 43% of respondents self-identified as bisexual, 48% self-identified as gay, and 7% self-identified as being straight (2% refused to provide a label).

The Cronbach alpha for the complete sample was .78. A subgroup of respondents ($n = 218$) completed a 1-year follow-up interview. Test-retest reliability for this subsample was .74.

Validity

In the sample described above, scores on the IGCS were positively correlated with 7-point Kinsey ratings of sexual orientation ($r = .58, p < .0001$) such that people with stronger involvement and identification with the gay community tended to rate themselves as more homosexual in orientation. Similarly, scores on the IGCS reliably differentiated between men who variously described their sexual orientation as either gay, bisexual, or straight ($Ms = 3.09$, 2.38, and 1.51, respectively), $F(2, 733) = 159.0, p < .0001$. In addition, men showing greater identification with the gay community were more "out" to others about their same-sex activity, were less self-homophobic, reported that their friends were more accepting of their sexual preferences, and were more oriented toward using gay bars as a social resource ($rs = .53, -.35, .56$, and $.47$, respectively, $ps < .0001$). Similar construct validity data are reported by Stokes et al. (1993), using an earlier version of this scale.

Of greater theoretical interest are data linking scores on the IGCS to differences in sexual behavior with men and women, and specific practices that place homosexually active men at increased risk for HIV infection. In our sample, we found that rates of sexual behavior with men and women were directly related to differences in identification and involvement with the gay community, with high scorers on the IGCS reporting more overall sexual behavior with men and low scorers reporting more sexual behavior with women in the past 6 months (McKirnan, Vanable, & Stokes, 1995). In comparison to men who were less identified with the gay community, high scorers on the IGCS were more likely to report having had unprotected anal contact with another man. However, when the sample was restricted to only those men who had any anal sex with men in the past 6 months, these differences were eliminated. These data suggest that men showing greater identification and involvement with the gay community are at increased risk for HIV as a direct function of their being more likely to have anal sex with men at all (for a discussion of related findings, see McKirnan, Stokes, Vanable, Burzette, & Doll, 1993; Vanable et al., 1993). A reversal in this pattern occurs for behaviors with women, with lower scores on the IGCS being associated with an increased likelihood of having unprotected vaginal or anal sex with a woman in the past 6 months. Again, these differences were eliminated when the sample was limited to only those men who had some sex with women in the past 6 months.

Other Information

Support for this research was provided through Cooperative Agreement Number U64/CCU506809-02 with the Centers for Disease Control and Prevention.

References

McKirnan, D. J., Stokes, J. P., Doll, L. S., & Burzette, R. G. (1995). Bisexually active men: Social characteristics and sexual behavior. *The Journal of Sex Research, 32*, 64-75.

McKirnan, D. J., Stokes, J. P., Vanable, P. A., Burzette, R. G., & Doll, L. S. (1993, June). *Predictors of unsafe sex among bisexual men: The role of gay identification.* Poster presentation to the IX International Conference on AIDS, Berlin.

McKirnan, D. J., & Vanable, P. A. (1995). [Centers for Disease Control Collaborative HIV Sero-Incidence Study]. Unpublished raw data.

McKirnan, D. J., Vanable, P. A., & Stokes, J. P. (1995). *HIV-risk sexual behavior among bisexually active men: The role of gay identification and social norms.* Manuscript submitted for publication.

Stokes, J. P., McKirnan, D. J., & Burzette R. G. (1993). Sexual behavior, condom use, disclosure of sexuality, and stability of sexual orientation in bisexual men. *The Journal of Sex Research, 30*, 202-213.

Vanable, P. A., McKirnan, D. J., Stokes, J. P., Taywaditep, K. J., & Burzette, R. G. (1993, November). *Subjective sexual identification among bisexually active men: Effects on sexual behavior and sexual risk.* Paper presented at the annual meeting of the Society for the Scientific Study of Sex, Chicago.

Exhibit

Identification and Involvement With the Gay Community Scale

Directions: This questionnaire concerns some of your general attitudes and experiences. For each question, circle the response that is most accurate for you personally. Answer the questions quickly, giving your first "gut reaction."

		Do not agree at all				Strongly agree
(1)	It is very important to me that at least some of my friends are bisexual or gay.	1	2	3	4	5
(2)	Being gay makes me feel part of a community.	1	2	3	4	5
(3)	Being attracted to men is important to my sense of who I am.	1	2	3	4	5
(4)	I feel very distant from the gay community.	1	2	3	4	5

For Questions 5-7, please think in terms of the last six months or so.

(5) How often do you read a gay or lesbian oriented paper or magazine, such as the *Advocate* or other local gay/bisexual papers?
    A = Never   C = Several times a month   E = Several times a week or daily
    B = Once a month or less   D = About once a week

(6) How often do you attend any gay or lesbian organizational activities, such as meetings, fund-raisers, political activities, etc.?
    A = Never   C = Several times a month   E = Several times a week or daily
    B = Once a month or less   D = About once a week

(7) How often do you go to a gay bar?
    A = Never   C = Several times a month   E = Several times a week or daily
    B = Once a month or less   D = About once a week

(8) About how many gay men would you call personal friends (as opposed to casual acquaintances)?
    A = None   C = 2 gay friends   E = 5 or more gay friends
    B = 1 gay friend   D = 3 or 4 gay friends

The Homosexual Information Scale and the Homosexual Distancing Scale

Joel W. Wells,[1] *University of Northern Iowa*

The development of these scales is described by Wells and Franken (1987).

[1]Address correspondence to Joel W. Wells, Department of DCFS, 229 Latham Hall, University of Northern Iowa, Cedar Falls, IA 50614-0332.

Reference

Wells, J. W., & Franken, M. L. (1987). University students' knowledge and attitudes toward homosexuality. *Journal of Humanistic Education and Development, 26*(2), 81-95.

Exhibit

The Homosexual Information Scale

1. In the last 25 years there has been an increase in homosexuality.
2. Most homosexual men and women want to be heterosexual.
3. Lesbian women and homosexual men report greater sexual satisfaction than do heterosexual men and women.
4. Most homosexuals want to encourage or entice others into a homosexual or gay lifestyle.
5. Heterosexual teachers, more often than homosexual teachers, seduce their students or sexually exploit them.
6. History reveals that a significant number of homosexuals have made important contributions to various societies.
7. Most other cultures view homosexuality more positively than do Americans.
8. Greece and Rome fell because of homosexuality.
9. Heterosexuals generally have a stronger sex drive than do homosexuals.
10. About one-half of the population of men and more than one-third of women have had a homosexual experience to the point of orgasm at some time in their lives.
11. Most homosexuals follow "masculine" or "feminine" behavior in their same-sex relationships.
12. The homosexual population includes a greater proportion of men than of women.
13. Heterosexual men and women commonly report homosexual fantasies.
14. If the media portrays homosexuality or lesbianism as positive, this could sway youths into becoming homosexual or desiring homosexuality as a way of life.
15. Homosexuals are usually identifiable by their appearance or mannerisms.
16. Homosexuals who live with a same-sex partner are usually reported to be as happy or happier than are married women and men.
17. Homosexuals do not make good role models for children and could do psychological harm to children with whom they interact as well as interfere with the normal sexual development of children.
18. Causation of sexual orientation is very complex and without a definite answer at this time.

The Homosexual Distancing Scale

1. I would feel self-conscious greeting a known homosexual in a public place.
2. I would patronize a business establishment with a homosexual ownership or management.
3. Homosexuals are more immoral than are heterosexuals.
4. I would be comfortable being with a homosexual of the same sex.
5. Homosexuals are inferior to heterosexuals in motivation, character, personal goals, and social traits.
6. A homosexual couple should be denied the right to obtain a marriage license.
7. If I were being interviewed for a job, I would not mind being interviewed by a homosexual.
8. I would sit next to a homosexual of the same sex in a classroom.
9. I would be more uncomfortable if a homosexual propositioned me than if a heterosexual propositioned me.
10. When seeking friendship, a person's sexual orientation would not matter.

11. I think that homosexuals have a quiet courage that most heterosexuals don't have.
12. I would vote for a qualified candidate in the public election regardless of sexual orientation.
13. A homosexual should be afforded equal rights and integrated into the mainstream of society.

Source. These scales are reprinted with permission of the author.

A Sexual Ideology Instrument

Ilsa L. Lottes,[1] *University of Maryland, Baltimore County*

The original purpose of the Sexual Ideology Instrument (SII) was to test Reiss's (1981, 1983, 1986) hypotheses about the sexual ideologies of Americans. Reiss proposed three sexual ideologies: traditional romantic, modern naturalistic, and abstinence. A *sexual ideology* is a coherent set of beliefs regarding what is appropriate, acceptable, desirable, and innate sexual behavior. A *tenet* is a specific belief of an ideology. The SII contains scales and specific items designed to measure attitudes toward the tenets of the three ideologies and toward the four controversial topics mentioned below.

The five tenet types in the Reiss ideologies are concerned with *gender role equality,* the value of *body-centered sexuality,* the *power of sexual emotions,* the importance of *coital focus* in sexual relations, and the necessity of love for satisfactory sex or the *love need in sex.* These are described more specifically in Table 1, in conjunction with the three ideologies. Reiss also claimed that adherents of each ideology would have predictable attitudes on the following four areas of public controversy: abortion, gender genetic differences, pornography, and homosexuality. The expected views, as linked to each ideology, are also indicated in Table 1. Although the SII was originally constructed to test hypotheses about sexual ideologies, its use would also be appropriate in studies that require assessment of a wide range of sexual attitudes. In addition, because the SII contains several small scales, the use of all or some of its scales would be appropriate in studies that assess many variables and where the length of the questionnaire is an important consideration.

[1]Address correspondence to Ilsa L. Lottes, Department of Sociology and Anthropology, University of Maryland, Baltimore County, 5401 Wilkens Avenue, Baltimore, MD 21228; email: lottes@umbc2.umbc.edu.

Table 1 Tenets and Attitudes of Sexual Ideologies

Tenet Type 1. Gender Role Equality

Traditional romantic:	Gender roles should be distinct and interdependent, with the male gender role as dominant.
Modern naturalistic:	Gender roles should be similar for males and females and should promote egalitarian participation in the society.

Tenet Type 2. Body-Centered Sexuality

Traditional romantic:	Body-centered sexuality is to be avoided by females.
Modern naturalistic:	Body-centered sexuality is of less worth than person-centered sexuality, but it still has a positive value for both genders.
Abstinence:	Body-centered sexuality is to be avoided by males and females.

Tenet Type 3. Power of Sexual Emotions

Traditional romantic:	Sexuality is a very powerful emotion and one that should be particularly feared by females.
Modern naturalistic:	One's sexual emotions are strong but manageable, by both males and females, in the same way as are other basic emotions.
Abstinence:	Sexuality is a very powerful emotion and one that should be feared by males and females.

Tenet Type 4. Coital Focus

Traditional romantic:	The major goal of sexuality is heterosexual coitus and that is where the man's focus should be placed.
Modern naturalistic:	The major goals of sexuality are physical pleasure and psychological intimacy in a variety of sexual acts, and this is so for both genders.

(continued)

Table 1 Continued

Tenet Type 5. Love Need in Sex

Traditional romantic:	Love redeems sexuality from its guilt, particularly for females.
Modern naturalistic:	A wide range of sexuality should be accepted without guilt by both genders providing it does not involve force or fraud.
Abstinence:	Love redeems sexuality from guilt for males and females.

Abortion

Traditional romantic and abstinence:	Laws should prohibit abortion.
Modern naturalistic:	Women should be allowed to make their own decisions about abortion.

Genetic Differences

Traditional romantic and abstinence:	Differences between men and women are due more to genetics than to social conditioning.
Modern naturalistic:	Differences between men and women are due more to social conditioning than to genetics.

Pornography

Traditional romantic and abstinence:	Pornography produces harmful effects for society.
Modern naturalistic:	Most pornography does not produce harmful effects for society.

Homosexuality

Traditional romantic and abstinence:	Homosexuality is not acceptable.
Modern naturalistic:	Homosexuality is acceptable

Description

The SII is a 72-item questionnaire containing 15 scales. The response options to each item are *strongly agree* (1), *agree* (2), *undecided* (3), *disagree* (4), or *strongly disagree* (5). The items are ordered so that items in any one scale are not grouped together. Tenet Types 2, 3, and 5 each requires a comparison of beliefs about males and females. Therefore, 15 pairs of equivalent male and female items are included. To reduce the tendency of respondents to give the same answer for pairs of equivalent items, they are placed on different pages. For the test sample, correlations between equivalent items ranged from .24 to .72, with the average equal to .56. Thus, for that sample, respondents in general did not answer these pairs of items identically.

Lottes (1983b) analyzed the psychometric properties of a preliminary version of the SII. The weakest items were eliminated. It was tested on a sample of 395 adults in the northeastern United States. This sample was composed of 259 students and 136 nonstudents, and it contained 60% females and 40% males. For the students, the mean ages of both the males and females were 22. For the nonstudents, the mean ages of the males and females were 31 and 40, respectively. The SII is appropriate to administer to adults.

Table 2 Reliability and Item Numbers of the Scales of the Sexual Ideology Instrument

Scale	Cronbach's alpha	Item numbers in scale[a]
Gender Role Equality[b]	.75	*1, 6, *11, 16, 24, *43, 51, *64
Body-Centered Sexuality		
Scale 1	.80	*35, *40, *50
Scale 2	.75	*7, *15, *30
Scale 3	.56	12, 13, 17
Scale 4	.64	2, 65
Power of Sexual Emotions		
Scale 1	.46	28, 34
Scale 2	.51	53, 60
Scale 3	.57	*3, *18, *23, *39, *52, *72
Coital Focus	.72	4, 19, *22, 44, *48, 56, *57, 63, *66
Love Need in Sex[c]		
Scale 1	.80	*5, 9, 20, 21, 33, 41, 55, *62, *68
Scale 2	.86	*8, 10, *25, *31, *32, *36, *37, *38, *42, *46, *49, *58, *67, *69, *71
Abortion	.65	29, *54, 70
Gender Genetic Differences	.52	27, 45, 61
Pornography	.63	26, *47, *59
Homosexuality	.81	14, *38, *67

a. The asterisk before a number indicates a reverse-scored item.

b. Items 6, 24, 51, and 64 of this scale are from National Opinion Research Center (1980).

c. Items 20, 41, 42, 55, 68, and 71 are from Weis and Slosnerick (1981).

Response Mode and Timing

The SII is distributed with an answer sheet, preferably for computer scoring. Respondents indicate the number reflecting their agreement or disagreement with each item. The SII requires an average of 30 minutes for completion.

Scoring

To determine the score for each scale, add the responses (coded 1-5) to the individual items of the scale. The reverse-scored items are indicated by an asterisk in Table 2.

For the Gender Role Equality and Coital Focus scales, a high score indicates support for the Modern Naturalistic tenets and a low score indicates support for the Traditional Romantic tenets.

For the four Body-Centered Sexuality scales, high scores on all scales indicate support for the Modern Naturalistic tenet, and low scores on all scales indicate support for the abstinence tenet. Low scores on Body-Centered Sexuality scales 1 and 3 and a high score on scale 2 indicate support for the Traditional Romantic tenet (i.e., the view that body-centered sexuality is acceptable for men but not women).

For the three Power of Sexual Emotions scales, high scores on all scales indicate support for the Modern Naturalistic tenet, and low scores on all scales indicate support for the Abstinence tenet. A high score for Power of Sexual Emotions scale 1 and a low score for scale 2 indicate support for the Traditional Romantic tenet (i.e., the view that men's sexual emotions are more powerful and unmanageable than women's).

For the two Love Need in Sex scales, high scores indicate support for the Modern Naturalistic tenet, and low scores indicate support for the Abstinence tenet. To determine support for the Traditional Romantic tenet, the results of Items 41 and 55 need to be compared. A high score for Item 41 and a low score for Item 55 would indicate support for the Traditional Romantic tenet (i.e., for the view that love is necessary for women but not men in sexual relations).

For the Abortion, Gender Genetic Differences, Pornography, and Homosexuality scales, high scores indicate, respectively, support for belief in (a) freedom of choice for abortion, (b) environment over heredity as the prime former of personality difference, (c) tolerant attitudes toward pornography, and (d) acceptance of homosexuality.

Reliability

The reliability of each scale was estimated by computing Cronbach's alpha. Listed in Table 2 are the 15 scales used in the SII, their items, and their reliabilities.

Validity

The construct validity of the 15 scales was generally supported by both interscale correlations and factor analysis. Exceptions were the Body-Centered Sexuality and the Love Need in Sex scales. Both high interscale correlations and factor analysis suggested that these two types of scales were measuring the same construct. However, Lottes (1983a) found significant differences in response to these two types of scales for young women students.

The construct validity was supported by examining (a) correlations with background variables of age, sex, and religiosity and (b) differences between scale means for men and women students and for women students and women nonstudents. Both correlations and differences between scale means, significant at the .001 level, were consistent with predictions suggested by previous research.

Further information concerning the reliability and validity of the scales is reported by Lottes (1983b).

References

Lottes, I. L. (1983a, April). *An investigation of the tenet patterns in the Reiss sexual ideologies.* Paper presented at the Eastern Region meeting of the Society for the Scientific Study of Sex, Philadelphia.

Lottes, I. L. (1983b). *Psychometric characteristics of a sexual ideology instrument.* Unpublished manuscript.

Lottes, I. L. (1985). The use of cluster analysis to determine belief patterns of sexual attitudes. *The Journal of Sex Research, 21,* 405-421.

National Opinion Research Center. (1980). *General social surveys, 1972-1980: Cumulative codebook.* Chicago: University of Chicago Press.

Reiss, I. L. (1981). Some observations on ideology and sexuality in America. *Journal of Marriage and the Family, 43,* 271-283.

Reiss, I. L. (1983). Sexuality: A research and theory perspective. In P. Houston (Ed.), *Sexuality and the family life span* (pp. 141-147). Iowa City: University of Iowa Press.

Reiss, I. L. (1986). *Journey into sexuality.* Englewood Cliffs, NJ: Prentice Hall.

Weis, D. L., & Slosnerick, M. (1981). Attitudes toward sexual and nonsexual extramarital involvements among a sample of college students. *Journal of Marriage and the Family, 43,* 349-358.

Exhibit

Sexual Ideology Instrument

Directions: Put your answers on SIDE 1, beginning with question 1. For each of the statements, indicate whether you *strongly agree* (SA) = 1, *agree* (A) = 2, are *undecided* (U) = 3, *disagree* (D) = 4, or *strongly disagree* (SD) = 5.

	SA	A	U	D	SD
	1	2	3	4	5

Remember: (1) Be sure that the number of the statement you are reading corresponds to the number you are marking on the answer sheet.
(2) Mark only one response for each statement.
(3) Respond the way you really feel, which may or may not be in agreement with the majority of public opinion.

_____ 1. I am in favor of laws that promote gender equality.

_____ 2. Women who emphasize sexual pleasure in their lives overlook life's more important pursuits.

_____ 3. Sexual emotions are strong but manageable by most males.

_____ 4. A mature man and woman should get their greatest sexual pleasure from intercourse rather than from some other sexual activity.

_____ 5. Having a physical attraction to someone would be sufficient for me to enjoy sex with that person.

_____ 6. A preschool child is likely to suffer if the mother works.

_____ 7. It is acceptable for a 16- to 17-year-old unmarried male to have sexual intercourse.

_____ 8. Masturbation is an acceptable activity for males.

_____ 9. I would feel very guilty if I had sexual relations with someone I did NOT love.

_____10. I would be very upset if my spouse had had many previous sexual relationships.

_____11. I hope that the family, social, and career roles of men and women become more alike.

_____12. Since many men seem to be unable to control their sex drive, it is important for women to be in control of theirs.

_____13. I do NOT respect women who appear in pornographic films or magazines.

_____14. Homosexuals should NOT be teaching school. It is too risky to allow the possibility of such a teacher taking advantage of or influencing the sexual orientation of even one student.

_____15. I approve of a man having premarital sex with someone he likes but is NOT in love with.

_____16. If a woman really loves her husband, she will want to include the vow "to obey" her husband in the marriage ceremony.

_____17. Women degrade themselves when they show obvious sexual interest in a man they are NOT in love with.

_____18. Men can have affairs that do NOT disrupt their lifestyle.

_____19. The primary goal of sexual activity between men and women should be intercourse.

_____20. A successful and satisfying sex partnership CANNOT be established unless the sex partners are quite willing to be sexually faithful to one another.

_____21. It would be difficult for me to enjoy sex with someone I did NOT love.

_____22. Orgasm resulting from manual genital stimulation by the sex partner can be as satisfying as intercourse.

_____23. Women can have affairs without significant emotional involvement.

_____24. It is more important for a wife to help her husband's career than to have one herself.

_____25. I approve of a woman having extra-marital sex WITH her husband's consent.

_____26. Pornography influences men to commit sexual crimes including rape.

_____27. Men are generally more interested in sex than women.

_____28. If women yield to their sexual feelings, these feelings will probably disrupt and dominate their lives in destructive ways.

_____29. The Supreme Court ruling making abortions legal should be reversed.

_____30. I approve of a man having premarital sex with someone he is strongly attracted to but knows only casually.

_____31. Group sex (sex involving more than two people) is an acceptable sexual activity for men and women.

_____32. John is married to Ann. John is strongly attracted to, but not in love with Mary. I approve of John and Mary having sexual relations.

_____33. Extra-marital sex is always wrong.

_____34. Sexuality is a very powerful force and females should do all they can to control it in their lives.

_____35. It is acceptable for a 16- to 17-year-old unmarried female to have sexual intercourse.

_____36. I approve of a man having extra-marital sex WITHOUT his wife's consent.

_____37. I would NOT object to my spouse having had a couple of previous sexual relationships.

_____38. I can accept and do NOT condemn homosexual activities for females.

_____39. Sexual emotions are strong but manageable by most females.

_____40. I approve of a woman having premarital sex with someone she likes but is NOT in love with.

_____41. A man CANNOT have a satisfactory and satisfying sex life without being in love with his sex partner.

_____42. Sexual intercourse with someone other than the regular sex partner can bring about an improvement in the sexual relationship of the established pair.

_____43. It would be best for our society if there were about an equal number of men and women in all high-level positions of government, business, and education.

_____44. To advocate an emphasis on sexual pleasure is to forget that the major purpose of sexual relations is procreation.

_____45. The innate differences in men's and women's strengths and weaknesses are the major source of satisfaction in male-female relationships.

_____46. I approve of a man having extra-marital sex WITH his wife's consent.

_____47. I enjoy looking at the pictures of nude men and women that appear in "Playgirl" and "Playboy" type magazines.

_____48. Oral or mouth-genital sex is a good substitute for intercourse.

_____49. Masturbation is an acceptable activity for females.

_____50. I approve of a woman having premarital sex with someone she is strongly attracted to but knows only casually.

_____51. It is much better for everyone involved if the man is the achiever outside the home and the woman takes care of the home and family.

_____52. Men can have affairs without significant emotional involvement.

_____53. If men yield to their sexual feelings, these feelings will probably disrupt and dominate their lives in destructive ways.

_____54. The decision about an abortion should be left up to a woman and her doctor.

_____55. A woman CANNOT have a satisfactory and satisfying sex life without being in love with her sex partner.

_____56. Having intercourse is the best way to end sex.

_____57. Anal intercourse is a good substitute for vaginal intercourse.

_____58. Ann is married to John. Ann is strongly attracted to, but not in love with Jim. I approve of Ann and Jim having sexual relations.

_____59. Nonviolent pornography is harmless to our society.

_____60. Sexuality is a very powerful force and males should do all they can to control it in their lives.

_____61. Men and women have different sexual needs that are based on differences in male and female anatomy and hormones.

_____62. Basically, I simply love sex and would enjoy making love to many different people.

_____63. It is a mistake to allow oral sex to become as important as intercourse in one's sex life.

_____64. A working mother can establish just as warm and secure a relationship with her children as a mother who is NOT employed.

_____65. Men who emphasize sexual pleasure in their lives overlook life's more important pursuits.

_____66. Sexual intercourse does NOT have to be the major focus of positive and pleasurable sexual activity for men and women.

_____67. I can accept and do NOT condemn homosexual activities for males.

_____68. Sexual intercourse is often best when enjoyed for its own sake, rather than for the purpose of expressing love.

_____69. I approve of a woman having extramarital sex WITHOUT her husband's consent.

_____70. Where abortions are legal, the father should have the right to veto the abortion.

_____71. Casual sexual intercourse with a variety of sex partners can be as satisfying and satisfactory as intercourse that is limited to an established sex partnership.

_____72. Women can have affairs that do NOT disrupt their lifestyle.

Sexual Polarity Scale

Donald L. Mosher[1] and James Sullivan, _University of Connecticut_

Sexual polarity is defined as a sexual ideology (a) consisting of a more or less organized set of ideas about sexuality that orders information about the ideals and aspirations in

[1]Address correspondence to Donald L. Mosher, 5051 North A1a, PH1-1, North Hutchinson Island, FL 34949; email: dlmosher@aol.com

a sexual world view; (b) polarizing into a left-wing (_naturalist_) and a right-wing (_jehovanist_) set of ideas; and (c) serving as a script, often shared by a community of believers, to interpret, to predict, to explain, to evaluate, or to control past, present, and future sexual scenes. The concepts of jehovanist and naturalist, introduced by Davis (1983), suggested the content of the items. Jehovanists believe that sex is dirty and aside from moderate intensity—marital coitus—threatens the dissolution of the individual's self and the destruction of the social order. Naturalists are modernists who place sex into a nonsacred, biological context of natural behavior that occurs commonly in humans across cultures and in other species of animals.

The Sexual Polarity Scale (SPS), in addition, contains selected items from Tomkins's (1965) Polarity Scale (TPS). Tomkins (1965) defined ideology as "any organized set of ideas about which humans are most passionate and for which there is no evidence and about which they are least certain" (p. 78). The left wing of the polarity, called *humanist*, is rooted in the view, introduced by Protagoras, of man as the measure of all things. The right wing of the polarity, called *normative*, is anchored to the Platonic conception of Ideas and Essences as the realm of reality and value. Humanists, who view people as basically good, view science as promoting human realization; government as promoting social welfare; and socialization as requiring unconditional love, sympathy, and play. Normatives, who view people as basically bad, view science as establishing truth, government as preserving law and order, and socialization as requiring conditional love to promote respect for rules and authority.

Description

The SPS consists of 30 forced-choice items measuring the sexual polarity of jehovanist or the naturalist ideology and 30 selected forced-choice items from the TPS measuring the polarity in worldviews of the normative or humanist ideology. The 60 items are randomly mixed. Thus, the scale measures a relative preference for a left-wing worldview (humanist ideology) and a left-wing sexual ideology (naturalist) or a right-wing worldview (normative ideology) and a right-wing sexual ideology (jehovanist).

Response Mode and Timing

Respondents can circle the letter of the preferred alternative in each pair or respond on a machine-scorable answer sheet. Approximately 13 minutes is required for completion.

Scoring

Alternatives assigned to the jehovanist ideology are scored 1, and naturalist alternatives are scored 0. The jehovanist item numbers and letters for that choice are as follows: 1a, 4b, 8a, 9b, 10b, 11a, 14a, 15b, 16b, 17b, 19b, 20a, 22b, 23b, 25b, 27b, 28b, 29a, 30b, 35a, 36a, 37b, 39b, 40a, 41b, 43b, 44a, 46b, 51b, and 52a.

Alternatives assigned to the normative ideology are scored 1, and humanist alternatives are scored 0. The nor-

mative item numbers and letters for that choice are as follows: 2b, 3b, 5a, 6b, 7b, 12a, 13a, 18a, 21b, 24a, 26b, 31a, 52b, 33a, 34a, 38b, 42b, 45b, 47b, 48b, 49a, 50b, 53a, 55b, 56b, 57a, 58a, 59b, and 60a. Scores for normative and jehovanist ideologies can range from 0, if only humanist and naturalist alternatives are selected, to 30, if only normative and jehovanist alternatives are selected.

Reliability

Internal consistency item analyses, from a sample of 140 male University of Connecticut undergraduates, were used to select 30 items from 40 items sampling the content of the sexual polarity and 30 items from the 59 items of the TPS. In the pool of 40 items measuring the sexual polarity, 37 items had discriminated the jehovanist/naturalist polarity at the .95 level of significance; for the TPS, 45 of 59 items significantly discriminated the normative/humanist polarity. The Cronbach alpha coefficient for the sexual jehovanist/humanist polarity was .86. The Cronbach alpha coefficient for Tomkins's normative/humanist polarity was .79.

Validity

Evidence of construct validity is limited to a study of 140 male undergraduates (Mosher & Sullivan, 1986). A pattern of significant Pearson correlations with other measures revealed a pattern that confirmed expectations. More jehovanist men, in comparison to more naturalist men, attended church more frequently, $r(138) = .23$; reported more involvement in church activities, $r(138) = .33$; scored higher on sex-guilt, $r(138) = .56$; had a normative rather than a humanist worldview, $r(138) = .36$; were more intolerant of ambiguity, $r(138) = .32$, and accepted more rape myths, $r(138) = .16$.

Tomkins (1965) summarized evidence from diverse experimental methods that supported the construct validity of the normative/humanist ideology. In addition to being more jehovanist, more normative men, in comparison to more humanist men, were more macho, $r(138) = .22$; intolerant of ambiguity, $r(138) = .20$; and had a higher proclivity to rape, $r(138) = .19$.

References

Davis, M. S. (1983). *Smut: Erotic reality/obscene ideology*. Chicago: University of Chicago Press.

Mosher, D. L., & Sullivan, J. (1986). *The development of a measure of sexual ideology: The polarity of jehovanist or naturalist*. Unpublished manuscript, University of Connecticut, Storrs.

Tomkins, S. S. (1965). Affect and the psychology of knowledge. In S. S. Tomkins & C. E. Izard (Eds.), *Affect, cognition, and personality* (pp. 72-97). New York: Springer.

Exhibit

Sexual Polarity Scale

Instructions: An ideology is an organized set of ideas that offers a worldview. An ideology can be concerned with theories of value, education, science, sex, or socialization. These are just a few examples. A sexual ideology is an organized set of ideas about sex reflecting the ideas and aspirations of the individual, society, and culture. In the 60 items that follow, polar or contrasting ideas are presented. Your task is to select the item in each pair which is closest to your personal point of view. If you prefer alternative (a) circle letter (a); if you prefer alternative (b) circle letter (b). Although your cooperation is appreciated, you are, of course, free not to answer any item.

1. a) Pornography is disgusting.
   b) So-called pornography can be enjoyable.
2. a) The most important aspect of science is that is enables man to realize himself by gaining understanding and control of the world around him.
   b) The most important aspect of science is that it enables man to separate the true from the false, the right from the wrong, reality from fantasy.
3. a) To assume that most people are well-meaning brings out the best in others.
   b) To assume that most people are well-meaning is asking for trouble.
4. a) Abandoning yourself to pleasure helps to produce orgasmic response.
   b) Sexual abandonment endangers the person's ability to control his or her own body.
5. a) No government should sanction legalized gambling. Ultimately this will undermine the very foundations of authority.
   b) Legalized gambling is at worst innocuous. At best it lends spice and zest to life.
6. a) What children demand should be of little consequence to their parents.
   b) What children demand, parents should take seriously and try to satisfy.
7. a) The most important thing in the world is to know yourself and be yourself.
   b) The most important thing in the world is to try to live up to the highest standards.
8. a) The sin of fornication can be a worse crime than murder.
   b) It is better to make love than to fight.
9. a) Homosexual teachers have no necessary affect on children's personality or sexual orientation.
   b) Homosexual teachers can corrupt a young mind.
10. a) Sexual fantasy is a way for a person to increase their erotic pleasure through the use of imagination.
    b) Too much thinking about sex is a sign of an impure mind that will be easy prey to sexual temptation.
11. a) Sex undermines the distinction between humans and animals, making people more bestial.
    b) Sex affirms the essential similarity of all of nature's creatures.
12. a) Juvenile delinquency is simply a reflection of the basic evil in human beings. It has always existed in the past and it always will.
    b) Juvenile delinquency is due to factors we do not understand. When we do understand these we will be able to prevent it in the future.
13. a) When man faces death he learns how basically insignificant he is.
    b) When man faces death he learns who he really is and how much he loved life.
14. a) Pornography pollutes the senses, the self, and the society.
    b) Erotica arouses the senses, frees the self, and purges false prudery from society.
15. a) The child molester deserves society's help, treatment, and rehabilitation.
    b) The child molester should receive their just deserts—punishment.
16. a) Scientific knowledge provides the best guide to leading a satisfying sex life.
    b) The Bible and religious leaders provide the best guide to leading a moral sex life.
17. a) Pornography is protected by the freedom of speech clause in the First Amendment.
    b) Pornography should not be protected by the First Amendment because it creates a clear and present danger to society.
18. a) The important thing in science is to be right and make as few errors as possible.
    b) The important thing in science is to strike out into the unknown—right or wrong.
19. a) Sexually explicit materials can be used in the classroom to educate young people about the facts of human sexuality.
    b) The danger of sex education in the classroom is that it will corrupt the minds of young people who are open to immoral influences.
20. a) Nudity at public beaches endangers the well-being of the young.
    b) Nudity at public beaches can lead to an appreciation of the human body as part of nature.
21. a) Great achievements require first of all great imagination.
    b) Great achievements require first of all severe self-discipline.

22. a) Engaging in a single homosexual act does not necessarily mean the person has, or will adopt, an identity as a homosexual.
   b) Engaging in a single homosexual act identifies a person as homosexual.
23. a) Although child pornography is distasteful, its influence is overrated.
   b) If child pornography is permitted in any form, civilization, as we know it, is doomed.
24. a) If human beings were really honest with each other, there would be a lot more antipathy and enmity in the world.
   b) If human beings were really honest with each other, there would be a lot more sympathy and friendship in the world.
25. a) Leaders in the public eye have no special moral obligations—they are fallible like all humans.
   b) Sexual morality is necessary in our clergy, government officials, and teachers to uphold the standards of society.
26. a) The beauty of theorizing is that it has made it possible to invent things which otherwise never would have existed.
   b) The trouble with theorizing is that it leads people away from the facts and substitutes opinion for truth.
27. a) Sometimes abortion is the best choice available to a young, unmarried woman.
   b) Abortion is immoral because it takes a human life.
28. a) Sex education in the schools, including teaching about contraception, is the most effective way to reduce teenage pregnancies.
   b) Sex education in the schools threatens to undermine the authority of the family and the morality of the community.
29. a) People should wash their hands and genitals after engaging in sexual relations
   b) Washing after sex destroys the relaxed mood that is created since it implies that sex is dirty.
30. a) The loss of control during sexual intercourse heightens orgasmic and interpersonal fulfillment.
   b) Sexual intercourse and orgasm resemble having an epileptic fit, lacking the gracefulness and beauty of more refined social interaction.
31. a) Imagination leads people into self-deception and delusions.
   b) Imagination frees people from the dull routines of life.
32. a) Thinking is responsible for all discovery and invention.
   b) Thinking keeps people on the straight and narrow.
33. a) Observing the world accurately enables human beings to separate reality from imagination.
   b) Observing the world accurately provides a human being with constant excitement and novelty.
34. a) Some people can only be changed by humiliating them.
   b) No one has the right to humiliate another person.
35. a) Sex is so powerful that it alters your moral character, making you more like your partner.
   b) Sex has no more power to alter personality or character than any other form of social interaction.
36. a) The wages of sexual sin is death.
   b) The wages of sexual guilt is sexual inhibition.
37. a) Marital sex can remain exciting if the couple is imaginative and uninhibited.
   b) Marriage is a good remedy for sexual temptation.
38. a) Those who err should be forgiven.
   b) Those who err should be corrected.
39. a) Consenting sex is a worthwhile moral end.
   b) Too often, sex leads people to relate to one another as means rather than as ends.
40. a) Oral and anal sex are more depraved than sexual intercourse.
   b) Oral and anal sex are as morally acceptable as intercourse as long as the couple agrees.
41. a) Any position a couple wants to use during intercourse is normal because preferences for positions vary from culture to culture.
   b) There are natural and unnatural positions for men and women to use during sexual intercourse.
42. a) Whenever a person has difficulty in deciding which of two things to do he should do that which will give him the greatest satisfaction. In the long run that will be the right choice.
   b) Whenever a person has difficulty in deciding which of two things to do he should do what he ought to do, whether it gives him satisfaction or not.
43. a) All of sex is natural, without necessarily having any cosmic or religious significance.
   b) Marital sex, and only marital sex, is sacred—to be regarded with wonder.
44. a) Human sex was set apart forever from animal sex by the divine act that created the human soul.
   b) Human sex is similar, biologically and behaviorally, to sex in primates like the apes.
45. a) Anger should be direct against the oppressors of mankind.
   b) Anger should be directed against those revolutionaries who undermine law and order.
46. a) Masturbation is a normal sexual behavior that has produced needless worries.
   b) At best, masturbation must be controlled; at worst, it is a sinful waste of human seed.
47. a) Familiarity, like absence, makes the heart grow fonder.
   b) Familiarity breeds contempt.
48. a) Reason is the chief means by which human beings make great discoveries.
   b) Reason has to be continually disciplined and corrected by reality and hard facts.

49. a) The changeableness of human feelings is a weakness in human beings.
    b) The changeableness of human feelings makes life more interesting.
50. a) There are a great many things in the world which are good for human beings and which satisfy them in different ways. This makes the world an exciting place and enriches the lives of human beings.
    b) There are a great many things which attract human beings. Some of them are proper, but many are bad for human beings, and some are degrading.
51. a) Psychology studies sexual behavior with the same scientific methods used to study other forms of experience and behavior.
    b) Psychology can only study the surface of sex, not its essence.
52. a) The Kinsey Reports are an example of poor science.
    b) The Kinsey Reports reduced irrational guilt by describing how common many sexual behaviors were.
53. a) Children should be seen and not heard.
    b) Children are entirely delightful.
54. a) For a human being to live a good life he must act like a good man, i.e., observe the rules of morality.
    b) For a human being to live a good life he must satisfy both himself and others.
55. a) Mystical experiences may be sources of insight into the nature of reality.
    b) So-called mystical experiences have most often been a source of delusion.
56. a) Man must always leave himself open to his own feelings—alien as they may sometimes seem.
    b) If sanity is to be preserved, man must guard himself against the intrusion of feelings which are alien to his nature.
57. a) There is no surer road to insanity than surrender to the feelings, particularly those which are alien to the self.
    b) There is a unique avenue to reality through the feelings, even when they seem alien.
58. a) Life sometimes smells bad.
    b) Life sometimes leaves a bad taste in the mouth.
59. a) The mind is like a lamp which illuminates whatever it shines on.
    b) The mind is like a mirror which reflects whatever strikes it.
60. a) Things are beautiful or ugly independent of what human beings think.
    b) Beauty and ugliness are in the eye of the beholder.

Influence Tactics Scale

Sara Steen,[1] *University of Washington*

The Influence Tactics Scale (Howard, Blumstein, & Schwartz, 1986) was developed as a measure of the various types of influence used within intimate relationships to gain compliance. Six distinct types of influence are included in the scale: manipulation, supplication, bullying, autocracy, disengagement, and bargaining. These types of influence are further distinguished as weak tactics (manipulation and supplication), strong tactics (bullying and autocracy), and neutral tactics (disengagement and bar-

gaining). By enabling researchers to distinguish between different influence techniques, this scale provides an important step toward a clearer understanding of the operation of power within intimate relationships.

Description

The Influence Tactics Scale consists of 21 items, broken down into six distinct types of influence. Respondents to the original survey were asked, "When your partner wants you to do something you do not want to do, how often does (he/she) do each of the following?" Responses were provided on a 9-point scale ranging from *always* to *never* for the 21 different influence tactics. The scale could also

[1]Address correspondence to Sara Steen, Department of Sociology, Box 353340, University of Washington, Seattle, WA 98195; email: ssteen@u.washington.edu.

be used to answer the question for the respondent (in terms of what influence tactics he or she would use if attempting to gain compliance from a partner). From the responses of each partner in 235 same-sex and cross-sex couples, a varimax factor analysis identified the six factors noted previously.

Response Mode and Timing

Respondents circle a number from 1 to 9 depending on the frequency of the partner's use (or their own use) of the tactic. The scale requires approximately 5 minutes to complete.

Scoring

Each of the 21 items is scored in the same direction, with a higher score indicating greater frequency of use of the influence tactic. When the tactics are combined, the scores are added to create an overall score for the influence category. The composition and range of scores for each of the categories of influence tactics is shown in Table 1.

Reliability

In a sample of 235 couples drawn from both homosexual (75 male couples, 62 female couples) and heterosexual (98 male-female couples) populations (Howard et al., 1986), the Cronbach alphas for the six scales were as follows: Manipulation = .60, Bullying = .82, Disengagement = .75, Supplication = .71, Autocracy = .72, and Bargaining = .55.

Validity

As predicted, Howard et al. (1986) found that the use of some influence tactics, specifically those classified as weak tactics, varied by sex role orientation and sex of partner (surprisingly, sex of actor did not have a significant effect). Controlling for structural factors, such as income,

Table 1 Composition and Range of Scores for Each Influence Tactic

Category	Influence strategies	Range
Manipulation (weak tactic)	Dropping hints, flattering, behaving seductively, reminding of past favors	4-36
Supplication (weak tactic)	Pleading, crying, acting ill, acting helpless	4-36
Bullying (strong tactic)	Making threats, insulting, becoming violent, ridiculing	4-36
Autocracy (strong tactic)	Insisting, claiming greater knowledge, asserting authority	3-27
Disengagement (neutral tactic)	Sulking, trying to make one's partner feel guilty, leaving the scene	3-27
Bargaining (neutral tactic)	Reasoning, offering to compromise, offering a trade-off	3-27

those individuals who were relatively less masculine than their partner (in both same-sex and cross-sex couples) were more likely to be perceived as using both weak techniques (Supplication $b = -.12$, $p < .05$) and neutral techniques (Bargaining $b = -.13$, $p < .05$). Individuals with male partners were also more likely to be perceived as using weak techniques (Manipulation $b = .19$, $p < .001$; Supplication $b = .11$, $p < .05$). These findings suggest that relational circumstances, specifically having a male partner and being relatively less masculine than one's partner, elicit the use of relatively weak influence tactics. The measures used help the researcher to explore the processes through which relationship factors shape the nature of interpersonal influence and control.

Reference

Howard, J. A., Blumstein, P., & Schwartz. P. (1986). Sex, power, and influence tactics in intimate relationships. *Journal of Personality and Social Psychology, 51,* 102-109.

Exhibit

Influence Tactics Scale

Instructions: The following activities are behaviors which sometimes occur in intimate relationships. The activities include ways in which your partner might attempt to convince you to engage in a behavior which you do not wish to engage in. Each item is to be rated on a 9-point scale depending on the frequency with which your partner engages in the behavior when he or she wishes to gain your compliance. A response of "1" indicates that your partner always responds in this way, while a response of "9" indicates that your partner never responds in this way. The scores in between indicate an intermediate level of response. Please circle your response directly on the sheet below.

When your partner wants you to do something you do not want to do how often does he/she do each of the following?

	Always								Never
a. Drop hints	1	2	3	4	5	6	7	8	9
b. Threaten	1	2	3	4	5	6	7	8	9
c. Flatter	1	2	3	4	5	6	7	8	9
d. Plead	1	2	3	4	5	6	7	8	9
e. Offer a "trade off"	1	2	3	4	5	6	7	8	9
f. Reason	1	2	3	4	5	6	7	8	9

g. Insist	1	2	3	4	5	6	7	8	9
h. Claim greater knowledge	1	2	3	4	5	6	7	8	9
I. Offer to compromise	1	2	3	4	5	6	7	8	9
j. Sulk	1	2	3	4	5	6	7	8	9
k. Try to make me feel guilty	1	2	3	4	5	6	7	8	9
l. Cry	1	2	3	4	5	6	7	8	9
m. Behave seductively	1	2	3	4	5	6	7	8	9
n. Assert authority	1	2	3	4	5	6	7	8	9
o. Insult	1	2	3	4	5	6	7	8	9
p. Leave the scene	1	2	3	4	5	6	7	8	9
q. Act ill	1	2	3	4	5	6	7	8	9
r. Become violent	1	2	3	4	5	6	7	8	9
s. Ridicule	1	2	3	4	5	6	7	8	9
t. Act helpless	1	2	3	4	5	6	7	8	9
u. Remind me of past favors	1	2	3	4	5	6	7	8	9

The Sexually Assertive Behavior Scale

Peter B. Anderson[1] and Maria Newton, *University of New Orleans*

The purpose of the Sexually Assertive Behavior Scale (SABS) is to assess women's behaviors and motives relative to initiating sexual contact.

Description

The SABS is a 19-item scale composed of six factors—Sexual Arousal, Hidden Motives, Verbal Pressure, Retaliation or Gain, Physical Force, and Exploitation. Factor 1 (Sexual Arousal) contains items that relate to mutually consenting sexual contact and attempts to arouse a partner. Factor 2 (Hidden Motives) is characterized by items relating to initiating sexual relationships with a man other than her partner to make her partner jealous, to hurt him, or to terminate their relationship. Factor 3 (Verbal Pressure) is composed of items related to verbally persuasive tactics. Factor 4 (Retaliation or Gain) is composed of items relating to initiating sexual contact with a partner out of anger, to retaliate for something done by a partner, or to gain favor. The two items on Factor 5 (Physical Force) relate to the threat and use of physical force. The final factor (Exploi-

tation) contains items related to initiating sexual contact while the partner was vulnerable.

The SABS was developed to assess a wide range of behaviors and motives relative to women initiating sexual contact. Thirteen of the items in the SABS were adapted from the Sexual Experiences Survey (SES) developed by Koss and Oros (1982). The SES is a self-report instrument using dichotomous (yes-no) responses to 13 questions that reflect various degrees of male sexual aggression and female victimization. For example, women responding to the SES were asked, "Have you had sexual intercourse when you didn't want to because a man used his position of authority (boss, teacher, camp counselor, supervisor) to make you?" This work was chosen for adaptation because it was previously tested and shown to have good internal consistency reliability (Cronbach's alpha = .74 for women, .89 for men), test-retest reliability of .93, and external validity established through face-to-face interview (Pearson r = .61, $p < .001$) (Koss & Gidycz, 1985).

In addition to the 13 items adapted from the SES for inclusion in the SABS, 13 more items were generated from a review of the literature on male sexual aggression and item suggestions by a panel of experts in sexual aggression. For example, "How many times have you attempted to have sexual contact with a man by taking advantage of a compromising position he was in (being where he did not belong

[1]Address correspondence to Peter B. Anderson, Department of Human Performance and Health Promotion, University of New Orleans, New Orleans, LA 70148; email: pbahp @jazz.ucc.uno.edu.

or breaking some rule)?" or "How many times have you attempted to have sexual contact with a man to get even with or hurt another man?" All items were worded to conform to the interviewing style used by Kinsey, Pomeroy, and Martin (1948), who assumed all respondents had engaged in each behavior mentioned and allowed for specific numerical responses (i.e., "How many times have you . . . ?" rather than "Have you ever . . . ?"). Also, we attempted to arrange the order of items in the SABS to ask what we judged to be the more comfortable questions first. Factor analysis of the original 26 items yielded a six-factor, 19-item solution accounting for 59.8% of the variance.

Response Mode and Timing

The SABS contains written instructions directing the respondents to write in the number of times they have initiated sexual contact as described in each question. Completion of the 19-item questionnaire typically takes approximately 5 minutes.

Scoring

Actual frequency counts are elicited for each question. To date, we have compiled and transformed the responses into dichotomous scores of 0 for those who reported no experience and 1 for those who reported engaging in the behavior or motive one or more times. One may also choose to create a response distribution per item and then subdivide the distribution into quartiles. Items contained in each subscale are Sexual Arousal (Items 1-5), Hidden Motives (Items 9-11), Verbal Pressure (Items 6-8), Retaliation or Gain (Items 12-14), Physical Force (Items 18-19), and Exploitation (Items 15-17).

Reliability

Anderson and Newton (1995) found that the Hidden Motives subscale demonstrated satisfactory reliability (al-

pha coefficient = .75). Internal consistency for the Sexual Arousal, Retaliation or Gain, and Verbal Pressure subscales was marginally acceptable (alphas = .64, .56, and .61 respectively). The Exploitation subscale (alpha = .43) yielded low reliability and should be interpreted with caution. The Physical Force subscale contained only two items (alpha = .58).

Validity

This instrument was reviewed for face and content validity, pretested, pilot tested, and reviewed twice by a panel of experts to establish consensual validation (Anderson, 1990). Construct validity, in relation to factor structure, was supported by the factor analyses (Anderson & Newton, 1995).

References

Anderson, P. B. (1990, November). *Aggressive sexual behavior by females: Incidence, correlates, and implications.* Paper presented at the annual meeting of the Mid-South Educational Research Association, New Orleans, LA.

Anderson, P., & Aymami, R. (1993). Reports of female initiation of sexual contact: Male and female differences. *Archives of Sexual Behavior, 22,* 335-343.

Anderson, P., & Newton, M. (1997). The Initiating Heterosexual Contact Scale: A factor analysis. *Sexual Abuse: A Journal of Research and Treatment, 9*(3), 179-186.

Kinsey, A., Pomeroy, W., & Martin, C. (1948). *Sexual behavior in the human male.* Philadelphia: Saunders.

Koss, M., & Gidycz, C. (1985). Sexual Experiences Survey: Reliability and validity. *Journal of Consulting and Clinical Psychology, 53,* 422-423.

Koss, M., & Oros, C. (1982). Sexual Experiences Survey: A research instrument investigating sexual aggression and victimization. *Journal of Consulting and Clinical Psychology, 50,* 455-457.

Exhibit

The Sexually Assertive Behavior Scale

This portion of the questionnaire is an attempt to discover some of the behavior that you employ in your sexual activity. Sexual contact is defined as fondling, kissing, petting, or intercourse. There are no right or wrong answers to the questions. Please answer as honestly as you can.

1. How many times have you had sexual contact (fondling, kissing, petting, or intercourse) with a man when you both wanted to?
2. How many times have you initiated sexual contact (fondling, kissing, petting, or intercourse) with a man?
3. In initiating sexual contact with a man, how many times have you overestimated the level of sexual activity he desired to have with you?
4. How many times have you attempted to have sexual contact with a man because you were so sexually aroused you did not want to stop?
5. How many times have you attempted to have sexual contact with a man by getting him sexually aroused?
6. How many times have you attempted to have sexual contact (fondling, kissing, petting, or intercourse) with a man by threatening to end your relationship?
7. How many times have you attempted to have sexual contact with a man by saying things that you didn't mean?
8. How many times have you attempted to have sexual contact with a man by pressuring him with verbal arguments?

9. How many times have you attempted to have sexual contact with a man in order to make another man jealous?
10. How many times have you attempted to have sexual contact with a man to get even with or hurt another man?
11. How many times have you attempted to have sexual contact with a man because you wanted to end a relationship with another man?
12. How many times have you attempted to have sexual contact with a man in a position of authority over you (boss, teacher, or supervisor) in order to better your situation or gain something?
13. How many times have you attempted to have sexual contact with a man because you were angry at him?
14. How many times have you attempted to have sexual contact with a man to retaliate for something he did to you?
15. How many times have you attempted to have sexual contact (fondling, kissing, petting, or intercourse) with a man to gain power or control over him?
16. How many times have you attempted to have sexual contact with a man while his judgment was impaired by drugs or alcohol?
17. How many times have you attempted to have sexual contact with a man by taking advantage of a compromising position he was in (being where he did not belong or breaking some rule)?
18. How many times have you attempted to have sexual contact with a man by threatening to use some degree of physical force (holding him down, hitting him, etc.)?
19. How many times have you attempted to have sexual contact with a man by using some degree of physical force?

Source. This scale is also published in "The Initiating Heterosexual Contact Scale: A Factor Analysis," 1997, *Sexual Abuse: A Journal of Research and Treatment,* 9(3), 179-186.

The Sexual Signaling Behaviors Inventory

Clinton J. Jesser,[1] *Northern Illinois University*

In 1975 I undertook some research, the main focus of which was to determine how college students signal their heterosexual partners when they want coitus. As background, two main streams of thought were involved. The first might be called "interaction theory." Specifically, the problem was how do people make transitions in the flow of interaction from one type of activity to another so that the actions of the actors (in this case two people) remain coparallel and understandable to each other? Obviously, communication is involved in this process, and the transition from doing whatever one is doing to preparing to engage in sex must be made somehow.

The second stream of thought revolves around the notion of gender subcultures, which includes the idea that in a society such as ours, where there is some polarization between what is preferred masculine and preferred feminine, we should find differences not only in how men and

women behave generally but also how they communicate—specifically, how they signal each other when they are interested in coitus. Both verbal and nonverbal, direct and indirect signals are possible, and it was expected that women would use more indirect signals than men (Doyle, 1985, p. 155).

Description

The instrument developed to probe this signaling behavior, the Sexual Signaling Behaviors Inventory (SSBI), refers to behavior in the inclusive sense—both verbal and nonverbal, direct and indirect. I developed the SSBI with the assistance of student discussion to sensitize myself to the whole range of behaviors that might be used and to develop the appropriate refinements in describing them.

Twenty items were finally used including an *other* category (Jesser, 1978). I regard this inventory as exploratory, because no other such inventory could be located in the published research literature.

The SSBI was included in a larger questionnaire in which some other areas of sexuality and sex role behaviors and

[1]Address correspondence to Clinton J. Jesser, Department of Sociology, Northern Illinois University, DeKalb, IL 60115-2891.

attitudes were queried and completed by 56 male and 97 female college students early in the semester in Sociology of Sex Roles classes at a large public midwestern university. In addition to the SSBI items, other items in the questionnaire included the following: "What is (usually or sometimes) the outcome (of using particular signals)?" "Which (signals) would you like to use (even if only sometimes)?" "Which ones does your partner usually use?" (checked in the right-hand column), and "What is the outcome? (usually, sometimes)," "Which (signals) do you wish s/he would use?" "Which (signals) do you wish s/he would not use?"

Response Mode and Timing

Respondents are allowed to check as many items as they wish using blanks in the left-hand column. Typically, the time required to complete the SSBI is less than a minute.

Reliability and Validity

To my knowledge, no formal reliability or validity checks of the SSBI have been made to date. It would appear that the SSBI could be used with many other types of respondents including homosexuals. A valuable visualization of all the results on the SSBI for the respondents only is given in Nass, Libby, and Fisher (1984, p. 101).

References

Doyle, J. A. (1985). *Sex and gender.* Dubuque, IA: William C. Brown.
Jesser, C. J. (1978). Male response to direct verbal sexual initiatives of females. *The Journal of Sex Research, 14,* 118-128.
Nass, G. D., Libby, R. W., & Fisher, M. P. (1984). *Sexual choices.* Monterey, CA: Wadsworth.

Exhibit

The Sexual Signaling Behaviors Inventory

Instructions: When you think your partner can be persuaded to have sex though s/he has not yet become aware of your desire, what do you usually do? Check all items that apply.

A. _____ ask directly
B. _____ use some code words with which (s)he is familiar
C. _____ use more eye contact
D. _____ use touching (snuggling, kissing, etc.)
E. _____ change appearance or clothing
F. _____ remove clothing
G. _____ change tone of voice
H. _____ make indirect talk of sex
I. _____ do more favors for the other
J. _____ set mood atmosphere (music, lighting, etc.)

K. _____ share a drink
L. _____ tease
M. _____ look at sexual material
N. _____ play games such as chase or light "roughhousing"
O. _____ make compliments ("I love you," "You're nice")
P. _____ use some force
Q. _____ use "suggestive" body movements or postures
R. _____ allow hands to wander
S. _____ lie down
T. _____ other (describe _____)

Source. This inventory was originally published in *The Journal of Sex Research, 14*(2), 118-128, May 1978. Reprinted with permission.

Depth of Sexual Involvement Scale

Marita P. McCabe[1] and John K. Collins, *Macquarie University*

The purpose of this instrument is to measure the depth or intimacy of desired and experienced sexual behaviors during various stages of heterosexual dating.

Description

A Guttman-type scale of 16 behaviors (Guttman, 1944) was constructed by extending the scale used by Collins (1974) with items from Luckey and Nass (1969). This scale was administered to 259 high school and university students who were asked to indicate which of 16 behaviors they would like to experience in a heterosexual dating relationship. The scale was reduced to 12 items by combining adjacent scale items that showed similar responses by males and females over a number of stages of dating. Examples of items that were combined were "hand holding" and "light embrace," redefined as "hand holding: holding hands or locking arms, generally while walking." Three other items that were combined were "necking," "deep kissing," and "general body contact." These were redefined as "necking: close body contact, with hugging and prolonged kissing." The final scale is a Guttman-type scale of 12 behaviors that could measure either the heterosexual desires or experiences of adolescents and young adults during dating.

The three stages of dating for which the instrument has been used are the first date (defined as "the first time you go out with a new dating partner to whom you are attracted"), several dates (defined as "when going out with a partner consistently, but both partners feeling free to go out with others"), and going steady (defined as "when both partners come to a mutual and implicit understanding that dating will exclude others"). The scale could also be used for other relationship stages.

Response Mode and Timing

Respondents circle *yes* if they have experienced (or want to experience) a particular behavior, and *no* if they have not experienced (or do not want to experience) a particular behavior at the stage of dating being studied. The length of time taken to complete the scale will depend on the number of aspects of the dating relationships under consideration, that is, the number of times the scale is administered. Any single administration of the scale requires an average of 3 minutes.

Scoring

Because the scale is of a Guttman type, a score may be obtained by determining the last item that received an af-

firmative response. Alternatively, the number of affirmative responses for each use of the scale may be totaled. Higher scores indicate a greater desire for, or experience of, sexual intimacy at the stage of dating being studied.

Reliability

McCabe and Collins (1984) reported test-retest reliability over an 8-week period with 61 student volunteers for behavior on a first date as .83; after several dates, .73; and when going steady, .96. For desires, over the same time period, the coefficient for the first date was .85; after several dates, .80; and when going steady, .78. McCabe and Collins also administered the scale to 2,001 volunteers ranging in age from 16 to 25 years to evaluate the scalability of the component items of each of the six uses of the scale. The coefficient of reproducibility exceeded .90 and the corresponding coefficient of scalability was greater than .70. These same data show the scale to be internally consistent and predominantly unidimensional with coefficient alpha exceeding .87 for each use of the scale.

Validity

Construct validity has been established by McCabe and Collins (1984). The scale was administered to 156 respondents ranging in age from 18 to 48 years. Results showed that as dating became more involved, the level of sexual activity both desired and experienced by males and females also increased. A further study of 259 respondents demonstrated that the desire for sexual experience was higher for males than for females until a committed relationship was established and that females desire greater sexual involvement with increasing age.

Criterion validity was demonstrated by McCabe and Collins (1984). Twenty-nine couples who were going steady at the time of testing were asked to indicate their desired level of sexual experience for this stage of dating. Results showed that 62% of couples indicated the same number of *yes* responses, with a total of 77% scoring within one *yes* response of their partners.

References

Collins, J. K. (1974). Adolescent data intimacy: Norms and peer expectations. *Journal of Youth and Adolescence, 3,* 317-328.

Collins, J. K., & McCabe, M. P. (1980). The influence of sex roles on psychobiological and psychoaffectional orientations to dating. In C. A. Rigg & L. B. Sherin (Eds.), *Adolescent medicine: Present and future concepts* (pp. 181-195). Chicago: Year Book Medical Publishers.

Guttman, L. (1944). A basis for scaling qualitative ideas. *American Sociological Review, 9,* 139-150.

[1]Address correspondence to Marita P. McCabe, School of Psychology, Deakin University, 221 Burwood Highway, Burwood, Victoria 3125, Australia; email: maritam@deakin.edu.au.

Luckey, E., & Nass, G. A. (1969). A comparison of sexual attitudes and behavior in an international sample. *Journal of Marriage and the Family, 31*, 364-379.

McCabe, M. P. (1982). The influence of sex and sex role on the dating attitudes and behavior of Australian youth. *Journal of Adolescent Health Care, 3*, 54-62.

McCabe, M. P., & Collins, J. K. (1981). Dating desires and experiences: A new approach to an old question. *Australian Journal of Sex, Marriage and the Family, 2*, 165-173.

McCabe, M. P., & Collins, J. K. (1983). The sexual and affectional attitudes and experiences of Australian adolescents during dating: The effects of age, church attendance, type of school and socio-economic class. *Archives of Sexual Behavior, 12, 525-539.*

McCabe, M. P., & Collins, J. K. (1984). Measurement of depth of desired and experienced sexual involvement at different stages of dating. *The Journal of Sex Research, 20*, 377-390.

Exhibit

Depth of Sexual Involvement Scale

The following instructions accompany the scale, depending on the purpose for which it is used.

Desire on First Date

This task is to determine what you *would like* at different stages in the dating relationship.

Indicate which of the following you *would like* on the FIRST DATE (i.e., the first time you go out with a new dating partner to whom you are attracted).

Circle the response which is applicable.

Behavior on First Date

Instructions as above, but "*would like*" is replaced by "*have never experienced.*"

Desires After Several Dates

Instructions as for Desires on First Date but "FIRST DATE" is replaced by "SEVERAL DATES" with the definition of this stage of dating given earlier in this chapter.

Behavior After Several Dates

Instructions as for Behavior on First Date but "FIRST DATE" is replaced by "SEVERAL DATES" with the definition of this stage of dating given earlier in this chapter.

Desires When Going Steady

Instructions as for Desires on First Date but "FIRST DATE" is replaced by "when GOING STEADY" with the definition of this stage of dating given earlier in this chapter.

Behavior When Going Steady

Instructions as for Behavior on First Date but "FIRST DATE" is replaced by "when GOING STEADY" with the definition of this stage of dating given earlier in this chapter.

Scale of Sexual Activities

1. Hand holding: holding hands or locking arms, generally while walking.
2. Light kissing: casual goodnight kiss on the lips.
3. Necking: close body contact, with hugging and prolonged kissing.
4. Light breast petting: caress of the girl's breasts outside the clothing.
5. Heavy breast petting: fondling or kissing of the girl's breasts under the clothing.
6. Light genital petting of the female: touching genital area of the girl, outside the clothing.
7. Heavy genital petting of female: touching genital area of the girl, under the clothing.
8. Manual stimulation of male genitals.
9. Oral stimulation of female genitals.
10. Oral stimulation of male genitals.
11. Petting of each other's genitals resulting in orgasm for one or both partners.
12. Intercourse.

Sexual Path Preferences Inventory

Donald L. Mosher,[1] *University of Connecticut*

In Mosher's (1980) sexual involvement theory, orgasmic response is potentiated by effective sexual stimulation that is subjectively experienced as pleasurable: (a) sensory signals, (b) the discrete affects of interest-excitement and enjoyment-joy, and (c) the cognitive interpretation and evaluation of sensory and affective pleasure as ordered by rules contained in facilitating sexual scripts. Effective sexual stimulation is a joint function of the optimal density of physical sexual stimulation and depth of involvement in the sexual episode. The *optimal density* of physical stimulation is a function of scripted rules for ordering information about the intensity times duration of sexual touching. *Involvement* is defined as a latent or theoretical construct consisting of a complex of interacting psychological processes that motivate and define the state of absorption in the sexual episode. The involvement complex consists of (a) the affects of interest-excitement and enjoyment-joy; (b) affect-cognition blends of anticipatory excitement and sexual pleasure with the sexual goal, image, and plan (i.e., the sexual motive) for the episode; and (c) the facilitating sexual scripts of involvement potential and path preference.

The Sexual Path Preferences Inventory measures involvement potential and path preferences. In addition, it measures, for couples, the compatibility of path preferences and potential involvement. Involvement is manifested as a state of absorption in the inherently acceptable affective scene of the sexual episode. To be involved or absorbed means the person is fully attending to or totally engrossed in the possibilities of the sexual image and plan and the unfolding actualities or expressive action, subject experience, and interpersonal engagement emergent in the present moment of the sexual episode. Depth of involvement in the sexual episode is a function of a deepening involvement within three (so far identified) general paths, or families of plans, that are distinguished conceptually as (a) the path of involvement in sexual role enactment, (b) the path of involvement in sexual trance, and (c) the path of involvement with the sex partner.

A *path* is defined as a general sexual script containing (a) the ordered set of rules for generating, predicting, interpreting, controlling, and evaluating a related family of sexual scenes and (b) its associated affect. The potentiality for deep involvement in a particular sexual scene is a function of (a) involvement potential; (b) multiple, highly valued path preferences; and (c) flexibility in responding to feedback from auxiliary information about the goodness of fit of the unfolding incidents and events to the sexual image and plan. *Involvement potential* is defined as a latent capacity, realized in an actual sexual scene, for absorption in

the sexual episode as a function of the total set of facilitating sexual scripts. *Path preference* is defined as a relative preference for a specific set of plans sharing a family resemblance, the three paths to involvement identified above. *Compatible involving path or paths* is defined as the sharing by a couple of one or more paths that are involving for them as individuals and on which they overlap, preferring the same specific features within the path. This inventory is appropriate for use in research on sexual involvement theory and for clinical use with clients experiencing sexual dysfunction.

Description

This inventory consists of 90, 7-point Likert-type items, arranged into 30 item triplets by categories, with response options labeled 0, *not at all true of (for) me* to 6, *extremely true of (for) me*. Each item triplet consists of an item from the sexual role enactment, sexual trance, and sex partner paths in categories that define path preference (e.g., sexual metaphors, mood, settings, sexual techniques, etc.). This novel item arrangement in sets of three is named a *limited comparison format* because respondents are encouraged to compare their responses within the set to delineate gradations in preference. The inventory is appropriate for use with sexually experienced adults who have had an opportunity to develop preferences.

Response Mode and Timing

Respondents rate each item on a 0 to 6 scale by circling a number on the test booklet or filling in a blank on a machine-scorable answer sheet. Approximately 20 minutes are required for completion.

Scoring

The sum of the scores for all 90 items measures involvement potential. The summed scores of the following 30 items measure Preference for the Path of Sexual Role Enactment: 1, 5, 9, 11, 13, 18, 19, 23, 26, 28, 33, 35, 38, 42, 44, 46, 49, 52, 55, 59, 62, 66, 68, 70, 74, 78, 80, 83, 86, and 90. The summed scores of the following 30 items measure Preference for the Path of Sexual Trance: 3, 4, 8, 12, 14, 16, 20, 24, 27, 29, 31, 36, 39, 40, 43, 47, 50, 54, 56, 60, 61, 65, 69, 72, 75, 77, 81, 84, 85, and 89. The summed scores of the following 30 items measure Preference for the Path of Partner Engagement: 2, 6, 7, 10, 15, 17, 21, 22, 25, 30, 32, 34, 37, 41, 45, 48, 51, 53, 57, 58, 63, 64, 67, 71, 73, 76, 79, 82, 87, and 88. An individual might have one, two, three, or no highly valued paths as defined by scores above 120 for a particular path. If each partner of a couple has completed the inventory independently, then indexes of compatibility of involving path

[1]Address correspondence to Donald L. Mosher, 5051 North A1a, PH1-1, North Hutchinson Island, FL 34949; email: dlmosher@aol.com.

preference can be scored. A score for Compatible Role Path is a count of the 30 items keyed above on which both members of the couple rated the same item as 5, 6, or 7 (i.e., it was true of them both). A score for Compatible Trance Path is a similar count of the 30 items keyed in that path that both members of the couple endorsed as true for them; likewise, a count is made for Compatible Partner Path. A sum of these three scores yields an index of Potential for Compatible Involvement.

Reliability

Cronbach alpha coefficients were computed on a sample of 100 sexually experienced adult men and women for Involvement Potential, alpha = .93; Preference for Role Path, alpha = .92; Preference for Trance Path, alpha = .86; and Preference for Partner Path, alpha = .91.

Validity

Sirkin (1985) found that 76 college men, M = 100.01, scored significantly higher on the Path of Role Enactment than 62 college women, M = 87.52, $t(136)$ = 2.72, $p <$ .01. For the women in the sample, Involvement Potential, Trance Path Preference, and Role Path Preference were significantly correlated (Mdn $r(60)$ = .43) with self-reports of sexual behavior, sexual pleasure, and sexual fantasy. Partner Path Preference was correlated, also for women, with reported sexual pleasure. For the men, there were only three significant correlations. Two were for Partner Path Preference and reports of sexual behavior, $r(74)$ = –.28,

and masturbation, $r(73)$ = .32 (i.e., men who scored higher on the Partner Path reported less sexual behavior with partners and more masturbation). Men scoring higher on the Role Path reported more sexual fantasy, $r(72)$ = .25.

Moreover, Sirkin (1985), using a method of guided sexual imagery, experimentally varied conditions of hypnotic trance induction with a relaxation control and a no-treatment control to test for a theoretically predicted interaction between the Path of Sexual Trance and hypnotic induction. Using ratings of sexual arousal as the dependent variable, men and women who scored above the median on the Path of Sexual Trance and who received the hypnotic trance induction reported significantly higher sexual arousal than all of the other respondents in various conditions, $t(136)$ = 2.83, $p <$ .01. Preference for the Trance Path was also associated, alone or in interaction with the other two path preferences, with reports of experiencing the positive affects of enjoyment-joy and interest-excitement during the guided sexual imagery. Furthermore, Involvement Potential, after partialing out the treatment effects, was predictive of greater depth of involvement in the guided imagery, more subjective sexual arousal across three measures, and more affective enjoyment and interest.

References

Mosher, D. L. (1980). Three dimensions of depth of involvement in human sexual response. *The Journal of Sex Research, 16*, 1-42.
Sirkin, M. I. (1985). *Sexual involvement theory, sexual trance, and hypnotizability: The experimental use of guided imagery.* Unpublished doctoral dissertation, University of Connecticut, Storrs.

Exhibit

Sexual Path Preferences Inventory

Instructions: This Inventory of Sexual Preferences provides you with an opportunity to clarify what your sexual preferences are. It consists of 90 items arranged into 30 triplets. Each set of three items is related to some aspect of a sexual episode between two partners. You are to respond to each of the 90 items as honestly as you can by rating your response on a 7-point scale where 0 means not at all true of (for) me, and 6 means extremely true of (for) me. Ratings of 1 through 5 represent ratings of disagreement/agreement that are intermediate between not at all true and extremely true. The items are arranged in sets of three to permit you to compare the intensity of agreement/disagreement among the set since they all relate to the same feature of the sexual situation. This limited comparison is often useful since people frequently most or least prefer one item in each set. In some instances it is possible that all items in a set may be not at all true or extremely true for you. Most often, there will be a gradation in preference. You may prefer or believe some items to be more characteristically true of you than others, and you may not prefer some items which are much less true for you than others. Rate each of the 90 items from 0 to 6 as you keep in mind the value of comparing items within the triplets.

Sexual metaphors

1. Sex is artful and dramatic play.
2. Sex is union.
3. Sex is trance.

Mood

4. My favorite mood for enjoying sex is like a tranquil meditative state or the relaxation that you might get from a massage or marijuana.
5. When I'm feeling that "All the world's a stage, and all the people are sex players," then I know I want to get it on.
6. When my heart is bursting with love, I know our sex will be bursting with loving pleasure.

Settings

7. I like to have sex in a romantic context in which my partner and I are feeling loved toward one another.
8. I could enjoy having sex in a setting close to nature (e.g., on a mountain top or by the ocean), if I knew that we were totally alone and sure of privacy.
9. I would enjoy having sex in a dramatic setting, like in an oriental harem or an elegant New Orleans brothel.

Sexual techniques

10. Regardless of contemporary views on sexual variety, for me nothing will replace my favorite position for coitus of being face to face with the one I love.
11. I enjoy having sexual intercourse in a wide variety of positions.
12. I prefer slow and rhythmic movement that permits me to really sense the shades and nuances of pleasure that can exist during sexual intercourse.

Sexual metaphors

13. Sex is a drama that begins with attraction, develops a plot filled with intrigue, mystery, and sex play, and ends in tumultuous climax worthy of an audience's applause.
14. Sex is a trip into your own sensory nerves and erotic images.
15. I consider sex to be the organ of love.

Mood

16. The most important aspect of my mood when I get into sex is that I be physically relaxed and mentally receptive.
17. To really want sex my mood must be one of really loving my partner.
18. I love serious sex play when I'm in a playful mood.

Settings

19. I believe that I would feel very excited by having secret sex in a semi-public place.
20. I like a setting for having sex that ensures total privacy.
21. I enjoy having sex in a place that has special meanings for me and my partner.

Sexual techniques

22. Ideally, all sexual techniques begin and build from kissing the face and lips.
23. I pride myself in being quite accomplished in the techniques of oral sex.
24. The most important thing about sexual technique is pacing and repetition that permits you and your partner to become absorbed into the sex.

Sexual style

25. My sexual style is affectionate and loving.
26. My sexual style is as varied as my mood suggests and my fantasies can create.
27. I concentrate on my inward sensations and experience during sex.

Ideal partner

28. Sexual skill and a flair for experimenting make an ideal sex partner.
29. An ideal sex partner flows with your mood and the situation rather than trying to dictate just how sex is to be done.
30. My ideal sex partner is my ideal love object.

Sex talk

31. If I talk during sex it's liable to be to say something like "oh, that feels so good, oh more, mmmh good, etc."
32. Most of all during sex I like to hear and say "I love you."
33. I really get off when my partner is urging, begging, or directing me by saying, for example, "fuck me, fuck me, fuck me!"

Sex fantasies

34. Sometimes I imagine that my partner through his/her sexual participation is pledging his/her love to me for life.
35. I can enjoy a wide range of sexual fantasies that create novelty in partners, activities, and settings.
36. I like to use my imagination to increase my absorption into the sensory experience of sex.

Sexual techniques

37. My sexual style concentrates on mutual pleasuring to bond us closer together.
38. Sexual variety is the spice of a love life.
39. When I have truly good sex I care less about what and how we are doing it sexually than I do about what I am sensing, feeling, and experiencing as a consequence.

Sexual style

40. For me the sexual experience is truly entrancing, and you would never know how intensely I am experiencing the sex by just looking at me.
41. In my sexual style I try to blend the romantic with the erotic to offer a full rich gift of sexual love.
42. I like to play different sexual roles and scripts that act out fantasies while having sex.

Ideal partner

43. I expect my sexual partner to help create and sustain an ambiance of sensual pleasure.
44. I like a partner who moans and writhes and is carried away by his/her passion.
45. I expect my sex partner to be truly sexually considerate and loving.

Sex talk

46. I can enjoy lusty sex talk that uses erotic language for erotic acts.
47. During sex I like little talk and more sensual friction.
48. Sex talk should be love talk.

Sex fantasies

49. I have several fantastic sex fantasies with dramatic and exciting plots that help turn me on during ordinary sex.
50. I may imagine how I look or how my own and my partner's sex organs look, etc., during sex to enhance my erotic pleasure.
51. Sometimes I imagine my partner is telling me how much he/she loves me during our lovemaking in ways that exceed the limits of mere words.

Ideal sex

52. Truly good sex for me usually entails a wide variety of sex practices and coital positions.
53. Good sex is the physical expression through sexual union of an interpersonal loving union.
54. Good sex for me is characterized by an intense involvement into the sensual and sexual sensation of the moment.

Music

55. Music to have sex by should have dramatic changes in rhythm, tempo, and volume while building to a lively crescendo.
56. Music to have sex by should be soft, low, and repetitive to form a rhythmic background that facilitates the flow without setting a pace to be followed.
57. Music to have sex by should be lyrical, romantic, and poetic in tone to match the partner's loving mood.

Orgasms

58. I most enjoy orgasms in which I seem to flow into my partner and lose myself in our union.
59. I love it when sex moves me to uninhibited self-expression that leaves me with no sense of control of my sounds, movements, and orgasm.
60. I most enjoy orgasms in which I experience sensations that are so intense that I actually lose consciousness or at least waking consciousness fades in the face of the culminative sensations and experience.

Ideal partner

61. An ideal sex partner knows exactly what I like and want now.
62. I enjoy a partner who is open to playing different roles so that we can create a novel and dramatic sexual script.
63. If a person cannot look me in the eye before, during and after sex, I suspect the attraction is to my body and not to me.

Sex fantasies

64. Most of my fantasies during sex are really memories of past shared moments in which we felt especially close and loving.
65. Sometimes I experience visual and auditory images that accompany the sensual sensory experience during sex.
66. Sometimes I imagine that I could enjoy sex on a stage surrounded by an admiring audience.

Ideal sex

67. The best sex for me is loving sex.
68. The best sex occurs when sexual expression becomes to ecstatic that it becomes nonvolitional and I lose all sense of conscious control.
69. When I'm having the best sex, my sex organs become alive and their sensations demand and direct the action.

Orgasms

70. I love it when my orgasms are nearly convulsive and I involuntarily scream in pleasure, and grab, and/or bite, or scratch.
71. To orgasm, I must be secure in my love for and from my partner.
72. During orgasms my awareness is flooded with intense sensations.

Emotions

73. Love is the predominant emotion in my sexual experience.
74. Excitement is the predominant emotion in my sexual experience.
75. Enjoyment is the predominant emotion in my sexual experience.

Meanings of sex

76. Sex is the merger of two into a unity of physical and spiritual love.
77. The meaning of sex is that it permits me to set aside my daily existence and to be transported into an underworld of sensations.
78. Sex when most meaningful is a cathartic drama that requires mastery and artful performance of one's sexual identity.

Sex fantasies

79. I sometimes imagine that my partner and I have been selected to symbolize the essence of love in a religious-like, sexual-spiritual ritual.
80. I can enjoy imagining that I am an amazingly successful porno film star and sex symbol in our culture.
81. I rarely have a sex fantasy with a plot; usually I only have a series of nonconnected, visual, sexual images of, for example, sex organs.

Ideal sex

82. The best sex occurs when I enter into a loving warm union with my partner, when we become two in one.
83. Sexual ecstasy is my criterion of good sex.
84. Good sex is total absorption into the sexual experience.

Orgasms

85. The moment of orgasm is a moment of total surrender to intense sensations.
86. The best orgasm is like an involuntary dramatic shock that overwhelms yet releases my sexual tension.
87. Orgasms are a unique moment of fusion in which my soul cries out its love through my body, and my longing for my partner is fulfilled.

Meanings of sex

88. Sharing sex with my partner can become a ritual that celebrates the profound meaning of life.
89. During sex I feel transported into another level of consciousness or plane of existence that gives me a new understanding of my life and the universe.
90. When I have a super sexual experience I feel as if I embody all men/women in a universal and timeless sexual ritual.

Source. This inventory is reprinted with permission of the author.

The Anticipated Sexual Jealousy Scale

Bram Buunk,[1] *University of Nijmegen*

Sexual jealousy can be defined as an aversive emotional reaction that occurs as the result of the partner's sexual attraction to a rival that is real, imagined, or considered likely to occur (Bringle & Buunk, 1985). In line with this definition, the Anticipated Sexual Jealousy Scale measures the degree to which the idea of sexual attraction felt by one's partner for another person evokes a negative emotional response. Because sexual attraction can be manifested in divergent ways, a range of sexually laden behaviors that could be exhibited by the partner are described, and the respondent's reaction to these hypothetical events is assessed. Another consideration behind the construction of the scale was that the negative emotional reactions to such events are not necessarily labeled as jealousy. Because the word *jealous* has a negative connotation in Western culture, individuals may resist labeling their feelings as such. Therefore, the word jealous is avoided in the scale: People are simply asked how bothered they would be. Furthermore, it was assumed that extradyadic sexual behaviors exhibited by the partner can evoke negative, neutral, and positive emotional reactions (see Buunk, 1981a) and that this should be reflected in the response code.

Description, Response Mode, and Timing

The scale consists of five items. The format for each item is the same: The respondents are asked how they would feel if their partner were to engage in flirting, light petting, falling in love, sexual intercourse, and a long-term sexual relationship with another person of the opposite sex. The nine response options range from *extremely bothered* to *extremely pleased*. The midpoint is described as *neutral*. Each of the possible answers is spelled out literally. The respondents circle the number corresponding with the answer that best fits their anticipated feelings. The scale usually requires no more than 1 or 2 minutes for completion.

Scoring

The items can simply be summed. No reverse scoring is necessary. Higher scores indicate a higher degree of jealousy.

Reliability

The Cronbach alpha of the scale was .94 in a sample more or less representative of the general Dutch population and consisting of people with diverse levels of sexual permissiveness (Buunk, 1978); .90 in a study of people who had all been involved in extramarital relationships (Buunk, 1982); .91 in a sample of people in sexually open marriages

(Buunk, 1981a); and .91 in a sample of undergraduate students (Buunk, 1981b). Over a 3-month period, test-retest reliability in the open marriage sample was $r(100) = .76, p < .001$.

Validity

There is considerable evidence for the concurrent validity of the Anticipated Sexual Jealousy Scale. Individuals who said they were presently less jealous than before scored significantly lower on the scale than people who indicated they were as jealous now as they had been in the past (Buunk, 1981a). The scale particularly discriminates between persons high and low in sexual permissiveness. The sample described above, consisting of people who had been involved in extramarital relationships, scored much lower on the scale than a sample of undergraduate students, $t(596) = 19.78, p < .001$, and also much lower than the sample more or less representative of the average population, $t(466) = 11.27, p < .001$.

Further evidence for the concurrent validity of the Anticipated Sexual Jealousy Scale is provided by the strong negative correlations that were found between this scale and a scale for extramarital behavioral intentions in three samples (Buunk, 1982). Finally, in the aforementioned sample of individuals from the average population, the scale showed a high correlation with a scale measuring moral disapproval of extramarital sex, $r(250) = .77, p < .001$.

Construct validity of the Anticipated Sexual Jealousy Scale has been established in several studies showing positive and rather high correlations with other scales measuring jealousy or related constructs. So a correlation of $r(218) = .56, p < .001$, was found with a scale measuring jealousy as a consequence of a spouse's real extramarital relationship that had occurred in the recent past (see Buunk, 1984). Additionally, in the sample of persons from the average population, a positive correlation was established with a scale measuring the desire for an exclusive relationship, $r(250) = .63, p < .01$. In the undergraduate student sample mentioned previously, the Anticipated Sexual Jealousy Scale correlated rather strongly, $r(380) = .59, p < .001$, with a scale based on the factor Threat to Exclusive Relationship, the first and main factor that was found in a factor analysis of jealousy related items by Hupka et al. (1985).

In the same study, Rubin's (1970) love scale correlated significantly with the scale described here, and his liking scale did not (Buunk, 1981a). These last findings support the construct validity of the Anticipated Sexual Jealousy Scale because the love scale—as opposed to the liking scale as conceptualized by Rubin—refers to the emotional bond in a relationship, and jealousy is supposed to stem from a threat to such a bond.

---

[1]Address correspondence to Bram Buunk, University of Nijmegen, Postbus 9104, 6500 HE Nijmegen, The Netherlands.

Final evidence for the validity of the Anticipated Sexual Jealousy Scale comes from the open marriage study. Here, among women, a high correlation was found between the scale and their jealousy as perceived by their husbands, $r(50) = .61$, $p < .001$. The same correlation among men was lower, but also significant, $r(50) = .39$, $p < .01$.

References

Bringle, R. G., & Buunk, B. (1985). Jealousy and social behavior: A review of person, relationship and situational determinants. In P. Shaver (Ed.), *Review of personality and social psychology* (Vol. 6). Beverly Hills, CA: Sage.

Buunk, B. (1978). Jaloezie 2. Ervaringen van 250 Nederlanders [Jealousy: Experiences of 250 Dutch people]. *Intermediair, 14*(11), 43-51.

Buunk, B. (1981a). Jealousy in sexually open marriages. *Alternative Lifestyles, 4*, 357-372.

Buunk, B. (1981b). Liefde, sympathie en jaloezie [Loving, liking and jealousy]. *Gedrag, Tijdschrift voor Psychologie, 9*, 189-202.

Buunk, B. (1982). Anticipated sexual jealousy: Its relationship to self-esteem, dependency, and reciprocity. *Personality and Social Psychology, 8*, 310-316.

Buunk, B. (1984). Jealousy as related to attributions for the partner's behavior. *Social Psychology Quarterly, 47*, 107-112.

Hupka, R. B., Buunk, B., Falus, G., Fulgosi, A., Ortega, E., Swain, R., & Tarabrina, N. V. (1985). Romantic jealousy and romantic envy. A seven-nation study. *Journal of Cross-Cultural Psychology, 16*, 423-446.

Rubin, Z. (1970). Measurement of romantic love. *Journal of Personality and Social Psychology, 16*, 265-273.

Exhibit

The Anticipated Sexual Jealousy Scale

How would you feel if your partner were to engage in the following behavior with another man/woman?

1. Flirting
   a. Extremely pleased
   b. Very pleased
   c. Fairly pleased
   d. Somewhat pleased
   e. Neutral
   f. Somewhat bothered
   g. Fairly bothered
   h. Very bothered
   i. Extremely bothered

2. Sexual intercourse[a]
3. Light petting
4. A long-term sexual relationship
5. Falling in love

Source. This scale is reprinted with permission of the author.

a. The nine response options are repeated for each item.

Acquisition of Sexual Information Test

Jerome B. Dusek,[1] *Syracuse University*

The purpose of the test is to assess student learning of information concerning the various aspects of human sexuality typically taught in a sex education class.

Description

The test was designed for use as an in-classroom assessment device, that is, for use as a classroom test of information learned. It also could be used as a screening device to assess knowledge of various aspects of sexuality, as was done by Monge, Dusek, and Lawless (1977). They reported substantial increases in knowledge from the pretest to the posttest for students enrolled in a sex education course but no increase for a control group. Although the test was constructed for use in a particular course, the course content was sufficiently general to render the test useful for a variety of sex education courses or purposes.

The test is composed of 50 items presented in a four-alternative multiple-choice format. The items were selected from a larger pool of items (100) written by secondary school teachers of sex education classes. The items were chosen to assess knowledge of both general developmental phenomena, such as stages of human development, and various aspects of adolescent sexuality, including birth control, the anatomy of the male and female reproductive systems, venereal disease, premarital sexual relations, and pregnancy.

To identify the aspects of sexuality measured, and the items defining each aspect, two independent raters were instructed to sort into categories items that seemed to measure similar aspects of human sexuality and to place all remaining items into an "other" category. The raters did this in a highly reliable manner (k = .94; Light, 1971). In other words, the two raters agreed on 48 of the 50 items. A consensus was reached on the placement of the two items on which there was disagreement.

This sort resulted in the four sexuality categories described. A total of 24 items were included in these categories. The remaining 26 items were identified as assessing knowledge of general aspects of human development.

Although the test was designed for use in a ninth-grade class, the vocabulary and length of the items and test make it suitable for both younger and older adolescents.

Response Mode and Timing

Respondents are instructed to read each item and each alternative and to circle the alternative that correctly answers the question. Students in upper grade levels may be

asked to answer the questions on an optical scanning answer sheet. The test is readily completed in a single class period (43 minutes) by ninth graders (Monge et al., 1977). It is of interest to note that this also was the case for the pretested students in the Monge et al. study. That these students were able to complete the test readily in a single class period without having been exposed formally to the material attests to the appropriateness of the test length.

Scoring

The correct responses for each item are indicated on the test. There are five major sections to the test. Twenty-four items measure knowledge in four areas of human sexuality: venereal disease (Items 5, 29, 32, 33, 48, and 50); birth control, sexual relations, and reproduction (Items 2, 7, 8, 25, 34, 39, and 43); male biological aspects of sexuality (Items 1, 14, 19, 21, 27, and 45); and female biological aspects of sexuality (Items 13, 16, 36, 40, and 49). The remaining 26 items assess knowledge of various general aspects of human development.

Reliability

The reliability information presented below comes from a study reported by Monge et al. (1977). The sample consisted of 379 students, including 182 students (88 males and 94 females) enrolled in a sex education course and 197 students (106 males and 91 females) not enrolled in a sex education course. All students attended the same school and were enrolled in other classes together. Of those enrolled in the course, 88 (44 males and 44 females) were pretested with the test. Of those not enrolled in the course, 78 (44 males and 34 females) were pretested. Pretesting was done prior to the beginning of the sex education course. All students completed the posttest 6 weeks following the pretest, that is, after the students enrolled in the course had completed the course. Because sex differences in performance on the test were minimal (cf. Monge et al., 1977), no breakdown of data is given by sex.

The most appropriate test-retest reliability estimates come from the data for the control group in the Monge et al. (1977) study. The test-retest correlation for the entire 50-item test was .65. For the 24 items assessing knowledge of various aspects of human sexuality the test-retest correlation was .68. The test-retest correlations for the four human sexuality subscales were as follows: Venereal Disease, .44; Birth Control, Sexual Relations, and Reproduction, .52; Male Biological Aspects of Sexuality, .60; and Female Biological Aspects of Sexuality, .60.

A total of six estimates of reliability for the 50-item test are available using the Kuder-Richardson formula 20 (K-R 20). On the pretest, the K-R 20 for the group enrolled in the course was .83, and the K-R 20 for the group not

[1] Address correspondence to Jerome B. Dusek, Department of Psychology, Syracuse University, Syracuse, NY 13244-2340; email: jbd@syr.edu.

enrolled in the course was .85. On the posttest the K-R 20 values for these two groups were .85 and .83, respectively. The K-R 20 values for the nonpretested experimental and control groups on the posttest were .89 and .83, respectively.

For the posttest scores, the K-R 20 values for those enrolled in the course and for those not enrolled in the course on the 24 items assessing knowledge of aspects of human sexuality were .80 and .80, respectively. The K-R 20 value for the entire posttest group on the 24 items assessing aspects of human sexuality also was .80.

The test-retest and K-R 20 values indicate the test is a suitably reliable instrument. The data are especially impressive when the lengths of the test and the subscales are considered. In all likelihood, the reliability values presented above are as high as could be obtained given the number of items on the test and the subscales (cf. Cronbach, 1970).

Validity

At the present time there is no information concerning the degree to which the gain in knowledge due to exposure to the course, which was clearly demonstrated (cf. Monge et al., 1977), altered adolescent sexual behavior. Extant validity data, then, are limited to the following.

First, the items on the test, and particularly those dealing with aspects of sexuality, have clear face or content validity (Cronbach, 1970). One need only read the pertinent items to determine that this is the case. This is the form of validity Cronbach notes in common in tests designed to evaluate educational programs.

Second, the test has a form of construct validity (cf. Cronbach, 1970) in that it has been demonstrated (cf. Monge et al., 1977) that students exposed to the substantive content assessed by the test evidence improvement in scores on the test and the human sexuality subscales and students not exposed to the content do not. That is, exposure to the treatment (viz., enrolled in a sex education course) has the expected facilitative effect on the test scores.

Other Information

The instrument described in this report was developed as part of a research project supported by Grant HD-06724 from the Center for Population Research of the National Institutes of Child Health and Human Development.

References

Cronbach, L. J. (1970). *Essentials of psychological testing* (3rd ed.). New York: Harper & Row.

Light, R. (1971). Measures of response agreement for qualitative data: Some generalizations and alternatives. *Psychological Bulletin, 76,* 365-377.

Monge, R. H., Dusek, J. B., & Lawless, J. (1977). An evaluation of the acquisition of sexual information through a sex education class. *The Journal of Sex Research, 13,* 170-184.

Exhibit

Acquisition of Sexual Information Test

1. The male reproductive system consists of
   a. one sex organ
   b. one sex organ and a system of glands*
   c. two glands
   d. two sex organs
2. The union of the egg and the sperm is the result of
   a. coitus*
   b. umbilicus
   c. abortion
   d. menstruation
3. Another word for esteem is
   a. respect*
   b. intimacy
   c. influence
   d. money
4. The type of family which is most common in our society is the
   a. nuclear family*
   b. procreated family
   c. extended family
   d. modified extended family
5. A venereal disease with three stages of infection is
   a. gonorrhea
   b. Wasserman
   c. syphilis*
   d. pustulus
6. The beginnings of a person's self-image of self-concept begins at what stage of development?
   a. early infancy
   b. late infancy*
   c. early childhood
   d. late childhood
7. The use of methods in sexual intercourse to prevent pregnancy is
   a. contraception*
   b. conception
   c. menopause
   d. sterility
8. The ovaries and the prostate gland both produce
   a. eggs
   b. sperm
   c. hormones*
   d. semen

9. Which is *not* true concerning merit system love?
   a. It is always conditional.
   b. It is based on the word "because."
   c. It is a free expression of love.*
   d. It has to be earned.

10. The first three phases of the family life cycle are
    a. adolescence, late adolescence, young adolescence
    b. early infancy, adolescence, and young adolescence
    c. early infancy, early adolescence, late adolescence
    d. infancy, childhood, adult*

11. The identification model for a three-year-old boy should be the
    a. mother
    b. father*
    c. both mother and father
    d. sister

12. A "nuclear" family refers to
    a. mother, father, children, aunts and uncles
    b. mother, father and grandparents
    c. mother, father and their children*
    d. the children only

13. Which is not a part of the female reproductive system?
    a. vagina
    b. seminal vesicles*
    c. ovaries
    d. uterus

14. Which is not a part of the male reproductive system?
    a. penis
    b. scrotum
    c. fallopian tube*
    d. vas deferens

15. Which of the following may *not* be a cause of homosexuality?
    a. unbalanced love of a boy for his mother
    b. an overbearing, domineering mother
    c. identification of a boy with his mother
    d. effects of a fast changing society*

16. The stopping of menstruation is known as
    a. masturbation
    b. menopause*
    c. menses
    d. masculinization

17. Which of the following statements is *not* true?
    a. Every child must have success at controlling his environment.
    b. A person who fails to learn autonomy will always be subject to what people think of him.
    c. The child should have rules and regulations concerning the best for his welfare.
    d. Parents should use punishment whenever necessary for their sake.*

18. The most important thing a child can learn during infancy is
    a. to play with others
    b. to trust people*
    c. to be creative
    d. to know yourself

19. In a large proportion of men over sixty what part of the male reproductive system may cause problems?
    a. prostate gland*
    b. vas deferens
    c. epididymis
    d. testes

20. Which of the statements below is *not* true of love?
    a. Love is respect.
    b. Love is mutual trust.
    c. Love is meeting or fulfilling a need.
    d. Love is physical attraction.*

21. Sperm are produced in the
    a. vas deferens
    b. penis
    c. testes*
    d. epididymis

22. The "complementary" theory of mate selections suggests that you should select a mate
    a. whose personality is highly similar to yours
    b. on the basis of physical attraction
    c. whose mental abilities are the same as yours
    d. whose personality provides satisfaction to your needs*

23. The traditional philosophy of childrearing concerns
    a. creativity
    b. self-expression
    c. individuality
    d. values*

24. A conscience begins to develop around the age of
    a. 4-5 years*
    b. 8-9 years
    c. 12-13 years
    d. 1-3 years

25. When a baby is born with the feet delivering first, it is called a
    a. cesarean birth
    d. natural birth
    c. posterior birth
    d. breech birth*

26. When a person achieves some measure of satisfaction of his basic needs, the person is then free to proceed to a new level which is
    a. self-fulfillment*
    b. material rewards
    c. more friends
    d. autonomy

27. The male sex glands produce a fluid known as
    a. sperm
    b. semen*
    c. lubinol
    d. urine

28. The type of learning which is usually unconscious is
    a. problem-solving
    b. conditioning
    c. "formal" learning
    d. internalization*
29. Gonorrhea can be detected through
    a. a blood test
    b. a smear test*
    c. an X-ray
    d. a urine test
30. Monogamy refers to a type of marriage which is
    a. the type of marriage in our society*
    b. an illegal type of marriage
    c. a marriage with many wives
    d. a marriage with many husbands
31. The most influential factor in a person's attitude toward sex is
    a. his peer group
    b. his parents*
    c. his close friends
    d. society
32. A disease which is not transmitted through direct sexual relations is
    a. gonorrhea
    b. syphilis
    c. congenital syphilis*
    d. spirochetes
33. One of the first symptoms of syphilis is a
    a. chancre sore*
    b. rash
    c. fever
    d. high blood pressure
34. Secondary sex characteristics develop during the stage of
    a. infancy
    b. childhood
    c. adolescence*
    d. young adulthood
35. According to Dr. Maslow, man's four most basic needs are for
    a. food, love, money, and esteem
    b. food, safety, love, and esteem*
    c. food, happiness, love, and esteem
    d. food, love, happiness, and status
36. The shedding of tissues and blood which has built up on the uterine wall is known as
    a. menstruation*
    b. menopause
    c. masturbation
    d. monopoly
37. Masturbation is *not*
    a. a form of releasing sexual energy
    b. practiced by both males and females
    c. good if it takes the place of normal sexual development*
    d. self-manipulation of the genitals
38. Masculinity is dependent upon
    a. involvement in athletics
    b. the amount of chest hair
    c. a person's self-image*
    d. society
39. The structure *through* which the unborn child receives the nutrients is called the
    a. placenta
    b. amniotic sac
    c. navel
    d. umbilical cord*
40. The female reproductive system consists of
    a. one ovary, a fallopian tube, and the uterus
    b. one ovary, two fallopian tubes, uterus, and cervix
    c. two ovaries, two fallopian tubes, uterus, and cervix*
    d. two ovaries, two fallopian tubes, uterus, and urethra
41. If a child does not move toward autonomy, then that child will
    a. doubt himself*
    b. feel responsible for himself
    c. not have respect for others
    d. become conceited
42. A doctor who takes care of babies after they have been delivered and are growing is known as the
    a. pediatrician*
    b. podiatrist
    c. psychiatrist
    d. obstetrician
43. From the third month of development until birth the unborn child is known as the
    a. embryo
    b. fetus*
    c. zygote
    d. sperm
44. Which of the following is *not* true of a "rejecting" environment?
    a. The children will tend to feel insecure.
    b. There may be an attitude of anger and aggression.
    c. Parents may have been rejected when they were children.
    d. The personality of the children will not be affected.*
45. The testes are located in a sac known as the
    a. amniotic sac
    b. scrotum*
    c. penis
    d. prostate
46. According to Dr. Sears's theory on punishment, there are positive conclusions which can be drawn. Which one of the following is *not* one of these conclusions?
    a. Punishment may be physical or nonphysical.
    b. Most people who punish severely were probably brought up in the same way.
    c. Punishment should be used as a training and controlling device.*
    d. Punishment is frequently an outlet for built-up emotions of the parents.

47. Giving freedom to a child in an amount that he can reasonably handle is essential to
    a. the development of a healthy personality*
    b. learning generativity
    c. becoming intimate with others
    d. developing integrity
48. Which is *not* an effect of gonorrhea?
    a. Men who are infected with gonorrhea will feel pain at urination.
    b. Sterility in the female may result.
    c. Blindness and destruction of tissue may result.
    d. An increase in body weight occurs.*
49. The ovary is the storage place for
    a. eggs*
    b. semen
    c. sperm
    d. lubinol
50. Which statement is *not* true concerning syphilis?
    a. It can be detected by a blood test.
    b. It can cause miscarriage or abortion of the fetus.
    c. Once the first sign of syphilis disappears the infection has ceased.*
    d. A baby can contract syphilis from the mother if she is infected.

*Indicates correct answer.

A 24-Item Version of the Miller-Fisk Sexual Knowledge Questionnaire

The Editors

The Sexual Knowledge Questionnaire (SKQ) was created to assess knowledge of reproductive physiology, contraceptive methods, and topics related to fertility and infertility. It was derived from a 49-item test developed by Miller and Fisk in 1969. Details concerning the derivation of the instrument were described by Gough (1974). An Italian translation and application of the test in Italy was published by Lazzari and Gough (1974). The items provide respondents with four multiple-choice options or a true-false response. It takes between 10 and 20 minutes to complete the test.

Additional information and a copy of the instrument may be obtained from the first editor.

References

Gough, H. G. (1974). A 24-item version of the Miller-Fisk Sexual Knowledge Questionnaire. *Journal of Psychology, 87,* 183-192.

Lazzari, R., & Gough, H. G. (1974). Une breve questionario sulle conoscenze sessuali per studi demografici, controllo delle nascite e problemi connessi. *Sessuolgia, 15*(3), 18-25.

The Sex Knowledge and Attitude Test

Harold I. Lief,[1] *Philadelphia, Pennsylvania*

The Sex Knowledge and Attitude Test (SKAT) was developed as a means of gathering information about sexual attitudes, sexual knowledge, and degree of experience in a variety of sexual behaviors (Miller & Lief, 1979). It was hoped that the SKAT would be of value as a teaching aid in courses dealing with human sexuality and serve as a research instrument for educators, social scientists, and health professionals. Since its publication in 1972, the SKAT has been administered to thousands of undergraduate, graduate, nursing, and medical students and other health professionals. The test has been used in many countries and has been translated into a variety of languages.

Description

The SKAT is an omnibus instrument: It consists of an attitudes section, a knowledge section, and two sections dealing with background data and sexual experiences. The SKAT contains 149 multiple-choice questions. Part I (Attitudes) is composed of 35 five-alternative, Likert-type items. Part II (Knowledge) contains 71 true/false items, and in Parts III and IV the number of response alternatives per item ranges from 2 to 10 (Table 1). In addition to item-response data, scores on four attitudinal scales and two knowledge scales may be obtained. The SKAT attitudinal scales are not designed to assess or to diagnose individuals as such. They should be used in a survey fashion—to describe groups of respondents.

Beginning in 1965, Lief and Reed assembled a pool of questionnaire items drawn primarily from three sources: (a) a survey of relevant literature, (b) clinical experience, and (c) socially controversial sex-related topic areas. This pool of questions gave the SKAT its essential character in the sense of content areas to be covered and item formats to be adopted. Several early decisions were made: (a) The SKAT would consist entirely of multiple-choice and true/false items and would be scorable; (b) there would be measurement of a number of variables through groups of items (e.g., scales); and (c) the SKAT would be potentially usable throughout the range of post-high school higher education.

A 180-item draft questionnaire was assembled. The preliminary version was administered to 834 students in three countries: 300 in England, 34 in Sweden, and 500 in the United States. These data led to the second experimental version (SKAT, Form I). During 1969-1970, the revised SKAT was completed by 2,274 medical students at 43 institutions. Examination of this second round of data led to the present SKAT.

Table 1 Content of the Sex Knowledge and Attitude Test

A. Part I—Attitudes (35 items)
  Topic areas
  1. Sexual activities outside marriage
  2. Sexual activities within marriage
  3. Sexual activities before marriage
  4. Sexual variance, causative agents, and remedial or punitive actions
  5. Auto eroticism: male, female, group
  6. Abortion: medical-legal aspects; personal freedom
B. Part II—Knowledge (71 items)
  Topic areas
  1. Physiological aspects
  2. Psychological aspects
  3. Social aspects
C. Part III—Basic Information (12 items)
  Topic areas
  1. Basic Information
    a. Age
    b. Sex
    c. Race
    d. Marital status
  2. Personal Background
    a. Father's occupation
    b. Parents' education status
    c. Religious affiliation
    d. Earliest sex education
D. Part IV—Frequency of Sexual Encounters (31 items)
  Topic areas
    a. Heterosexual encounters
    b. Dating, etc.
    c. Autoerotic activities

The 1972 version of the SKAT represents essentially an abridgement of the previous experimental versions. At the same time, it stands as the outcome of more than 7 years of continuous research, development, and deliberation.

The development of the SKAT attitudinal scales. The final form and item composition of the attitudinal section of the SKAT (Form 2) is the direct result of an empirical analysis of the 50 attitudinal items contained in its predecessor, the SKAT (Form I). Factor analysis (with oblique rotation) of the item responses of 1,137 freshmen through senior medical students (oblique solution for simple loadings), using the simplest criterion for determining the number of factors to rotate (the number of eigenvalues above 1), identified four factors underlying the Attitudes section of the SKAT (Form I): Liberalism (renamed Heterosexual Relations), Acceptance of Sexual Myths, Abortion, and Autoeroticism. Scale scores on these factors were obtained by summing within each scale those items that had factor loadings above

---

[1]Address correspondence to Harold I. Lief, Wayne Counseling Center, 987 Old Eagle Road, Suite 719, Wayne, PA 19087.

.30. Internal consistency reliability was estimated for each of these scales through the calculation of alpha coefficients. These results were cross-validated with a separate sample of 1,137 freshmen through senior medical students. Although there was very little shrinkage upon cross-validation, several of the scale reliabilities were fairly low (.50-.70). The current revision of the Attitudes section of the SKAT (Form 2) was undertaken in an attempt to further refine the empirically derived scales from the SKAT (Form I).

Because the SKAT was conceived as an instrument for describing groups rather than individuals, it was concluded that the number of items per scale could be relatively small (with a consequent loss in reliability of individual scores). With the items from the SKAT (Form I) as a nucleus, new items were constructed.

In the fall of 1971, the SKAT (Form 2) was administered to 850 freshmen through senior medical students in 16 medical schools throughout the United States. Respondents within this group were randomly assigned to either the experimental or the cross-validation samples. The results confirmed the four factors developed from the SKAT (Form I). The item means, standard deviations, and item-scale correlations of those items loading significantly on each factor in the SKAT (Form 2) are presented in Table 2. Item statistics were based on complete data within a scale. Repeating the process articulated earlier, scale scores were calculated for each of the four scales for all members of the experimental sample, and internal consistency reliability estimates (coefficient alpha) were computed. These results were then verified on the cross-validation sample. The raw scale score means, standard deviations, sample sizes, and coefficient alpha reliability estimates for each scale in both the experimental and cross-validation samples are presented in Table 3.

The data presented in Table 3 are clear evidence for the high stability and internal consistency of the SKAT (Form 2) attitudinal scale scores. The varying number of subjects within each scale is the result of incomplete data.

Table 2 Item Statistics for the Sex Knowledge and Attitude Test (Form 2) Attitudes Questions

Question	Scale	Direction[a]	M	SD	Item-total correlation
1	SM	F	3.40	1.17	.50
2	SM	F	3.51	0.98	.48
3	HR	F	2.89	1.22	.52
4	A	R	3.88	1.24	.78
5	SM	F	3.86	1.05	.56
6	M	R	3.63	0.91	.72
7	HR	F	3.98	1.11	.79
8	SM	F	3.88	0.99	.53
9	M	F	4.11	0.88	.77
10	HR	R	3.27	1.07	.76
11	A	F	4.12	1.10	.71
12	M	F	4.20	0.85	.76
13	A	R	3.21	1.40	.64
14	SM	F	4.31	0.83	.54
15	A	R	3.39	1.24	.65
16	HR	F	4.04	1.12	.81
17	SM	F	4.21	0.82	.55
18	A	R	3.22	1.36	.69
19	M	F	4.26	0.81	.74
22	A	F	4.66	0.66	.42
23	HR	R	3.54	1.10	.75
24	M	R	2.45	0.85	.59
25	A	F	3.11	1.08	.46
26	SM	F	3.91	0.88	.57
27	HR	R	4.10	1.01	.77
29	SM	F	4.05	0.81	.56
30	SM	F	3.53	0.89	.55
31	A	F	4.22	1.02	.69
32	M	F	3.31	0.97	.62
33	HR	F	3.54	1.11	.70
34	HR	R	2.81	1.06	.53
35	M	R	3.58	0.93	.71

Note. Questions 20, 21, and 28 are not included in the scoring. SM = Sexual Myths; HR = Heterosexual Relations; A = Abortion; M = Masturbation/ Autoeroticism.

a. R = reverse scored; F = scored forward.

The knowledge section. Part II combines 21 true/false items chosen specifically for the heuristic (teaching) value and 50 true/false questions selected on the basis of purely psychometric considerations. Those items designated as teaching items were selected from the larger item pool using the following criteria. First, any item designated as a teaching item had to be one that the authors considered all medical or graduate students should know, but that previous research had indicated that at least 10% failed to answer correctly. In most cases, over 25% of these students failed to answer correctly the teaching items. Second, the content of any item designated as a teaching item had to be of such a nature that it could serve as the focal point for either a lecture or a group discussion.

Items included in the 50-question sex knowledge test were selected using purely psychometric criteria: item dif-

Table 3 Raw Score Means, Standard Deviation, Sample Sizes, and Coefficient Alpha Reliability Estimates for the Sex Knowledge and Attitude Test (Form 2) Attitudinal Scales

	Experimental sample				Cross-validation sample			
Scale designation	M	SD	N	α	M	SD	N	α
Heterosexual Relations	28.10	6.41	420	.86	28.35	6.19	420	.86
Sexual Myths	34.72	4.62	422	.71	334.82	4.48	420	.68
Abortion	29.70	6.08	423	.80	29.99	5.66	418	.77
Autoeroticism	25.65	4.20	424	.81	25.63	4.55	418	.84

ficulties ranging from .25 to .75, point biserial correlations of .30 or greater, and each item adding a positive increment to the consistency of the overall test.

The raw correct score mean of the 50-item knowledge test, based on the entire sample of 851 medical students, is 38.81. The 50-item test has a standard deviation of 5.78 and a standard error of measurement of 2.75. The reliability (K-R 21) has been estimated to be .87.

Response Mode, Timing, and Scoring

On average, it takes about 30 minutes to complete the SKAT, less if only Parts I and II are used, as is often done. In the Attitudes section, respondents circle the number indicating their agreement or disagreement with each statement. The Knowledge section involves true/false responses. A scoring sheet for the true/false part of the test is supplied to the investigator. The scoring sheet differentiates the test items from the teaching items as well as indicates whether the item is true or false. On the section dealing with Attitudes, 14 of the 35 items are reverse scored (see Table 2).

With regard to missing data, the procedure adopted is to compute no Attitudes scale score when an individual has omitted more than one of the items within a scale. When one item is omitted, the mean of the answered item values is added to the sum of the answered items to obtain a total raw score estimate. Researchers using the scales should bear in mind that the scales in the SKAT must be regarded as ordinal measures only. That is, scale scores serve to order groups of students in higher-than or lower-than relationships on the dimensions measured by the scales.

As an aid to both classroom teachers and researchers, two scores can be used for each subject on the SKAT, Part II. One represents the total number of correctly answered items for all 71 items in Part II, and the other is a T score derived by standardization of the number of items correctly answered on the 50-item sex knowledge test.

Reliability and Validity

Internal consistency estimates (coefficient alpha), based on a sample of 425 medical students in 15 medical schools, are .86 for Heterosexual Relations, .71 for Sexual Myths, .80 for Abortion, and .81 for Autoeroticism. These reliabilities were used to calculate the standard error of measurement presented in Table 2.

Evidence for the construct validity of the SKAT Attitudes and Knowledge scales comes from two general types of evidence: (a) correlations between the SKAT scales and selected items within the SKAT, and (b) studies in which the SKAT was administered to respondents before and after some intervention expected to alter sexual attitudes and/or knowledge. Correlational studies based on a sample of 850 medical students demonstrated construct validity (Miller & Lief, 1979). Each of the four Attitudes scales is related to other SKAT responses in a way that supports the meaning and interpretation of the scales. For example, liberal attitudes about heterosexual relationships are associated with greater numbers of coital partners ($r = .39$) and a greater rejection of conservative social values ($r = .48$). An increased tendency to reject sexual myths is related to greater

sexual knowledge ($r = .57$). Conservative attitudes about abortion are significantly associated with the Catholic religious preference ($r = .34$), and liberal attitudes toward masturbation are associated with greater frequency of masturbation in senior high school ($r = .23$). With a sample of 850, correlations of .10 are significant, $p < .01$.

Evidence for the validity of the Knowledge scale is more difficult to obtain from such an internal analysis of item interrelationships because it is less clear how one's knowledge about sexuality should relate to sexual values or behavior. It is noteworthy, however, that the highest correlation involving the Knowledge scale is that between the Knowledge scale and the Sexual Myths scale.

The second type of evidence for the construct validity of the SKAT scales, that obtained from SKAT testing before and after an intervention designed to change attitudes and/or knowledge, may be found in a number of published studies. Most, but not all, studies demonstrate an increase in sexual knowledge and liberalization of sexual attitudes as measured by the SKAT following educational experiences designed to produce such changes. Several relevant references are included in the list of references.

Other Information

About 35,000 medical students had taken the SKAT by 1979 when computer analysis was no longer included as a direct service to researchers. Since that time, it has been impossible to estimate the number of people who have taken the test, but there is no doubt that many thousands more have been given the SKAT. Not only has it been given to medical students, its primary population, but college students and their parents, nursing students, graduate students, graduate nurses, a variety of health professionals, handicapped adults, public school teachers, and even spouse-abused women have taken the test, and it has been administered to American, English, Swedish, Israeli, Arab, Colombian, Spanish, Indian, and Japanese medical students (and this list is probably not complete).

The SKAT is no longer available directly from the author. It is available on the Internet. The Web site is www.itgworld. com. The program is available on diskette. It is currently priced at $95 for a single-station license, $199 for a 5-station license, $295 for a 10-station license, and $495 for a site license. These prices are for having the program shipped. If it is downloaded from the Web site, the single station is discounted. Prices and additional information can be obtained from either the Web site or by email at the following address: dan@itgworld.com.

References

Alzate, H. (1974). A course in human sexuality in a Colombian medical school. *Journal of Medical Education, 49,* 438-443.

Alzate, H. (1982). Effect of formal sex education on the sexual knowledge and attitudes of Colombian medical students. *Archives of Sexual Behavior, 11,* 201-204.

Bernard, H. S., & Schwartz, A. J. (1977). Impact of a human sexuality program on sex related knowledge, attitudes, behavior and guilt of college undergraduates. *Journal of the American College Health Association, 25,* 182-185.

Boss, J. R., & McKillip, J. (1979). Program evaluation in sex education: Outcome assessment of sexual awareness weekend workshops. *Archives of Sexual Behavior, 8,* 507-522.

Ebert, R. K., & Lief, H. I. (1975). Why sex education for medical students? In R. Green (Ed.), *Human sexuality: A health practitioner's text* (pp. 1-6). Baltimore: Williams and Wilkins.

Elstein, M., Dennis, K. J., & Buckingham, M. A. (1977). Sexual knowledge and attitudes of Southampton medical students. *The Lancet, 2,* 495-497.

Elstein, M., Gordon, A. D. G., & Buckingham, M. S. (1977). Sexual knowledge and attitudes of general practitioners in Wessex. *British Medical Journal, 1,* 369-371.

Garrard, J., Alden, L., & Chilgren, R. A. (1972). Student allocation of time in a semioptional medical curriculum. *Journal of Medical Education, 47,* 460-466.

Garrard, J., Vatkus, A., & Chilgren, R. A. (1972). Evaluation of a course in human sexuality. *Journal of Medical Education, 47,* 772-778.

Garrard, J., Vatkus, A., Held, J., & Chilgren, R. A. (1976). Follow-up effects of a medical school course in human sexuality. *Archives of Sexual Behavior, 5,* 331-340.

Golden, J. S., & Liston, E. G. (1972). Medical sex education: The world of illusion and the practical realities. *Journal of Medical Education, 47,* 761-771.

Hadorn, D., & Grant, I. (1976). Evaluation of a sex education workshop. *British Journal of Medical Education, 10,* 378-381.

Hoch, Z., Kubat (Seidenros), H., & Brandes, J. M. (1977). Results of the Sexual Knowledge and Attitude Test of medical students in Israel. In R. Gemme & C. C. Wheeler (Eds.), *Progress in sexology* (pp. 467-482). New York: Plenum.

Hoch, Z., Kubat (Seidenros), H., Fisher, M., & Brandes, J. M. (1978). Background in sexual experience of Israeli medical students. *Archives of Sexual Behavior, 7,* 429-441.

Johnson, M. N., & Boren, Y. (1982). Sexual knowledge and spouse abuse: A cultural phenomenon. *Issues in Mental Health Nursing, 4,* 217-231.

Kraeger, S. M. (1977). Sexuality and disability. *ARN Journal (Association of Rehabilitation Nurses), 2,* 8-14.

Lamberti, J. W., & Chapel, J. L. (1977). Development and evaluation of a sex education program for medical students. *Journal of Medical Education, 52,* 582-586.

Lief, H. I. (1971). Sex education in medical schools. *Journal of Medical Education, 46,* 373-374.

Lief, H. I. (1974). Sexual knowledge, attitudes and behavior of medical students: Implications for medical practice. In W. Abse, E. Nash, & L. Louden (Eds.), *Marital and sexual counseling in medical practice* (pp. 474-494). Hagerstown, MD: Harper and Row.

Lief, H. I. (1978). Sex education in medicine: Retrospect and prospect. In N. Rosenzweig & F. Pearsall (Eds.), *Sex education for the health professional* (pp. 22-36). New York: Grune & Stratton.

Lief, H. I., & Ebert, R. K. (1975). A survey of sex education in United States medical schools. In *Education and treatment in human sexuality: The training of health professionals.* (World Health Organization Technical Report Series 572)

Lief, H. I., & Payne, T. (1975). Sexuality: Knowledge and attitudes. *American Journal of Nursing, 75,* 2026-2029.

Lief, H. I., & Reed, D. M. (1972). *Sex Knowledge and Attitude Test technical manual.* Philadelphia: Marriage Council of Philadelphia.

Marcotte, D. B., & Kilpatrick, D. G. (1974). Preliminary evaluation of sex education course. *Journal of Medical Education, 49,* 703-705.

Marcotte, D. B., Kilpatrick, D. G., & Willis, A. (1977). The Sheppe and Hain study revisited: Professional students and their knowledge and attitudes about human sexuality. *Journal of Medical Education, 11,* 201-204.

Marcotte, D. B., & Logan, C. (1977). Medical sex education allowing attitude alteration. *Archives of Sexual Behavior, 6,* 155-162.

McNab, W. L. (1976). Sexual attitude development in children and the parents' role. *Journal of School Health, 46,* 537-542.

Miller, W. R., & Lief, H. I. (1976). Masturbatory attitudes, knowledge and experience: Data from the Sex Knowledge and Attitude Test (SKAT). *Archives of Sexual Behavior, 5,* 447-467.

Miller, W. R., & Lief, H. I. (1979). The Sex Knowledge and Attitude Test (SKAT). *Archives of Sexual Behavior, 5,* 282-287.

Mims, F. H., Brown, L., & Kubow, R. (1976). Human sexuality course evaluation. *Nursing Research, 25,* 187-191.

Mims, F. H., Yeawork, R., & Hornstein, S. (1974). Effectiveness of an interdisciplinary course in human sexuality. *Nursing Research, 23,* 278-253.

Moracco, J., & Zeidan, M. (1982). Assessment of sex knowledge and attitudes of non-Western medical students. *Psychology: A Quarterly Journal of Human Behavior, 19,* 13-21.

Payne, T. (1976). Sexuality of nurses: Correlation of knowledge, attitudes and behavior. *Nursing Research, 25,* 286-292.

Ray, R. E., & Kirkpatrick, B. R. (1983). Two time formats for teaching human sexuality. *Teaching of Psychology, 10,* 84-88.

Robinson, S. (1984). Effects of sex education program on intellectually handicapped adults. *Australia and New Zealand Journal of Developmental Disabilities, 10,* 21-26.

Rosenberg, P., & Chilgren, R. (1973). Sex education discussion groups in a medical setting. *International Journal of Group Psychotherapy, 23,* 23-41.

Schnarch, D. M. (1981). Impact of sex education on medical students' projections of patients' attitudes. *Journal of Sex & Marital Therapy, 7,* 141-155.

Schnarch, D. M. (1982). The role of medical students' stereotype of physicians in sex education. *Journal of Medical Education, 57,* 922-930.

Schnarch, D. M., & Jones, K. (1981). Efficacy of sex education courses in medical schools. *Journal of Sex & Marital Therapy, 7,* 307-317.

Smith, P. B., Flaherty, C., Webb, L. J., & Mumford, D. M. (1984). Long-term effects of human sexuality training programs for public school teachers. *Journal of School Health, 54,* 157-159.

Williams, A. M., & Miller, W. R. (1978). The design and use of assessment instruments and procedures for sexuality curricula. In N. Rosenzweig & F. P. Pearsall (Eds.), *Sex education for the health professional* (pp. 137-146). New York: Grune & Stratton.

Sexual Knowledge, Experience, Feelings, and Needs Scale

Marita P. McCabe,[1] *Deakin University*

The Sexual Knowledge, Experience, Feelings, and Needs Scale (SexKen) is designed to evaluate the knowledge, experience, feelings, and needs of respondents in a range of sexual areas. There are four parallel versions of the scale: for people from the general population (SexKen), for people with mild intellectual disability (SexKen-ID), for people with physical disability (SexKen-PD), and for caregivers of people with disabilities (SexKen-C). The development of these parallel forms allows the similarities and differences in the sexuality of different groups of respondents to be evaluated and also the report of people with disabilities to be contrasted with the report of their caregivers. The measures may be completed as either a questionnaire or interview.

Description

Each of the versions of SexKen consists of 13 subscales. Within each subscale there are questions on the knowledge, experience, feelings, and needs of respondents as they relate to that area of sexuality. The number of items within each of these areas is different for each subscale, because the need for questions in each of these areas is different for the various aspects of sexuality. The subscales, with the number of questions in each area, are summarized in Table 1.

The first version of the scale to be developed was SexKen-ID. The reason for its development was the lack of an instrument that adequately evaluated the sexuality of people with mild intellectual disability across a broad range of areas. The scale was designed to focus on sexual knowledge, experience, feelings, and needs. SexKen-ID was generally intended to be administered as an interview. The areas covered by the scale and the original questions included in the scale came from a review of the sexuality literature and other sexuality scales, mainly those developed for the general population. The original scale was tested with five people with mild intellectual disability, and feedback was obtained from professionals working in the sexuality area, carestaff working with people with intellectual disability, and academics who specialized in psychometrics.

The revised scale and the parallel SexKen and SexKen-C versions of the scale, which were designed for the general population and caregiver assessment of the sexuality of people with intellectual disability, were administered to 25 people with mild intellectual disability, 39 volunteer students, and 10 carestaff working with people with intellectual disability (Szollos & McCabe, 1995). SexKen and SexKen-C were completed as questionnaire measures and

Table 1 Description of the Subscales, Areas, and Range of Scores for the Sexual Knowledge, Experience, Feelings, and Needs Scale (SexKen, SexKen-ID, SexKen-PD, SexKen-C)

Subscale	Area	Range of scores
Friendship (23 items)	Knowledge (1 item)	0-2
	Experience (13)	5-22
	Feelings (4)	4-20
	Needs (5)	5-25
Dating and Intimacy (16 items)	Knowledge (2 items)	0-4
	Experience (4)	3-9
	Feelings (6)	4-11
	Needs (4)	4-20
Marriage (16 items)	Knowledge (2 items)	0-4
	Experience (0)	—
	Feelings (13)	6-10
	Needs (1)	1-5
Body Part Identification (21 items)	Knowledge (21 items)	0-42
	Experience (0)	—
	Feelings (0)	—
	Needs (0)	—
Sex and Sex Education (16 items)	Knowledge (1 item)	0-2
	Experience (7)	6-27
	Feelings (5)	5-25
	Needs (3)	3-15
Menstruation (16 items)	Knowledge (11 items)	0-22
	Experience (2)	2-4
	Feelings (2)	2-10
	Needs (1)	1-5
Sexual Interaction (52 items)	Knowledge (21 items)	0-42
	Experience (15)	8-31
	Feelings (14)	8-31
	Needs (2)	2-10
Contraception (19 items)	Knowledge (9 items)	0-18
	Experience (8)	4-11
	Feelings (1)	1-5
	Needs (1)	1-5
Pregnancy, Abortion, and Childbirth (24 items)	Knowledge (15 items)	0-30
	Experience (3)	—
	Feelings (4)	4-20
	Needs (2)	2-10
Sexually Transmitted Diseases (19 items)	Knowledge (11 items)	0-22
	Experience (2)	1-2
	Feelings (4)	4-20
	Needs (2)	2-10

(continued)

[1]Address correspondence to Marita P. McCabe, School of Psychology, Deakin University, 221 Burwood Highway, Burwood, Victoria 3125, Australia; email: maritam@deakin.edu.au.

Table 1 Continued

Subscale	Area	Range of scores
Masturbation (16 items)	Knowledge (3 items)	0-6
	Experience (6)	4-20
	Feelings (6)	5-25
	Needs (1)	1-5
Homosexuality (10 items)	Knowledge (1 item)	0-2
	Experience (1)	1-5
	Feelings (6)	4-20
	Needs (2)	2-10

SexKen-ID was administered as an interview. From this study, it was clear that some items in the scale were not readily understood by people with mild intellectual disability. Items in the scale were altered or removed to address the problems in relevance and comprehension that were evident from this study.

Modified versions of SexKen-ID and SexKen were used to evaluate the sexuality of people with mild intellectual disability and a student population in two further studies (McCabe & Cummins, 1996; McCabe, Cummins, & Reid, 1994). Analysis of responses and discussions with respondents led to further modification of the scales. SexKen-ID was restructured so that it comprised three separate interviews. The subscales were organized so that they ranged from the least intrusive to the most intrusive subscales in successive interviews. Interview 1 comprised the subscales of Friendship, Dating and Intimacy, Marriage, and Body Part Identification; Interview 2 comprised Sex and Sex Education, Menstruation, Sexual Interaction, Contraception, and Pregnancy, Abortion, and Childbirth; and Interview 3 comprised Sexually Transmitted Diseases, Masturbation, and Homosexuality. There were knowledge questions at the end of each interview to determine whether respondents had sufficient knowledge to proceed to the next interview. SexKen and SexKen-C were also reorganized, but remained as questionnaire measures, with the subscales in the same order as for SexKen-ID. A further parallel questionnaire measure was developed for people with physical disability (SexKen-PD).

SexKen, SexKen-ID, and SexKen-PD have been used to gather data over the past 2 years among people from the general population ($n = 100$), people with mild intellectual disability ($n = 60$), and people with physical disability ($n = 60$). Test-retest data have been collected on 30 people in each group. These data are available from the author.

Response Mode and Timing

Each of the SexKen measures may be completed as either an interview or questionnaire measure. However, SexKen-ID is designed to be completed as an interview, and SexKen, SexKen-C, and SexKen-PD are designed as questionnaire measures. If completed as a questionnaire, the measure takes about 1 hour to complete. SexKen-ID is divided into three interviews, with each interview taking about 1 hour to complete.

Scoring

Whether completed as an interview or questionnaire, the experience, feelings, and needs items are either *yes/no* (scored as 1 or 2) responses or are scored on a 5-point Likert-type scale (ranging from 1 to 5). The knowledge questions are open ended, with responses scored 0, 1, or 2 depending on the accuracy of the responses. The nature of the acceptable responses for each question was determined through pilot work. Some items are categorical (e.g., what do you do with your friends?) and do not contribute to the total score. All other items are scored in the same direction. A total score is obtained for each area within each subscale. The range of scores for each subarea and each subscale is listed in Table 1.

Reliability and Validity

Data have been gathered on people with mild intellectual disability, physical disability, and the general population, which will allow the internal consistency of each of the scales and the test-retest reliability of the scales to be evaluated.

The validity of the scale has been ensured through the initial development of the scale with close attention being paid to the wording of items (Sigelman, Budd, Winer, Schoenrock, & Martin, 1982). Subsequent modification of the scale has been based on feedback from professionals working with people with intellectual disability, psychometricians, and respondents from each group who completed the various versions of the scale. There have been three revisions of the scale based on data collected over the past 7 years. It is not possible to assess the validity of the scale using another measure of sexuality because no other psychometrically sound measure of sexuality has been developed for people with disabilities or their carestaff.

Other Information

Any version of the scale, along with the scoring code, can be purchased from the author for a cost of U.S. $10. This single version can then be duplicated.

References

McCabe, M. P., & Cummins, R. A. (1996). The sexual knowledge, experience, feelings and needs of people with mild intellectual disability. *Education and Training in Mental Retardation and Developmental Disabilities, 31,* 13-22.

McCabe, M. P., Cummins, R. A., & Reid, S. B. (1994). An empirical study of the sexual abuse of people with intellectual disability. *Journal of Sexuality and Disability, 12,* 297-306.

Sigelman, C., Budd, E. C., Winer, J. L., Schoenrock, C. J., & Martin, P. W. (1982). Evaluating alternative techniques of questioning mentally retarded persons. *American Journal of Mental Deficiency, 86,* 511-518.

Szollos, A., & McCabe, M. P. (1995). The sexuality of people with mild intellectual disabilities: Perceptions of clients and caregivers. *Australia and New Zealand Journal of Developmental Disabilities, 20,* 205-222.

Dyadic Sexual Regulation Scale

Joseph A. Catania,[1] *University of California, San Francisco*

The Dyadic Sexual Regulation Scale (DSR) measures the extent to which an individual perceives sexual activity to be regulated from an internal versus an external locus of control. In developing a locus of control scale specific to the dyadic sexual situation, we sought to develop a scale that assesses perceptions of the ability to emit behaviors that (a) influence the acquisition and termination of sexual rewards, (b) affect events between these latter two points, and (c) prevent or avoid aversive sexual encounters. Moreover, the scale would reflect control flexibility, which is generally defined as an individual's ability either to relinquish or to accept control, dependent on the variant nature of social/sexual interactions.

Description

The DSR is an 11-item, respondent- or interviewer-administered, Likert-type scale with 7 points (1 = *strongly disagree*, 7 = *strongly agree*). The scale items were derived from open-ended interviews about sexual attitudes with heterosexual and homosexual couples. Five items are reversed (Items 2, 5, 6, 8, 10) for counter-balancing purposes. A shortened five-item interviewer-administered form of the DSR is also available.

Response Mode and Timing

All forms of the scale are available in English and Spanish. The expanded form is self-administered; the briefer revised form is interviewer administered. Both forms take 1-2 minutes to complete.

Scoring

After reversing the reverse-worded items, total scores are computed so that higher scores indicate a greater degree of internal control. Sum across scores to obtain total score. Scale scores range from 11 (external) to 77 (internal).

Reliability and Validity

The DSR has been administered to varied populations, including college students; national urban probability samples constructed to adequately represent White, Black, and Hispanic ethnic groups; and high-HIV-risk-factor groups (Catania, Coates, Kegeles, et al., 1992; Catania, Coates, Stall, et al., 1992). The DSR has also been administered to respondents from introductory psychology classes at a university recruited to participate in a sexual survey study that assessed locus of control in sexual contexts (Catania,

McDermott, & Wood, 1984). The college-age analyses (Catania et al., 1984) examined only heterosexuals who had a current, regular sexual partner. Sample 1 consisted of 151 White students (59 males and 92 females) with a mean age of 27. Sample 2 consisted of 27 males and 43 females with similar demographic features as Sample 1. Reliability was good (Cronbach's alpha = .74 in Sample 1, .83 in Sample 2). A principal component analysis with varimax rotation was conducted on the DSR items for Sample 1. There were no item loadings beyond the first factor greater than .30, and the first factor accounted for 95% of the variance. Test-retest reliability was .77, with a 2-week interval. The DSR revealed convergent validity with the Nowicki-Strickland Adult Internal-External Control Scale (NSLC; Nowicki & Duke, 1974) ($r = .19$, $p < .05$, $df = 149$) (Catania et al., 1984). The DSR was found to be related with each dyadic measure of sexual activity. The scale was not found to be related to monadic activities (i.e., masturbation), further supporting the concurrent validity of the DSR with locus of control. Internality with regard to sexual activity is associated with higher frequencies of intercourse, oral sex from partner, orgasms with partner, sexual relations, affectionate behaviors, and sexual satisfaction, and with lesser anxiety in sexual situations. DSR was not found to be related to gender. In contrast, the NSLC was more weakly associated with each criterion.

The five-item, shortened version of the DSR was administered to respondents recruited to participate in the 1990-1991 National AIDS Behavior Survey (NABS)[2] longitudinal cohort study, which was composed of three interlaced samples designed to oversample African Americans and Hispanics for adequate representation (Catania, Coates, Kegeles, et al., 1992). The interlaced samples included a national sample, an urban sample of 23 cities with high prevalences of AIDS cases, and a special Hispanic urban sample. The revised version of the DSR was administered to 4,620 respondents between the ages of 18 and 49. Reliability was good (Cronbach's alpha = .62 for total sample). Means, standard deviations, range, median, and reliabilities are given for White, Black, and Hispanic groups, males and females, and levels of education for both national and urban, high-risk city samples in Table 1. The shortened five-item version was also administered to 954 respondents who participated in the third wave of the AIDS in Multiethnic Neighborhoods (AMEN)[3] study (Catania, Coates, Stall, et al., 1992). The AMEN study is a longitudinal study

---

[1]Address correspondence to Joseph A. Catania, Center for AIDS Prevention Studies, University of California, San Francisco, 74 New Montgomery, Suite 600, San Francisco, CA 94105.

[2]For further details on sample construction and weighting of the NABS study, see Catania, Coates, Stall, et al. (1992).
[3]For further details on sample construction and weighting of the AMEN cohort study, see Catania, Coates, Kegeles, et al. (1992).

Table 1 Normative Data for the Dyadic Sexual Self-Regulation Scale

	N	Mean	SD	Range	Mdn	Alpha
			NABS[a] study (Wave 2)			
National sample	1,022	15.62	2.83	15.0	16.0	.59
High-risk cities	3,598	15.37	2.86	15.0	15.0	.57
Ethnicity						
White						
National sample	747	15.75	2.75	15.0	16.0	.61
High-risk cities	1,565	15.62	2.68	15.0	16.0	.61
Black						
National sample	162	15.23	2.99	14.0	15.0	.47
High-risk cities	1,181	15.18	3.06	15.0	15.0	.52
Hispanic						
National sample	90	15.45	3.03	14.0	15.65	.61
High-risk cities	764	14.98	3.20	15.0	15.0	.60
Gender						
Male						
National sample	410	15.37	2.65	14.0	15.0	.86
High-risk cities	1,553	15.24	2.77	15.0	15.0	.56
Female						
National sample	612	15.85	2.98	15.0	16.0	.61
High-risk cities	2,043	15.53	2.94	15.0	16.0	.58
Education						
< 12 years						
National sample	82	14.74	2.89	12.0	15.0	.38
High-risk cities	483	14.76	3.12	15.0	15.0	.53
= 12 years						
National sample	273	15.75	2.93	13.0	16.0	.59
High-risk cities	807	15.41	2.96	15.0	16.0	.54
> 12 years						
National sample	668	15.71	2.76	15.0	16.0	.59
High-risk cities	2,308	15.54	2.72	15.0	16.0	.58
			AMEN[b] study			
Total	954	15.08	3.01	15.0	15.0	.58
Ethnicity						
White	418	15.14	2.88	13.0	15.0	.63
Black	238	15.0	13.24	15.0	15.0	.53
Hispanic	229	14.98	3.08	15.0	15.0	.55
Gender						
Male	410	15.22	2.74	15.0	15.0	.52
Female	544	14.98	3.20	15.0	15.0	.61
Education						
< 12 years	109	15.44	.330	13.0	16.0	.57
= 12 years	213	14.64	3.21	15.0	15.0	.54
> 12 years	626	15.26	2.86	14.0	15.0	.59

Note. Because weights for probability of selection are used, all frequencies may not sum to equal total frequencies.

a. National AIDS Behavior Survey.

b. AIDS in Multiethnic Neighborhoods.

(three waves) in which the distribution of HIV, sexually transmitted diseases, related risk behaviors, and their correlates across social strata were examined. Respondents ranged from 20 to 44 years of age and included White (418), African American (124), and Hispanic (229) ethnic groups. Reliability was moderate (Cronbach's alpha = .59). The mean, standard deviation, median, range, and reliabilities of ethnic groups, gender, and levels of education are provided in Table 1.

References

Catania, J. A., Coates, T., Kegeles, S., Thompson-Fullilove, M., Peterson, J., Marin, B., Siegel, D., & Hulley, S. (1992). Condom use in multi-ethnic neighborhoods of San Francisco: The population-based AMEN (AIDS in Multi-Ethnic Neighborhoods) study. *American Journal of Public Health, 82,* 284-287. (See also Erratum, June 1992, 82, 998)

Catania, J. A., Coates, T., Peterson, J., Dolcini, M., Kegeles, S., Siegel, D., Golden, E., & Fullilove, M. (1993). Changes in condom use among Black, Hispanic, and White heterosexuals in San Francisco: The AMEN cohort survey. *The Journal of Sex Research, 30,* 121-128.

Catania, J. A., Coates, T. J., Stall, R., Turner, H., Peterson, J., Hearst, N., Dolcini, M. M., Hudes, E., Gagnon, J., Wiley, J., & Groves, R. (1992). Prevalence of AIDS-related risk factors and condom use in the United States. *Science, 258,* 1101-1106.

Catania, J. A., McDermott, L. J., & Wood, J. A. (1984). The assessment of locus of control: Situational specificity in the sexual context. *The Journal of Sex Research, 20,* 310-324.

Nowicki, S., & Duke, M. (1974). A Locus of Control Scale for non-college as well as college adults. *Journal of Personality Assessment, 38,* 136-137.

Exhibit

Dyadic Sexual Regulation Scale

Instructions: The following statements describe different things people do and feel about sex. Please tell me how much you agree or disagree with these statements.

	1	2	3	4	5	6	7	
Strongly agree						Strongly disagree		

1. I often take the initiative in beginning sexual activity.
2. If my sexual relations are not satisfying there is little I can do to improve the situation.
3. I have sexual relations with my partner as often as I would like.
4. My planning for sexual encounters leads to good sexual experiences with my partner.
5. I feel that it is difficult to get my partner to do what makes me feel good during sex.
6. I feel that my sexual encounters with my partner usually end before I want them to.
7. When I am not interested in sexual activity I feel free to reject sexual advances by my partner.
8. I want my partner to be responsible for directing our sexual encounters.
9. I find it pleasurable at times to be the active member during sexual relations while my partner takes a passive role.
10. I would feel uncomfortable bringing myself to orgasm if the stimulation my partner was providing was inadequate.
11. During some sexual encounters I find it pleasurable to be passive while my partner is the active person.

Note. Items 2, 3, 4, 5, and 6 make up the brief revised form. Items 3 and 8 are reworded in the short form as follows: 3. You have sexual relationships as often as you like. Do you agree or disagree? 8. Your sexual partner makes most of the decisions about when the two of you will have sex. Do you agree or disagree?

The Juvenile Love Scale: A Child's Version of the Passionate Love Scale

Elaine Hatfield,[1] *University of Hawaii at Manoa*

Hatfield and Walster (1978) defined passionate love as "a state of intense longing for union with another. Reciprocated love (union with the other) is associated with fulfillment and ecstasy. Unrequited love (separation) with emptiness, anxiety, or despair. A state of profound physiological arousal" (p. 9). Other names for this emotion are "puppy love," "a crush," "lovesickness," "obsessive love," "infatuation," or "being in love." It includes components of sexual desire.

[1]Address correspondence to Elaine Hatfield, Department of Psychology, University of Hawaii at Manoa, 2430 Campus Road, Honolulu, HI 96822; email: elaineh@.uhcc.hawaii.edu.

Description

The Juvenile Love Scale (JLS) is designed to measure passionate love in children from 3 to 18 years of age. The JLS is an exact equivalent of the Passionate Love Scale (PLS), which measures this emotion in adolescents and adults. (A detailed description of the PLS is provided elsewhere in this volume.) The JLS and the PLS tap cognitive, emotional, and behavioral indicants of "desire for union." The JLS, like the PLS, comes in a short version (15 items) and a long version (30 items). Only the short version is shown in the exhibit.

Researchers have used two techniques in administering the JLS.

If children are very young. The first step in administering the JLS is to make sure the children understand the concepts of "boyfriend" and "girlfriend" (almost all do), the 15 test items (almost all do), and how to use the response scale.

The response scale is explained first. Essentially, one wants to teach children that when the experimenter makes a statement, they can indicate how much they agree via a 9-point scale. This is done in the following way: Children are shown a large "ruler." Its dimensions are 4 × 20 inches. It is divided into nine blocks. The first block is labeled (1) *agree very little*. The last block is labeled (9) *agree very much*. The experimenter then conducts several tests to teach children how to respond via the scale. First, the children are given nine buildings and asked to put them in order. (The buildings are made from piles of checkers, and range from one to nine checkers in height.) Generally, all children can do this. This gives some confidence that even the youngest children can grasp the idea of "more" and "less." Then children are taught how to use the checkers to answer some questions. The experimenter explains: "I want you to use these checker buildings to tell me how much you agree with what I say. Suppose I say, 'I like my birthday.' Do you agree with that? Would you say so too?" The experimenter allows time for the children to answer. Then he or she proceeds: "Show me by touching one of the checker buildings *how much* you like your birthday. If you think birthdays are great, if you agree very much, you would choose that one (9). If you think they're awful, if you agree very little, you would choose that one (1). If you are right in the middle about how you feel, you would choose one of those (3-5)." More examples follow—How do children feel about cleaning their rooms? Eating breakfast? The experimenter then proceeds to administer the JLS. Researchers such as Greenwell (1983) have found that even children as young as 3 or 4 years of age have no trouble understanding this scale. (For more information of these procedures, see Greenwell.)

If children are older. Most researchers have found that once children are 7 or 8 years old, one can simply follow the same procedure used in administering the PLS to adolescents and adults.

Response Mode and Timing

Respondents either put a block in the appropriate square (if they are very young) or circle the number indicating how true each statement is for them (if they are older). The JLS is generally given individually. Once children are 7 or 8, it can be given in groups. How long it takes to explain the scale to children depends on the child. Usually, the short (15 items) version of the JLS takes approximately 25 minutes, and the long version (30 items) takes 40 minutes to complete.

Scoring

The individual items are simply summed to produce a total score.

Reliability

Greenwell (1983) provided statistical evidence that the JLS and PLS are unidimensional and reliable and produce comparable results when taken by children or adults. She also provided evidence that both scales reflect a real-world experience called "being in love." She argued that the JLS and PLS measure a single entity—passionate love. A principal components factor analysis revealed that one major factor accounts for most of the variance. In various samples, the first factor accounted for between 38% to 53% of the variance (see Greenwell, 1983, for tables of eigenvalues). The scales are internally consistent and reliable. In various samples, coefficient alphas were found to range from .94 to .98. Children and adolescents receive virtually identical scores on both scales. This is not surprising because the scales are designed to be identical, differing only in the difficulty of their language. In various populations, the JLS and PLS were found to correlate .88 for children and .87 for adults.

Greenwell (1983) also provided information on item-by-item correspondences. She found items highly intercorrelated. She also correlated each item with its own scale total, the other scale total, and the combined total of all 60 items (i.e., she used the long version of both the JLS and the PLS). All items correlated highly with all totals, with 67 items in the .25 to .50 range, 221 in the .51 to .75 range, and 59 in the .76 to 1.00 range. It is clear from these analyses that the JLS and the PLS are virtually equivalent measures of passionate love.

Finally, Greenwell (1983) provided evidence that both scales reflect the real-world experience of "being in love." For example, she asked children and adolescents to describe their feelings for a person whom they currently love, had loved in the past, or (if they had never been in love) who was as close as they had come to being in love. She found that people who had experienced passion did score higher on both the JLS and the PLS than did those who had never been in love. (For more information on the JLS, see Hatfield, Schmitz, Cornelius, & Rapson, 1986, who provided information on the JLS scores typically secured by boys and girls, from 4 to 18 years of age.)

References

Greenwell, M. E. (1983). *Development of the Juvenile Love Scale.* Unpublished master's thesis, University of Hawaii at Manoa, Honolulu.

Hatfield, E., Schmitz, E., Cornelius, J., & Rapson, R. L. (1986). Passionate love: How early does it begin? *Journal of Psychology and Human Sexuality, 1,* 111-111.

Hatfield, E., & Sprecher, S. (1986). Measuring passionate love in intimate relations. *Journal of Adolescence, 9,* 383-410.

Hatfield, E., & Walster, G. W. (1978). *A new look at love.* Lantham, MA: University Press of America.

Exhibit

The Juvenile Love Scale

1. I feel like things would always be sad and gloomy if I had to live without _____ forever.
2. Did you ever keep thinking about _____ when you wanted to stop and couldn't?
3. I feel happy when I am doing something to make _____ happy.
4. I would rather be with _____ than anybody else.
5. I'd feel bad if I thought _____ liked somebody else better than me.
6. I want to know all I can about _____.
7. I'd like _____ to belong to me in every way.
8. I'd like it a lot if _____ played with me all the time.
9. If I could, when I grow up I'd like to marry (live with) _____.
10. When _____ hugs me my body feels warm all over.
11. I am always thinking about _____.
12. I want _____ to know me, what I am thinking, what scares me, what I am wishing for.
13. I look at _____ a lot to see if he (she) likes me.
14. When _____ is around I really want to touch him (her) and be touched.
15. When I think _____ might be mad at me, I feel really sad.

Possible answers range from

	1	2	3	4	5	6	7	8	9	
	Agree very little							Agree very much		

Source. This scale is reprinted with permission of the author.

The Passionate Love Scale

Elaine Hatfield, [1] *University of Hawaii at Manoa*

Hatfield and Walster (1978) defined passionate love as "a state of intense longing for union with another. Reciprocated love (union with the other) is associated with fulfillment and ecstasy. Unrequited love (separation) with emptiness, anxiety, or despair. A state of profound physiological arousal" (p. 9).

This emotion has sometimes been labeled "puppy love," "a crush," "lovesickness," "obsessive love," "infatuation," or "being in love." It includes a component of sexual desire. The Passionate Love Scale (PLS) is designed to measure this emotion.

Description

The PLS is a 15- or 30-item Likert-type scale (9 points) with response options ranging from *not at all true* to *definitely true.* It taps cognitive, emotional, and behavioral indicants of "longing for union."

Cognitive components. Cognitive components consist of the following:

[1]Address correspondence to Elaine Hatfield, Department of Psychology, University of Hawaii at Manoa, 2430 Campus Road, Honolulu, HI 96822; email: elaineh@uhcc.hawaii.edu.

1. Intrusive thinking or preoccupation with the partner: Items 5, 19, and 21.
2. Idealization of the other or of the relationship: Items 7, 9, and 15.
3. Desire to know the other and be known: Item 10 measures the desire to know: Item 22 measures the desire to be known.

Emotional components. Emotional components consist of the following:

1. Attraction to other, especially sexual attraction. Positive feelings when things go well: Items 16, 18, and 29.
2. Negative feelings when things go awry: Items 1, 2, 8, 20, 28, and 30.
3. Longing for reciprocity—passionate lovers not only love, but they want to be loved in return: Item 14.
4. Desire for complete and permanent union: Items 11, 12, 23, and 27.
5. Physiological arousal: Items 3, 13, 17, and 26.

Behavioral components. A passionate lover's desire for union may be reflected in a variety of behaviors:

1. Actions toward determining the other's feelings: Item 24.
2. Studying the other person: Item 4.
3. Service to the other: Items 6 and 25.
4. Maintaining physical closeness. (We had hoped to include some items designed to measure lovers' efforts to get *physically* close to the other, but lovers did not endorse such items, and they were dropped from the final version of the scale.)

Response Mode and Timing

Respondents circle the number indicating how true each statement is for them. The PLS can be given either individually or in large groups. The short version takes approximately 15 minutes to complete; the long version takes approximately 30 minutes.

Scoring

The individual items are simply summed to produce a total score.

Reliability

A series of studies indicate that the PLS is highly reliable. For example, Hatfield and Sprecher (1986) gave the PLS to 120 men and women at the University of Wisconsin. They attempted to determine whether the PLS is (a) unidimensional; (b) reliable, as indicated by a measure of internal consistency; (c) uncontaminated by a social desirability bias; and (d) correlated with other indicants of love and intimacy. They found that the PLS is a highly reliable scale. Coefficient alpha was .94. The shorter version of the PLS had only a slightly lower coefficient alpha, .91.

The PLS appears to be unidimensional. The responses to the PLS were subjected to principal components factoring, with multiple correlations used as communality esti-

mates. After rotation, one major factor explained 70% of the variance (eigenvalue = 12.24). The results suggest that the scale is uncontaminated by a social desirability bias. The correlation between the PLS and Crowne and Marlowe's (1964) Social Desirability Scale was nonsignificant (r = .09).

Validity

If the PLS is valid, it should be related to other variables in ways expected by past theoretical and empirical work. The PLS was highly correlated with other measures of love and intimacy. (See Easton, 1985; Hatfield, Schmitz, Cornelius, & Rapson, 1988; Hatfield & Sprecher, 1986; Sullivan, 1985; Sullivan & Landis, 1984, for additional information on the reliability and validity of the PLS.)

From the results of a number of studies, researchers have suggested that almost everyone is capable of loving passionately. Men and women (Easton, 1985), of widely varying ages (Hatfield et al., 1988; Traupmann & Hatfield, 1981), of varying intellectual capacities, mentally ill or healthy, of varying ethnic groups (Easton, 1985) seem capable of falling in love. However, the question as to whether there are sex and ethnic group differences in the readiness to love has long intrigued scientists. Men and women may not fall in love with equal frequency or intensity. Society encourages men and women to have somewhat different attitudes toward love, sex, and the desire for intimacy. When sex differences are found to exist (and often they are not), it is generally women who seem to love more passionately (see DeLamater, 1982; Peplau, 1983).

Various ethnic groups may also differ in the emotions they feel and express in close relationships. Easton (1985) provides information on PLS scores typically secured by men and women of various ethnic groups.

References

Crowne, D. P., & Marlowe, D. (1964). *The approval motive: Studies in evaluative dependence.* New York: Wiley.

DeLamater, J. (1982, August). *Gender differences in sexual scenarios.* Paper presented at the meeting of the American Sociological Association, San Francisco.

Easton, M. (1985). *Love and intimacy in a multi-ethnic setting.* Unpublished doctoral dissertation, University of Hawaii at Manoa, Honolulu.

Hatfield, E., Schmitz, E., Cornelius, J., & Rapson, R. L. (1988). Passionate love: How early does it begin? *Journal of Psychology and Human Sexuality, 1,* 35-51.

Hatfield, E., & Sprecher, S. (1986). Measuring passionate love in intimate relations. *Journal of Adolescence, 9,* 383-410.

Hatfield, E., & Walster, G. W. (1978). *A new look at love.* Lantham, MA: University Press of America.

Peplau, L. A. (1983). Roles and gender. In H. H. Kelley, E. Berscheid, A. Christensen, J. H. Harvey, T. L. Husted, G. Levinger, E. McClintock, L. Peplau, & D. R. Peterson (Eds.), *Close relationships* (pp. 220-264). New York: Freeman.

Sullivan, B. O. (1985). *Passionate love: A factor analytic study.* Unpublished manuscript, University of Hawaii at Manoa, Honolulu.

Sullivan, B. O., & Landis, D. (1984, August/September). *The relationship of sexual behaviors and attitudes cross-culturally.* Paper presented at the VII Congress of the International Association for Cross-Cultural Psychology, Acapulco, Mexico.

Traupmann, J., & Hatfield, E. (1981). Love and its effect on mental and physical health. In R. Forgel, E. Hatfield, S. Kiesler, & E. Shanas (Eds.), *Aging: Stability and change in the family* (pp. 253-274). New York: Academic Press.

Exhibit

The Passionate Love Scale

In this section of the questionnaire you will be asked to describe how you feel when you are passionately in love. Some common terms for this feeling are passionate love, infatuation, love sickness, or obsessive love.

Please think of the person whom you love most passionately *right now*. If you are not in love right now, please think of the last person you loved passionately. If you have never been in love, think of the person whom you came closest to caring for in that way. Keep this person in mind as you complete this section of the questionnaire. (The person you choose should be of the opposite sex if you are heterosexual or of the same sex if you are homosexual.) Try to tell us how you felt at the time when your feelings were the most intimate.

All of your answers will be strictly confidential.

1. Since I've been involved with _____, my emotions have been on a roller coaster.

1   2   3   4   5   6   7   8   9[a]

Not at all true   Definitely true

2. I would feel despair if _____ left me.
3. Sometimes my body trembles with excitement at the sight of _____.
4. I take delight in studying the movements and angles of _____'s body.
5. Sometimes I feel I can't control my thoughts; they are obsessively on _____.
6. I feel happy when I am doing something to make _____ happy.
7. I would rather be with _____ than anyone else.
8. I'd get jealous if I thought _____ were falling in love with someone else.
9. No one else could love _____ like I do.
10. I yearn to know all about _____.
11. I want _____ —physically, emotionally, mentally.
12. I will love _____ forever.
13. I melt when looking deeply into _____'s eyes.
14. I have an endless appetite for affection from _____.
15. For me, _____ is the perfect romantic partner.
16. _____ is the person who can make me feel the happiest.
17. I sense my body responding when _____ touches me.
18. I feel tender toward _____.
19. _____ always seems to be on my mind.
20. If I were separated from _____ for a long time, I would feel intensely lonely.
21. I sometimes find it difficult to concentrate on work because thoughts of _____ occupy my mind.
22. I want _____ to know me—my thoughts, my fears, and my hopes.
23. Knowing that _____ cares about me makes me feel complete.
24. I eagerly look for signs indicating _____'s desire for me.
25. If _____ were going through a difficult time, I would put away my concerns to help him/her out.
26. _____ can make me feel effervescent and bubbly.
27. In the presence of _____, I yearn to touch and be touched.
28. An existence without _____ would be dark and dismal.
29. I possess a powerful attraction for _____.
30. I get extremely depressed when things don't go right in my relationship with _____.

Source. This scale is reprinted with permission of the author.

Note. Items 2, 5, 6, 7, 8, 10, 11, 14, 15, 17, 19, 22, 24, 29, and 30 constitute the short version of the Passionate Love Scale.

a. This response scale follows each item.

The Desired Loving Behaviors Scale

Martin Heesacker,[1] Mary B. Smith, and Alvin Lawrence, *University of Florida*

The purpose of the Desired Loving Behaviors Scale (DLBS) is to understand what behaviors individuals want from romantic partners to feel loved. Sexual behaviors constitute one of four factor analytically derived subscales of the DLBS. The DLBS can be used as a research instrument as well as in clinical applications, such as marital or couples counseling.

Description

The DLBS is a 39-item, paper-and-pencil measure. Items were developed in two steps. In the first step, anonymous, volunteer undergraduate students were asked to list answers to the following questions: "What do you want your partner to DO to make you feel loved?" and "What do you want your partner to SAY to make you feel loved?" Responses were compiled, and redundant items were removed, leaving 158 items, which were corrected for grammar and made gender neutral. In the second step, 302 female and 157 male anonymous, collegiate volunteers indicated how often they would like their partners to do or say each of these 158 items for them to feel loved. They rated each item on a 5-point Likert-type scale with values of *never* (1), *rarely* (2), *sometimes* (3), *often* (4), and *always* (5). Results were factor analyzed, with a principal components analysis and scree test suggesting four factors. Oblique rotation resulted in 39 items achieving simple structure on the four factors. These factors were labeled Relationship Support (10 items), Scripting (10 items), Sex (10 items), and Caring Actions (9 items).

Response Mode and Timing

Respondents read the following: "What do you want your partner to DO or SAY to make you feel loved? USE THE FOLLOWING SCALE TO INDICATE HOW OFTEN YOU WOULD LIKE YOUR PARTNER TO DO OR SAY THE FOLLOWING THINGS IN ORDER FOR YOU TO FEEL LOVED." Respondents then indicate their responses directly on the questionnaires or on answer sheets. The DLBS requires approximately 8 minutes to complete.

Scoring

Each subscale is scored by calculating the mean. The Relationship Support subscale includes Items 2, 8, 9, 12, 13, 16, 19, 20, 23, and 30. The Scripting subscale includes Items 1, 3, 15, 18, 25, 26, 27, 35, 36, and 38. The Sex subscale includes Items 5, 7, 11, 14, 21, 22, 31, 32, 34, and

39. The Caring Actions subscale includes Items 4, 6, 10, 17, 24, 28, 29, 33, and 37.

Reliability

Test-retest reliability for a sample of 158 college students across a 26-day interval for the DLBS as a whole was $r = .65$. Test-retest reliability scores for the subscales were as follows: Relationship Support, $r = .55$; Scripting, $r = .57$; Sex, $r = .59$; and Caring Actions, $r = .55$; all $ps < .0001$.

Internal consistency reliability was calculated using Cronbach's alpha: overall scale alpha = .91, Relationship Support alpha = .90, Scripting alpha = .90, Sex alpha = .91, and Caring Actions alpha = .78. These coefficients indicate adequate internal consistency reliability for the overall scale and for the subscales.

Validity

To validate the DLBS, we conducted a study calculating the discrepancy between what people desired (using the DLBS) and what they actually received (using DLBS items with modified instructions). Then we correlated the magnitude of that discrepancy with relationship satisfaction. As predicted, satisfaction decreased as the magnitude of the discrepancy increased. In another study, we found that failed relationships had significantly higher discrepancy scores than intact relationships, across all four subscales. Also, as predicted, in a cross-lag panel analysis we found that overall discrepancy significantly predicted satisfaction 26 days later ($r = -.51$, $p < .0001$; Smith & Heesacker, 1996). Satisfaction was also a significant predictor of discrepancy 26 days later ($r = -.38$, $p < .0001$), and as predicted, at a significantly smaller magnitude, $t(169) = 2.43$, p (one-tailed) $< .01$. The patterns of correlations for the four subscales, individually, were similar to this overall pattern of correlations.

Other Information

The DLBS may be used in couples counseling to generate discussion regarding the types of behaviors partners would like to feel loved. In addition, the discrepancy between DLBS scores and what people perceive they actually get can also be useful in couples counseling. Inspection of items and scales for those with the greatest discrepancies is likely to suggest areas for productive behavior change. For example, one partner in a couple may be providing a surfeit of loving behaviors in one subscale area and a dearth in another. Through inspection of the direction and magnitude of discrepancies, action may be redirected to produce a more satisfying result for one's partner, in some cases with no increase in the overall effort exerted. Such change is, in turn, likely to improve one's self-efficacy as a romantic

[1]Address correspondence to Martin Heesacker, Department of Psychology, University of Florida, Gainesville, FL 32611-2250; email: heesack@psych.ufl.edu.

partner and relationship satisfaction for both members of the couple.

References

Heesacker, M., & Lawrence, A. (1994, August). Men, women, and behaviors they desire from a partner in order to feel loved. In J. Robertson & G. Good (Chairs), *Men, masculinity, and psychological services*. Symposium conducted at the annual meeting of the American Psychological Association, Los Angeles.

Smith, M. B., & Heesacker, M. (1996). *Accurate provision of desired loving behaviors and relationship satisfaction: A cross-lag panel study*. Manuscript in preparation.

Exhibit

The Desired Loving Behaviors Scale

While considering your current relationship or while considering your most recent previous relationship, please answer the following questions. What do you want your partner to DO or SAY to make you feel loved?

Use the following scale to indicate how often you would like your partner to do or say the following things in order for you to feel loved.

1 = Never   2 = Rarely   3 = Sometimes   4 = Often   5 = Always

1. Tell me that I make them happier than anyone else.
2. Make our relationship a mutual project.
3. Say to me, "You mean so much to me."
4. Do my laundry every once in a while.
5. Tell me what he/she likes and dislikes in bed.
6. Put a note on my car.
7. Seduce me.
8. Be a good listener to me.
9. Spend time talking with me.
10. Leave a rose on my pillow.
11. Be open to trying new sexual positions.
12. Help me through rough times.
13. Be a good communicator.
14. Take a more active role in sex and foreplay.
15. Say that he/she wants to marry me.
16. Create a feeling of security between us.
17. Cook a special meal just for the two of us.
18. Say, "I love you with all my heart and soul."
19. Accept my imperfections.
20. Remember my birthday.
21. Good sex.
22. Say to me, "Let's make love."
23. Be supportive of me and my decisions.
24. Make a tape of corny love songs.
25. Talk about our future together.
26. Say to me, "I enjoy spending time with you more than any other person.
27. Say to me, "I want to be with you forever."
28. Take walks with me during the day.
29. Write poems.
30. Be sympathetic to my feelings.
31. Have sex in strange places.
32. Oral sex.
33. Make me cookies and brownies.
34. Encourage me to keep going during sex.
35. Say to me, "You are the best thing that ever happened to me."
36. Say to me, "I'll always love you."
37. Change his/her religion.
38. Say to me, "I think that we make a great couple."
39. Initiate sex.

Gender Identity and Erotic Preference in Males

Kurt Freund and Ray Blanchard,[1] *Clarke Institute of Psychiatry*

This test package includes seven scales. Six of these are concerned with the assessment of erotic preference and erotic anomalies; one is concerned with the assessment of gender identity. This last instrument, in its present form and in earlier versions, has a longer history in the published literature than the other six. All seven instruments are intended for use with adult males.

The Feminine Gender Identity Scale (FGIS, see Exhibit 1) was developed to measure that "femininity" occurring in homosexual males (Freund, Langevin, Satterberg, & Steiner, 1977; Freund, Nagler, Langevin, Zajac, & Steiner, 1974). There were two reasons to develop a special instrument to measure this attribute rather than rely on conventional masculinity-femininity tests. First, conventional masculinity-femininity tests are usually assembled from items that are differentially endorsed by males and females. Such differential endorsement may reflect other differences between the sexes besides gender identity (e.g., body build and upbringing). Moreover, femininity in homosexual males need not be identical with what psychologically differentiates males from females. Therefore, rather than using biological females as a reference group, Freund identified the "feminine" behavioral patterns and self-reports of homosexual male-to-female transsexuals as the extreme of that femininity observable in homosexual males. Accordingly, feminine gender identity in males was conceived as a continuous variable, inferable from the extent of an individual's departure from the usual male pattern of behavior toward the pattern typical of male-to-female transsexuals.

The second reason for developing a new instrument was that conventional masculinity-femininity scales did not include those items pointed out by the classical sexologists (e.g., Hirschfeld and Krafft-Ebing) as indicative of femininity in homosexual males (e.g., whether, as a child, the individual had preferred to be in the company of males or females; whether he had preferred girls' or boys' games and toys). In Freund's clinical experience, such developmental items seemed to be of particular importance.

The item content of the six erotic interest scales was derived from Freund's clinical experience. The Androphilia and Gynephilia Scales (see Exhibits 2 and 3) were originally assembled to measure the extent of bisexuality reported by androphilic males and to measure the erotic interest in other persons reported by patients with cross-gender identity problems. The term *androphilia* refers to erotic attraction to physically mature males, and *gynephilia*, to erotic attraction to physically mature females. The Heterosexual Expe-

rience Scale (Exhibit 4) was intended to assess sexual experience with women, as opposed to sexual interest in them. The Fetishism, Masochism, and Sadism Scales (Exhibits 5-7) were constructed from face-valid items as self-report measures of these anomalous erotic preferences.

The interested reader should note the availability of certain closely related instruments. We have developed a companion instrument for the FGIS, the Masculine Gender Identity Scale for Females (Blanchard & Freund, 1983), presented elsewhere in this volume. Modifications of the Androphilia and Gynephilia Scales specifically intended for male patients with gender identity disorders have been developed by Blanchard (1985a, 1985b). Blanchard (1985a) includes a scale for measuring *cross-gender* fetishism (roughly *transvestism*), also reprinted in this volume.

Description

All seven scales are presented in full (see Exhibits 1-7). Most of the scales are a mixture of dichotomous and multiple-choice items. The number of items in each scale is summarized in Table 1, along with the types and numbers of subjects used in item analysis, the alpha reliability of each scale, and the proportion of total variance accounted for by the largest single factor found with principal components analysis.

With the exception of the FGIS, all scales are appropriate for any adult male with sufficient reading comprehension. Part A of the FGIS, which was constructed by selecting items differentially endorsed by adult gynephiles and (nontranssexual) androphiles, may also be administered by any adult male.

Parts B and C of the FGIS were constructed from items differentially endorsed by transsexual and nontranssexual homosexuals. Part B consists of three items, which also appear on the Androphilia Scale, and which presuppose homosexuality. Part B in only appropriate for homosexual respondents; hence, the full scale (Parts A, B, and C) may be administered only to homosexual respondents: androphilic transsexuals, androphiles, homosexual hebephiles (men who erotically prefer pubescent males), or homosexual pedophiles (men who erotically prefer male children). Part C consists of items aimed at transsexualism and is appropriate for males presenting with any cross-gender syndrome, including transvestism.

Response Mode and Timing

Respondents check one and only one response option for each item. The shortest scale takes only a few minutes to complete; the longest (the full FGIS) takes about 15 minutes. Respondents are permitted to ask for clarification on any item whose meaning they do not understand.

[1]Address correspondence to Ray Blanchard, Gender Identity Clinic, Clarke Institute of Psychiatry, 250 College Street, Toronto M5T 1R8, Ontario, Canada; email: blanchardr@cs.clarke-inst.on.ca.

Table 1 Psychometric Information

Scale[a]	N of items	Respondents used in item analysis[b]	N of respondents	Alpha[c]	% Variance[d]
FGI(A)	19	CGI patients, andro patients, courtship disorder, sadists	743	.93	43.8
FGI(BC)	10	CGI patients, andro patients	332	.89	51.4
Andro	13	CGI patients, andro controls, andro patients, homo pedohebe	437	.93	59.8
Gyne	9	CGI patients, hetero controls, andro controls, andro patients, homo pedohebe, hetero pedohebe	605	.85	40.4
Het Exp	6	As above	606	.82	47.8
Fetish	8	CGI patients, hetero controls, andro controls, homo pedohebe, hetero pedohebe, courtship disorder, sadists, hyperdominants, masochists	444	.91	59.6
Maso	11	As above	491	.83	33.7
Sadism	20	As above	491	.87	28.0

Note. The FGI Scale data were prepared for this table by Blanchard. The data for the other six scales are from Freund, Steiner, and Chan (1982).

a. FGI(A), Feminine Gender Identity Scale for Males–Part A; FGI(BC), Feminine Gender Identity Scale for Males–Parts B and C combined; Andro, Androphilia Scale; Gyne, Gynephilia Scale; Het Exp, Heterosexual Experience Scale; Fetish, Fetishism Scale; Maso, Masochism Scale; Sadism, Sadism Scale.

b. CGI, patients with cross-gender identity; courtship disorder, patients with voyeurism, exhibitionism, toucherism, frotteurism, obscene telephone calling, or the preferential rape pattern; pedohebe, pedophiles of hebephiles; hyperdominants, borderline sadists.

c. Alpha reliability coefficient.

d. Percentage of total variance accounted for by the strongest principal component.

Scoring

Scoring weights for each response option of each item follow that option in parentheses in the exhibits. The total scores for each scale (and for the three subscales of the FGIS) are obtained by totaling the respondent's scores for each item in that scale (or subscale). For all scales, high scores indicate that the relevant attribute (e.g., sadism, feminine gender identity) is strongly present, and low scores indicate that it is absent.

Reliability

The alpha reliability coefficient of each scale is presented in Table 1. Test-retest reliabilities have never been computed.

Validity

The main line of evidence for the construct validity of the FGIS is the demonstration of reliable group differences among heterosexual, nontranssexual homosexual, and transsexual homosexual males. Two studies have cross-validated Part A of the most recent version of the FGIS (Freund et al., 1977) and have also shown the relative insensitivity of the scale to socioeconomic variables. Freund, Scher, Chan, and Ben-Aron (1982) found no difference in the FGIS scores of gynephilic prisoners (whose modal education was less than high school graduation) and gynephilic university students; both groups produced lower FGIS scores than a sample of androphilic volunteers, who, in turn, scored lower than androphilic male-to-female transsexuals.

Part A scores on the FGIS have also been shown to enter into orderly relationships with a variety of other sexological variables and questionnaire measures. Freund, Scher, et al. (1982) found a positive correlation between the degree of homosexuals' femininity and the age group to which they

are most attracted sexually. The androphilic respondents in this study produced higher FGIS scores than the homosexual hebephiles or pedophiles. The homosexual pedophiles did not differ in feminine gender identity from gynephiles. Freund and Blanchard (1983) found that those androphiles who produced the highest (most feminine) FGIS scores also tended to report the worst childhood relationships with their fathers. Blanchard, McConkey, Roper, and Steiner (1983) found a high negative correlation (–.71) between Part A of the FGIS and retrospectively reported boyhood aggressiveness, defined as a generalized disposition to engage in physically combative or competitive interactions with male peers.

Freund et al. (1977) reported a moderate correlation (+.46) between Part A of the FGIS and the MMPI Masculinity-Femininity (Mf) Scale, and Hooberman (1979) reported a similar correlation (+.52) between Part A of the 1974 version of the FGIS and the femininity scale of the Bem Sex-Role Inventory (BSRI; Bem, 1981). Hooberman did not report the correlation between the FGIS and the BSRI masculinity scale; presumably, it was lower and not statistically significant. Guloien (1983) found a statistically significant negative correlation (–.20) between Part A of the FGIS and Jackson's (1974) social desirability scale in a mixed sample of heterosexual and homosexual male university students; Blanchard, Clemmensen, and Steiner (1985) found a significant positive correlation (+.37) between Part A and the Crowne and Marlowe (1964) Social Desirability Scale among male patients at a gender identity clinic, most of whom were seeking sex reassignment surgery.

Freund, Scher, et al. (1982) found that the Gynephilia and Heterosexual Experience Scales differentiated between two groups of androphiles, one claiming considerable, the other only minimal, bisexuality. The two scales discriminated between groups about equally well. Freund, Steiner, and Chan (1982) reported good agreement between clinicians' assessment of erotic partner preference (heterosexual vs. homosexual) and assessment by means of the Androphilia and Gynephilia Scales. They also found, among the various syndromes of cross-gender identity that they investigated, group differences in all seven measures presented here. Of particular interest was the confirmation they obtained with the Sadism, Masochism, and Fetishism Scales of their clinical impression that these anomalies tend to be differentially associated with heterosexual-type cross-gender identity.

References

Bem, S. L. (1981). *Bem Sex-Role Inventory professional manual*. Palo Alto, CA: Consulting Psychologists Press.

Blanchard, R. (1985a). Research methods for the typological study of gender disorders in males. In B. W. Steiner (Ed.), *Gender dysphoria: Development, research, management* (pp. 227-257). New York: Plenum.

Blanchard, R. (1985b). Typology of male-to-female transsexualism. *Archives of Sexual Behavior, 14*, 247-261.

Blanchard, R., Clemmensen, L. H., & Steiner, B. W. (1985). Social desirability response set and systematic distortion in the self-report of adult male gender patients. *Archives of Sexual Behavior, 14*, 505-516.

Blanchard, R., & Freund, K. (1983). Measuring masculine gender identity in females. *Journal of Consulting and Clinical Psychology, 51*, 205-214.

Blanchard, R., McConkey, J. G., Roper, V., & Steiner, B. W. (1983). Measuring physical aggressiveness in heterosexual, homosexual, and transsexual males. *Archives of Sexual Behavior, 12*, 511-524.

Crowne, D. P., & Marlowe, D. (1964). *The approval motive: Studies in evaluative dependence*. New York: Wiley.

Freund, K., & Blanchard, R. (1983). Is the distant relationship of fathers and homosexual sons related to the sons' erotic preference for male partners, or to the sons' atypical gender identity, or to both? *Journal of Homosexuality, 9*, 7-25.

Freund, K., Langevin, R., Satterberg, J., & Steiner, B. W. (1977). Extension of the Gender Identity Scale for Males. *Archives of Sexual Behavior, 6*, 507-519.

Freund, K., Nagler, E., Langevin, R., Zajac, A., & Steiner, B. W. (1974). Measuring feminine gender identity in homosexual males. *Archives of Sexual Behavior, 3*, 249-260.

Freund, K., Steiner, B. W., & Chan, S. (1982). Two types of cross-gender identity. *Archives of Sexual Behavior, 11*, 49-63.

Freund, K., Scher, H., Chan, S., & Ben-Aron, M. (1982). Experimental analysis of pedophilia. *Behavior Research & Therapy, 20*, 105-112.

Guloien, E. H. (1983). *Childhood gender identity and adult erotic orientation in males*. Unpublished master's thesis, University of Guelph, Guelph, Ontario.

Hooberman, R. E. (1979). Psychological androgyny, feminine gender identity, and self-esteem in homosexual and heterosexual males. *The Journal of Sex Research, 15*, 306-315.

Jackson, D. (1974). *Personality research form manual*. Goshen, NY: Research Psychologist's Press.

Exhibit 1

Feminine Gender Identity Scale for Males

Part A

1. Between the ages of 6 and 12, did you prefer
   a. to play with boys (0)
   b. to play with girls (2)
   c. didn't make any difference (0)
   d. not to play with other children (1)
   e. don't remember (1)

2. Between the ages of 6 and 12, did you
   a. prefer boys' games and toys (soldiers, football, etc.) (0)
   b. prefer girls' games and toys (dolls, cooking, sewing, etc.) (2)
   c. like or dislike both about equally (1)
   d. had no opportunity to play games or with toys (1)

3. In childhood, were you very interested in the work of a garage mechanic? Was this
   a. prior to age 6 (0)
   b. between ages 6 and 12 (0)
   c. probably in both periods (0)
   d. do not remember that I was very interested in the work of a garage mechanic? (1)

4. Between the ages of 6 and 14, which did you like more, romantic stories or adventure stories?
   a. liked romantic stories more (2)
   b. liked adventure stories more (0)
   c. it did not make any difference (1)

5. Between the ages of 6 and 12, did you like to do jobs or chores which are usually done by women?
   a. yes (2)
   b. no (0)
   c. don't remember (1)

6. Between the ages of 13 and 16, did you like to do jobs or chores which are usually done by women?
   a. yes (2)
   b. no (0)
   c. don't remember (1)

7. Between the ages of 6 and 12, were you a leader in boys' games or other activities?
   a. more often than other boys (0)
   b. less often than other boys (1)
   c. about the same, or don't know (0)
   d. did not partake in children's games and/or other activities (1)

8. Between the ages of 6 and 12, when you read a story did you imagine that you were
   a. the male in the story (cowboy, detective, soldier, explorer, etc.) (0)
   b. the female in the story (the girl being saved, etc.) (2)
   c. the male sometimes and the female other times (1)
   d. neither the male nor the female (1)
   e. did not read stories (1)
9. In childhood or at puberty, did you like mechanics magazines? Was this
   a. between ages 6 and 12 (0)
   b. between ages 12 and 14 (0)
   c. probably in both periods (0)
   d. do not remember that I liked mechanics magazines (1)
10. Between the ages of 6 and 12, did you wish you had been born a girl instead of a boy
    a. often (2)
    b. occasionally (1)
    c. never (0)
11. Between the ages of 13 and 16, did you wish you had been born a girl instead of a boy
    a. often (2)
    b. occasionally (1)
    c. never (0)
12. Since the age of 17, have you wished you had been born a girl instead of a boy
    a. often (2)
    b. occasionally (1)
    c. never (0)
13. Do you think your appearance is
    a. very masculine (0)
    b. masculine (0)
    c. a little feminine (1)
    d. quite feminine (2)
14. In childhood, did you sometimes imagine yourself a well-known sports figure, or did you wish you would become one? Was this
    a. prior to age 6 (0)
    b. between ages 6 and 12 (0)
    c. probably in both periods (0)
    d. do not remember such fantasies (1)
15. In childhood fantasies did you sometimes wish you could go hunting big game? Was this
    a. prior to age 6 (0)
    b. between ages 6 and 12 (0)
    c. probably in both periods (0)
    d. do not remember such fantasies (1)
16. In childhood fantasies did you sometimes imagine yourself as being a policeman or soldier? Was this
    a. prior to age 6 (0)
    b. between ages 6 and 12 (0)
    c. probably in both periods (0)
    d. do not remember that I had such a fantasy (1)
17. In childhood was there ever a period in which you wished you would, when adult, become a dressmaker or dress designer?
    a. prior to age 6 (1)
    b. between ages 6 and 12 (1)
    c. probably in both periods (1)
    d. do not remember having this desire (0)
18. In childhood fantasies did you sometimes imagine yourself driving a racing car? Was this
    a. prior to age 6 (0)
    b. between ages 6 and 12 (0)
    c. probably in both periods (0)
    d. do not remember having this fantasy (1)
19. In childhood did you ever wish to become a dancer? Was this
    a. prior to age 6 (1)
    b. between ages 6 and 12 (1)
    c. probably in both periods (1)
    d. do not remember having this desire (0)

Part B

20. What kind of sexual contact with a male would you have preferred on the whole, even though you may not have done it?
    a. inserting your privates between your partner's upper legs (thighs) (0)
    b. putting your privates into your partner's rear end (0)
    c. you would have preferred one of those two modes but you cannot decide which one (0)
    d. your partner putting his privates between your upper legs (thighs) (1)
    e. your partner putting his privates into your rear end (2)
    f. you would have preferred one of these two latter modes but you cannot decide which one (1)
    g. you would have liked all four modes equally well (1)
    h. you would have preferred some other mode of sexual contact (1)
    i. had no desire for physical contact with males (*exclude subject*)
21. What qualities did you like in males to whom you were sexually attracted?
    a. strong masculine behavior (2)
    b. slightly masculine behavior (1)
    c. rather feminine behavior (0)
    d. did not feel sexually attracted to males (*exclude subject*)
22. Would you have preferred a partner
    a. who was willing to have you lead him (0)
    b. who was willing to lead you (2)
    c. you didn't care (1)
    d. did not feel sexually attracted to males (*exclude subject*)

Part C

23. Between the ages of 6 and 12, did you put on women's underwear or clothing
    a. once a month or more, for about a year or more (2)
    b. (less often, but) several times a year for about 3 years or more (1)
    c. very seldom did this during this period (0)
    d. never did this during this period (0)
    e. don't remember (0)
24. Between the ages of 13 and 16, did you put on women's underwear or clothing
    a. once a month or more, for about a year or more (2)
    b. (less often, but) several times a year for about 2 years or more (1)
    c. very seldom did this during this period (0)
    d. never did this during this period (0)
25. Since the age of 17, did you put on women's underwear or clothing
    a. once a month or more, for at least a year (2)
    b. (less often, but) several times a year for at least 2 years (1)
    c. very seldom did this during this period (0)
    d. never did this during this period (0)
26. Have you ever wanted to have an operation to change you physically into a woman?
    a. yes (2)
    b. no (0)
    c. unsure (1)
27. If you have ever wished to have a female body rather than a male one, was this
    a. mainly to please men but also for your own satisfaction (2)
    b. mainly for your own satisfaction but also to please men (2)
    c. entirely for your own satisfaction (2)
    d. entirely to please men (1)
    e. about equally to please men and for your own satisfaction (2)
    f. have never wanted to have a female body (0)
28. Have you ever felt like a woman
    a. only if you were wearing at least one piece of female underwear or clothing (1)
    b. while wearing at least one piece of female underwear or clothing and only occasionally at other times also (1)
    c. at all times and for at least 1 year (female clothing or not) (2)
    d. never felt like a woman (0)
29. When completely dressed in male clothing (underwear, etc.) would you
    a. have a feeling of anxiety because of this (2)
    b. have no feeling of anxiety but have another kind of unpleasant feeling because of this (2)
    c. have no unpleasant feelings to do with above (0)

Source. This scale was originally published in "Extension of the Gender Identity Scale of Males" by K. Freund, R. Langevin, J. Satterberg, and B. W. Steiner, 1977, *Archives of Sexual Behavior, 6*, 515-519. Copyright 1977 by Plenum Publishing Corporation. Reprinted by permission.

Exhibit 2

Androphilia Scale

1. About how old were you when you first made quite strong efforts to see males who were undressed or scantily dressed?
    a. younger than 12 (1)
    b. between 12 and 16 (1)
    c. older than 16 (1)
    d. never (0)
2. About how old were you when you first felt sexually attracted to males?
    a. younger than 6 (1)
    b. between 6 and 11 (1)
    c. between 12 and 16 (1)
    d. older than 16 (1)
    e. never (0)
3. Since what age have you been sexually attracted to males only?
    a. younger than 6 (1)
    b. between 6 and 11 (1)
    c. between 12 and 16 (1)
    d. older than 16 (1)
    e. never (0)
4. Since the age of 16, have you ever fallen in love with a person of the male sex?
    a. yes (1)
    b. no (0)
5. How old were you when you first kissed a male because you felt sexually attracted to him?
    a. younger than 12 (1)
    b. between 12 and 16 (1)
    c. older than 16 (1)
    d. never (0)
6. Since age 12, how old were you when you first touched the privates of a male to whom you felt sexually attracted?
    a. between 12 and 16 (1)
    b. older than 16 (1)
    c. never (0)
7. What kind of sexual contact with a male would you have preferred on the whole, even though you may not have done it?

a. inserting your privates between your partner's upper legs (thighs) (1)

b. putting your privates into your partner's rear end (1)

c. you would have preferred one of those two modes but you cannot decide which one (1)

d. your partner putting his privates between your upper legs (thighs) (1)

e. your partner putting his privates into your rear end (1)

f. you would have preferred one of those two latter modes but you cannot decide which one (1)

g. you would have liked all four modes equally well (1)

h. you would have preferred some other mode of sexual contact (1)

i. had no desire for physical contact with males (0)

8. What qualities did you like in males to whom you were sexually attracted?
   a. strong masculine behavior (1)
   b. slightly masculine behavior (1)
   c. rather feminine behavior (1)
   d. did not feel sexually attracted to males (0)

9. Would you have preferred
   a. male homosexual partners (1)
   b. male partners who were not homosexual (1)
   c. had no preference (1)
   d. did not feel sexually attracted to males (0)

10. Since age 18, how old was the oldest male to whom you could have felt sexually attracted?
    a. younger than 6 (1)
    b. between 6 and 11 (1)
    c. between 12 and 16 (1)
    d. between 17 and 19 (1)
    e. between 20 and 30 (1)
    f. between 31 and 40 (1)
    g. between 41 and 50 (1)
    h. older than 50 (1)
    i. did not feel sexually attracted to males (0)

11. Would you have preferred a partner
    a. who was willing to have you lead him (1)
    b. who was willing to lead you (1)
    c. you didn't care (1)
    d. did not feel sexually attracted to males (0)

12. Since age 16 and up to age 25 (or younger if you are less than 25) how did the preferred age of male partners change as you got older?
    a. became gradually younger (1)
    b. became gradually older (1)
    c. remained about the same (1)
    d. never felt attracted to males (0)

13. Since age 16, have you ever been equally, or more, attracted sexually by a male age 17 and over than by females at 17-40?
    a. yes (1)
    b. no (0)

Exhibit 3

Gynephilia Scale

1. Since the age of 17 when you went dancing, was this to
   a. mainly meet girls at the dance (1)
   b. mainly meet male friends at the dance (0)
   c. mainly because you liked dancing itself (0)
   d. never went dancing since age 17 (0)

2. How old were you when you first tried (on your own) to see females 13 or older naked or dressing or undressing (including strip-tease, movies or pictures)?
   a. younger than 12 (1)
   b. between 12 and 16 (1)
   c. older than 16 (1)
   d. never (0)

3. Since age 13, have you ever fallen in love with or had a crush on a female who was between the ages of 13-40?
   a. yes (1)
   b. no (0)

4. Have you ever desired sexual intercourse with a female age 17-40?
   a. yes (1)
   b. no (0)

5. How do you prefer females age 17-40 to react when you try to come into sexual contact (not necessarily intercourse) with them?
   a. cooperation on the part of the female (1)
   b. indifference (1)
   c. a little resistance (1)
   d. considerable resistance (1)
   e. you don't care (0)
   f. do not try to come into sexual contact with females age 17-40 (0)

6. Do you prefer females of age 17-40
   a. who have no sexual experience (1)
   b. who have had a little experience (1)
   c. who have had considerable experience (1)
   d. you don't care how much experience (1)
   e. not enough interest in females age 17-40 to know (0)

7. Between 13 and 16, when you first saw females 13 or over in the nude (or dressing or undressing) including strip-tease, movies or pictures, did you feel sexually aroused?
   a. very much (1)
   b. mildly (1)
   c. not at all (0)
   d. never saw females 13 or over in the nude, dressing or undressing (including striptease, movies or pictures) (0)

8. When you have a wet dream (reach climax while dreaming), do you always, or almost always, dream of a female age 17-40?
   a. yes (1)   c. don't remember any wet dreams (0)
   b. no (0)
9. In your sexual fantasies, are females age 17-40 always, or almost always involved?
   a. yes (1)   c. haven't had such fantasies (0)
   b. no (0)

Exhibit 4

Heterosexual Experience Scale

1. Since age 13, how old were you when you first kissed a female age 13-40 who seemed to be interested in you sexually?
   a. between the ages 13-16 (1)   c. 26 or older (1)
   b. between the ages 17-25 (1)   d. never after age 12 (0)
2. Since age 13, how old were you when you first petted (beyond kissing) with a female age 13-40 who seemed to be interested in you sexually?
   a. between the ages 13-16 (1)   c. 26 or older (1)
   b. between the ages 17-25 (1)   d. never after age 12 (0)
3. Have you ever attempted sexual intercourse with a female age 17-40?
   a. yes (1)   c. no, and you are 25 or younger (0)
   b. no, and you are older than 25 (0)
4. When did you first have sexual intercourse with a female age 17-40?
   a. before age 16 (1)   d. never, and you are older than 25 (0)
   b. between 16 and 25 (1)   e. never, and you are 25 or younger (0)
   c. 26 or older (1)
5. When did you first get married or begin living common-law?
   a. before 30 (1)   d. never married or had common-law relations, and you are
   b. between 30-40 (1)   older than 30 (0)
   c. age 41 or older (1)   e. never, and you are 30 or younger (0)
6. Was there any period of 14 days or less when you had sexual intercourse with a female age 17-40 more than 5 times?
   a. yes (1)   c. no, and you are 25 or younger (0)
   b. no, and you are older than 25 (0)

Exhibit 5

Fetishism Scale

1. Do you think that certain inanimate objects (velvet, silk, leather, rubber, shoes, female underwear, etc.) have a stronger sexual attraction for your than for most other people?
   a. yes (1)   b. no (0)
2. Has the sexual attractiveness of an inanimate (not alive) thing ever increased if it had been worn by, or had been otherwise in contact with
   a. a female (1)   e. a female or male person equally (1)
   b. a male (1)   f. contact between a person and a thing never increased its
   c. preferably a female but also when in contact or having   sexual attractiveness (1)
      been in contact with a male (1)   g. do not feel sexually attracted to any inanimate thing (0)
   d. preferably a male but also when in contact or having
      been in contact with a female (1)
3. Did the sexual attractiveness to you of such a thing ever increase if you wore it or were otherwise in contact with it yourself?
   a. yes (1)   c. have never been sexually attracted to inanimate things (0)
   b. no (0)
4. Were you ever more strongly sexually attracted by inanimate things than by females or males?
   a. yes (1)   b. no (0)

5. What was the age of persons who most increased the sexual attractiveness for you of a certain inanimate object by their contact with it?
   a. 3 years or younger (1)
   b. between 4 and 6 years (1)
   c. between 6 and 11 years (1)
   d. between 12 and 13 years (1)
   e. between 14 and 16 years (1)
   f. between 17 and 40 years (1)
   g. over 60 years (1)
   h. contact between a person and a thing never increased its sexual attractiveness (1)
   i. have never been sexually attracted to inanimate things (0)
6. Is there more than one kind of inanimate thing which arouses you sexually?
   a. yes (1)
   b. no (1)
   c. have never been sexually attracted to inanimate things (0)
7. Through which of these senses did the thing act most strongly?
   a. through the sense of smell (1)
   b. through the sense of taste (1)
   c. through the sense of sight (1)
   d. through the sense of touch (1)
   e. through the sense of hearing (1)
   f. have never been sexually attracted to inanimate objects (0)
8. At about what age do you remember first having a special interest in an inanimate thing which later aroused you sexually?
   a. younger than 2 (1)
   b. between 2 and 4 (1)
   c. between 5 and 7 (1)
   d. between 8 and 10 (1)
   e. between 11 and 13 (1)
   f. older than 13 (1)
   g. have never been sexually attracted to inanimate objects (0)

Exhibit 6

Masochism Scale

1. If you were insulted or humiliated by a person to whom you felt sexually attracted, did this ever increase their attractiveness?
   a. yes (1)
   b. no (0)
   c. unsure (0)
2. Has imagining that you were being humiliated or poorly treated by someone ever excited you sexually?
   a. yes (1)
   b. no (0)
3. Has imagining that you had been injured by someone to the point of bleeding ever excited you sexually?
   a. yes (1)
   b. no (0)
4. Has imagining that someone was causing you pain ever aroused you sexually?
   a. yes (1)
   b. no (0)
5. Has imagining that someone was choking you ever excited you sexually?
   a. yes (1)
   b. no (0)
6. Has imagining that you have become dirty or soiled ever excited you sexually?
   a. yes (1)
   b. no (0)
7. Has imagining that your life was being threatened ever excited you sexually?
   a. yes (1)
   b. no (0)
8. Has imagining that someone was imposing on you heavy physical labor or strain ever excited you sexually?
   a. yes (1)
   b. no (0)
9. Has imagining a situation in which you were having trouble breathing ever excited you sexually?
   a. yes (1)
   b. no (0)
10. Has imagining that you were being threatened with a knife or other sharp instrument ever excited you sexually?
    a. yes (1)
    b. no (0)
11. Has imagining that you are being tied up by somebody ever excited you sexually?
    a. yes (1)
    b. no (0)

Exhibit 7

Sadism Scale

1. Did you ever like to read stories about or descriptions of torture?
   a. yes (1)
   b. no (0)
2. Did you usually re-read a description of torture several times?
   a. yes (1)
   b. no (0)
   c. don't remember (0)

3. Were you
   a. very interested in descriptions of torture (1)   c. not at all interested (0)
   b. a little interested (0)   d. never read such descriptions (0)
4. Between the ages of 13 and 16, did you find the sight of blood
   a. exciting (1)   c. unpleasant (0)
   b. only pleasant (1)   d. did not affect you in any way (0)
5. Has beating somebody or imagining that you are doing so ever excited you sexually?
   a. yes (1)   b. no (0)
6. Have you ever tried to tie the hands or legs of a person who attracted you sexually?
   a. yes (1)   b. no (0)
7. Has cutting or imagining to cut someone's hair ever excited you sexually?
   a. yes (1)   b. no (0)
8. Has imagining that you saw someone bleeding ever excited you sexually?
   a. yes (1)   b. no (0)
9. Has imagining someone being choked by yourself or somebody else ever excited you sexually?
   a. yes (1)   b. no (0)
10. Has imagining yourself or someone else imposing heavy physical labor or strain on somebody ever excited you
    sexually?
    a. yes (1)   b. no (0)
11. Has imagining that someone was being ill-treated in some way by yourself or somebody else ever excited you
    sexually?
    a. yes (1)   b. no (0)
12. Has imagining that you or someone else were causing pain to somebody ever excited you sexually?
    a. yes (1)   b. no (0)
13. Has imagining that you or somebody else were threatening someone's life ever excited you sexually?
    a. yes (1)   b. no (0)
14. Has imagining that someone other than yourself was crying painfully ever excited you sexually?
    a. yes (1)   b. no (0)
15. Has imagining that someone other than yourself was dying ever excited you sexually?
    a. yes (1)   b. no (0)
16. Has imagining that you or someone else were making it difficult for somebody to breathe ever excited you sexually?
    a. yes (1)   b. no (0)
17. Has imagining that you or someone else were tying up somebody ever excited you sexually?
    a. yes (1)   b. no (0)
18. Has imagining that you or somebody else were threatening someone with a knife or other sharp instrument ever
    excited you sexually?
    a. yes (1)   b. no (0)
19. Has imagining that someone was unconscious or unable to move ever excited you sexually?
    a. yes (1)   b. no (0)
20. Has imagining that someone had a very pale and still face ever excited you sexually?
    a. yes (1)   b. no (0)

The Stereotypes About Male Sexuality Scale

William E. Snell, Jr.,[1] *Southeast Missouri State University*

Cognitive approaches to human sexuality have recently received considerable attention. However, there has been a paucity of instruments designed to deal with the types of cognitive beliefs that might influence sexual feelings and behaviors. Snell and his colleagues attempted to address this concern through the development and validation of the Stereotypes About Male Sexuality Scale (SAMSS; Snell, Belk, & Hawkins, 1986, 1990; Snell, Hawkins, & Belk, 1988). The SAMSS is an objective self-report questionnaire that is designed to measure 10 distinctive stereotypic beliefs about males and their sexuality (cf. Zilbergeld, 1978; Chap. 4): (a) Inexpressiveness, (b) Sex Equals Performance, (c) Males Orchestrate Sex, (d) Always Ready for Sex, (e) Touching Leads to Sex, (f) Sex Equals Intercourse, (g) Sex Requires Erection, (h) Sex Requires Orgasm, (i) Spontaneous Sex, and (j) Sexually Aware Men. The 10 subscales on the SAMSS can be used in research as individual-tendency measures of stereotypes about males and their sexuality.

Description

The SAMSS consists of 60 items. Individuals respond to the 60 items on the SAMSS using a 5-point Likert-type scale: *agree* (+2); *slightly agree* (+1); *neither agree nor disagree* (0); *slightly disagree* (–1); and *disagree* (–2).

Response Mode and Timing

Individuals typically indicate their responses on a computer scan sheet by darkening in a response ranging from A (*agree*) to E (*disagree*). The questionnaire usually takes about 20-25 minutes to complete.

Scoring

Individuals respond to the 60 statements on the SAMSS using a 5-point Likert-type scale. The items are recoded so that A = +2, B = +1, C = 0, D = –1, and E = –2, so that the anchors range from *agree* (+2) to *disagree* (–2). The items assigned to each subscale are as follows: (a) Inexpressiveness (1, 11, 21, 31, 41, 51); (b) Sex Equals Performance (2, 12, 22, 32, 42, 52); (c) Males Orchestrate Sex (3, 13, 23, 33, 43, 53); (d) Always Ready for Sex (4, 14, 24, 34, 44, 54); (e) Touching Leads to Sex (5, 15, 25, 35, 45, 55); (f) Sex Equals Intercourse (6, 16, 26, 36, 46, 56); (g) Sex Requires Erection (7, 17, 27, 37, 47, 57); (h) Sex Requires Orgasm (8, 18, 28, 38, 48, 58); (i) Spontaneous Sex (9, 19, 29, 39, 49, 59); and (j) Sexually Aware Men (10, 20, 30, 40, 50, 60). Higher subscale scores thus correspond to greater agreement with the 10 cognitive beliefs measured by the SAMSS.

Reliability

The alpha values for these 10 subscales range from a low of .63 to a high of .93 with an average of .80 (Snell et al., 1986).

Validity

Snell et al. (1990) reported the results of two investigations involving the SAMSS. In the first study, the relationship between the SAMSS and two gender role measures were examined. The results were that the restrictive emotionality aspect of the masculine role was strongly associated with stereotypic beliefs about male sexuality (Doyle, 1989; Gould, 1982; Gross, 1978; Herek, 1987; Mosher & Anderson, 1986; Mosher & Sirkin, 1984). Other gender role preferences and behaviors were also found to be positively associated with conventional "performance" approaches to male sexuality. In the second investigation, counseling trainees were asked to describe how mentally healthy adult men and women would respond to the SAMSS. The responses of both male and female in-training counselors indicated that they expected mentally healthy males (a) to reject inhibited, control, and constant readiness approaches to the expression of male sexuality and (b) to express greater disagreement toward defining male sexuality only in terms of sexual intercourse and toward viewing males as inherently knowledgeable about sex. These results thus provide evidence for the importance of the SAMSS and a cognitive approach to the study of male sexuality. Finally, the SAMSS has been found to correlate significantly and negatively with the use of bilateral social influence strategies (Snell et al., 1988), thus providing evidence for the validity of the SAMSS in that conventional beliefs about sex, as measured by the SAMSS, were expected to be associated with the use of selfish (vs. bilateral) influence strategy use with an intimate partner.

References

Doyle, J. A. (1989). *The male experience* (2nd ed.). Dubuque, IA: Brown.

Gould, R. (1982). Sexual functioning in relation to the changing roles of men. In K. Solomon & N. Levy (Eds.), *Men in transition: Theory and therapy* (pp. 165-173). New York: Plenum.

Gross, A. E. (1978). The male role and heterosexual behavior. *Journal of Social Issues, 34*(1), 87-107.

Herek, G. M. (1987). On heterosexual masculinity: Some psychical consequences of the social construction of gender and sexuality. In M. S. Kimmel (Ed.), *Changing men: New directions in research on men and masculinity* (pp. 68-82). Newbury Park, CA: Sage.

[1]Address correspondence to William E. Snell, Jr., Department of Psychology, Southeast Missouri State University, One University Plaza, Cape Girardeau, MO 63701; email: wesnell@semovm.semo.edu.

Mosher, D. L., & Anderson, R. D. (1986). Macho personality, sexual aggression, and reactions to guided imagery of realistic rape. *Journal of Research in Personality, 20,* 77-94.

Mosher, D. L., & Sirkin, M. (1984). Measuring a macho personality constellation. *Journal of Research in Personality, 18,* 150-163.

Snell, W. E., Jr., Belk, S. S., & Hawkins, R. C. II. (1986). The Stereotypes About Male Sexuality Scale (SAMSS): Components, correlates, antecedents, consequences, and counselor bias. *Social and Behavioral Sciences Documents, 16,* 10. (Ms. No. 2747)

Snell, W. E., Jr., Belk, S. S., & Hawkins, R. C. II (1990). Cognitive beliefs about male sexuality: The impact of gender roles and coun-

selor perspectives. *Journal of Rational-Emotive Therapy, 8,* 249-265.

Snell, W. E., Jr., Hawkins, R. C. II, & Belk, S. S. (1988). Stereotypes about male sexuality and the use of social influence strategies in intimate relationships. *Journal of Social and Clinical Psychology, 7,* 42-48.

Tiefer, L. (1987). In pursuit of the perfect penis: The medicalization of male sexuality. In M. Kimmel (Ed.), *Changing men: New directions in research on men and masculinity* (pp. 165-184). Newbury Park, CA: Sage.

Zilbergeld, B. (1978). *Male sexuality.* Boston: Little, Brown.

Exhibit

The Stereotypes About Male Sexuality Scale

Instructions: We would like to know something about people's beliefs about male sexuality. For this reason we are asking you to respond to a number of items that deal with male sexuality, indicating the extent to which you disagree/agree with the statements. For each of the items on this page, you will be indicating your answer on the computer-scorable answer sheet by darkening in the number (or letter) that corresponds to your response. Your response should be based on the sorts of things that you believe about male sexuality. Use the following scale to indicate your degree of agreements/disagreement with each item:

A	B	C	D	E
Agree	Slightly agree	Neither agree nor disagree	Slightly disagree	Disagree

There are no right or wrong answers. Your choices should be a description of your own personal beliefs.

1. Men should not be held.
2. Most men believe that sex is a performance.
3. Men generally want to be the guiding participant in sexual behavior.
4. Most men are ready for sex at any time.
5. Most men desire physical contact only as a prelude to sex.
6. The ultimate sexual goal in men's mind is intercourse.
7. Lack of an erection will always spoil sex for a man.
8. From a man's perspective, good sex usually has an "earthshaking" aspect to it.
9. Men don't really like to plan their sexual experiences.
10. Most men are sexually well-adjusted.
11. Only a narrow range of emotions should be permitted to men.
12. Men are almost always concerned with their sexual performance.
13. Most men don't want to assume a passive role in sex.
14. Men usually want sex, regardless of where they are.
15. Among men, touching is simply the first step toward sex.
16. Men are not sexually satisfied with any behavior other than intercourse.
17. Without an erection a man is sexually lost.
18. Quiet, lazy sex is usually not all that satisfying for a man.
19. Men usually like good sex to "just happen."
20. Most men have healthy attitudes toward sex.
21. A man who is vulnerable is a sissy.
22. In sex, it's a man's performance that counts.
23. Sexual activity is easier if the man assumes a leadership role.
24. Men are always ready for sex.
25. A man never really wants "only" a hug or caress.
26. Men want their sexual experiences to end with intercourse.
27. A sexual situation cannot be gratifying for a man unless he "can get it up."

28. Sexual climax is a necessary part of men's sexual behavior.
29. Most men yearn for spontaneous sex that requires little conscious effort.
30. In these days of increased openness about sex, most men have become free of past inhibiting ideas about their sexual behavior.
31. A man should be careful to hide his feelings.
32. Men's sexuality is often goal-orientated in its nature.
33. Sex is a man's responsibility.
34. Most men come to a sexual situation in a state of constant desire.
35. Men use physical contact as a request for sex.
36. Men believe that every sexual act should include intercourse.
37. Any kind of sexual activity for a man requires an erection.
38. Satisfying sexual activity for a man always includes increasing excitement and passion.
39. A satisfying sexual experience for a man does not really require all that much forethought.
40. Most men have progressive ideas about sex.
41. It is unacceptable for men to reveal their deepest concerns.
42. Men usually think of sex as work.
43. A man is supposed to initiate sexual contact.
44. Men are perpetually ready for sex.
45. Many men are dissatisfied with any bodily contact which is not followed by sexual activity.
46. Many men are only interested in sexual intercourse as a form of sexual stimulation.
47. An erection is considered by almost all men as vital for sex.
48. Men's sexual desire is often "imperative and driven" in nature.
49. Men consider sex artificial if it is preplanned.
50. In these days of wider availability of accurate information, most men are realistic about their sexual activities.
51. Intense emotional expressiveness should not be discussed by men.
52. Sex is a pressure-filled activity for most men.
53. Men are responsible for choosing sexual positions.
54. Men usually never get enough sex.
55. For men, kissing and touching are merely the preliminaries to sexual activity.
56. During sex, men are always thinking about getting to intercourse.
57. Without an erection, sexual activity for a man will end in misery.
58. Sexual activity must end with an orgasm for a man to feel satisfied.
59. For men, natural sex means "just doing it instinctively."
60. Most men have realistic insight into their sexual preferences and desires.

Source. This scale is reprinted with permission of the author.

The Marriage Expectation Scale

Gabriele D. Jones,[1] *University of Southern Mississippi*

The Marriage Expectation Scale (MES; Jones & Nelson, 1996) was developed to measure expectations of marriage among college students who were not married and had not previously been married. The items assess expectations regarding three different aspects of marriage: intimacy, equality, and compatibility. The scale measures whether the respondent conforms to pessimistic, realistic, or idealistic expectations about marriage. Researchers (e.g., Larson, 1988) have asserted that the high divorce rate in America may stem from marital dissatisfaction associated with unrealistic expectations about marriage. Typically, children of divorce still long for, and seek out, a positive marriage even though they witnessed unhappiness in their parents' relationship. They feel that "it won't happen to me" (Jones & Nelson, 1996) and may even deny the realities of what makes marriages work. Hence, they exhibit idealistic expectations of marriage. Wallerstein (1987), in a 10-year follow-up study, found that participants still believed in romantic love, despite the fact that they witnessed divorce between their parents. Additionally, if a person witnessed large degrees of conflict in his or her parents' relationship (Grych & Fincham, 1990; Markland & Nelson, 1993) he or she may display pessimistic expectations of marriage, avoiding dating and viewing future marriage in a bleak manner (Jones & Nelson, 1996). Although the MES was originally developed to compare expectations of marriage among college students from intact and nonintact homes (Jones & Nelson, 1996) and can be used in similar research designs, it can also be used as an individual difference measure to aid in premarital counseling.

Description

The MES is a 40-item, self-report questionnaire that is answered using a 5-point Likert-type scale ranging from 1 (*strongly disagree*) to 5 (*strongly agree*). Three main dimensions of marriage are assessed: intimacy, equality, and compatibility. These dimensions were established after a careful review of the literature, and interviews with married people. The items that assess intimacy include statements about emotional closeness, communication, and sexual relations. Equality items cover issues of homemaking, family, friends, and children. The items that assess compatibility include statements regarding the personality and attractiveness of the future spouse, as well as activities and recreation within the envisioned marriage.

[1]Address correspondence to Gabriele D. Jones, Department of Psychology, Southern Station Box 5025, University of Southern Mississippi, Hattiesburg, MS 39406; email: gjones@ ocean.st.usm.edu.

Response Mode and Timing

While completing the scale, respondents are instructed to imagine what their future marriages will-be like. Respondents report their answers by circling the appropriate number from 1 to 5 for each item. However, because of the recoding scheme, it is recommended that the respondent record the responses on an answer sheet that can be scored by a computer. The MES requires approximately 10 minutes to complete.

Scoring

Several items (4, 18, 23, 28, 30, 35, 38) on the scale are reversed. Generally, lower scores indicate pessimistic expectations of marriage, and higher scores indicate idealistic expectations of marriage. Scores in the midrange indicate realistic expectations of marriage. Specific profiles for the three categories were obtained by a panel of experts in the field, based on item content. For each item, panel members determined whether each point on the scale represented pessimistic, realistic, or idealistic attitudes. Based on ratings by the panel, each item was recoded (see Table 1) from a 5-point scale to a 3-point scale, with pessimistic responses coded as 1, realistic responses coded as 2, and idealistic responses coded as 3. Therefore, total scores could range from 40 to 120. In a recent study, 307 participants responded to the scale (Jones & Nelson, 1996). Scores ranged from 63 to 110. Those who scored in the highest quartile of all scores were considered to be "idealistic," and students who scored in the lowest quartile were considered to be "pessimistic." Participants who scored in the middle 50% were considered to be "realistic." In terms of raw scores, the profiles were classified as follows: 0-85, pessimistic; 86-96, realistic; and 97-120, idealistic.

Reliability

A pilot study of the MES was carried out prior to the Jones and Nelson (1996) study. This sample consisted of 59 college students. Cronbach's alpha for the total scale (Items 1-40) was .80. Notably, the coefficient for the MES in the Jones and Nelson study that used 307 college students was comparable at .79. The MES performed as well as the two other scales (Love Attitudes Scale; Hendrick & Hendrick, 1986; and the Dean Romanticism Scale; Dean, 1961) in the study with regard to internal consistency.

Validity

As expected, Jones and Nelson (1996) found that scores on the MES were significantly positively correlated with scores on a measure of romanticism, the Dean Romanticism Scale (Dean, 1961). In other words, as scores on the MES went from pessimistic to realistic to idealistic, scores on the

Table 1 Recoding Scheme for the Marriage Expectation Scale

Recode	Item number
1 = 1, 2 = 1, 3 = 1, 4 = 2, 5 = 3	1
1 = 1, 2 = 1, 3 = 2, 4 = 2, 5 = 3	5, 6, 8, 12, 13 15, 16, 19, 20, 25, 34
1 = 1, 2 = 1, 3 = 2, 4 = 3, 5 = 3	2, 9, 17
1 = 1, 2 = 2, 3 = 2, 4 = 2, 5 = 3	7, 10, 14
1 = 1, 2 = 2, 3 = 2, 4 = 3, 5 = 3	3, 11, 21, 22, 24, 26, 27, 29, 31, 32, 33, 36, 37, 39, 40
1 = 3, 2 = 3, 3 = 2, 4 = 1, 5 = 1	18, 28, 35, 38
1 = 3, 2 = 3, 3 = 2, 4 = 2, 5 = 1	4, 23, 30

Dean Romanticism Scale went up, indicating higher degrees of romanticism. Results from the Jones and Nelson study suggest the MES is a noteworthy scale that may be useful in future research. The MES's strong positive relationship to romanticism also indicates the scale's validity, because romanticism has been previously linked to unrealistic and ideal expectations (Larson, 1988). Hendrick and Hendrick (1986) reported that the Love Attitudes Scale was "adequate in its present form as a research instrument" (p. 400). Because the MES performed just as well as the Love Attitudes Scale and the Dean Romanticism Scale on internal consistency, results suggest that the scale is reliable and valid.

Other Information

Much appreciation is expressed to Eileen Nelson, Virginia Andreoli Mathie, and Donna Sundre of James Madison University for their assistance in the development of the MES.

References

Dean, D. G. (1961). Romanticism and emotional maturity: A preliminary study. *Marriage and Family Living, 23*, 44-45.

Grych, J. H., & Fincham, F. D. (1990). Marital conflict and children's adjustment: A cognitive-contextual framework. *Psychological Bulletin, 108*, 267-290.

Hendrick, C., & Hendrick, S. (1986). A theory and method of love. *Journal of Personality and Social Psychology, 50*, 392-402.

Jones, G. D., & Nelson, E. S. (1996). Expectations of marriage among college students from intact and non-intact homes. *Journal of Divorce and Remarriage, 26*, 171-189.

Larson, J. H. (1988). The marriage quiz: College students' beliefs in selected myths about marriage. *Family Relations, 37*, 3-11.

Markland, S. R., & Nelson, E. S. (1993). The relationship between familial conflict and the identity of young adults. *Journal of Divorce and Remarriage, 20*, 193-209.

Wallerstein, J. S. (1987). Children of divorce: Report of a 10-year follow-up of early latency-age children. *American Journal of Orthopsychiatry, 57*, 199-211.

Exhibit

The Marriage Expectation Scale

Strongly disagree	Disagree	Neutral	Agree	Strongly agree
1	2	3	4	5

Please respond to the following statements using the above scale. Simply mark the response that first comes to your mind. There are no "right" or "wrong" answers, and the statements may be interpreted differently according to the individual. Please mark your answers on the computer-scored sheet using a No. 2 pencil. *Imagining what your future marriage might be like*, mark the response that first comes to mind. Thank you!

1. My marriage will be more intense than any of my other close relationships.
2. We will both place the same amount of emphasis on sex.
3. My partner and I will be similar in our habits of cleanliness.
4. Keeping the finances straight will be difficult.
5. Asking each other for help will not be a problem.
6. My partner will be quite attractive.
7. We will have certain household chores that each of us will do.
8. Time alone will not be as important as time together.
9. Maintaining romantic love will be a key factor to our marital happiness.
10. My spouse will want to have children at the same time I do.
11. My partner will absolutely be willing to "follow me" to another city if I'm promoted.
12. Our marital satisfaction will be reflected by our sex life.
13. My partner will have a great sense of humor.
14. We will both be willing to see a marriage counselor if necessary.

15. My spouse and I will be quite affectionate with each other.
16. Having children will improve marital satisfaction for both of us.
17. My spouse will instinctively know what I want and need to be happy.
18. My partner will have trouble understanding me.
19. It will not bother me if my spouse loses his or her "shape."
20. My partner will cherish me.
21. My partner will always listen to me.
22. I will be able to change my partner by pointing out his/her shortcomings.
23. We will get angry with each other.
24. Sex will always be exciting.
25. We will always express feelings openly.
26. We will always agree about whose side of the family we will spend holidays with.
27. Decisions will be made together at all times.
28. I will be suspicious of my partner's fidelity.
29. All our fights will be resolved quickly.
30. My partner will forget important dates such as our anniversary.
31. My spouse will automatically like my side of the family.
32. We will share equally the household chores.
33. My spouse will always consult me when making decisions.
34. We will always have extreme emotional closeness.
35. My spouse and I will argue a lot.
36. My partner and I will eat meals together all the time.
37. We will share all of the same interests.
38. I will have trouble getting along with the in-laws.
39. My partner will agree with me if I tell him or her to change something about him/herself.
40. My spouse will never be attracted to people of the opposite sex.

The GRIMS: A Psychometric Instrument for the Assessment of Marital Discord

The Editors

The Golombok Rust Inventory of Marital Status (GRIMS) is a companion questionnaire to the Golombok Rust Inventory of Sexual Satisfaction (GRISS). It is a short, 28-item scale, for the assessment of the quality of a relationship. It is identical for men and women. It is a Likert-type (4-point) scale with response options labeled *strongly disagree* (SD), *disagree* (D), *agree* (A), and *strongly agree* (SA). The scale requires less than 10 minutes for completion. It has a split-half reliability of .92 for men and .90 for women. Diagnostic validity was obtained by Rust and Golombok (1985). The copyright of the GRIMS is held by the authors, and the scale may be obtained from John Rust, the senior author, at the Department of Psychology, Goldsmiths College, Lewisham Way, New Cross SE16, 6NW, London, England, or the first editor of this *Handbook*. Permission must be sought for reproduction. However, widespread use is encouraged by the authors.

References

Bennun, I. (1985). Prediction and responsiveness in behavioral marital therapy. *Behavioural Psychotherapy, 13,* 186-201.
Bennun, I., Rust, J., & Golombok, S. (1985). The effects of marital therapy. *Scandinavian Journal of Behaviour Therapy, 14,* 65-72.
Rust, J., Bennun, I., Crowe, M., & Golombok, S. (1986). The Golombok Rust Inventory of Marital Status. *Sexual and Marital Therapy, 1,* 55-60.
Rust, J., & Golombok, S. (1985). The validation of the Golombok Rust Inventory of Sexual Satisfaction. *British Journal of Clinical Psychology, 24,* 63-64.
Rust, J., & Golombok, S. (1986a). *The Golombok Rust Inventory of Sexual Satisfaction.* Windsor, UK: NFER-Nelson.
Rust, J., & Golombok, S. (1986b). The GRISS: A psychometric instrument for the assessment of sexual dysfunction. *Archives of Sexual Behavior, 15,* 153-165.

The Male Role Norms Inventory

Ronald F. Levant,[1] *Harvard Medical School*
Jeffrey Fischer, *University of Florida, Gainesville*

The Male Role Norms Inventory (MRNI; Levant et al., 1992) was developed to measure masculinity ideology—"beliefs about the importance of men adhering to culturally defined standards for male behavior" (Pleck, 1995, p. 19). Theoretically, masculinity ideology derives from the "gender role strain paradigm" (Pleck, 1995) and is congruent with the "social constructionist" perspective on men and masculinity (Kimmel, 1987). The MRNI assesses "traditional" masculinity ideology—that constellation of male role ideals that held sway in the United States in the postwar era—and conceptualizes it as a multidimensional construct, in which each dimension represents a norm for male behavior. The gender role strain paradigm argues that there is no single standard for masculinity nor is there an unvarying masculinity ideology. Rather, because masculinity is a social construction, ideals of manhood may differ for people of different social classes, races, ethnic groups, genders, sexual orientations, life stages, and historical eras. Variations in masculinity ideology may be reflected in the differential endorsement of the various norms of traditional masculinity ideology, as well as in the overall rejection of traditional norms and the endorsement of nontraditional norms.

Description

The MRNI has been revised from its original form (Levant et al., 1992) using an approach designed to maximize item to subscale correlations for each subscale. It now consists of 57 items, grouped into eight subscales. The first seven subscales represent the norms of traditional masculinity ideology: Avoidance of Femininity, Rejection of Homosexuals, Self-Reliance, Aggression, Achievement/Status, Attitudes Toward Sex, and Restrictive Emotionality. The eighth subscale is new and assesses Nontraditional Attitudes Toward Masculinity. There is also a Total Traditional Scale, which is an average of the scores on the seven traditional subscales. The items, presented in a random sequence, consist of normative statements to which respondents indicate the degree of their agreement or disagreement on 7-point Likert-type scales, ranging from *strongly disagree* (1) to *strongly agree* (7), with 4 being the neutral point (*neither agree nor disagree*). The MRNI has been translated into Chinese, Spanish, and Russian.

Response Mode and Timing

Respondents can circle the number from 1 to 7 corresponding to their degree of agreement or disagreement with

the item, but the more common scoring approach is to mark the answers on separate machine-scorable sheets. The MRNI requires approximately 25 minutes to complete.

Scoring

To obtain subscale scores, first compute a raw score by adding up the scores on the items for that scale and then divide the raw score by the number of items for that subscale, as follows: Avoidance of Femininity = $(5 + 26 + 28 + 33 + 36 + 41 + 47)/7$; Rejection of Homosexuals = $(1 + 8 + 27 + 42)/4$; Self-Reliance = $(6 + 10 + 19 + 21 + 38 + 50 + 56)/7$; Aggression = $(12 + 17 + 32 + 49 + 52)/5$; Achievement/Status = $(2 + 3 + 13 + 18 + 24 + 37 + 55)/7$; Attitudes Toward Sex = $(9 + 14 + 39 + 40 + 43 + 46 + 51 + 54)/8$; Restrictive Emotionality = $(11 + 16 + 20 + 35 + 44 + 45 + 57)/7$; Nontraditional Attitudes = $(4 + 7 + 15 + 22 + 23 + 25 + 29 + 30 + 31 + 34 + 48 + 53)/12$. To obtain the Total Traditional Scale score, add up the raw scores on the seven traditional subscales and divide by 57.

Reliability

Levant and Majors (1996) assessed 320 European American and 371 African American male and female college students, and Levant, Wu, and Fischer (1996) studied 399 U.S. and 394 Chinese (PRC) male and female college students. The Cronbach alphas were, respectively: Avoidance of Femininity (.77, .82), Rejection of Homosexuals (.54, .58), Self-Reliance (.54, .51), Aggression (.52, .65), Achievement/Status (.67, .69), Attitudes Toward Sex (.69, .81), Restrictive Emotionality (.75, .81), Nontraditional Attitudes Toward Masculinity (.57, .56), and Total Traditional Scale (.84, .88).

Validity

Levant and Fischer (1995) evaluated the discriminant and convergent validity of the MRNI, attempting to demonstrate that it was not associated with a closely related but theoretically distinct measure (the short form of the Personal Attributes Questionnaire, or PAQ, Spence & Helmreich, 1978) and that it is associated with theoretically congruent measures (the Masculine Gender Role Stress Scale, or MGRSS, Eisler & Skidmore, 1987; and the Gender Role Conflict Scale-I, or GRCS-I, O'Neil, Helms, Gable, David, & Wrightsman, 1986). The MRNI (Total Traditional Scale, or TTS) was not related to the PAQ in a college student sample (for males, $N = 97$, $r = .06$ with the M, or masculinity, Scale; for females, $N = 220$, $r = .08$ with the F, or femininity, Scale). This is consistent with the

―――――――――
[1]Address correspondence to Ronald F. Levant, 1093 Beacon Street, Suite 3C, Brookline, MA 02146; email: rlevant@aol.com.

proposition of the strain paradigm that ideology is a fundamentally different construct than gender role orientation as assessed by the PAQ (Pleck, Sonenstein, & Ku, 1993). In another sample of 190 male undergraduates, the MRNI (TTS) correlated with the MGRSS ($r = .52, p < .001$) and the GRCS-I ($r = .52, p < .001$). These results are consistent with the strain paradigm, in which the MGRSS and the GRCS-I are viewed as measures of discrepancy strain, and predicted to be associated with masculinity ideology (Pleck, 1995).

Levant and Fischer (1995) also found support for the concurrent validity of several of the MRNI subscales. An analysis of the pattern of subscale correlations revealed that the MRNI Restrictive Emotionality subscale correlated with the MGRSS Emotional Inexpressiveness Scale ($r = .46, p < .001$) and with the GRCS-I Restrictive Emotionality Scale ($r = .40, p < .001$); that the MRNI Aggression and Status subscales correlated with the GRCS-I Success, Power, and Competition Scale ($r = .35, p < .001; r = .35, p < .01$, respectively); and that the MRNI Rejection of Homosexuals subscale correlated with the GRCS-I Restrictive Affectionate Behavior Between Men Scale ($r = .49, p < .001$).

Levant et al. (1992), Levant and Majors (1996), Levant, Majors, and Kelly (1996), and Massoth, Breed, Broderick, Callaghan, and Montello (1996) found MRNI scores to vary in theoretically meaningful ways by gender, age, marital status, culture, and race. Maxton (1994) found MRNI scores of midlife males to be significantly correlated with their scores on the Fear of Intimacy Scale (Descutner & Thelen, 1991). Silvestri and Lowe (1995) found that midlife male alcoholics were less traditional than were the college students reported in Levant et al. (1992), and nearly as nontraditional as a comparison sample of midlife women. Massoth, Broderick, Festa, and Montello (1996) found a sample of gay men scored less traditionally on all but the self-reliance subscale than a sample of predominantly heterosexual, White college students (reported in Levant & Majors, 1996). Finally, Massoth et al. found a sample of men with head injuries scored less traditionally on the Aggression subscale and more traditionally on the Rejection of Homosexuals subscale.

Other Information

In the exhibit, Items 4, 21, 26, 32, 45, 48, 50, and 52 were borrowed or adapted from the Brannon Masculinity Scale (Brannon & Juni, 1984). Items 43, 46, and 54 were borrowed or adapted from the Stereotypes About Male Sexuality Scale (Snell, Belk, & Hawkins, 1996).

References

Brannon, R., & Juni, S. (1984). A scale for measuring attitudes about masculinity. *Psychological Documents, 14*(1). (University Microfilms No. 2612)

Descutner, C., & Thelen, M. (1991). Development and validation of a Fear of Intimacy Scale. *Psychological Assessment, 3*, 218-225.

Eisler, R. M., & Skidmore, J. R. (1987). Masculine Gender Role Stress: Scale development and component factors in the appraisal of stressful situations. *Behavior Modification, 11*, 123-136.

Kimmel, M. S. (1987). Rethinking "masculinity": New directions in research. In M. S. Kimmel (Ed.), *Changing men: New directions in research on men and masculinity* (pp. 9-24). Newbury Park, CA: Sage.

Levant, R. F., & Fischer, J. (1995). [The construct validity of the Male Role Norms Inventory]. Unpublished raw data.

Levant, R. F., Hirsch, L., Celentano, E., Cozza, T., Hill, S., MacEachern, M., Marty, N., & Schnedeker, J. (1992). The male role: An investigation of norms and stereotypes. *Journal of Mental Health Counseling, 14*, 325-337.

Levant, R. F., & Majors, R. G. (1996). *An investigation into variations in the construction of the male gender role among young African-American and European-American women and men.* Manuscript submitted for publication.

Levant, R. F., Majors, R. G., & Kelley, M. L. (1996). *Masculinity ideology among young African-American and European-American women and men: A replication and extension.* Manuscript submitted for publication.

Levant, R. F., Wu, R., & Fischer, J. (1996). Masculinity ideology: A comparison between U.S. and Chinese young men and women. *Journal of Gender, Culture, and Health, 1*, 217-220.

Massoth, N., Breed, S., Broderick, C., Callaghan, E., & Montello, N. (1996). *An investigation of regional differences among college students in masculinity ideology as measured by the Male Role Norms Inventory.* Manuscript submitted for publication.

Massoth, N., Broderick, C., Festa, J., & Montello, N. (1996). *A comparison of gay and head-injured males with normative data on the Male Role Norms Inventory.* Manuscript submitted for publication.

Maxton, R. A. (1994). How do men in mid-life conceptualize masculinity, and how do these conceptualizations relate to intimacy? (Doctoral dissertation, Boston University, 1994). *Dissertation Abstracts International, 54*, B4432.

O'Neil, J. M., Helms, B. J., Gable, R. K., David, L., & Wrightsman, L. S. (1986). Gender Role Conflict Scale: College men's fear of intimacy. *Sex Roles, 14*, 335-350.

Pleck, J. H. (1995). The gender role strain paradigm: An update. In R. F. Levant & W. S. Pollack (Eds.), *A new psychology of men* (pp. 11-32). New York: Basic Books.

Pleck, J. H., Sonenstein, F. L., & Ku, L. C. (1993). Masculinity ideology and its correlates. In S. Oskamp & M. Costanzo (Eds.), *Gender issues in contemporary society* (pp. 85-100). Newbury Park, CA: Sage.

Silvestri, S., & Lowe, L. (1995, October). *Male role norms of alcoholic men.* Paper presented at the annual conference on Psychopathology, Psychopharmacology, Substance Abuse, and Culture.

Snell, W. E., Jr., Belk, S. S., & Hawkins, R. C., II. (1996). The Stereotypes About Male Sexuality Scale (SAMSS): Components, correlates, antecedents, consequences, and counselor bias. *Social and Behavioral Science Documents, 16*(1, 9).

Spence, J. T., & Helmreich, R. L. (1978). *Masculinity and femininity: Their psychological dimensions, correlates, and antecedents.* Austin: University of Texas Press.

Exhibit

Male Role Norms Inventory

Thank you for your help with our study! We are exploring the roles of men in our society and are very interested in your opinions. Please answer the brief demographic questions on this page, and then complete the questionnaire by circling the number which indicates your level of agreement or disagreement with each statement. We would like this survey to remain anonymous, so please do not put your name on the questionnaire.

Again, we appreciate your cooperation.

Code: _____
Age (Years & months): _____   *Sex:* M F
Race: _____
Marital status:
   Single   Married   Separated   Divorced
   Widowed   Living with significant other
Where would you place your family's socioeconomic status?
   Upper class   Middle class   Lower class

Strongly disagree	Disagree	Slightly disagree	No opinion	Slightly agree	Strongly agree	Agree
1	2	3	4	5	6	7

1. It is disappointing to learn that a famous athlete is gay.[a]
2. If necessary a man should sacrifice personal relationships for career advancement.
3. A man should do whatever it takes to be admired and respected.
4. A boy should be allowed to quit a game if he is losing.
5. A man should prefer football to needlecraft.
6. A man should never count on someone else to get the job done.
7. Men should be allowed to kiss their fathers.
8. A man should not continue a friendship with another man if he finds out that the man is a homosexual.
9. Hugging and kissing should always lead to intercourse.
10. A man must be able to make his own way in the world.
11. Nobody likes a man who cries in public.
12. It is important for a man to take risks, even if he might get hurt.
13. Men should make the final decision involving money.
14. It is important for a man to be good in bed.
15. It is OK for a man to ask for help changing a tire.
16. A man should never reveal worries to others.
17. Boys should be encouraged to find a means of demonstrating physical prowess.
18. A man should try to win at any sport he participates in.
19. Men should always be realistic.
20. One should not be able to tell how a man is feeling by looking at his face.
21. A man who takes a long time and has difficulty making decisions will usually not be respected.
22. Men should be allowed to wear bracelets.
23. A man should not force the issue if another man takes his parking space.
24. In a group, it's up to the man to get things organized and moving ahead.
25. A man should love his sex partner.
26. It is too feminine for a man to use clear nail polish on his fingernails.
27. Being called "faggot" is one of the worst insults to a man or boy.
28. Jobs like firefighter and electrician should be reserved for men.
29. When physically provoked, men should not resort to violence.
30. A man should be able to openly show affection to another man.
31. A man doesn't need to have an erection in order to enjoy sex.
32. When the going gets tough, men should get tough.
33. Housework is women's work.
34. It is not particularly important for a man to control his emotions.
35. Men should not be too quick to tell others that they care about them.
36. Boys should prefer to play with trucks rather than dolls.
37. It's OK for a man to buy a fast, shiny sports car if he wants, even if he may have to stretch beyond his budget.

38. A man should never doubt his own judgment.
39. A man shouldn't have to worry about birth control.
40. A man shouldn't bother with sex unless he can achieve an orgasm.
41. A man should avoid holding his wife's purse at all times.
42. There are some subjects which men should not talk about with other men.
43. Men should always take the initiative when it comes to sex.
44. Fathers should teach their sons to mask fear.
45. Being a little down in the dumps is not a good reason for a man to act depressed.
46. A man should always be ready for sex.
47. Boys should not throw baseballs like girls.
48. If a man is in pain, it's better for him to let people know than to keep it to himself.
49. Men should get up to investigate if there is a strange noise in the house at night.
50. A man should think things out logically and have good reasons for what he does.
51. For a man, sex should always be spontaneous, rather than a pre-planned activity.
52. A man who has no taste for adventure is not very appealing.
53. It is not important for men to strive to reach the top.
54. For men, touching is simply the first step toward sex.
55. A man should always be the major provider in his family.
56. A man should be level-headed.
57. Men should be detached in emotionally charged situations.

Source. This scale was originally published in "Masculinity Ideology: A Comparison Between U.S. and Chinese Young Men and Women," by R. F. Levant, R. Wu, and J. Fischer, 1996, *Journal of Gender, Culture, and Health, 1,* 217-220. Reprinted with permission.

a. Each item is followed by a 7-point scale.

Hypermasculinity Inventory

Donald L. Mosher,[1] *University of Connecticut*

The Hypermasculinity Inventory was developed to measure a macho personality constellation consisting of three components: (a) callous sexual attitudes toward women, (b) violence as manly, and (c) danger as exciting. The construct of the macho personality is viewed as a script—a set of rules, magnified by affect, for predicting, interpreting, controlling, and evaluating a family of related scenes—developed through socialization and enculturation. It is assumed that parents' use of contempt and humiliation to control their son's fear and distress during childhood, together with the boy's excitement and pride in mastery of fear and distress, produces a boy who is unusually receptive to the socially inherited script of macho as warrior and hero deserving dominion over inferiors.

[1]Address correspondence to Donald L. Mosher, 5051 North A1a, PH1-1s, North Hutchinson Island, FL 34949; email: dlmosher@aol.com.

Description

The Hypermasculinity Inventory consists of 30 forced-choice items that can be divided into three 10-item subscales: (a) Callous Sexual Attitudes, (b) Violence as Manly, and (c) Danger as Exciting. The latent variable, the macho personality pattern, is a relatively homogeneous factor (Mosher & Sirkin, 1984) and should be used as a single scale unless the nature of the research indicates the wisdom of considering subscale scores.

Response Mode and Timing

Respondents circle the number of the preferred alternative in each pair or respond on a machine-scorable answer sheet. Approximately 13 minutes are required for completion.

Scoring

The score for macho is the number of macho alternatives selected from 30 forced-choice pairs. The number of the macho alternative is italicized following the item-pair numbers that appear after the subscale designation. Callous Sexual Attitudes: 4-*2*, 9-*1*, 11-*2*, 13-*1*, 14-*2*, 15-*1*, 24-*1*, 25-*1*, 26-*2*, and 28-*2*; Violence as Manly: 3-*2*, 6-*2*, 8-*2*, 12-*2*, 18-*2*, 19-*1*, 20-*1*, 21-*1*, 29-*1*, and 30-*1*; and Danger as Exciting: 1-*2*, 2-*1*, 5-*1*, 7-*1*, 10-*1*, 16-*1*, 17-*2*, 22-*2*, 23-*2*, and 27-*2*.

Reliability

Mosher and Sirkin (1984), with a sample of 135 college men, reported a Cronbach alpha of .89, a mean of 11.03, and a standard deviation of 6.79 for the macho score from the 30 forced-choice items. The respective means, standard deviations, and Cronbach alpha coefficients for the three subscales were as follows: Callous, 3.33, 2.63, and .79; Violence, 3.84, 2.84, and .79; and Danger, 3.87, 2.44, and .71.

Validity

The Hypermasculinity Inventory is a theoretical extension of earlier research on callous sexual attitudes toward women (Kier, 1972; Mosher, 1971a, 1971b), which provided some evidence for the validity of that construct. Scores from the Hypermasculinity Inventory were significantly correlated with self-reported drug use, aggressive behavior and dangerous driving following alcohol consumption, delinquent behavior during the high school years (Mosher & Sirkin, 1984), and aggressive sexual behavior (Mosher & Anderson, 1986). Construct validity of the Hypermasculinity Inventory as a measure of a macho personality pattern was supported by a predicted pattern of correlations with the Jackson (1974) *Personality Research Form* (Mosher & Sirkin, 1984) and by macho men's reports of less affective disgust, anger, fear, distress, shame, contempt, and guilt while imagining committing realistic, violent rape (Mosher & Anderson, 1986).

References

Jackson, D. N. (1974). *Personality Research Form–Form E*. Goshen, NY: Research Psychologist's Press.

Kier, R. G. (1942). *Sex, individual differences, and film effects on responses to sexual films*. Unpublished doctoral dissertation, University of Connecticut, Storrs.

Mosher, D. L. (1971a). Psychological reactions to pornographic films. In *Technical report of the Commission on Obscenity and Pornography: Erotica and social behavior* (Vol. 8, pp. 255-312). Washington, DC: Government Printing Office.

Mosher, D. L. (1971b). Sex callousness toward women. In *Technical report of the Commission on Obscenity and Pornography: Erotica and social behavior* (Vol. 8, pp. 313-325). Washington, DC: Government Printing Office.

Mosher, D. L., & Anderson, R. D. (1986). Macho personality, sexual aggression, and reactions to guided imagery of realistic rape. *Journal of Research in Personality, 20*(2), 77-94.

Mosher, D. L., & Sirkin, M. (1984). Measuring in a macho personality constellation. *Journal of Research in Personality, 18*, 150-164.

Exhibit

Hypermasculinity Inventory

Instructions: This inventory consists of 30 forced-choice items designed to measure controversial attitudes and beliefs. It is arranged in a forced-choice format in which you are asked to select one of two alternatives as true or more true for you. Sometimes it may be difficult to agree with either alternative as neither may seem very desirable to you. Or, it may be that you agree with both alternatives, but you are still asked to select the one item that most represents you and your opinion. The forced-choice format solves some technical problems of measurement, but it is not always subjectively comfortable to complete. Although you are, of course, free to refuse to answer any item, the scientific purposes of the research are best fulfilled through your cooperation. In addition, the language used in some of the alternatives might be considered offensive or even obscene by some men. Others may find the language representative of comments overheard in all male groups. It is not the authors' intent to offend anyone's sensibility or to endorse any of the alternative attitudes and beliefs herein as scientifically or socially valid. Rather, the intent of the inventory is to measure your personal preferences in order to investigate personality, attitudes, and behavior in a domain specific to men.

Before being asked to complete this inventory, a competent and ethical researcher will have obtained your informed consent and provided for anonymity or confidentiality of responses. Your debriefing should specifically refer to the nature of this inventory and respond to any concerns, attitudes, or feelings inspired by it. Please use the accompanying answer sheet to record your answers.

1.
   1. After I've gone through a really dangerous experience my knees feel weak and I shake all over.
   2. After I've gone through a really dangerous experience I feel high.
2.
   1. I'd rather gamble than play it safe.
   2. I'd rather play it safe than gamble.
3.
   1. Call me a name and I'll pretend not to hear you.
   2. Call me a name and I'll call you another.

4. 1. Fair is fair in love and war.
    2. All is fair in love and war.
5. 1. I like wild, uninhibited parties.
    2. I like quiet parties with good conversations.
6. 1. I hope to forget past unpleasant experiences with male aggression.
    2. I still enjoy remembering my first real fight.
7. 1. Some people tell me I take foolish risks.
    2. Some people have told me I ought to take more chances.
8. 1. So-called effeminate men are more artistic and sensitive.
    2. Effeminate men deserve to be ridiculed.
9. 1. Get a woman drunk, high, or hot and she'll let you do whatever you want.
    2. It's gross and unfair to use alcohol and drugs to convince a woman to have sex.
10. 1. I like fast cars and fast women.
    2. I like dependable cars and faithful women.
11. 1. So-called prick teasers should be forgiven.
    2. Prick teasers should be raped.
12. 1. When I have a few drinks under by belt, I mellow out.
    2. When I have a few drinks under my belt, I look for trouble.
13. 1. Any man who is a man needs to have sex regularly.
    2. Any man who is a man can do without sex.
14. 1. All women, even women's libbers, are worthy of respect.
    2. The only woman worthy of respect is your own mother.
15. 1. You have to fuck some women before they know who's boss.
    2. You have to love some women before they know you don't want to be boss.
16. 1. When I have a drink or two I feel ready for whatever happens.
    2. When I have a drink or two I like to relax and enjoy myself.
17. 1. Risk has to be weighed against possible maximum loss.
    2. There is no such thing as too big a risk, if the payoff is large enough.
18. 1. I win by not fighting.
    2. I fight to win.
19. 1. It's natural for men to get into fights.
    2. Physical violence never solves an issue.
20. 1. If you're not prepared to fight for what's yours, then be prepared to lose it.
    2. Even if I feel like fighting, I try to think of alternatives.
21. 1. He who can, fights; he who can't, runs away.
    2. It's just plain dumb to fist fight.
22. 1. When I'm bored I watch TV or read a book.
    2. When I'm bored I look for excitement.
23. 1. I like to drive safely avoiding all possible risks.
    2. I like to drive fast, right on the edge of danger.
24. 1. Pick-ups should expect to put out.
    2. So-called pick-ups should choose their men carefully.
25. 1. Some women are good for only one thing.
    2. All women deserve the same respect as your own mother.
26. 1. I only want to have sex with women who are in total agreement.
    2. I never feel bad about my tactics when I have sex.
27. 1. I would rather be a famous scientist than a famous prizefighter.
    2. I would rather be a famous prizefighter than a famous scientist.
28. 1. Lesbians choose a particular lifestyle and should be respected for it.
    2. The only thing a lesbian needs is a good, stiff cock.
29. 1. If you are chosen for a fight, there's no choice but to fight.
    2. If you are chosen for a fight, it's time to talk your way out of it.
30. 1. If you insult me, be prepared to back it up.
    2. If you insult me, I'll try to turn the other cheek.

Negative Attitudes Toward Masturbation

Donald L. Mosher,[1] *University of Connecticut*

Abramson and Mosher (1975) developed an inventory, Attitudes Toward Masturbation, as a measure of negative attitudes toward masturbation, to measure the construct of masturbation-guilt (Mosher, 1979b; Mosher & Vonderheide, 1985). Although the inventory is regarded as a homogeneous measure, a factor analysis conducted for descriptive purposes found three factors: (a) positive attitudes toward masturbation, (b) false beliefs about the harmful nature of masturbation, and (c) personally experienced negative affects associated with masturbation (Abramson & Mosher, 1975). Masturbation-guilt is regarded as a script—a set for rules for ordering a coassembled family of scenes—learned scenes in which the negative affects of guilt, disgust, shame, and fear have reciprocally interacted with cognitions about masturbation (including general fantasies and sex myths). Masturbation-guilt, as a script, predicts, interprets, regulates, and evaluates conduct in scenes entailing masturbation or in scenes associatively linked through family resemblance of affect, objects, or scene features to past of imagined masturbatory scenes.

Description

This inventory is a 30-item (10 of which have reversed scoring), 5-point Likert-type scale anchored by *not at all true* and *extremely true*. Because items were taken from college respondents' responses to open-ended questions about the consequences of masturbation (Abramson, 1973), the items are useful with educated populations of men and women.

Response Mode and Timing

Respondents can circle the number indicating the relative truth of the statement for them, but the more common scoring has had them indicate response choices on machine-scorable answer sheets. The scale requires approximately 7 minutes to complete.

Scoring

The 10 items with reversed scoring are 3, 5, 8, 11, 13, 14, 17, 22, 27, and 29. To obtain an index of masturbation-guilt, scores are summed to yield a score from 30 to 150.

Reliability

A corrected split-half reliability of .75 was reported for the original sample of 198 male and female college students (Abramson & Mosher, 1975). A Cronbach alpha of .94 was found for a sample of 186 college women (Mosher & Vonderheide, 1985).

Validity

The scale has successfully predicted decreased frequency and lower percentage of orgasm to masturbatory behavior (Abramson & Mosher, 1975; Mosher & O'Grady, 1979); less subjective sexual arousal and more negative affective responses to explicit films of male and female masturbation (Mosher & Abramson, 1977); less positive projective stories to films of masturbation (Abramson & Mosher, 1979); less subjective sexual arousal and more negative affects to films of male homosexuality and male masturbation (Mosher & O'Grady, 1979); less pelvic vasocongestion, as measured by thermography, in women reading an erotic story (Abramson, Perry, Rothblatt, Seeley, & Seeley, 1981); more negative affect when recalling a memory of past masturbation (Green & Mosher, 1985); and more negative attitudes toward contraceptives and avoidance of selecting the diaphragm as a method of birth control (Mosher & Vonderheide, 1985). Although masturbation-guilt and sex-guilt (Mosher, 1966, 1968, 1979a) can be viewed as measuring a latent construct of *guilt over sexuality,* there is also evidence of discriminant validity from sex-guilt (which is a more general sexual script) in a number of the studies cited above.

References

Abramson, P. R. (1973). The relationship of the frequency of masturbation to several aspects of behavior. *The Journal of Sex Research, 9,* 132-142.

Abramson, P. R., & Mosher, D. L. (1975). The development of a measure of negative attitudes toward masturbation. *Journal of Consulting and Clinical Psychology, 43,* 485-490.

Abramson, P. R., & Mosher, D. L. (1979). Am empirical investigation of experimentally induced masturbatory fantasies. *Archives of Sexual Behavior, 8,* 24-39.

Abramson, P. R., Perry, L. B., Rothblatt, A., Seeley, T. T., & Seeley, D. M. (1981). Negative attitudes toward masturbation and pelvic vasocongestion: A thermographic analysis. *Journal of Research in Personality, 15,* 497-509.

Green, S. E., & Mosher, D. L. (1985). A causal model of arousal to erotic fantasies. *The Journal of Sex Research, 21,* 1-23.

Mosher, D. L. (1966). The development and multitrait-multimethod matrix analysis of three measures of three aspects of guilt. *Journal of Consulting Psychology, 30,* 35-39.

Mosher, D. L. (1968). Measurement of guilt in females by self-report inventories. *Journal of Consulting and Clinical Psychology, 32,* 690-695.

Mosher, D. L. (1979a). The meaning and measurement of guilt. In C. E. Izard (Ed.), *Emotions in personality and psychopathology* (pp. 105-129). New York: Plenum.

Mosher, D. L. (1979b). Negative attitudes toward masturbation in sex therapy. *Journal of Sex & Marital Therapy, 5,* 315-333.

[1]Address correspondence to Donald L. Mosher, 5051 North A1a, PH1-1, North Hutchinson Island, FL 34949; email: dlmosher@aol.com.

Mosher, D. L., & Abramson, P. R. (1977). Subjective sexual arousal to films of masturbation. *Journal of Consulting and Clinical Psychology, 45,* 796-807.

Mosher, D. L., & O'Grady, K. E. (1979). Homosexual threat, negative attitudes toward masturbation, sex guilt, and male's sexual and affective reactions to explicit sexual films. *Journal of Consulting and Clinical Psychology, 47,* 860-873.

Mosher, D. L., & Vonderheide, S. G. (1985). Contributions of sex guilt and masturbation guilt to women's contraceptive attitudes and use. *The Journal of Sex Research, 21,* 24-39.

Exhibit

Attitudes Toward Masturbation

The following 30 items sample diverse opinions and attitudes about masturbation. Masturbation means stimulating your own genitals to enjoy the pleasurable sensations or experience orgasm. Answers are to be marked on the separate answer sheet. Marking 1 means the item is *not at all true for you;* marking 2 means it is *somewhat untrue;* marking 3 means you are *undecided;* marking 4 means it is *somewhat true;* marking 5 means it is *strongly true for you.*

1. People masturbate to escape feelings of tension and anxiety.
2. People who masturbate will not enjoy sexual intercourse as much as those who refrain from masturbation.
3. Masturbation is a private matter which neither harms nor concerns anyone else.
4. Masturbation is a sin against yourself.
5. Masturbation in childhood can help a person develop a natural, healthy attitude toward sex.
6. Masturbation in an adult is juvenile and immature.
7. Masturbation can lead to homosexuality.
8. Excessive masturbation is physically impossible, as it is a needless worry.
9. If you enjoy masturbating too much, you may never learn to relate to the opposite sex.
10. After masturbating, a person feels degraded.
11. Experience with masturbation can potentially help a woman become orgasic in sexual intercourse.
12. I feel guilty about masturbating.
13. Masturbation can be a "friend in need" when there is no "friend in deed."
14. Masturbation can provide an outlet for sex fantasies without harming anyone else or endangering oneself.
15. Excessive masturbation can lead to problems of impotence in men and frigidity in women.
16. Masturbation is an escape mechanism which prevents a person from developing a mature sexual outlook.
17. Masturbation can provide harmless relief from sexual tension.
18. Playing with your own genitals is disgusting.
19. Excessive masturbation is associated with neurosis, depression, and behavioral problems.
20. Any masturbation is too much.
21. Masturbation is a compulsive, addictive habit which once begun is almost impossible to stop.
22. Masturbation is fun.
23. When I masturbate, I am disgusted with myself.
24. A pattern of frequent masturbation is associated with introversion and withdrawal from social contacts.
25. I would be ashamed to admit publicly that I have masturbated.
26. Excessive masturbation leads to mental dullness and fatigue.
27. Masturbation is a normal sexual outlet.
28. Masturbation is caused by an excessive preoccupation with thoughts about sex.
29. Masturbation can teach you to enjoy the sensuousness of your own body.
30. After I masturbate, I am disgusted with myself for losing control of my body.

Postcoronary Sexual Activity

The Editors

The purpose of this instrument is to examine correlations between knowledge of cardiac problems and sexual activity of wives of men who have had heart attacks, and the wife's anxiety. The questionnaire includes items requesting demographic data and information regarding the husband's heart attack, a knowledge scale, and an anxiety inventory. Respondents are asked to indicate the truth or falsity of 16 general statements concerning normal and abnormal physiological responses to sexual arousal and exertion, the relative cardiac costs of different types of exercise, and the influence of emotional and other factors concerning postcoronary sexual functioning and activity.

Speilberger's (1970) State-Trait Anxiety Inventory was adapted to measure degree of anxiety felt in a specific situation. Wives are asked to use "when thinking about sexual relations with your husband" as the situation about which to report their anxiety.

Reference

Speilberger, C. (1970). *State-Trait Anxiety Inventory (STAI) manual*. Palo Alto, CA: Consulting Psychologists' Press.

Weinstein, S. A., & Como, J. (1980). The relationship between knowledge and anxiety about postcoronary sexual activity among wives of postcoronary males. *The Journal of Sex Research, 16,* 316-324.

The Adolescent Menstrual Attitude Questionnaire

Janice M. Morse,[1] *Pennsylvania State University*
Dianne Kieren, *University of Alberta*
Joan L. Bottorff, *University of British Columbia*

The Adolescent Menstrual Attitude Questionnaire (AMAQ) is an age-appropriate, 5-point Likert-type instrument designed to measure adolescent attitudes toward menstruation. The scale is available in two forms, one for premenarcheal and the other for postmenarcheal girls. Each form consists of 58 items (43 parallel items and 11 unique items). Factor analysis revealed six subscales: Positive Feelings, Negative Feelings, Openness Toward Menarche, Living With Menstruation, Acceptance of Menarche, and Menstrual Symptoms.

Description

The initial scales were developed from a qualitative study of 135 adolescents (Morse & Doan, 1987). Content analysis of these data revealed five dimensions: a negative re-

sponse to menstruation, a natural/accepting response to menstruation, an excited/anticipatory response toward menstruation and maturing, a response to menstrual symptoms, and a response to managing symptoms. The original 93-item pool for the Pre- and Postmenarcheal scales was developed from these qualitative data, ensuring the language was age appropriate. The scale was reviewed by seven experts in adolescence or menstruation for appropriateness (Lynn, 1986), and seven items were discarded.

The two 86-item instruments were tested on all consenting girls enrolled in Grades 6-9 in 49 randomly selected schools in a major Canadian city (Morse, Kieren, & Bottorff, 1993). A total of 860 premenarcheal girls and 1,013 postmenarcheal girls completed the questionnaires. Discriminant analysis revealed that 22 items primarily distinguished between the pre- and postmenarcheal respondents, but that parallel versions would impair the validity of the scale. Thus, the final versions of each scale consist of 58 items, with 47 items common to both forms (Items 1-47), and 11 unique items (Items 48-58).

[1]Address correspondence to Janice M. Morse, Pennsylvania State University, 307 East Health & Human Development, University Park, PA 16802; email: jmm17@email.psu.edu.

Principal components factor analysis with orthogonal varimax rotation of the factor analysis resulted in a six-factor solution for both pre- and postmenarcheal data. The subscales replicated the dimensions identified by Morse and Doan (1987), confirming construct validity. Managing Menstruation, however, was identified as two subscales in this analysis: Living With Menstruation and Openness Toward Menstruation.

Response Mode and Timing

The AMAQ is available in machine-readable format and takes approximately 30 minutes to complete. Respondents are seated so they cannot view one another's answers, are given both forms (the pre- and the postmenarcheal), and asked to select the appropriate form to complete.

Scoring

Items are scored 1 for *strongly disagree* to 5 for *strongly agree,* with the exception of the reversed items. Reversed items common to both scales are as follows: 1, 3, 5, 6, 7, 8, 10, 11, 16, 17, 18, 20, 23, 25, 27, 29, 30, 31, 33, 34, 35, 38, 41, 42, and 44. Those items that are also reversed on the Premenarcheal Scale only are: 48, 50, 52, 53, 55, 56, and 57. On the Postmenarcheal Scale additional reversed items are: 48, 49, 53, 54, 57, and 58. Subscale items are listed in Table 1.

Reliability

Total test reliability was .91 for the Premenarcheal Scale and .90 for the Postmenarcheal Scale. Reliability for each subscale was estimated using coefficient alpha to determine internal consistency and the Spearman-Brown prophecy formula to estimate reliabilities of scales with equal length, which, in this case, projected to 18 items. These ranged from .79 to .93 for subscales on the Premenarcheal form and from .83 to .90 for subscales on the Postmenarcheal form (Morse et al., 1993).

Validity

Using discriminant analysis, 90% of the cases were correctly identified—91% of the premenarcheal and 88% of the postmenarcheal respondents. A Wilks's lambda of 0.40 supports the hypothesis that the responses of the two samples are unique.

As previously discussed, validity of the subscales was supported by comparing the results of the factor analysis with the results of the content analysis from the previous qualitative study. The factor structure is shown in Table 1. Additionally, factor analysis comparing the pre- and postmenarcheal data revealed that the factors loaded in different order, providing additional evidence that there is a qualitative difference between the pre- and the postmenarcheal girls.

Other Information

Additional information regarding scale development can be found in Morse et al. (1993). Normative scores for the

Table 1 Items and Percentage Variance Contributed for Each Factor Structure: Pre- and Postmenarcheal Versions

Factor (no. of items)	Items	% Variance
Positive feelings		
Pre (12)	2, 4, 15, 21, 24, 26, 28, 32, 43, 45, 47, 55	17
Post (11)	2, 4, 21, 24, 26, 28, 32, 43, 45, 47, 52	15
Negative feelings		
Pre (17)	1, 5, 6, 7, 8, 10, 11, 18, 23, 27, 33, 41, 42, 44, 48, 52, 57	7
Post (18)	1, 5, 6, 7, 8, 10, 11, 18, 23, 33, 39, 40, 41, 42, 44, 49, 54, 57	7
Living with menstruation		
Pre (10)	12, 17, 25, 29. 35, 46, 50, 53, 54, 56	5
Post (8)	12, 17, 25, 29, 35, 46, 53, 58	3
Openness		
Pre (6)	3, 9, 16, 22, 38, 39	3
Post (5)	3, 9, 16, 22, 38	2
Acceptance of menarche		
Pre (8)	13, 19, 36, 37, 40, 49, 51, 58	3
Post (7)	13, 15, 19, 27, 36, 37, 55	4
Menstrual symptoms		
Pre (5)	14, 20, 30, 31, 34	3
Post (9)	14, 20, 30, 31, 34, 48, 50, 51, 56	6

total scale and for each subscale by age and by grade have also been published (Morse & Kieren, 1993). The scale also has been used to explore readiness for menstruation (see Kieren, in press; Kieren & Morse, 1992).

Permission to use the AMAQ may be obtained from J. Morse. Copyright permissions may be obtained from Taylor & Francis, Inc., 1101 Vermont Ave., NW, Ste. 200, Washington, DC 20005.

We acknowledge the assistance of G. Ewing, J. Innes, G. Ewing, P. Donahue, and B. McMahaffey, University of Alberta, and H. Doan, York University, in the development of these scales. Support was provided by a grant from the University of Alberta Central Research Fund to J. Innes.

References

Kieren, D. K. (in press). Developmental factors and pre- and post-menarcheal menstrual attitudes. *Canadian Home Economics Journal.*

Kieren, D. K., & Morse, J. M. (1992). Preparation factors and menstrual attitudes of pre- and post-menarcheal girls. *Journal of Sex Education and Therapy, 18,* 155-174.

Lynn, M. R. (1986). Determination and quantification of content validity. *Nursing Research, 35,* 382-385.

Morse, J. M., & Doan, H. M. (1987). Growing up at school: Adolescents' response to menarche. *Journal of School Health, 57,* 385-389.

Morse, J. M., & Kieren, D. (1993). The Adolescent Menstrual Attitude Questionnaire, Part II: Normative scores. *Health Care for Women International, 14,* 63-76.

Morse, J. M., Kieren, D., & Bottorff, J. (1993). The Adolescent Menstrual Attitude Questionnaire, Part 1: Scale construction. *Health Care for Women International, 14,* 39-62.

Exhibit

The Adolescent Menstrual Attitude Questionnaire[a]

Answer this questionnaire if you *have* or *have had* your period.

Grade _____ Age _____

Birthdate _____

Have you had your first period?   Yes   No

If yes, your age when your first period started: Years _____   Months _____

Instructions

Next is a questionnaire concerning how girls feel about *menstruation,* which is another word for your *period.* We will be asking you to indicate how much you agree, or disagree, with each statement, like this:

1. I think boys should be told everything about girls' periods.

    SD means that you *strongly* disagree with the statement.
    D means that you disagree with the statement, but you do not strongly disagree.
    N means that you don't care, are not sure, or do not know.
    A means that you agree with the statement.
    SA means that you *strongly* agree with the statement.

Now, think about the statement, and fill in the circle next to the statement that is *your own opinion.* There are no right or wrong answers. We are only interested in what *you* think. You do not have to answer any question that you do not want to. If you decide not to answer any questions at all, that's fine too, but we ask you to go to the other activity room.

Please *do not* put your name on this form. These answers are your own personal opinions, and we consider your feelings private.

1. When I am having my period, I am scared that the boys will find out.
2. It makes me feel very happy to know that I am menstruating.
3. I have not told anyone that my periods have started.
4. I was happy when I found out about menstruation.
5. I worry that one day I might not notice that I'm bleeding.
6. Most girls are bothered by buying pads or tampons at school or at a store.
7. Just the fact that I have my period makes me uncomfortable.
8. I was scared stiff when my first period started.
9. I often talk about periods with my friends.
10. I worry a lot about my periods starting unexpectedly.
11. Girls do not like to be seen putting pads in the garbage.
12. It is normal for girls to menstruate.
13. I do not feel any different than usual when I menstruate.
14. Girls who say they feel sick when they have their periods are just making excuses.
15. I will feel okay when I get my period.
16. When I talk with my friends about periods, I feel uncomfortable about it.
17. When girls have their period, they should be allowed to stay home.
18. Girls worry a lot that blood will leak through their clothes.
19. I quickly got used to having my periods.
20. Menstruating girls are grumpy and tense.
21. I couldn't wait to get my first period.
22. I like to talk about periods with my friends.

23. It's embarrassing to ask questions about periods.
24. When I have my period, I feel good.
25. Girls with periods should avoid exercise.
26. I feel excited when I get my period.
27. I feel scared because I don't know what is happening when I have my period.
28. I feel very grown up when I have my period.
29. When girls have their periods, they should not shampoo their hair.
30. Girls are often grouchy when they have their periods.
31. When I get my period, I feel sick.
32. I feel pleased when I think of having a period.
33. I am terrified that people will find out when I have my period.
34. Girls feel moody when they get their period.
35. Girls who get cramps with their period should worry that something is wrong with them.
36. Coping with periods is easy.
37. Most girls understand what is happening to their body when they get a period.
38. Girls feel uncomfortable studying about menstruation at school.
39. I feel it's OK to discuss periods with boys.
40. Girls do not mind buying pads.
41. I feel people can tell when I have my period.
42. Every time someone mentions "period," I get nervous.
43. I am glad I have grown mature enough to menstruate.
44. Most girls find that getting a pad from a machine in a public washroom is very embarrassing.
45. I feel special when I have my period.
46. It is OK to swim when you have your period.
47. I feel proud when I have my period.
48. Cramps during my period are very painful.
49. When you have your period, it is important to act cool so no one will know.
50. Girls get severe backaches with their periods.
51. When girls get their periods, they often feel like throwing up.
52. When I began having my period, I changed into a woman.
53. It's OK to miss school if you have cramps with your period.
54. I feel ugly and gross when I have my period.
55. When I am menstruating, I feel the same.
56. Girls cry more easily when they have their period.
57. Girls dislike touching themselves to change their pads or tampons.
58. When girls get their periods, they should be excused from gym.

Have you thought of anything you would like to ask us?

The Adolescent Menstrual Attitude Questionnaire (premenstrual version)

Answer this questionnaire if you have *never had* your period.

1. When I have my period, I will be scared that the boys will find out.
2. It will make me feel very happy to know that I am finally menstruating.
3. I will not tell anyone when my period starts.
4. I was happy when I found out about menstruation.
5. I worry that one day I might not notice that I'm bleeding.
6. Most girls are bothered by buying pads or tampons at school or at a store.
7. I think I will feel uncomfortable when I have my period.
8. I am scared stiff at the thought of my period starting.
9. I often talk about periods with my friends.
10. I worry a lot about my periods starting.
11. Girls do not like to be seen putting pads in the garbage.
12. It is normal for girls to menstruate.
13. I will not feel any different than usual when I menstruate.

14. Girls who say they feel sick when they have their periods are just making excuses.
15. I will feel okay when I get my period.
16. When I talk with my friends about periods, I feel uncomfortable about it.
17. When girls have their period, they should be allowed to stay home.
18. Girls worry a lot that blood will leak through their clothes.
19. I will get used to periods very quickly.
20. Menstruating girls are grumpy and tense.
21. I look forward to getting my period.
22. I like to talk about periods with my friends.
23. It's embarrassing to ask questions about periods.
24. When I get my period, I will feel good.
25. Girls with periods should avoid exercise.
26. I will feel excited when I get my period.
27. I feel scared because I don't know what will happen when I get my period.
28. I will feel very grown up when I have my period.
29. When girls have their periods, they should not shampoo their hair.
30. Girls are often grouchy when they have their periods.
31. When I get my period, I expect I will feel sick.
32. I feel pleased when I think of starting my period.
33. When I start having my period, I am terrified that people will find out.
34. I expect to feel moody when I get my period.
35. Girls who get cramps with their period should worry that something is wrong with them.
36. Coping with periods is easy.
37. Most girls understand what is happening to their body when they get a period.
38. Girls feel uncomfortable studying about menstruation at school.
39. I feel it's OK to discuss periods with boys.
40. Girls do not mind buying pads.
41. When I get my period, I will worry that people will be able to tell.
42. Every time someone mentions "period," I get nervous.
43. I am glad I am growing mature enough to menstruate.
44. Most girls find that getting a pad from a machine in a public washroom is very embarrassing.
45. I will feel special when I get my period.
46. It is OK to swim when you have your period.
47. I will feel proud when I get my period.
48. The thought of getting my period is hard to get used to.
49. I do not care if my period starts or not.
50. I think I will walk differently when I am menstruating.
51. Getting my period will be no big deal.
52. I think periods are very dirty.
53. Girls who have their periods should not take a bath.
54. When girls have their periods, they should shower more frequently.
55. Having a period is a big nuisance.
56. Girls avoid talking to anyone about their concerns regarding periods.
57. I will feel shocked when my period begins.
58. Most girls understand exactly what to do when they get their first period.

Source. From *Health Care for Women International*, 1993, 14(1), 39-62, 63-76, published by Taylor & Francis, Inc., Washington, DC. Reproduced with permission. All rights reserved.

a. The formatting of the machine-readable form has been altered for this display. Also, only the text of the 58 items for the premenstrual version of the questionnaire is shown.

Hurlbert Index of Sexual Narcissism

David F. Hurlbert,[1] *Adult and Adolescent Counseling Center*

The Hurlbert Index of Sexual Narcissism (HISN) is described by Hurlbert, Apt, Gasar, Wilson, and Murphy (1994).

[1]Address correspondence to David F. Hurlbert, Adult and Adolescent Counseling Center, 619 North Main, Belton, TX 76513.

Reference

Hurlbert, D. F., Apt, C., Gasar, S., Wilson, N. E., & Murphy, Y. (1994). Sexual narcissism: A validation study. *Journal of Sex & Marital Therapy, 20,* 24-34.

Exhibit

Hurlbert Index of Sexual Narcissism

1. In sex, I like to be the one in charge.
2. My partner has difficulty understanding my sexual needs.
3. In general, most people take sex too seriously.
4. When it comes to sex, I consider myself a knowledgeable person.
5. In a close relationship, sex is an entitlement.
6. I believe I have a special style of making love.
7. I think people have the right to do anything they please in sex.
8. My partner tends to place too many emotional demands on me.
9. Pleasing yourself in sex is most important because it is hard to please someone sexually if you do not know how to please yourself first.
10. A relationship can keep one from engaging in a lot of fulfilling sexual activities.
11. Not enough people have sex for fun anymore.
12. I have no sexual inhibitions.
13. Too much relationship closeness can interfere with sexual pleasure.
14. In certain situations, sexually cheating on a partner is justifiable.
15. I think I am better at sex than most people my age.
16. In a close relationship, I would expect my partner to fulfill my sexual wishes.
17. My partner seldom gives me the sexual praise I deserve.
18. In a relationship where I commit myself, sex is a right.
19. In order to have a good sexual relationship, at least one partner needs to take charge.
20. Relationships that are too close are often too demanding.
21. When it comes to sex, not enough people live for the moment.
22. I know some pretty unique sexual techniques.
23. Emotional closeness can easily get in the way of sexual pleasure.
24. Couples should leave a relationship when they find sex to no longer be enjoyable.
25. In a close relationship, if a sexual act feels good, it is right.

Source. This index was originally published in "Sexual Narcissism: A Validation Study," by D. F. Hurlbert, C. Apt, N. E. Wilson, and Y. Murphy, 1994, *Journal of Sex & Marital Therapy, 20,* 24-34. Reprinted with permission.

Note. Respondents are asked to write in their choices. Scoring is based on the following choices: SA = *I strongly agree* (+4); A = *I agree* (+3); U = *I am undecided* (+2); D = *I disagree* (+1); SD = *I strongly disagree* (+0). Scores range from 0 to 100, with higher scores corresponding to greater sexual narcissism.

Topless Behavior Attitude Scale

Edward S. Herold[1] and Bruna Corbesi, *University of Guelph*
John Collins, *Macquarie University*

In some cultural contexts, it is acceptable for women not to wear a swimsuit top in public, whereas in other cultural contexts it is not acceptable. However, even in countries where there is acceptance of topless behavior on public beaches, there can still be a lack of agreement concerning the norms of propriety about going topless. For example, in Australia it is acceptable for women to go topless at some beaches but not at others. Even at beaches where going topless is accepted, many women choose not to go topless. Our objective was to develop a topless attitude scale that would capture the key attitudinal issues regarding topless behavior.

Description and Response Mode

The scale is an eight-item Likert type (4-point), with response options labeled from *strongly agree* to *strongly disagree*. Respondents are asked to circle the number indicating their agreement or disagreement with each item.

[1]Address correspondence to Edward S. Herold, Department of Family Studies, College of Family and Consumer Studies, University of Guelph, Ontario N1G 2W1, Canada; email: eherold@facs.uoguelph.ca.

Timing and Scoring

The scale requires an average of 2-3 minutes for completion. Negatively worded items are recoded by reversing their scores. The eight items are summed to produce an overall score. Higher scores indicate more favorable attitudes about women's topless behavior.

Reliability and Validity

With a sample of 116 female psychology students attending Macquarie University in Sydney, Australia, Herold, Corbesi, and Collins (1994) found that the Cronbach alpha coefficient of reliability was .79. Validity was indicated by significant correlations with two measures of topless behavior. The scale had a Pearson correlation of .48 with the behavioral measure of whether the women had ever been topless at a public beach and a correlation of .52 with an index combining different situations of going topless.

Reference

Herold, E. S., Corbesi, B., & Collins, J. (1994). Psychosocial aspects of female topless behavior on Australian beaches. *The Journal of Sex Research, 31,* 133-142.

Exhibit

Topless Behavior Attitude Scale

1. Women should have the same right to go topless as men.
2. Going topless has nothing to do with sex.
3. Going topless gives women a sense of personal freedom.
4. Going topless is a sign of decaying moral values.
5. Topless women are more likely to arouse sexual feelings in men.
6. Going topless is a greater sign of liberation for women.
7. Women who go topless are more likely to be sexually assaulted.
8. Topless women are exhibitionists.

Causal Attribution for Coital Orgasm Scale

Joseph W. Critelli,[1] *North Texas State University*
Charles F. Bridges, *Terrill State Hospital, Terrill, Texas*
Victor E. Loos, *Galveston Family Institute*

The Causal Attribution for Coital Orgasm Scale is designed to evaluate causal attributions for orgasm and nonorgasm during sexual intercourse.

Description

This scale was developed to evaluate attributions of coital outcomes, along the two major attributional dimensions identified by Weiner (1979; Weiner & Kukla, 1970): internal versus external, and stable versus unstable. The scale uses a paired-comparison forced-choice format as suggested by McMahan (1973), Weiner, Nierenberg, and Goldstein (1976), and Girodo, Dotzenroth, and Stein (1981). The labels in the questionnaire were judged to translate most adequately Weiner's notions of ability (internal-stable), effort (internal-unstable), task difficulty (external-stable), and luck (external-unstable). For both orgasmic and nonorgasmic coital outcomes, respondents are presented with every possible pairing of causal attributions. With four attributional categories (internal-stable, internal-unstable, external-stable, external-unstable), this yields two sets of six forced-choice options. Whether respondents refer to simultaneous clitoral stimulation does not seem to affect causal attributions (Loos, Bridges, & Critelli, 1987). The scale is designed for use with women who have had at least 15 coital contacts and have experienced coital orgasm at least one time.

Response Mode and Timing

Respondents place a check mark in front of the one choice in each pair of choices that they believe is more accurate for them. The questionnaire requires no more than 10 minutes to complete.

Scoring

One point is credited for each check mark; no points are given for unchecked items. For both Question I (orgasm) and Question II (nonorgasm), items are summed to form an attributional score (ranging from 0 to 3) for each of the four causal categories, as follows: internal-stable (1a + 4b + 5b); internal-unstable (1b + 2a + 6a); external-stable (2b + 3a + 5a); and external unstable (3b + 4a + 6b). The two underlying causal dimensions are formed by summing across quadrants, as follows: locus of control

(internal-stable + internal-unstable); stability (internal-stable + external-stable).

Reliability

The paired-comparison forced-choice format has been used reliably in a number of other studies investigating Weiner's four categories of causal attribution (Girodo et al., 1981; McMahan, 1973; Weiner & Kukla, 1970; Weiner et al., 1976) and is a standard method of assessing attributions in achievement-motivation situations (Crandall, Katkovsky, & Crandall, 1965). Girodo et al. reported a test-retest reliability ranging from .65 to .78 ($p < .001$) for success and failure ascriptions, and a high internal consistency of causal preferences across the four causal categories, with Kendall's tau ranging from .22 ($p < .05$) to .70 ($p < .001$).

Validity

Construct validity for Weiner's four attributional categories has been established in numerous studies in which respondents were asked to explain spontaneously the causes of certain imagined and real outcomes (Frieze, 1976; Weiner, 1979; Weiner, Russell, & Lerman, 1978; Wong & Weiner, 1981). The Causal Attribution for Coital Orgasm Scale has been used successfully to differentiate between attributional styles of women with high and low orgasm frequency (Bridges, 1981; Loos et al., 1987).

References

Bridges, C. F. (1981). *Orgasm consistency, causal attribution, and inhibitory control.* Unpublished master's thesis, North Texas State University, Denton.

Crandall, V. C., Katkovsky, W., & Crandall, V. J. (1965). Children's beliefs in their own control of reinforcements in intellectual-academic achievement situations. *Child Development, 46,* 91-109.

Frieze, I. H. (1976). Causal attributions and information seeking to explain success and failure. *Journal of Research in Personality, 10,* 293-305.

Girodo, M., Dotzenroth, S. E., & Stein, S. J. (1981). Causal attribution bias in shy males: Implications for self-esteem and self-confidence. *Cognitive Therapy and Research, 5,* 325-338.

Loos, V. E., Bridges, C. F., & Critelli, J. W. (1987). Weiner's attribution theory and female orgasmic consistency. *The Journal of Sex Research, 23,* 348-361.

McMahan, I. D. (1973). Relationships between causal attributions and expectancy of success. *Journal of Personality and Social Psychology, 28,* 108-114.

Weiner, B. (1979). A theory of motivation for some classroom experiences. *Journal of Educational Psychology, 71,* 3-25.

---

[1]Address correspondence to Joseph W. Critelli, Department of Psychology, North Texas State University, P.O. Box 13587, Denton, TX 76203-3587.

Weiner, B., & Kukla, A. (1970). An attributional analysis of achievement motivation. *Journal of Personality and Social Psychology, 15,* 1-20.

Weiner, B., Nierenberg, R., & Goldstein, M. (1976). Social learning (locus of control) versus attributional (causal stability) interpretations of expectancy of success. *Journal of Personality, 44,* 52-68.

Weiner, B., Russell, D., & Lerman, D. (1978). Affective consequences of causal ascriptions. In J. H. Harvey, W. J. Ickes, & R. F. Kidd (Eds.), *New directions in attribution research* (Vol. 1, pp. 59-90). Hillsdale, NJ: Lawrence Erlbaum.

Wong, T. P., & Weiner, B. (1981). Why people ask "why" questions, and the heuristics of attributional search. *Journal of Personality and Social Psychology, 40,* 650-663.

Exhibit

Causal Attributions for Coital Outcome Scale

I. Complete the following sentence by placing a check mark in front of the ONE CHOICE IN EACH PAIR of choices which you believe is MORE ACCURATE FOR YOU. Please response to *all six choices.*

When I have an orgasm *during coitus,* it is typically because: (Select one answer from each pair.)

1. a) _____ I am typically sexually responsive.
   OR
   b) _____ I particularly wanted to have an orgasm.
2. a) _____ I particularly wanted to have an orgasm.
   OR
   b) _____ My partner is a good lover.
3. a) _____ My partner is a good lover.
   OR
   b) _____ It was a matter of luck.
4. a) _____ It was a matter of luck.
   OR
   b) _____ I am typically sexually responsive.
5. a) _____ My partner is a good lover
   OR
   b) _____ I am typically sexually responsive.
6. a) _____ I particularly wanted to have an orgasm.
   OR
   b) _____ It was a matter of luck.

II. Complete the following sentence by placing a check mark in front of the ONE CHOICE IN EACH PAIR of choices which you believe is MORE ACCURATE FOR YOU. Please respond to *all six choices.*

When I *do not* have an orgasm *during coitus,* it is typically because: (Select one answer from each pair.)

1. a) _____ I am typically sexually unresponsive.
   OR
   b) _____ I did not particularly want to have an orgasm.
2. a) _____ I did not particularly want to have an orgasm.
   OR
   b) _____ My partner is not a good lover.
3. a) _____ My partner is not a good lover.
   OR
   b) _____ It was a matter of luck.
4. a) _____ It was a matter of luck.
   OR
   b) _____ I am typically sexually unresponsive.
5. a) _____ My partner is not a good lover.
   OR
   b) _____ I am typically sexually unresponsive.
6. a) _____ I did not particularly want to have an orgasm.
   OR
   b) _____ It was a matter of luck.

The Relationship Between Mode of Female Masturbation and the Achievement of Orgasm in Coitus

Michael Israel,[1] *Los Angeles*

This instrument assesses the relationship between masturbatory behavior and orgasmic capacity in coitus for women. Because masturbation is typically an individual's first sexual experience, and is certainly one of the most common expressions of sexuality, the link between masturbation and sexual activity with a partner is potentially important.

In 1953, Kinsey, Pomeroy, Martin, and Gebhard suggested that there was a positive correlation between ability to masturbate to orgasm and the capacity to achieve orgasm during coitus. Since Kinsey's time, the research results have been contradictory on this point. However, the belief in the salience of the relationship between the capacities for coital and masturbatory orgasm is so well entrenched that it forms the basis for the treatment of choice for women experiencing anorgasmia. The treatment strategy involves instruction in masturbatory techniques using direct clitoral stimulation (Barbach, 1974; Kaplan, 1974; LoPiccolo & Lobitz, 1972). The goal of the treatment strategy is for the acquired ability to achieve orgasm via masturbation to generalize to coitus.

The majority of girls learn to masturbate by self-discovery, using methods that are often chance events (Katchadourian & Lunde, 1972; Kinsey et al., 1953). For example, a young girl may first become aware of "sexual" feelings while pressing against sheets, rocking in a chair, sliding down a pole, or exploring her genitals. Although the significance of these sensations may not be immediately apparent to her, she may persevere in the acts long enough to experience initial orgasm. The manner in which she initially learns to masturbate may have a bearing on her later coital orgasmic capacity.

A number of investigators have reported that the instructional treatment for anorgasmia is quite efficacious (Barbach, 1974; Kaplan, 1974; LoPiccolo & Lobitz, 1972). The explanatory concepts of generalization or transfer of training and increased perceptions of bodily process, though, do not fully answer the question of how masturbatory experiences relate to coital orgasmic capacity.

The instrument was designed to answer the following questions: (a) Can women who masturbate be classified into two distinct categories—direct or indirect masturbators—on the basis of their masturbatory behavior? (b) What is the persistence of the initially learned masturbatory style over time? (c) Do women with different masturbatory styles and women who do not masturbate require different amounts of clitoral stimulation to achieve orgasm during coitus, prefer clitoral or vaginal stimulation as a means of achieving orgasm, and/or exhibit differential coital orgasmic capacities?

Description

The self-report questionnaire consists of 55 items, 50 of which are cast in an objective format including bipolar adjective checklists, multiple-choice, and Likert-type scale items. The other 5 items are of an open-ended nature. The number of possible response categories and their levels, on the objective questions, varies as appropriate.

The items on the questionnaire address six general areas as follows: demography; masturbatory history; current masturbatory practices; sexual history relative to intercourse; current sexual behaviors relative to masturbation, intercourse, and sexual satisfaction; and body image relative to the respondents' attitude toward their bodies.

Demographic data. Demographic data collected include age; marital status; educational, occupational, and income level; degree of religious devoutness; and religious upbringing.

Masturbatory history. Data regarding age and method of initial masturbatory practices are collected. This is done to determine whether age covaries with initial masturbatory experiences through direct or indirect means and to determine the persistence of the preferred masturbatory mode (direct or indirect).

Current masturbatory practices. Current masturbatory practices are investigated to determine (a) whether direct or indirect methods of masturbation are employed, (b) how frequently the respondent masturbates, and (c) the degree of psychological comfort experienced as a masturbating adult.

Sexual history. Sexual history data include age of first coital experience and latency of first coital orgasm. Sexual history data are collected as a means of ascertaining whether direct and indirect masturbators exhibit differential sexual histories.

Current sexual behavior. Current sexual behaviors assessed include frequency of current masturbation, frequency of intercourse, and degree of sexual satisfaction.

[1]Address correspondence to Michael Israel, 1715 Westridge Road, Los Angeles, CA 90049; email: 74143.3715@compuserve.com.

The intent of these items is to determine if direct and indirect masturbators indicate different levels of sexual activity and satisfaction.

Body image. Items relative to the respondents' attitudes toward their bodies are included to determine whether these variables relate to masturbatory activity and sexual responsiveness.

A pretest of the questionnaire was conducted to ascertain (a) whether the language of the items was clear and comprehensible; (b) whether respondents would be willing to answer the questions asked on the instrument fully and completely, and, if not, which items were to be reworded or eliminated; and (c) whether the responses appear to be consistent with the investigator's impressions of the respondents in an informal interview.

The respondents in the pilot study and in subsequent investigations have all been either graduate students, middle-class housewives, or professional women. I believe that the instrument could be appropriately administered to any woman, although some wording would have to be changed for administration to women who are lesbian or bisexual.

Response Mode and Timing

The instrument has typically been administered to respondents in groups. Other methods of administration are, however, certainly appropriate. Completion of the instrument usually requires about 20 minutes.

All responses to the items of the questionnaire are indicated on the instrument itself. Respondents are instructed to check the appropriate box (or boxes) that apply for each objective item. Space is provided, on the instrument, for the respondents to write in their responses to the open-ended items.

Scoring

The scoring of the instrument is generally quite straightforward and self-explanatory. No scale scores are calculated, and no items need to be recast. Depending on which items are of interest to the investigator, the data are simply analyzed as reported. There is one exception.

Calculation of masturbatory style. One of the primary purposes of the instrument is to identify, for purposes of analysis, the masturbatory style, either direct or indirect, of the respondent. Direct masturbation is defined as direct

digital manipulation of the clitoris or the use of a vibrator in the genital area. The use of a vibrator is subsumed under direct methods because it provides high-intensity stimulation equal to that provided by digital manipulation.

Indirect masturbation is defined as indirect stimulation of the clitoris during masturbation through stimulation of an adjacent area (e.g., rubbing the thighs together or pressing on the pubic area).

Because the mode of masturbatory activity, either direct or indirect, is not directly asked of the respondents, it is necessary for the investigator to infer the preferred mode by an examination of the obtained self-report data. The decision rule followed in making this clinical judgment is as follows. Question 3 in Part II of the instrument lists 13 different methods of masturbation, and the respondent is asked to indicate the frequency with which she employs each method on a 5-point scale ranging from *always* to *never.*

If the respondent indicates either direct or clitoral stimulation via "rubbing my clitoris" or the use of an electronic vibrator at least "frequently," she is classified as a direct masturbator. If any of the other methods are employed, the individual is classified as a indirect masturbator. In cases where more than one method is indicated, as least one indirect and one direct, the decision is made on the frequency of the methods employed. That is, a woman who "frequently" rubbed her thighs together and "seldom" rubbed her clitoris is classified as an indirect masturbator.

Reliability and Validity

No reliability or validity data are presently available.

References

Barbach, L. (1974). Group treatment for preorgasmic women. *Journal of Sex & Marital Therapy, 1,* 139-145.

Kaplan, H. S. (1974). *The new sex therapy.* New York: Brunner/Mazel.

Katchadourian, H., & Lunde, D. (1972). *Fundamentals of human sexuality.* New York: Holt, Rinehart & Winston.

Kinsey, A. C., Pomeroy, W. B., Martin, C. E., & Gebhard, P. H. (1953). *Sexual behavior in the human female.* Philadelphia: Saunders.

Leff, J. J., & Israel, M. (1983). The relationship between mode of female masturbation and achievement of orgasm in coitus. *Archives of Sexual Behavior, 12,* 227-236.

LoPiccolo, J., & Lobitz, W. C. (1972). The role of masturbation in the treatment of primary orgasmic dysfunction. *Archives of Sexual Behavior, 2,* 163-171.

Exhibit

Mode of Masturbation and Coital Orgasm

Many of these questions are highly personal and sensitive. All of the material will be kept confidential. Your cooperation in answering these questions is greatly appreciated. Please leave *blank* any question that does not apply to you.

I. Personal History
   1. Age: _____
   2. Marital status:
      _____ Single   _____ Divorced   _____ Separated   _____ Widowed   _____ Married

3. If not married, are you living with a sexual partner?
   _____ Yes _____ No
4. Number of children: _____
5. Husband's or partner's occupation: _____
6. Your occupation: _____
7. Husband's or partner's education level:
   _____ High school _____ Some college _____ B.A. _____ Graduate school
8. Your educational level:
   _____ High school _____ Some college _____ B.A. _____ Graduate school
9. I consider myself:
   _____ Very religious _____ Somewhat religious _____ Not very religious
10. My religious upbringing was:
   _____ Very religious _____ Somewhat religious _____ Not very religious
11. Husband's or partner's income level:
   _____ Under $5000 _____ $5000-10,000 _____ $10,000-15,000 _____ $15,000-20,000
   _____ $20,000-30,000 _____ $30,000-40,000 _____ $40,000-50,000 _____ Over $50,000
12. Personal income level:
   _____ Under $5000 _____ $5000-10,000 _____ $10,000-15,000 _____ $15,000-20,000
   _____ $20,000-30,000 _____ $30,000-40,000 _____ $40,000-50,000 _____ Over $50,000
13. Ethnic group:
   _____ Caucasian _____ Black _____ Latin American _____ Asian _____ Other: (specify) _____
14. Length of marriage or current sexual relationship if applicable: _____
15. Length of previous marriage if applicable: _____
16. How do you feel about your body?
   _____ I like it a lot _____ I think it is OK _____ I don't have any feelings about it
   _____ I dislike it somewhat _____ I don't like it at all
17. Have you ever masturbated?
   _____ Yes _____ No _____ Not sure
18. Have you achieved orgasm?
   a. with masturbation? _____ Yes _____ No _____ Not sure
   b. with intercourse? _____ Yes _____ No _____ Not sure
   c. with manual or oral stimulation? _____ Yes _____ No _____ Not sure

Note. Stop at this point if you have never had an orgasm and return the questionnaire. Thank you.

19. Age you began masturbating: _____
20. Age you first achieved orgasm with masturbation: _____
21. What ways did you first begin? (Indicate those that apply):
   _____ Rubbing thighs together   _____ Pillow between legs
   _____ Object inserted in vagina   _____ Rubbing against sheets
   _____ Pulling on inner-outer lips   _____ Pressure on pubic area
   _____ Rubbing clitoris   _____ Sliding down a tree
   _____ Sliding down a pole   _____ Horseback riding
   _____ Use of vibrator   _____ Rocking back and forth
   _____ Other: (specify) _____
22. What ways did you first achieve orgasm? (Indicate those that apply):
   _____ Rubbing thighs together   _____ Pillow between legs
   _____ Object inserted in vagina   _____ Rubbing against sheets
   _____ Pulling on inner-outer lips   _____ Pressure on pubic area
   _____ Rubbing clitoris   _____ Sliding down a tree
   _____ Sliding down a pole   _____ Horseback riding
   _____ Use of vibrator   _____ Rocking back and forth
   _____ Other: (specify) _____
23. Which of the following ways do you feel caused you to achieve your first orgasm?
   _____ Rubbing thighs together   _____ Pillow between legs
   _____ Object inserted in vagina   _____ Rubbing against sheets
   _____ Pulling on inner-outer lips   _____ Pressure on pubic area
   _____ Rubbing clitoris   _____ Sliding down a tree
   _____ Sliding down a pole   _____ Horseback riding
   _____ Use of vibrator   _____ Rocking back and forth
   _____ Other: (specify) _____

24. How soon after you first began sexual intercourse did you achieve orgasm?
   _____ Within one month   _____ 2-6 months
   _____ 6 months-1 year   _____ Later than 1 year
   _____ Never

II. Current Sexual Behavior
  1. On the average, how long does it take you to achieve orgasm when you masturbate?
     _____ Less than 1 minute   _____ 5-10 minutes   _____ 15-30 minutes
     _____ 30-45 minutes   _____ Over 45 minutes
  2. On the average, how often do you masturbate?
     _____ More than once a day   _____ 4-6 times a week   _____ 3 times a week
     _____ Twice a week   _____ Once every 2 weeks   _____ Once a month
     _____ Once every two months   _____ Once a year
  3. I prefer to masturbate to orgasm by:
     A. Rubbing my thighs together[a]   H. Horseback riding
     B. With a pillow between my legs   I. Sliding down a tree
     C. By inserting an object in my vagina J. Sliding down a pole
     D. Pulling on my inner-outer lips   K. Using a vibrator
     E. Rubbing my clitoris   L. Rocking back and forth
     F. Rubbing against sheets   M. Other: (specify) _____
     G. Pressure on pubic area
  4. Has there been a change in the way you masturbate since you first began and the way you do now?
     _____ Yes   _____ No   _____ Not sure
     If yes, please specify how: _____
  5. Do you have any fantasies when you masturbate?
     _____ Always   _____ Frequently _____ Occasionally   _____ Seldom   _____ Never
  6. Do you have any fantasies when you masturbate to orgasm?
     _____ Always   _____ Frequently _____ Occasionally   _____ Seldom   _____ Never
  7. Fantasy: Indicate *any* that apply:
     _____ I am being watched.
     _____ I am watching others having sexual relations.
     _____ I am undergoing pain.
     _____ I am tied up during sex.
     _____ I am being forced by my partner to do some act I do not wish to do.
     _____ I am taking off my clothes in front of many men.
     _____ I am being overwhelmed by an uncontrollable force.
     _____ I am having relations with someone who is forbidden to me either by law or custom (e.g., a close relative or priest).
     _____ I am making love to a specific person I know (e.g., a friend).
     _____ I am making love to someone I do not know (e.g., a film star).
     _____ I am having sex with someone appreciably younger.
     _____ I am having sex with my husband or lover.
     _____ I am engaging in sexual acts that I do not do in reality.
     _____ I am having sexual relations with an animal.
     _____ I am having sex with two men.
     _____ I am having sex with another woman and a man.
     _____ I am having sex with another woman.
     _____ He is tied up during sex.
     _____ I am being raped by many men.
     _____ I am initiating a young boy.
     _____ Other: (specify) _____
  8. Indicate your favorite fantasy: _____
  9. Has there been any change in your fantasy or fantasies over time; If so, please specify: _____
 10. Describe your feelings about having fantasies while masturbating:
     _____ Comfortable   _____ Somewhat comfortable   _____ No feelings   _____ Somewhat uncomfortable
     _____ Uncomfortable
 11. Do you feel guilty about the content of your fantasies?
     _____ Yes   _____ No   _____ Not sure
 12. Do you believe your fantasies contribute to your achieving orgasm?
     _____ Yes   _____ No   _____ Not sure

Note. If you are not currently having sexual relations with a partner, please answer the following questions as your sexual relations used to be.

 13. Do you have fantasies during sexual relations with a partner?
     _____ Always   _____ Frequently _____ Occasionally   _____ Rarely   _____ Never
 14. Are your fantasies with a partner different from those that you engage in during masturbation?
     _____ Always   _____ Frequently _____ Occasionally   _____ Rarely   _____ Never
 15. Describe your feelings about having fantasies while having sexual relations:
     _____ Comfortable   _____ Somewhat comfortable   _____ No feelings   _____ Somewhat uncomfortable
     _____ Uncomfortable

16. Do you feel guilty about the content of your fantasies during sexual relations?
_____ Always _____ Frequently _____ Occasionally _____ Rarely _____ Never

17. How often do you have intercourse?
_____ More than once a day _____ Once a day _____ 4-6 times a week
_____ 3 times a week _____ Twice a week _____ Once a week
_____ Once every two months _____ Once a year _____ Never

18. Do you achieve orgasm during intercourse?
_____ Yes _____ No _____ Not sure

19. What percentage of the time do you achieve orgasm during intercourse?
_____ 100% _____ 75% _____ 50% _____ 25% _____ 10%

Note. Many women reach orgasm by their partner stimulating their clitoris either manually or orally. Some women reach orgasm before or after intercourse with their partner's stimulation.

20. Do you achieve orgasm *before* and/or *after* sexual intercourse by partner's assistance?
_____ Always _____ Frequently _____ Occasionally _____ Seldom _____ Never

21. Do you engage in oral-genital contact?
_____ Yes _____ No

22. Do you achieve orgasm *during* intercourse by manual or other stimulation applied to your clitoris by yourself or by your partner?
_____ Always _____ Frequently _____ Occasionally _____ Seldom _____ Never

23. Are you comfortable nude and exposing your body during sexual activity?
_____ Comfortable _____ Somewhat comfortable _____ No feelings _____ Somewhat uncomfortable
_____ Uncomfortable

24. Do you describe your sexual responsiveness as:
_____ Considerably above average _____ Above average _____ Average
_____ Slightly below average _____ Quite below average

25. Are you comfortable talking about sex in the company of others?
_____ Comfortable _____ Somewhat comfortable _____ No feelings
_____ Somewhat uncomfortable _____ Uncomfortable

26. How often would you prefer to have sexual intercourse?
_____ More than once a day _____ Once a day _____ 4-6 times a week
_____ 3 times a week _____ Twice a week _____ Once a week
_____ Once every two months _____ Once a year _____ Never

27. How often does your partner prefer to have sexual intercourse?
_____ More than once a day _____ Once a day _____ 4-6 times a week
_____ 3 times a week _____ Twice a week _____ Once a week
_____ Once every two months _____ Once a year _____ Never

28. What method of birth control do you use?
_____ Pill _____ IUD _____ Diaphragm _____ Condom _____ Foam _____ Rhythm
_____ Sterilization _____ No method _____ Withdrawal

29. Describe when you notice the greatest amount of sexual arousal during the menstrual cycle:
_____ During menstruation _____ The week after menstruation stops
_____ During the middle of the cycle _____ The week before menstruation begins
_____ No difference noted during the cycle

30. Do you prefer clitoral or vaginal stimulation to achieve orgasm?
_____ Clitoral is the most important _____ Clitoral is somewhat more important
_____ Clitoral and vaginal stimulation are equally important _____ Vaginal is somewhat more important
_____ Vaginal is the most important

31. Do you ask your partner for clitoral stimulation?
_____ Yes _____ No _____ Occasionally

32. Are you comfortable asking your partner for clitoral stimulation?
_____ Comfortable _____ Somewhat comfortable _____ No feelings
_____ Somewhat uncomfortable _____ Uncomfortable

33. In terms of sexual responsiveness:
A. I consider the *quality of the emotional relationship* between me and my partner a most important part of my sexual enjoyment.[a]
B. I consider the *technical proficiency* of my partner (how good he is at making love) a most important part of my sexual enjoyment.

C. I consider *adequate bodily contact* a most important part of my sexual enjoyment.

D. I consider the *potency of my partner* (his ability to get and keep an erection) a most important part of my sexual enjoyment.

E. I consider *having different partners* a most important part of my sexual enjoyment.

F. I consider *other* (please specify) a most important part of my sexual enjoyment. _____

A questionnaire of this type may evoke many feelings. Try to answer the next two questions to the best of your ability.

34. Describe your feelings of comfort while reading this questionnaire:

_____ Comfortable _____ Somewhat comfortable _____ No feelings _____ Somewhat uncomfortable _____ Uncomfortable

35. Describe your feelings of sexual arousal while reading this questionnaire:

_____ Aroused _____ Somewhat aroused _____ No feelings _____ Slightly aroused _____ Not aroused at all

Source. This questionnaire is reprinted with permission of the author.

a. Five response options (*always, frequently, occasionally, seldom,* and *never*) are provided for each item.

Perceived Effect of an Ostomy

Barbara Pieper,[1] *Wayne State University*
Carol Mikols, *West Branch, Michigan*

Because of an alteration in body image, an ostomy may adversely affect a person's life. The Perceived Effect of an Ostomy questionnaire (PEO) measures a person's concerns about having a fecal-producing stoma (colostomy or ileostomy). Items explore concerns about the ostomy and its care; the effect on self, work, home, and other activities; and the effect on sexuality.

Description

The PEO is a 46-item questionnaire developed after reviewing the ostomy literature about patients' concerns. Historically, themes about ostomy concerns have focused on (a) the ostomy and its care; (b) participation in work, home, and leisure activities; (c) sexuality; and (d) body image. Additional ostomy concerns include odor, adjustments in clothing, appliance fit and leakage, appliance care, and diet (Deeny & McCrea, 1991; Druss, O'Connor, Prudden, & Stern, 1968; Druss, O'Connor, & Stern, 1969; Eardley et al., 1976; Rheame & Gooding, 1991). The effect of an ostomy on work, home, and leisure activities varies.

Some have noted that only a small percentage of persons with an ostomy resumed all former leisure and household activities (Eardley et al., 1976). Others have reported that persons with an ostomy feel less restricted in leisure, social, or family activities (Martinsson, Gosefsson, & Ek, 1991; McLeod et al., 1986). Fear of the diagnosis (e.g., cancer), loss of wholeness, inconvenience, and fear of the future are other concerns (Coe & Kluka, 1988). Sexual problems have been associated with ostomy surgery (Eardley et al., 1976; Gloechner & Starling, 1982; Thomas, Madden, & John, 1984; Thomas, Turner, & Madden, 1988). Sexual function is a common concern after ostomy surgery (Dlin, 1978). Moods, coping, and body image may be adversely affected (Druss et al., 1969; Keltikangs-Jarvinen, Lovin, & Moller, 1984; Padilla & Grant, 1985).

The PEO was developed for use with persons who have a colostomy or ileostomy. Slight modification (e.g., change *stool* to *urine*) of some items would make it appropriate for persons who have an urostomy. The PEO has 17 items related to the ostomy and its care; 10 items related to the home, work, and other activities; 12 items related to self and image; and 7 items related to sexuality.

[1]Address correspondence to Barbara Pieper, College of Nursing, Wayne State University, 5557 Cass Avenue, Detroit, MI 48202; email: piepwin@mail.ic.net.

Response Mode and Timing

Each item is rated on a 7-point Likert-type scale, which ranges from 1, *minimal/not a concern,* to 7, *very great concern.* A participant is asked to visualize a ladder with steps going from 1 at the bottom to 7 at the top. He or she selects the step on the ladder that represents his or her level of concern for each item. A respondent may complete the form alone. If the person has difficulty reading, the items can be read and the person allowed to verbalize level of concern.

The PEO can be completed within 15 minutes. It has been administered prior to and after discharge from the hospital. Prior to discharge, but after all ostomy patient teaching had been done, respondents rated their concerns, from how they perceived the ostomy would affect them. After discharge, ostomates rated concerns as to current occurrence.

Scoring

The PEO may be examined as separate items or as a total score. A higher rating of an item signifies greater concern. Total scores may range from 46 to 322. Higher total scores reflect greater overall concern about the ostomy affecting the person's life. Factor analysis has not been done to define subscores because the sample size was small.

Reliability

Sixty-seven ostomates completed the PEO predischarge; 50 of these persons completed it postdischarge. Subject loss related to an inability to contact the person (e.g., moving, going on vacation, disconnected telephone), not a refusal to continue participation in the study. The participants were 50 men and 17 women, who ranged in age from 18 to 78 years (M = 42.3 years, SD = 18.9). They were African American (n = 43) or Caucasian (n = 24) and had a colostomy (n = 56) or ileostomy (n = 11). The ostomy was created due to disease (n = 36), gunshot injury (n = 28), or accident (n = 3). The stoma was either temporary (n = 48) or permanent (n = 19).

The predischarge PEO was administered prior to discharge from the hospital, but after all ostomy teaching had been done by an enterostomal therapy nurse (nurses who are experts in the care of a person who has an ostomy). It had a coefficient alpha of .97. The postdischarge PEO was administered at least 2 weeks after discharge (M = 7 weeks, SD = 5 weeks), but prior to any additional surgery. The postdischarge PEO had a coefficient alpha of .97.

Validity

The PEO was reviewed for content by three enterostomal therapy nurses. Content validity was deemed appropriate. The instrument has not been factor analyzed.

Other Information

The top one third of the pre- and postdischarge PEO items were examined. Eight concerns remained high pre- and postdischarge (fear of stool leaking, odor, participation in sports, needing further treatment, wearing a pouch, change in body appearance, changing a pouch, and participating in sexual love play and intercourse; Pieper & Mikols, 1996). Five sexuality items were in the top one third of the concerns prior to discharge: interest in sex, participating in sexual love play and intercourse, ability to have sex, satisfaction after sexual intercourse, and relationship with spouse or girl/boyfriend. One item remained in the top third after discharge: participating in sexual love play and intercourse. Total PEO scores did not differ significantly by reason of stoma construction (disease or injury), temporary versus permanent ostomy, or pre- to postdischarge (Pieper & Mikols, 1996). Women had significantly higher total PEO scores (M = 162, SD = 80) than men (M = 114, SD = 47), $F(1, 42)$ = 5.66, p = .02.

The PEO has been used in only one research study. Additional psychometric testing must be done. This instrument has the potential to identify a patient's concerns during hospitalization, in an outpatient clinic, or at home. Teaching and counseling may then be tailored to the patient's specific need.

References

Coe, M., & Kluka, S. (1988). Concerns of clients and spouses regarding ostomy surgery for cancer. *Journal of Enterostomal Therapy, 15,* 232-239.

Deeny, P., & McCrea, H. (1991). Stoma care: The patient's perspective. *Journal of Advanced Nursing, 16,* 39-46.

Dlin, M. (1978). Emotional aspects of colostomy and ileostomy. *Psychosomatics, 4,* 214-218.

Druss, R. G., O'Connor, J. P., Prudden, J. F., & Stern, L. O. (1968). Psychologic response to colectomy. *Archives in General Psychiatry, 18,* 53-59.

Druss, R. G., O'Connor, J. P., & Stern, L. O. (1969). Psychologic response to colectomy: II. Adjustment to a permanent colostomy. *Archives in General Psychiatry, 20,* 419-427.

Eardley, A., George, W. D., Davis, F., Schofield, P. F., Wilson, M. C., Wakefield, J., & Sellwood, R. A. (1976). Colostomy: The consequences of surgery. *Clinical Oncology, 2,* 277-283.

Gloechner, M. R., & Starling, J. R. (1982). Providing sexual information to ostomy patients. *Diseases of Colon and Rectum, 25,* 575-599.

Keltikangs-Jarvinen, L., Loven, E., & Moller, C. (1984). Psychic factors determining the long-term adaptation of colostomy and ileostomy patients. *Psychotherapeutics & Psychosomatics, 41,* 153-159.

Martinsson, E. S., Gosefsson, M., & Ek, A. C. (1991). Working capacity and quality of life after undergoing ileostomy. *Journal of Advanced Nursing, 16,* 1035-1041.

McLeod, R. S., Lavery, I. C., Leatherman, J. R., Maryland, P. H., Fazio, V. W., Gagelman, D. G., & Weakley, F. L., (1986). Factors affecting quality of life with conventional ileostomy. *World Journal of Surgery, 10,* 474-480.

Padilla, G. V., & Grant, M. M. (1985). Quality of life as a cancer nursing outcome variable. *Advances in Nursing Science, 8,* 45-60.

Pieper, B., & Mikols, C. (1996). Predischarge and postdischarge concerns of persons with an ostomy. *Journal of Wound, Ostomy, and Continence Nursing, 23*(2), 105-109.

Rheame, A., & Gooding, B. A. (1991). Social support, coping strategies, and long-term adaption to ostomy among self-help group members. *Journal of Enterostomal Therapy, 18,* 11-15.

Thomas, C., Madden, F., & John, D. (1984). Psychosocial morbidity the first three months following stoma surgery. *Journal of Psychosomatic Research, 28,* 251-257.

Thomas, C., Madden, F., & John, D. (1987). Physiological effects of stoma: I. Psychosocial morbidity one year after surgery. *Journal of Psychosomatic Research, 31,* 311-316.

Thomas, C., Turner, P., & Madden, F. (1988). Coping and outcome of stoma surgery. *Journal of Psychosomatic Research, 32,* 457-467.

Exhibit

Perceived Effect of an Ostomy

Directions prior to discharge:

Now that you are getting ready to go home from the hospital, I would like you to tell me *how concerned you are about living with your ostomy.* Read and rate each item in terms of how concerned you are about it. To help you with the rating, think of a ladder. The bottom of the ladder is a 1; you have little concern about the item. The top of the ladder is a 7; you are very concerned about the item. Circle the number that best shows where you are on the ladder. There are no right or wrong answers.

Directions for postdischarge:

Now that you are home from the hospital, I would like you to tell me *about your concerns now of living with an ostomy.* Read and rate each item in terms of how concerned you are about it. To help you with the rating, think of a ladder. The bottom of the ladder is a 1; you have little concern about the item. The top of the ladder is a 7; you are very concerned about the item. Circle the number that best shows where you are on the ladder. There are no right or wrong answers.

Perceived Effect of an Ostomy

		Minimal/ Not a concern						Very Great Concern	Item Classification[a]
1.	My feeling like a whole person	1	2	3	4	5	6	7	3
2.	My feeling embarrassed	1	2	3	4	5	6	7	3
3.	My feelings of myself as a man/woman	1	2	3	4	5	6	7	4
4.	My ability to get along with people	1	2	3	4	5	6	7	3
5.	My moods	1	2	3	4	5	6	7	3
6.	My need to rely on others	1	2	3	4	5	6	7	2
7.	My self-worth	1	2	3	4	5	6	7	3
8.	My interest in life	1	2	3	4	5	6	7	3
9.	My social life	1	2	3	4	5	6	7	2
10.	My ability to tell others what I have	1	2	3	4	5	6	7	3
11.	My ability to work outside the home	1	2	3	4	5	6	7	2
12.	My feeling alone	1	2	3	4	5	6	7	3
13.	My looking after myself in other people's homes	1	2	3	4	5	6	7	1
14.	How I will cope in the days to come	1	2	3	4	5	6	7	3
15.	Change in body appearance	1	2	3	4	5	6	7	3
16.	Wearing a pouch	1	2	3	4	5	6	7	1
17.	Changing the pouch	1	2	3	4	5	6	7	1
18.	Cleaning my skin	1	2	3	4	5	6	7	1
19.	My fear of leaking stool	1	2	3	4	5	6	7	1
20.	Touching the stoma	1	2	3	4	5	6	7	1
21.	Odor	1	2	3	4	5	6	7	1
22.	Looking at my stool or feces	1	2	3	4	5	6	7	1
23.	Passing gas	1	2	3	4	5	6	7	1
24.	Taking time in the bathroom	1	2	3	4	5	6	7	1
25.	What I can eat	1	2	3	4	5	6	7	1
26.	Going out to eat	1	2	3	4	5	6	7	2
27.	Ability to care for my children/grandchildren	1	2	3	4	5	6	7	2
28.	Ability to do housework	1	2	3	4	5	6	7	2
29.	My budget	1	2	3	4	5	6	7	2

		Minimal/ Not a concern						Very Great Concern	Item Classification
30.	My clothing	1	2	3	4	5	6	7	1
31.	My ability to take a bath or shower	1	2	3	4	5	6	7	1
32.	Carrying supplies when I leave the house	1	2	3	4	5	6	7	1
33.	Knowing where to buy supplies	1	2	3	4	5	6	7	1
34.	My ability to participate in sports	1	2	3	4	5	6	7	2
35.	Going to a movie	1	2	3	4	5	6	7	2
36.	Changing my sleep	1	2	3	4	5	6	7	1
37.	Taking care of personal business such as shopping or banking	1	2	3	4	5	6	7	2
38.	Needing to have further treatment	1	2	3	4	5	6	7	1
39.	Thoughts of death	1	2	3	4	5	6	7	3
40.	My energy level	1	2	3	4	5	6	7	3
41.	Relationship with spouse or girl/boyfriend	1	2	3	4	5	6	7	4
42.	Ability to hug and kiss	1	2	3	4	5	6	7	4
43.	Interest in sex	1	2	3	4	5	6	7	4
44.	Participating in sexual love play/intercourse	1	2	3	4	5	6	7	4
45.	Ability to have sex	1	2	3	4	5	6	7	4
46.	Satisfaction after sexual intercourse	1	2	3	4	5	6	7	4

a. Item classification: 1 = ostomy; 2 = home, work, leisure activities; 3 = self-image; 4 = sexuality. This information is not typed on the copy given to respondents.

Sexual Socialization Instrument

Ilsa L. Lottes,[1] *University of Maryland, Baltimore County*
Peter J. Kuriloff, *University of Pennsylvania*

The purpose of the Sexual Socialization Instrument is to measure permissive sexual influences of parents and peers on adolescents and young adults. The term *permissive* here means acceptance of nonmarital sexual interactions. A permissive influence is one that would encourage sexual involvement in a wide variety of relationships—from casual to long term. A nonpermissive influence is one that discourages casual sexual encounters and promotes either abstinence or sex for individuals only in loving, long-term relationships.

Description

The Sexual Socialization Instrument was developed for use in a longitudinal study investigating the relationships among background variables; residential and social affiliations; and the attitudes, values, and sexual experiences of university students. The items of this instrument were included in a questionnaire completed by 557 first-year students (48% female) in 1987 and 303 of these same students (55% female) in 1991 when they were seniors.

The Sexual Socialization Instrument consists of two scales, the Parental Sexual Socialization Scale and the Peer Sexual Socialization Scale. When the Sexual Socialization Instrument was given to first-year students, short forms of the parental and peer scales, containing four items (numbered 1, 3, 19 and 20) and six items (numbered 2, 4, 5, 8, 15, and 18), respectively, were used. To improve the internal

[1]Address correspondence to Ilsa L. Lottes, Department of Sociology and Anthropology, University of Maryland, Baltimore County, 5401 Wilkens Avenue, Baltimore, MD 21228; email: lottes@umbc2.umbc.edu.

consistency reliability of both scales for the second administration of the questionnaire to seniors, the number of items in the parental and peer scales was increased to eight (numbered 1, 3, 6, 9, 12, 16, 19, and 20) and 12 (numbered 2, 4, 5, 7, 8, 10, 11, 13, 14, 15, 17, and 18), respectively. These versions of the scales are referred to as long forms. The response options to each item are one of the 5-point Likert-type choices: *strongly agree* (1), *agree* (2), *undecided* (3), *disagree* (4), and *strongly disagree* (5).

If one is interested in an overall measure of sexual socialization from parents and peers, the items of the parental and peer scales can be combined to form such a measure as was done by Bell et al. (1992), Bell, Lottes, and Kuriloff (1995), and Kuriloff, Lottes, and Bell (1995).

Response Mode and Timing

Respondents can circle the number from 1 to 5 corresponding to their degree of agreement or disagreement with each item, or if computer scoring is available, machine-scorable answer sheets can be provided for responses. The instrument requires about 5 minutes for completion.

Scoring

Eleven of the 20 items are scored in the reverse direction: Items 1, 4, 6, 8, 11, 13, 14, 15, 16, 18, and 19. For reverse direction items, recoding for scoring needs to transform all 5s to 1s and 4s to 2s and vice versa before responses to the items are summed to give a scale score. For the long form of the Parental Sexual Socialization Scale, scores can range from 8 to 40, and for the short form of this scale scores can range from 4 to 20. For the long form of the Peer Sexual Socialization Scale, scores can range from 12 to 60, and for the short form of this scale scores can range from 6 to 30. The higher the score, the more permissive the parental or peer influence for respondents.

Reliability

In a sample of 557 first-year college students (Lottes & Kuriloff, 1994), Cronbach alphas for the short forms of the Parental and Peer Sexual Socialization Scales were both .60.

Test-retest reliabilities comparing first-year students with a sample of 303 college seniors were .55 and .47, respectively. In this sample of 303 seniors, Cronbach alphas for the short forms of the parental and peer scales were .73 and .70, respectively, and alphas for the long forms of these scales were .78 and .85, respectively (Kuriloff & Lottes, 1994).

Validity

The construct validity of the Parental and Peer Sexual Socialization Scales was supported by statistically significant results for predicted correlations and group differences. As expected, Lottes and Kuriloff (1994) found that men reported significantly higher scores on both the short and long forms of the parental and peer scales. Also, as expected, future fraternity members as first-year students reported significantly higher scores on the short form of the peer scale than did first-year male students who remained independent. Similarly, compared with nonfraternity senior men, senior fraternity men reported significantly higher scores on the long form of the Peer Sexual Socialization Scale (Lottes & Kuriloff, 1994). In addition, the short forms of the Parental and Peer Sexual Socialization Scales were found to be positively significantly correlated with number of sex partners and negatively significantly correlated with age at first intercourse.

References

Bell, S. T., Kuriloff, P. J., Lottes I. L., Nathanson, J., Judge, T., & Fogelson-Turet, K. (1992). Rape and callousness in college freshmen: An empirical investigation of a sociocultural model of aggression towards women. *Journal of College Student Development, 33,* 454-461.

Bell, S. T., Lottes, I. L., & Kuriloff, P. J. (1995). *Understanding rape callousness in college students: Results of a panel study.* Manuscript submitted for publication.

Kuriloff, P. J., Lottes, I. L., & Bell, S. T. (1995). *The socialization of sexual misconduct in college students.* Manuscript submitted for publication.

Lottes, I. L., & Kuriloff, P. J. (1994). Sexual socialization differences by gender, Greek membership, ethnicity, and religious background. *Psychology of Women Quarterly, 18,* 203-219.

Exhibit

Sexual Socialization Instrument

Directions: Below you will see five numbers corresponding to five choices. Choose the response that best describes your degree of agreement/disagreement with each statement. Write or shade in only one response for each statement. Because all responses will remain anonymous you can respond truthfully with no concerns about anyone connecting responses with individuals.

Strongly agree (1)   Agree (2)   Undecided (3)   Disagree (4)   Strongly disagree (5)

_____ 1. My mother would have felt okay about my having sex with many different people.
_____ 2. I am uncomfortable around people who spend much of their time talking about their sexual experiences.
_____ 3. My father would have felt upset if he'd thought I was having sex with many different people.
_____ 4. Among my friends, men who have the most sexual experience are the most highly regarded.
_____ 5. My friends disapprove of being involved with someone who was known to be sexually easy.

_____ 6. According to my parents, having sexual intercourse is an important part of my becoming an adult.
_____ 7. Most of my friends don't approve of having multiple sexual partners.
_____ 8. My friends and I enjoy telling each other about our sexual experiences.
_____ 9. My parents stress that sex and intimacy should always be linked.
_____ 10. Most of my friends believe that you should only have sex in a serious relationship.
_____ 11. Among my friends alcohol is used to get someone to sleep with you.
_____ 12. My parents would disapprove of my being sexually active.
_____ 13. My friends approve of being involved with someone just for sex.
_____ 14. My friends brag about their sexual exploits.
_____ 15. My friends suggest dates to each other who are known to be sexually easy.
_____ 16. My parents encourage me to have sex with many people before I get married.
_____ 17. Among my friends, people seldom discuss their sexuality.
_____ 18. Among my friends, women who have the most sexual experience are the most highly regarded.
_____ 19. My father would have felt okay about my having casual sexual encounters.
_____ 20. My mother would only have approved of me having sex in a serious relationship.

Reiss Male and Female Premarital Sexual Permissiveness Scales

Ira L. Reiss,[1] *University of Minnesota*

This instrument measures the level of premarital sexual permissiveness that an individual accepts. The original format does so in two scales, one for female respondents and one for male respondents. The scale is a cumulative-type scale and fits all Guttman scaling requirements. It precisely places a person from low to high on the premarital sexual permissiveness dimension defined by the questions in the scale.

Description

The original scale is composed of 12 questions: 4 are concerned with kissing, 4 with petting, and 4 with "full sexual relations" or coitus. The four questions in each of these three behavioral areas focus on the degree of affectionate involvement in the relationship: not feeling *particularly affectionate, strong affection, love,* and finally *engagement.* These four degrees of involvement are asked about for each of the three behavioral areas. In the United States and in Western societies in general, the degree of affection-

ate involvement does alter the degree of acceptance of a particular sexual behavior. Therefore, to construct the dimension of premarital sexual permissiveness in ways appropriate for Western culture, it is necessary to combine these behavioral and affectionate aspects in each question. These questions have a definite advantage over those that simply ask if one accepts coitus, as is done in the one question used in the General Social Survey administered by the National Opinion Research Center.

The original instrument is designed in two forms, one for females and one for males. Respondents should answer the form of their own gender first and, if egalitarian measures are desired, they should also answer the form for the other gender. The full scale for each gender has 12 questions, but if desired, one may break it up into three separate scales of four questions each, measuring kissing, petting, and coital permissiveness.

The original scales have been used on people as young as 12 and as old as 90. For the very young and for very low-permissive groups, the full set of questions can be used. However, for those in senior high school and beyond, one need only use Questions 10, 11, and 12. This is so because the key questions with which this age group is concerned revolve around the acceptability of coitus under the affectionate conditions asked about in those three questions.

[1]Address correspondence to Ira L. Reiss, Department of Sociology, University of Minnesota, 267 19th Avenue South, Minneapolis, MN 55455-0412; email: reiss001@atlas.socsci.umn.edu.

Another alternative form that is widely used is to ask Questions 6 and 7, as well as Questions 10, 11, and 12 (Reiss, 1967, Chap. 2). That five-item version is called the "universal scale order" in that it selects all the questions from the original 12 that have always scaled in the same order in all samples tested. This five-item universal scale has been used a great deal, and it adds a measure of attitudes toward petting if that is desired (Whitbeck, Simons, & Kao, 1994).

In 1989 the Short-Form of these scales was published (Reiss, 1989). Instead of two 12-item scales, the Short-Form uses just four questions, and it focuses on measuring permissiveness in premarital sexual intercourse. In addition, the questions are not gender specific because research has shown that in most cases only small differences occur in responses to the different gender wording. This Short-Form has some advantages over simply using the coital questions from the original scale. First, the Short-Form asks the original Questions 10, 11, and 12 in a non-gender-specific fashion and thus cuts the number of questions in half. Second, the Short-Form adds one question concerning the acceptance of coitus under conditions of moderate affection. Adding this question produces a more evenly spaced dimension of affection: going from *love* to *strong affection* to *moderate affection* to *without much affection*. The Short-Form has been tested on college students in both the United States and Sweden (Schwartz & Reiss, 1995). As spelled out below, it was found to compare favorably with the original format on all measures of reliability and validity.

Response Mode and Timing

All the questions are asked with three degrees of agreement and three degrees of disagreement. Nevertheless, when computing the Guttman scales, I combine all degrees of agreement into one category of agreement and all degrees of disagreement into one category of disagreement. I still suggest keeping the subdivisions in the questionnaire because respondents seem to be more comfortable answering the questions when presented with degrees of choice, particularly because there is no neutral choice given.

The average respondent can answer all 24 questions in about 5 minutes. Respondents circle the degree of agreement or disagreement they have with each item. The four-item Short-Form is answered very quickly, usually in less than 1 minute.

Scoring

As noted above, the answers are dichotomized and scaled using any standard Guttman scaling program. Guttman scaling is a very quick and straightforward method of scaling. It is included in some forms of SPSS and described in a number of books on scaling as well as by the author (Reiss, 1967, Appendix E).

Reliability

Both the original scale and the Short-Form met all Guttman scale reliability criteria. In both formats, the coefficient of reproducibility was well above the 90% level required, and the coefficient of scalability was well above the 65% level required (Reiss, 1964b, 1967, Appendix D; Schwartz & Reiss, 1995). Similar results have been reported by others, both in the United States and in other industrialized countries (Reiss & Miller, 1979; Walsh, Zey-Ferrell, & Tolone, 1976; Whitbeck et al., 1994).

Validity

Construct validity in the original format was established by finding the expected differences between parents and college students, Whites and Blacks, and males and females (Reiss, 1967). The scale has been compared favorably with other similar scales (Hampe & Ruppel, 1974). In the Short-Form, the results fit precisely what was expected when comparing Swedish and American college students. For example, Swedish students were much more acceptant of Question 4 than were American students (Schwartz & Reiss, 1995).

Other Information

The original format has been used since 1959 by a large number of researchers in this country and abroad. The Short-Form version resembles very closely the original format, and thus comparisons with earlier research can still be made. Other scales cannot be so easily compared with prior research. If there is a shortage of space, a researcher can use just Questions 3 and 4 from the Short-Form. In the Swedish/American comparisons those were the key distinguishing questions (Schwartz & Reiss, 1995).

I would be interested in receiving a summary of any findings from the use of the scales.

References

Hampe, G., & Ruppel, H. (1974). The measurement of premarital sexual permissiveness: A comparison of two Guttman scales. *Journal of Marriage and the Family, 36,* 451-464.

Reiss, I. L. (1964a). Premarital sexual permissiveness among Negroes and Whites. *American Sociological Review, 29,* 688-698.

Reiss, I. L. (1964b). The scaling of premarital sexual permissiveness. *Journal of Marriage and the Family, 26,* 188-198.

Reiss, I. L. (1965). Social class and premarital sexual permissiveness: A reexamination. *American Sociological Review, 30,* 747-756.

Reiss, I. L. (1967). *The social context of premarital sexual permissiveness.* New York: Holt, Rinehart & Winston.

Reiss, I. L. (1989). Is this my scale? Responses to a revision of the Reiss PSP Scale. *Journal of Marriage and the Family, 51,* 1079-1080.

Reiss, I. L., & Miller, B. C. (1979). Heterosexual permissiveness: A theoretical analysis. In W. Burr, R. Hill, I. Nye, & I. Reiss (Eds.), *Contemporary theories about the family* (Vol. 1). New York: Free Press.

Schwartz, I., & Reiss, I. L. (1995). The scaling of premarital sexual permissiveness revisited: Test results of Reiss's new short-form version. *Journal of Sex and Marital Therapy, 21,* 78-86.

Walsh, R. H., Zey-Ferrell, M., & Tolone, W. L. (1976). Selection of reference group, perceived reference group permissiveness, and personal permissiveness attitudes and behavior: A study of two consecutive panels (1967-1971; 1970-1974). *Journal of Marriage and the Family, 38,* 495-507.

Whitbeck, L. B., Simons, R. L., & Kao, M. (1994). The effects of divorced mothers' dating behaviors and sexual attitudes on the sexual attitudes and behaviors of their adolescent children. *Journal of Marriage and the Family, 56,* 615-621.

Exhibit

Reiss Male and Female Premarital Sexual Permissiveness Scale

Original Format

First decide whether you agree or disagree with the view expressed. Then circle the degree of your agreement or disagreement with the views expressed in each question. We are not interested in your tolerance of other people's beliefs. Please answer these questions on the basis of how YOU feel toward the views expressed. Your name will never be connected with these answers. Please be as honest as you can. Thank you.

We use the words below to mean just what they do to most people but some may need definitions:

Love means the emotional state which is more intense than strong affection and which you would define as love.

Strong affection means affection which is stronger than physical attraction, average fondness, or "liking"—but less strong than love.

Petting means sexually stimulating behavior more intimate than kissing and simple hugging, but not including full sexual relations.

Male standards

I believe that kissing is acceptable for the male before marriage:

1. When he is engaged to be married.
   Agree: 1) Strong, 2) Medium, 3) Slight
   Disagree: 1) Strong, 2) Medium, 3) Slight
   (This six-way choice follows every question.)
2. When he is in love.
3. When he feels strong affection for his partner.
4. Even if he does not feel particularly affectionate toward his partner.

I believe that petting is acceptable for the male before marriage:

5. When he is engaged to be married.
6. When he is in love.
7. When he feels strong affection for his partner.
8. Even if he does not feel particularly affectionate toward his partner.

I believe that full sexual relations are acceptable for the male before marriage:

9. When he is engaged to be married.
10. When he is in love.
11. When he feels strong affection for his partner.
12. Even if he does not feel particularly affectionate toward his partner.

(The Female Standards questions are the same as the Male Standards except that the gender references are changed.)

Short-Form

1. I believe that premarital sexual intercourse is acceptable if one is in a love relationship.
   Agree: Strong,   Medium,   Slight
   Disagree: Strong,   Medium,   Slight
   (The same choices follow each question.)
2. I believe that premarital sexual intercourse is acceptable if one is in a relationship involving strong affection.
3. I believe that premarital sexual intercourse is acceptable if one is in a relationship involving moderate amounts of affection.
4. I believe that premarital sexual intercourse is acceptable even if one is in a relationship without much affection.

Source. These scales are reprinted with permission of the author.

Premarital Sexual Permissiveness Scale

Susan Sprecher,[1] *Illinois State University*

The purpose of the Premarital Sexual Permissiveness Scale (Sprecher, 1989; Sprecher, McKinney, Walsh, & Anderson, 1988) is to assess attitudes about premarital sexual behavior under different relationship conditions. It is a more precise way to assess premarital sexual attitudes than a single-item question (e.g., "Do you approve of sexual intercourse before marriage?") because the acceptability of sexual behavior is likely to depend on the emotional commitment of the relationship. The scale was modeled after the Reiss (1964, 1988) Premarital Permissiveness Scale, which measures the acceptability of sexual behavior at different levels of affection (no affection, strong affection, in love, and engaged). However, in this scale, the acceptability of sexual behavior is assessed for stages that are commonly recognized as labels marking the progression of relationship development. For a discussion of the relative merits of the two scales, see Reiss (1989) and Sprecher, McKinney, Walsh, and Anderson (1989).

Description

The scale can be administered in its full version (15 items; 3 sexual behaviors crossed by 5 relationship stages) or in a brief format (e.g., in several of my recent studies only attitudes about sexual intercourse were assessed). In the full version, the three sexual behaviors are heavy petting (touching of genitals), sexual intercourse, and oral-genital sex. The five relationship stages are first date, casually dating, seriously dating, pre-engaged, and engaged.

Participants can receive only one version of the scale or could receive several versions. If the researcher is interested in standards unmarried adults have for their own premarital sexual behaviors, only one version, with the items referring to "me" (e.g., "I believe that sexual intercourse is acceptable for me on a first date"), need be administered. However, sexual standards can be assessed for any number of targets (e.g., a male, a female, a close same-sex friend). If the researcher wants to compare standards for one target (e.g., a male) with standards for another target (e.g., a female), he or she may use either a within-participants design or a between-participants design. In a within-participants design, participants complete all versions of the scale (e.g., both the male and female versions), perhaps presented in a random order. In a between-participants design, participants receive only one version (randomly assigned) and a comparison is made between the scores of the groups who received the different targets (e.g., male vs. female). The advantage of the second method is that demand characteristics or social desirability biases related to gender are likely to be less problematic because it will be less obvious

to the participants that between-gender comparisons will be made.

The scale is most appropriately used for young, unmarried adults because they are the particular population for whom premarital sexual attitudes (for self or for others) are most salient. However, the scale could be used with other populations as well. For example, the items could be modified to refer to "my son or daughter" and administered to parents of teenagers or young college-age adults.

Response Mode and Timing

Participants respond to each item on a 6-point scale. They can agree *strongly, moderately,* or *slightly,* or disagree *strongly, moderately,* or *slightly.* Responses are recoded to range from 1 = *disagree strongly* to 6 = *agree strongly* so that the higher number indicates more agreement.

The scale can be administered on its own or as part of a larger questionnaire. One version of the scale takes less than 5 minutes to complete.

Scoring

Analyses can be conducted on the separate items of the scale and/or for total indexes (means or sums) created from the items. The primary index that can be computed is an overall total score, either the sum of or mean of all items included in one version of the scale (i.e., all items that refer to attitudes about the same target). Also, three "permissiveness by type of sexual activity" indexes can be created by collapsing (adding or averaging) the responses for each sexual behavior across types of relationships, and five "permissiveness by type of relationship" indexes can be created by collapsing the responses for each relationship stage across types of sexual activities. These indexes created from subparts of the scale allow the investigator to examine how standards depend on the type of relationship and the type of sexual behavior (such results are presented in Sprecher et al., 1988). Finally, a difference score can be calculated between how respondents answer one version of the scale (e.g., a male version) and how they answer another version (e.g., a female version). This difference score can be used as a dependent variable in analyses to determine what factors are associated with the adherence of a double standard (Sprecher & Hatfield, 1996).

Reliability

The scale has Guttman-like qualities for the items assessing acceptability of each sexual behavior across relationship stages. That is, an increasing proportion of participants approve of each sexual behavior as the relationship stage identified in the item moves from first date to engagement, with the greatest increases occurring among the first three stages—first date, casually dating, and seriously dating (e.g.,

[1]Address all correspondence to Susan Sprecher, Department of Sociology and Anthropology, Illinois State University, Normal, IL 61790-4660; email: sprecher@rs6000.cmp.ilstu.edu.

Sprecher et al., 1988). The scale also has high internal consistency. Analyses of unpublished data for the five-item subscale measuring attitudes about sexual intercourse yielded a Cronbach's alpha of .76 in one sample (N = 1,627) and .81 in a second sample (N = 2,512).

Validity

Construct validity is evidenced by findings of expected differences between male and female participants (e.g., Sprecher, 1989; Sprecher et al., 1988). Furthermore, in unpublished data, the subscale of acceptability of sexual intercourse was found to be significantly and positively correlated with sexual permissiveness items included in another established sexual permissiveness scale, the Sociosexuality Orientation Scale (Simpson & Gangestad, 1991). Although very little published data are available on the reliability and validity of the scale, this information has been published on its predecessor, the Reiss Premarital Sexual Permissiveness Scale (e.g., Reiss, 1964, 1967, 1988).

Other Information

If the researcher has the space for only a few items of the scale, my suggestion is that he or she includes the three items that ask about the acceptability of sexual intercourse during first date, casual dating, and serious dating.

References

Reiss, I. L. (1964). The scaling of premarital sexual permissiveness. *Journal of Marriage and the Family, 26*, 188-198.

Reiss, I. L. (1967). *The social context of premarital sexual permissiveness.* New York: Holt, Rinehart & Winston.

Reiss, I. L. (1988). Reiss Male and Female Premarital Sexual Permissiveness Scale. In C. M. Davis, W. L. Yarber, & S. L. Davis (Eds.), *Sexuality-related measures: A compendium* (pp. 233-235). Lake Mills, IA: Davis, Yarber, and Davis.

Reiss, I. L. (1989). Is this my scale? Responses to a revision of the Reiss PSP Scale. *Journal of Marriage and the Family, 51*, 1079-1080.

Simpson, J. A., & Gangestad, S. W. (1991). Individual differences in sociosexuality: Evidence for convergent and discriminant validity. *Journal of Personality and Social Psychology, 60*, 870-883.

Sprecher, S. (1989). Premarital sexual standards for different categories of individuals. *The Journal of Sex Research, 26*, 232-248.

Sprecher, S., & Hatfield, E. (1996). Premarital sexual standards among U.S. college students: Comparison with those of Russian and Japanese students. *Archives of Sexual Behavior, 25*, 261-288.

Sprecher, S., McKinney, K., Walsh, R., & Anderson, C. (1988). A revision of the Reiss Premarital Sexual Permissiveness Scale. *Journal of Marriage and the Family, 50*, 821-828.

Sprecher, S., McKinney, K., Walsh, R., & Anderson, C. (1989). Reply to Ira Reiss's comment. *Journal of Marriage and the Family, 51*, 1080-1082.

Exhibit

Premarital Sexual Permissiveness Scale

Following are the items for *sexual intercourse* in reference to *the self.*

Directions: For each of the following statements, indicate to what extent you agree or disagree with it. These statements concern what you think is appropriate behavior *for you.*

1) Agree strongly
2) Agree moderately
3) Agree slightly
4) Disagree slightly
5) Disagree moderately
6) Disagree strongly

_____ 1. I believe that sexual intercourse is acceptable for me on a first date.

_____ 2. I believe that sexual intercourse is acceptable for me when I'm casually dating my partner (dating less than one month).

_____ 3. I believe that sexual intercourse is acceptable for me when I'm seriously dating my partner (dating almost a year).

_____ 4. I believe that sexual intercourse is acceptable for me when I am pre-engaged to my partner (we have seriously discussed the possibility of getting married).

_____ 5. I believe that sexual intercourse is acceptable for when I'm engaged to my partner.

The researcher may also ask about the acceptability of other sexual behaviors. For example, the researcher may include similar items that ask about acceptability of *heaving petting (e.g., touching of genitals)* and *oral-genital sex* for the five different relationship stages, as was done in Sprecher et al. (1988). Furthermore, the researcher may ask about acceptability of sexual behaviors for different targets—for example, for a male and a female (see Sprecher, 1989; Sprecher et al., 1988). An example item to measure standards for a female would be: "I believe that sexual intercourse is acceptable for a female who is seriously dating her partner." An example item from the male version is: "I believe that sexual intercourse is acceptable for a male who is engaged to his partner."

Attitudes Toward Sexual Permissiveness

The Editors

This instrument, designed by Weaver and Arkoff (1965), is intended as a general measure of permissiveness toward sexual behavior. Two separate, three-item forms were developed using a 5-point Likert-type technique. A mixed sample of college students and older adults was used in construction of the scales. Both forms are included in the article.

Reference

Weaver, H. B., & Arkoff, A. (1965). Measurement of attitudes concerning sexual permissiveness. *Social Science, 40,* 163-168.

Intimate Relationship Scale

Susan E. Hetherington,[1] *University of Maryland School of Nursing*

To assess perceived changes in intimacy and sexuality in postpartum couples, I developed the Intimate Relationship Scale (IRS) described by Hetherington and Soeken (1990). The scale measures changes in intimacy and sexuality on three dimensions: personal, physical, and cognitive. The personal or emotional component includes such areas as satisfaction from sexual activities, desire for sex and touching, and feelings of sexual fulfillment. The physical dimension examines such aspects of the relationship as touching, holding, stroking, and sexual intercourse. The cognitive or intellectual dimension relates to communication between the couples in the form of quiet conversations or talks about sex.

Although developed for assessment of postpartum couples (Fischman [Hetherington], Rankin, Soeken, & Lenz, 1986), the IRS, with modifications to the introductory phase, has been used to assess changes in intimacy and sexuality during or after other medical, surgical, or stressful events. For example, the IRS has been used with pregnant couples (Higgins, 1988), posthysterectomy patients (Biddle, Hetherington, & Soeken, 1987), and breast cancer patients (Denicoff & Hetherington, 1995). The IRS introductory phrase was modified to read, "Since my/my spouse's pregnancy . . . ," or "Since my/my partner's mastectomy . . . ," or "Since my/my partner's chemotherapy treatment program. . . ."

Description

The IRS is a 12-item Likert-type scale with five response options ranging from *much less* to *much more*. The items were developed based on a review of the literature and were examined by nurse-midwives for content validity.

Psychometric evaluation of the IRS was performed through item analysis and factor analysis of data provided by a sample of 194 couples. Because the sample consisted of couples, analyses were conducted separately for mothers and fathers. Scale and item characteristics for mothers and fathers were similar. All items had acceptable corrected item-total correlations (> .25) and the internal consistency of the IRS was $\alpha = .87$ and $\alpha = .86$ for mothers and fathers, respectively. Among mothers, all interitem correlations were positive with an average of $r = .36$. Among fathers, one pair of items (numbers 2 and 11) correlated negatively. However, the average interitem correlation was $r = .34$.

Factor analysis was performed to aid in further understanding how the items relate to one another and to determine if interpretable and reliable subscales corresponding to the hypothesized dimensions could be empirically verified. Three factors did emerge, accounting for 62% and 65% of the variance for mothers and fathers, respectively. All items had positive factor loadings between .27 and .81 on the first unrotated factor suggesting that the entire scale can be used to measure intimate relationship behavior. Ten of the 12 items for mothers and 9 of the 12 for fathers had loadings above .50.

Because the hypothesized factors were thought to be related and because of the internal consistency of the scale,

[1]Address correspondence to Susan E. Hetherington, 5209 E. Woodspring Drive, Tucson, AZ 85712-1364.

oblique rotation was used. The average intercorrelation between the three rotated factors was $r = .37$ for mothers and $r = .29$ for fathers. A stringent criterion of .45 was used when examining the factor loadings. Item 4, "Since the birth of the baby, I derive satisfaction from our sexual activities," emerged as a "global" item. Its correlation with the remainder of the scale was $r = .67$ and $r = .64$ for mothers and fathers, respectively.

The resulting three factors corresponded to the hypothesized dimensions: personal or emotional, physical, and cognitive or communication. For mothers, the emotional factor emerged as the first factor accounting for 41.3% of the variance, whereas for fathers, the physical factor was first accounting for 41% of the variance.

Response Mode and Timing

Respondents circle the response options that best describe their perception of changes in lovemaking having occurred to them since the birth of the baby. The scale requires an average of 5 minutes for completion.

Scoring

Responses are totaled across the items so that a higher score indicates a greater degree of positive change. For all items except one, the responses range from (1) *much less* to (5) *much more*. Responses for Item 2 range from (1) *much more* to (5) *much less*.

Reliability

The IRS was pilot tested with 17 clients of several certified nurse-midwives. No one refused to complete the instrument or indicated any discomfort with the specific questionnaire items. A coefficient alpha of .93 was obtained for an 18-item version of the scale, which, because of the limited data, may have been overdetermined. Six items were deleted from the scale because of redundancy. A pilot test of the 12-item tool was conducted using 37 middle-class patients from several practices of certified nurse-midwives. An equally high alpha of .94 was obtained with this sample.

The final version of the IRS was mailed to 93 couples at 4 months postpartum and achieved response rates of 73% (68) for women and 60% (56) for men. Another mailing to 235 couples at 12 months postpartum had somewhat lower response rates: 54% (126) for women and 46% (109) for men. Reliability coefficients, as measured by Cronbach's alpha, at 4 and 12 months postpartum were .85 and .87 for mothers and .85 and .86 for fathers, respectively, demonstrating a high measure of internal consistency for the 12 items in the IRS. Because test-retest reliability is appropriate for traits or characteristics that do not change across time, and because the IRS is designed to measure changes in intimacy and sexuality, this test was not used.

The three subscales were subject to reliability analysis to determine if they could be used as separate scales. Despite the small number of items on each subscale, all reliability coefficients were above .64. Corrected item-total correlations within each subscale were above $r = .30$ and averaged above $r = .40$ across the subscales. These favorable results suggest that the total scale score as well as individual subscale scores can be computed to measure intimate relationship behavior and its components.

Validity

Only content or face validity data are available (see above).

Other Information

Notification to the author of the tool's use and the results obtained would be appreciated.

References

Biddle, K. J., Hetherington, S. E., & Soeken, K. L. (1987). Posthysterectomy effects on sexuality and intimacy. In *Proceedings from the 21st International Congress* (pp. 87-90). The Hague: International Confederation of Midwives.

Denicoff, A. M., & Hetherington, S. H. (1995). *Assessment of changes in sexuality in women with breast cancer.* Unpublished manuscript.

Fischman, S. (Hetherington), Rankin, E. A., Soeken, K. L., & Lenz, E. R. (1986). Changes in sexual relationships in postpartum couples. *Journal of Obstetric, Gynecologic, and Neonatal Nursing, 15,* 58-63.

Hetherington, S. H., & Soeken, K. L. (1990). Measuring changes in intimacy and sexuality: A self-administered scale. *Journal of Sex Education and Therapy, 16,* 155-163.

Higgins, P. G. (1988). Changes in intimacy behaviors in antepartum couples. *Journal of Nursing Science and Practice, 1*(4), 17-21.

Exhibit

Intimate Relationship Scale

Name or number _____ Please circle: Mother or Father   Date _____

Many couples experience changes in their patterns of lovemaking from before the pregnancy occurred to after the birth of the baby. We would appreciate it very much if you would share with us some of the ways these changes may or may not have occurred to you. Please *underline* the phrase that most accurately completes each statement, and give as honest an account of your own feelings and beliefs at this time as possible. Feel free to add additional comments in the space provided. Your answers will be held in strictest confidence.

If you have not resumed sex, please indicate why, and then return this form without filling out the attached questions. Otherwise, please complete the following questions. Thank you.

1. Since the birth of the baby, the frequency that my spouse and I are having sex is:
    (1) much less   (2) less   (3) unchanged   (4) more   (5) much more[a]
2. Since the birth of the baby, my feelings of fatigue interfere with our making love:
3. Since the birth of the baby, my spouse and I find time for quiet conversation:
4. Since the birth of the baby, I derive satisfaction from our sexual activities:
5. Since the birth of the baby, my desire to touch and hold is being satisfied:
6. Since the birth of the baby, my spouse initiates sexual activity which leads to intercourse:
7. Since the birth of the baby, my feelings of sexual fulfillment are:
8. Since the birth of the baby, my feelings of closeness to my spouse are:
9. Since the birth of the baby, my desire to be held, touched, and stroked by my spouse is:
10. Since the birth of the baby, my desire for sexual intercourse is:
11. Since the birth of the baby, my comfort in talking with my spouse about sex is:
12. Since the birth of the baby, I initiate sexual activity which leads to intercourse:
13. Does your baby sleep in your bedroom?   _____ Yes   _____ No
14. I worry that our lovemaking will wake up the baby:
    (1) not at all   (2) hardly ever   (3) occasionally   (4) most of the time   (5) all the time.
15. Number of children in your home: _____   Ages: _____
16. To your best recollection, how long after the baby's birth did you and your spouse resume sexual intercourse? Please indicate in number of weeks.
    _____ Weeks after the baby's birth.
17. How satisfying was it for you?
    (1) very satisfying   (2) satisfying   (3) okay   (4) not satisfying   (5) very unsatisfying
18. What kind of contraception, if any, are you using now? _____

Women only answer Questions 19-24.
19. Type of delivery: _____ Vaginal   _____ C-section
20. Episiotomy: _____ Yes _____ No
21. Vaginal tears: _____ Yes _____ No
22. Since the birth of the baby, my experience of physical discomfort with sexual intercourse has been:
23. Since the birth of the baby, my physical strength is:
24. Since the birth of the baby, my feelings of satisfaction with my bodily appearance are:

Source. This scale is reprinted with permission of the author.

a. Items 2-12 and 22-24 are also followed by these response options.

Attitudes Toward Rape Questionnaire and Rape Knowledge Test

The Editors

These instruments, developed by Feild (1978), measure attitudes toward the act of rape, the rape victim, the rapist, and factual knowledge of rape.

The attitude instrument contains 32 items (half positively phrased, half negatively phrased) to which participants are asked to respond using a 6-point Likert-type scale ranging from *strongly agree* to *strongly disagree*. Undergraduate students were used in scale development. Items are included in the article. Examples of items are as follows: "A woman can be raped against her will," "A woman can be responsible for preventing her rape," "Most women

secretly desire to be raped," and "The reason most rapists commit rape is for sex."

The knowledge instrument has 14 multiple-choice items that reflect empirical data on rape. Scores are based on the total number of questions answered correctly, with a higher score indicating more knowledge about rape.

Reference

Feild, H. S. (1978). Attitudes toward rape: A comparative analysis of police, rapists, crisis counselors, and citizens. *Journal of Personality and Social Psychology, 36,* 156-179.

Rape Supportive Attitude Scale

Ilsa L. Lottes,[1] *University of Maryland, Baltimore County*

The purpose of the Rape Supportive Attitude Scale is to measure attitudes that are hostile to rape victims, including false beliefs about rape and rapists. Seven beliefs measured by this scale are (a) women enjoy sexual violence, (b) women are responsible for rape prevention, (c) sex rather than power is the primary motivation for rape, (d) rape happens only to certain kinds of women, (e) a woman is less desirable after she has been raped, (f) women falsely report many rape claims, and (g) rape is justified in some situations. Researchers (Burt, 1980; Marolla & Scully, 1982; Russell, 1975; Williams & Holmes, 1981) have found support for the views that these beliefs not only promote rape but also hinder and prolong the recuperative process for survivors of a rape.

Description

The Rape Supportive Attitude Scale was developed from a pool of 40 items from the rape attitude measures of Barnett and Feild (1977), Burt (1980), Koss (1981), and Wheeler and Utigard (1984). The 20 items selected for the scale meet two criteria: (a) The items have content validity (i.e., they assess one of the seven victim-callous beliefs listed above), and (b) the items have high item-total scale correlations and high factor loadings on the same factor. The response options for each item are one of the five Likert-type scale choices: *strongly disagree* (1), *disagree* (2), *undecided* (3), *agree* (4), or *strongly agree* (5).

The Rape Supportive Attitude Scale was administered to two college student samples in the northeastern United States (Lottes, 1991). Students completed the scale in their regularly scheduled classes. For both samples, the 20 scale items were randomly distributed in a questionnaire containing 70 other items requiring similar Likert-type responses. The first sample consisted of 98 males and 148 females from education, health, and sociology classes at two universities. The second sample consisted of 195 males and 195 females from business, engineering, English, education, history, mathematics, physics, political science, and sociology classes at three universities. The majority of the students in both samples were single and in the 19- to 22-year-old age range. The Rape Supportive Attitude Scale is appropriate to administer to adults.

Response Mode and Timing

Two response modes are possible. If a machine-scorable sheet is used, respondents should shade in the circle of the number indicating their agreement or disagreement with

each item. If a machine-scorable sheet is not used, then the numbers 1 through 5 need to be included next to each item and the respondents should circle the number indicating their agreement or disagreement with each item. The 20-item scale takes about 10 minutes to complete.

Scoring

All of the items are scored in the same direction. To break up any response set, the 20 items of this scale can be randomly placed among Likert-type items assessing other characteristics. To determine each respondent's score for the scale, add the responses (coded 1 through 5) to the 20 items. The higher the score, the more rape supportive or victim-callous attitudes are supported by a respondent.

Reliability

For the first sample of 246 college students, the Cronbach alpha was .91. For the second sample of 390 students, the Cronbach alpha also was .91.

Validity

For both college student samples, respectively ($n = 246$ and $n = 390$), scores for the Rape Supportive Attitude Scale were significantly correlated ($p < .001$) in the predicted direction with (a) nonegalitarian gender role beliefs ($r = .58, r = .64$), traditional attitudes toward female sexuality ($r = .50, r = .42$), (c) adversarial sexual beliefs ($r = .65, r = .70$), (d) *arousal to sexual violence* ($r = .32, r = .37$), and (e) nonacceptance of homosexuality ($r = .25, r = .34$). For males in both samples, the Rape Supportive Attitude Scale was significantly correlated ($p < .001$) in the predicted direction with the Hypermasculinity Inventory of Mosher and Sirkin (1984) ($r = .44, r = .52$, respectively). Finally, for both samples, the correlations of sex with the scale ($r = .36, r = 35$, respectively) were significant ($p < .001$) and in the predicted direction. Males indicated more victim-callous attitudes than females.

A principal components analysis of the data from both samples revealed that a single, dominant factor emerged, accounting for 37% of the variance in each case. In both analyses, all items loaded on this factor at .39 or greater.

Other Information

Bell et al. (1992) found that a 12-item subset (containing Items 2, 3, 4, 5, 6, 7, 11, 12, 13, 15, 17, and 19) of the Rape Supportive Attitude Scale produced an alpha of .77 for a sample of 521 first-year university students. As seniors, 300 of the original first-year student sample completed a questionnaire containing the 12-item subset. Test-retest reliability was .53 and the Cronbach alpha for the senior sample was .76 (Bell, Lottes, & Kuriloff, 1995).

[1]Address correspondence to Ilsa L. Lottes, Department of Sociology and Anthropology, University of Maryland, Baltimore County, 5401 Wilkens Avenue, Baltimore, MD 21228; email: lottes@umbc2.umbc.edu.

Construct validity of this shortened Rape Supportive Attitude Scale was supported by significant correlations in the predicted directions between this scale and measures of feminist attitudes, male dominant attitudes, liberalism, and social conscience for both the first-year student and senior samples (Bell et al., 1992; Bell et al., 1995). For both samples, men reported significantly higher ($p < .001$, t test) scores on the Rape Supportive Attitude Scale than did women (Bell et al., 1992; Bell et al., 1995).

References

Barnett, N. J., & Feild, H. S. (1977). Sex differences in university students' attitudes toward rape. *Journal of College Student Personnel, 18*, 93-96.

Bell, S., Kuriloff, P., Lottes, I., Nathanson, J., Judge, T., & Fogelson-Turet, K. (1992). Rape callousness in college freshmen: An empirical investigation of a sociocultural model of aggression towards women. *Journal of College Student Development, 33*, 454-461.

Bell, S., Lottes, I., & Kuriloff, P. (1995). *Understanding rape callousness in college students: Results of a panel study*. Manuscript submitted for publication.

Burt, M. R. (1980). Cultural myths and supports for rape. *Journal of Personality and Social Psychology, 38*, 217-230.

Koss, M. P. (1981). *Hidden rape on a university campus* (Grant No. R01MH31618). Rockville, MD: National Institute of Health.

Lottes, I. L. (1991). Belief systems: Sexuality and rape. *Journal of Psychology and Human Sexuality, 4*, 37-59.

Marolla, J., & Scully, D. (1982). *Attitudes toward women, violence, and rape: A comparison of convicted rapists and other felons* (Grant No. R01MH33013-01A1). Rockville, MD: National Institute of Health.

Mosher, D. L., & Sirkin, M. (1984). Measuring a macho personality constellation. *Journal of Research in Personality, 18*, 150-163.

Russell, D. (1975). *The politics of rape*. New York: Stein and Day.

Wheeler, J. R., & Utigard, C. N. (1984, June). *Gender, stereotyping, rape attitudes, and acceptance of interpersonal violence*. Paper presented at the combined annual meeting of the Society for the Scientific Study of Sex and the American Association of Sex Educators, Counselors, and Therapists, Boston.

Williams, J. E., & Holmes, K. A. (1981). *The second assault, rape and public attitudes*. Westport, CT: Greenwood.

Exhibit

Rape Supportive Attitude Scale

Directions: Write all of your responses on the computer answer sheet. Use a No. 2 lead pencil. To indicate your opinion about each statement, shade in the number corresponding to one of the five circles. Indicate whether you *strongly disagree* (1), *disagree* (2), are *undecided* or *have no opinion* (3), *agree* (4), or *strongly agree* (5).

Strongly disagree (1)   disagree (2)   Undecided (3)   Agree (4)   Strongly agree (5)

Remember: Be sure that the statement you are reading corresponds to the statement number you are marking on the answer sheet. Mark only one response for each statement.

1. Being roughed up is sexually stimulating to many women.
2. A man has some justification in forcing a female to have sex with him when she led him to believe she would go to bed with him.
3. The degree of a woman's resistance should be the major factor in determining if a rape has occurred.
4. The reason most rapists commit rape is for sex.
5. If a girl engages in necking or petting and she lets things get out of hand, it is her fault if her partner forces sex on her.
6. Many women falsely report that they have been raped because they are pregnant and want to protect their reputation.
7. A man has some justification in forcing a woman to have sex with him if she allowed herself to be picked up.
8. Sometimes the only way a man can get a cold woman turned on is to use force.
9. A charge of rape two days after the act has occurred is probably not rape.
10. A raped woman is a less desirable woman.
11. A man is somewhat justified in forcing a woman to have sex with him if he has had sex with her in the past.
12. In order to protect the male, it should be difficult to prove that a rape has occurred.
13. Many times a woman will pretend she doesn't want to have intercourse because she doesn't want to seem loose, but she's really hoping the man will force her.
14. A woman who is stuck-up and thinks she is too good to talk to guys deserves to be taught a lesson.
15. One reason that women falsely report rape is that they frequently have a need to call attention to themselves.
16. In a majority of rapes the victim is promiscuous or had a bad reputation.
17. Many women have an unconscious wish to be raped, and may then unconsciously set up a situation in which they are likely to be attacked.
18. Rape is the expression of an uncontrollable desire for sex.
19. A man is somewhat justified in forcing a woman to have sex with him if they have dated for a long time.
20. Rape of a woman by a man she knows can be defined as a "woman who changed her mind afterwards."

Sexual Assault Treating/Reporting Attitudes Survey

Vetta L. Sanders Thompson[1] and Sharon West Smith,
University of Missouri–St. Louis

The Sexual Assault Treatment/Reporting Attitudes Survey is a 46-item survey designed to assess community attitudes on a variety of issues related to sexual assault. The survey consists of three sections: demographic data, sexual assault treatment and reporting attitudes, and vignette responses.

The first section of the survey elicits demographic data. Participants are asked to report age, sex, income, education, and marital status. The second section of the survey examines attitudes related to decisions to report or seek treatment in cases of sexual assault. The survey addresses knowledge of both short- and long-term effects of rape and child sexual abuse, attitudes toward the need for treatment, preferences for who provides treatment, and expectations and fears related to entering the treatment process. In addition, concerns regarding the involvement of the judicial system and various social service agencies are addressed.

The third section of the instrument is based on a prior survey (Howard, 1988). It consists of 10 vignettes, depicting either child molestation or rape. Three vignettes depict the sexual molestation of a female child; three, the sexual molestation of a male child; three, the rape of a female; and one vignette depicts the rape of a male by a stranger. Participants read each vignette and indicate whether a sexual assault has occurred, the need for treatment, type of treatment, and treatment source preferred. They also indicate the extent to which there is victim responsibility for the incident described using a 5-point rating scale.

A copy of this instrument may be obtained from the Health and Psychosocial Instruments database, Behavioral Measurement Database Services, P.O. Box 110287, Pittsburgh, PA 15232-0787.

[1]Address correspondence to Vetta L. Sanders Thompson, Department of Psychology, University of Missouri–St. Louis, 8001 Natural Bridge Road, St. Louis, MO 63121-4499; email: svlsand.@umslvma.umsl.edu.

Reference

Howard, J. (1988). A structural approach to sexual attitudes. *Sociological Perspectives, 31,* 88-121.

Exhibit

Sexual Assault Treating/Reporting Attitudes Survey (sample items)

Do you believe there are detrimental or bad effects for a child who has been sexually abused or molested?

If your child were sexually abused or molested, would you seek treatment or counseling (beyond medical treatment)?

Which of the following do you think/feel might be long-term effects of child sexual abuse or molestation:

If a family member or friend were raped or sexually assaulted, would you recommend that they seek treatment or counseling (beyond medical treatment)?

Would you be more likely to seek treatment if you knew that there would be no police or judicial involvement?

Can males be sexually molested or raped?

Where would you go for help or treatment?

The Multidimensional Sexual Approach Questionnaire

William E. Snell, Jr.,[1] *Southeast Missouri State University*

The Multidimensional Sexual Approach Questionnaire (MSAQ; Snell, 1992) is a self-report questionnaire designed to assess several different ways in which people can approach their sexual relationships (e.g., from a caring vs. an exchange perspective). More specifically, the MSAQ was developed to measure eight separate approaches to sexual relations (cf. Hughes & Snell, 1990): (a) a passionate, romantic approach to sexual relations; (b) a game-playing approach to sexual relations; (c) a companionate, friendship approach to sexual relations; (d) a practical, logical, and shopping-list approach to a sexual partner and a sexual relationship; (e) a dependent, possessive approach to sexual relations; (f) an altruistic, selfless, and all-giving approach to sexual partners and sexual relations; (g) a communal approach to sex (i.e., a sensitive approach to sexual relations that emphasizes caring and concern for a partner's sexual needs and preferences); and (h) an exchange approach to sex (i.e., a quid pro quo approach to sex, where a sexual partner "keeps tabs" on the sexual activities and favors that he or she does for a partner, expecting to be repaid in an exchange fashion at some time in the future of the relationship). Snell (1992) found significant relationships between the ways that people approach their sexual relations, as measured by the MSAQ, and both their sexual and love attitudes. Other findings reported by Snell revealed that several demographic and psychosocial variables (e.g., dating status) were also associated with the sexual styles measured by the MSAQ.

Description

The MSAQ consists of 56 items. In responding to the MSAQ, respondents are asked to indicate how much they agree or disagree with each statement. A 5-point Likert-type scale is used to collect data on the responses, with each item being scored from +2 to –2: *agree* (+2), *slightly agree* (+1), *neither agree nor disagree* (0), *slightly disagree* (–1), and *disagree* (–2). To create subscale scores, the items on each subscale are summed. Higher positive (vs. negative) scores thus correspond to the tendency to approach one's sexual relations in the manner described by each respective MSAQ subscale. A varimax factor analysis with an orthogonal rotation extracted eight factors that corresponded to the eight approaches measured by the MSAQ.

[1]Address correspondence to William E. Snell, Jr., Department of Psychology, Southeast Missouri State University, One University Plaza, Cape Girardeau, MO 63701; email: wesnell@semovm.semo.edu.

Response Mode and Timing

Respondents indicate their answers on a computer scan sheet by darkening in a response from A to E. The questionnaire usually takes 15-20 minutes to complete.

Scoring

For purposes of analyses, the statements are keyed so that A = 2, B = 1, C = 0, D = –1, and E = –2 (no items are reverse scored). This procedure results in six subscale scores, based on the sum of the items assigned to a particular subscale (i.e., add up the seven item scores). An overall scale score for the MSAQ is not particularly useful. The MSAQ subscales are coded so that a higher score indicates greater agreement with the respective MSAQ statements. Subscale scores can range from –14 to 14. The items assigned to each subscale are (a) a passionate, romantic approach to sexual relations (Items 1-7); (b) a game-playing approach to sexual relations (Items 8-14); (c) a companionate, friendship approach to sexual relations (Items 15-21); (d) a practical, logical, and shopping-list approach to a sexual partner and a sexual relationship (Items 22-28); (e) a dependent, possessive approach to sexual relations (Items 29-35); (f) an altruistic, selfless, and all-giving approach to sexual partners and sexual relations (Items 36-42); (g) sexual communion and a sensitive approach to sexual relations that emphasizes caring and concern for a partner's sexual needs and preferences (Items 43-48); and (h) sexual exchange (Items 49-56).

Reliability

To examine the internal reliability of the subscales on the MSAQ, Cronbach alpha coefficients were computed for males and females, separately and in combination (Snell, 1992). The results clearly indicated that the subscales on the MSAQ have high internal reliability among both males and females. Specifically, the Cronbach alphas ranged from a low of .72 for males and .73 for females to a high of .92 for males and .85 for females (average for males = .80, average for females = .78).

Validity

As expected, Snell (1992) found that males who took a friendly, companionate approach to their sexual relations were characterized by sexual possessiveness, selflessness, and sensitivity. Not surprisingly, it was also found that among males a game-playing sexual style was directly related to a logical, rational way of approaching their sexual relations. In contrast, females who approached sex as a game were less likely to engage in friendly, companionate sexual relations. Other results reported by Snell indicated that males reported higher scores than females on the measure of the altruistic sexual style (a selfless, all-giving approach to sexual relations). In contrast, females, relative to males, were more rejecting of an exchange approach to sex. Men's and women's scores on the remaining MSAQ subscales were quite similar; they endorsed a romantic, companionate, and communal approach to their sexual relations, while disavowing a game-playing sexual style. A final set of results reported by Snell examined the impact of sexual attitudes on the way that people approach their sexual relations (i.e., their sexual styles). As expected, sexually permissive attitudes were found to be positively associated with a game-playing approach to sex; people with sexually responsible attitudes toward contraceptives ap-

proached their sexual relations with a sensitive, caring sexual style; and a sexual attitude favoring idealized communal sex, as measured by the Sexual Attitudes Scale (Hendrick & Hendrick, 1987), was positively and strongly associated with all of the following MSAQ sexual styles: passionate, companionate, possessive, selfless, and caring approaches to sex.

References

Hendrick, S. S., & Hendrick, C. (1987). Multidimensionality of sexual attitudes. *The Journal of Sex Research, 23,* 502-526.

Hughes, T. G., & Snell, W. E., Jr. (1990). Communal and exchange approaches to sexual relations. *Annals of Sex Research, 3,* 149-164.

Snell, W. E., Jr. (1992, April). *Sexual styles: A multidimensional approach to sexual relations.* Paper presented at the annual meeting of the Southwestern Psychological Association, Austin, TX.

Exhibit

The Multidimensional Sexual Approach Questionnaire

Instructions: Listed below are several statements that reflect different attitudes about sex. For each statement fill in the response on the answer sheet that indicates how much you agree or disagree with that statement. Some of the items refer to a specific sexual relationship, while others refer to general attitudes and beliefs about sex. Whenever possible, answer the questions with your current partner in mind. If you are not currently dating anyone, answer the questions with your most recent partner in mind. If you have never had a sexual relationship, answer in terms of what you think your responses would most likely be in a future sexual relationship. For each statement:

A	=	Strongly *agree* with the statement.
B	=	Moderately *agree* with the statement.
C	=	Neutral—*Neither* agree nor disagree.
D	=	Moderately *disagree* with the statement.
E	=	Strongly *disagree* with the statement.

1. I was sexually attracted to my partner immediately after we first met.
2. I feel a strong sexual "chemistry" toward my partner.
3. I have a very intense and satisfying sexual relationship with my partner.
4. I was sexually meant for my partner.
5. I became sexually involved rather quickly with my partner.
6. I have a strong sexual understanding of my partner.
7. My partner fits my notion of the ideal sexual partner.
8. I try to keep my partner a little uncertain about my sexual commitment to him/her.
9. I believe that what my partner doesn't know about my sexual activity won't hurt him/her.
10. I have not always told my partner about my previous sexual experiences.
11. I could end my sexual relationship with my partner rather easily and quickly.
12. My partner wouldn't like hearing about some of the sexual experiences I've had with others.
13. When my partner becomes too sexually involved with me, I want to back off a little.
14. I like playing around with a number of people, including my partner and others.
15. The sexual relationship between myself and my partner started off rather slowly.
16. I had to "care" for my partner before I could make love to him/her.
17. I expect to always be a friend of my sexual partner.
18. The sex I have with my partner is better because it was preceded by a long friendship.
19. I was a friend of my sexual partner before we became lovers.
20. The sex my partner and I have is based on a deep friendship, not something mystical and mysterious.
21. Sex with my partner is highly satisfying because it developed out of a good friendship.
22. Before I made love with my partner, I spent some time evaluating her/his career potential.
23. I planned my life in a careful manner before I chose my sexual partner.
24. One of the reasons I chose my sexual partner is because of our similar backgrounds.
25. Before I made love with my sexual partner, I considered how s/he would reflect on my family.
26. It was important to me that my sexual partner be a good parent.
27. I thought about the implications for my career before I made love with my sexual partner.

28. I didn't have sex with my partner until after I had considered our hereditary backgrounds.
29. When sex with my partner isn't going right, I become upset.
30. If my sexual relationship with my partner ended, I would become extremely despondent and depressed.
31. Sometimes I am so sexually attracted to my partner that I simply can't sleep.
32. When my partner sexually ignores me, I feel really sick.
33. Since my partner and I started having sex, I have not been able to concentrate on anything else.
34. If my partner became sexually involved with someone else, I wouldn't be able to take it.
35. If my partner doesn't have sex with me for a while, I sometimes do stupid things to get her/his sexual attention.
36. If my partner were having a sexual difficulty, I would definitely try to help as much as I could.
37. I would rather have a sexual problem myself than let my partner suffer through one.
38. I could never be sexually satisfied unless first my partner was sexually satisfied.
39. I am usually willing to forsake my own sexual needs in order to let my partner achieve her/his own sexual needs.
40. My partner can use me the way s/he chooses in order for him/her to be sexually satisfied.
41. When my partner is sexually dissatisfied with me, I still accept him/her without reservations.
42. I would do practically any sexual activity that my partner wanted.
43. It would bother me if my sexual partner neglected my needs.
44. If I were to make love with a sexual partner, I'd take that person's needs and feelings into account.
45. If a sexual partner were to do something sensual for me, I'd try to do the same for him/her.
46. I expect a sexual partner to be responsive to my sexual needs and feelings.
47. I would be willing to go out of my way to satisfy my sexual partner.
48. If I were feeling sexually needy, I'd ask my sexual partner for help.
49. If a sexual partner were to ignore my sexual needs, I'd feel hurt.
50. I think people should feel obligated to repay an intimate partner for sexual favors.
51. I would feel somewhat exploited if an intimate partner failed to repay me for a sexual favor.
52. I would probably keep track of the times a sexual partner asked me for a sensual pleasure.
53. When a person receives sexual pleasures from another, s/he ought to repay that person right away.
54. It's best to make sure things are always kept "even" between two people in a sexual relationship.
55. I would do a special sexual favor for an intimate partner, only if that person did some special sexual favor for me.
56. If my sexual partner performed a sexual request for me, I would probably feel that I'd have to repay him/her later on.
57. I responded to the following items based on:
    (A) A current sexual relationship,
    (B) A past sexual relationship,
    (C) An imagined sexual relationship.

The Sexual Relationship Scale

William E. Snell, Jr.,[1] *Southeast Missouri State University*

Clark and Mills (1979) proposed a theory of relationship orientation based on the rules governing the giving and receiving of benefits. An exchange-relationship orientation was defined as one in which benefits are given on the assumption that a similar benefit would be reciprocated. The recipient of a benefit in such a relationship presumably in-curs a debt to make a suitable, comparable return. By contrast, a communal-relationship orientation was defined by Clark and Mills as one in which benefits are given on the assumption that they are in response to some need. In communal relationships, concern for a partner's welfare mediates interpersonal giving rather than anticipation of a reciprocated benefit. Sexual relationships may also be viewed from a communal perspective that emphasizes caring and concern for a partner's sexual needs and preferences, or else from an exchange perspective that emphasizes a quid pro quo approach to sexual relations. The

[1]Address correspondence to William E. Snell, Jr., Department of Psychology, Southeast Missouri State University, One University Plaza, Cape Girardeau, MO 63701; email: wesnell@semovm.semo.edu.

Sexual Relationship Scale (SRS; Hughes & Snell, 1990) is an objective self-report instrument that was designed to measure communal and exchange approaches to sexual relationships. More specifically, the SRS was developed to assess chronic dispositional differences in the type of orientation that people take toward their sexual relations. Some individuals take a communal approach to their sexual relations in which they feel responsible for and involved in their partner's sexual satisfaction and welfare. They want to respond to their partner's sexual needs and desires. In this sense, they contribute to their partner's sexual satisfaction and welfare to please the partner and to demonstrate a desire to respond to that person's sexual welfare. Moreover, people who take a communal approach to sexual relations also expect their partner to be responsive and sensitive to their own sexual welfare and needs. In contrast, those who approach sexual relations from an exchange orientation do not feel any special responsibility for their partner's sexual satisfaction and welfare. Nor do they feel any inherent need or desire to be attuned to or responsive to their partner's sexual pleasure. Rather, they give sexual pleasure only in response to sexual benefits they have received in the past or have been promised in the future. An exchange approach to sexual relations often involves sexual debts and obligations. The individuals involved in this type of sexual relationship are usually concerned with how many sexual favors they have given and received, and the comparability of these sexual exchanges. To examine these ideas, the SRS was developed to measure exchange and communal approaches to sexually intimate relations. The SRS was based on the Communal Orientation scale developed by Clark, Ouellette, Powell, and Milberg (1987) and the Exchange Orientation scale developed by Clark, Taraban, Ho, and Wesner (1989) and was intended to represent an extension of their ideas.

Description

The SRS consists of 24 items arranged in a 5-point Likert-type format, in which respondents rate how characteristic the SRS items are of them from (A) *not at all characteristic of me* to (E) *very characteristic of me*.

Response Mode and Timing

Typically, individuals respond to the items on the SRS by indicating their responses on a computer scan sheet, using a response range from A to E. The questionnaire usually takes about 10-15 minutes to complete.

Scoring

People are asked to respond to the SRS items by indicating how much each statement describes them, using a 5-point Likert-type scale: (0) *not at all characteristic of me,* (1) *slightly characteristics of me,* (2) *somewhat characteristic of me,* (3) *moderately characteristic of me,* and (4) *very characteristic of me.* The SRS items are coded so that A = 0, B = 1, C = 2, D = 3, and E = 4. Items 6, 8, 10, and 18 are reverse coded so that 0 = 4, 1 = 3, 2 = 2, 3 = 1, and 4 = 0. The SRS consists of two subscales, each containing eight separate items. The labels and items for these two subscales are (a) The Exchange Approach to Sexual Rela-

tions (Items 2, 6, 8, 10, 12, 14, 16, and 18) and (b) The Communal Approach to Sexual Relations (Items 1, 3, 4, 9, 13, 15, 21, and 24). Finally, the eight items on each subscale are summed so that higher scores indicate a stronger communal and exchange approach, respectively, to sexual relations.

Reliability

The internal consistency of the two SRS subscales was determined by computing Cronbach alpha coefficients for both females and males, as well as for the combined group of respondents (Hughes & Snell, 1990). For the sexual communion subscale, the coefficients were .77 for males, .79 for females, and .78 for both together. The coefficients for the sexual exchange subscale were .59 for males, .67 for females, and .67 for both. These findings indicate that the two subscales had sufficient internal consistency to justify their use in research. Other analyses have revealed that among females the two SRS subscales are essentially orthogonal to one another (Hughes & Snell, 1990).

Validity

Factor analysis (a principal components factor analysis with oblique rotation) was performed on the SRS items to determine whether the statements on the SRS would form two separate clusters. Because several items were unrelated to the initial factor solutions, they were first deleted and the same factor analysis procedure was reconducted. The pattern matrix loadings for the females clearly provided support for the expected two-factor structure, with conceptually similar items loading together (the results for the males were less clear, given the small sample size). Factor I consisted of sexual communion items (eigenvalue = 4.81, percent of variance = 20%), and Factor II contained sexual exchange items (eigenvalue = 2.98, percent of variance = 12%).

Hughes and Snell (1990) also found that males reported significantly higher scores than females on the sexual exchange subscale, but no difference was found for the sexual communion subscale. Further evidence for the validity of the SRS was obtained by correlating the SRS subscales with Clark's Communal and Exchange Orientation scales. The sexual communion subscale was significantly and positively correlated with the Communal Orientation scale for females and for the respondents as a whole. Significant and positive correlations were also found between the sexual exchange orientation subscale and scores on the Exchange Orientation scale for males, females, and both together. In addition, the SRS was found to be related to relationship satisfaction. Among males, a significant negative relationship was found between an exchange approach to sexual relations and their relationship satisfaction. The analysis for the females, in contrast, revealed a statistically significant positive correlation between relationship satisfaction and a communal approach to sexual relations.

These patterns of correlations thus provide preliminary evidence for the construct validity of the SRS, in that (a) those individuals characterized by a stronger communal approach to their sexual relations were expected to report greater satisfaction with their intimate relationships and to approach their partners with a more caring and companionate perspective, and (b) those individuals characterized by an exchange approach to their sexual relations were expected to have a similar exchange approach to their adult romantic relationships and to report less satisfaction with their romantic relationships.

References

Clark, M. S., & Mills, J. (1979). Interpersonal attraction in exchange and communal relationships. *Journal of Personality and Social Psychology, 37,* 12-24.

Clark, M. S., Ouellette, R., Powell, M. C., & Milberg, S. (1987). Recipient's mood, relationship type, and helping. *Journal of Personality and Social Psychology, 53,* 94-103.

Clark, M. S., Taraban, C., Ho, J., & Wesner, K. (1989). *A measure of exchange orientation.* Unpublished manuscript, Carnegie Mellon University, Pittsburgh, PA.

Hughes, T., & Snell, W. E., Jr. (1990). Communal and exchange approaches to sexual relations. *Annals of Sex Research, 3,* 149-163.

Exhibit

The Sexual Relationship Scale

Instructions: Listed below are several statements that concern the topic of sexual relationships. Please read each of the following statements carefully and decide to what extent it is characteristic of you. Some of the items refer to a specific relationship. Whenever possible, answer the questions with your current partner in mind. If you are not currently dating anyone, answer the questions with your most recent partner in mind. If you have never had a relationship, answer in terms of what you think your responses would most likely be. Then, for each statement fill in the response on the answer sheet that indicates how much it applies to you by using the following scale:

A	=	*Not at all* characteristic of me.
B	=	*Slightly* characteristic of me.
C	=	*Somewhat* characteristic of me.
D	=	*Moderately* characteristic of me.
E	=	*Very* characteristic of me.

Note: Remember to respond to all items, even if you are not completely sure. Your answers will be kept in the strictest confidence. Also, please be honest in responding to these statements.

1. It would bother me if my sexual partner neglected my needs.
2. When I make love with someone I generally expect something in return.
3. If I were to make love with a sexual partner, I'd take that person's needs and feelings into account.
4. If a sexual partner were to do something sensual for me, I'd try to do the same for him/her.
5. I'm not especially sensitive to the feelings of a sexual partner.
6. I don't think people should feel obligated to repay an intimate partner for sexual favors. (R)
7. I don't consider myself to be a particularly helpful sexual partner.
8. I wouldn't feel all that exploited if an intimate partner failed to repay me for a sexual favor. (R)
9. I believe sexual lovers should go out of their way to be sexually responsive to their partner.
10. I wouldn't bother to keep track of the times a sexual partner asked for a sensual pleasure. (R)
11. I wouldn't especially enjoy helping a partner achieve their own sexual satisfaction.
12. When a person receives sexual pleasures from another, s/he ought to repay that person right away.
13. I expect a sexual partner to be responsive to my sexual needs and feelings.
14. It's best to make sure things are always kept "even" between two people in a sexual relationship.
15. I would be willing to go out of my way to satisfy my sexual partner.
16. I would do a special sexual favor for an intimate partner, only if that person did some special sexual favor for me.
17. I don't think it's wise to get involved taking care of a partner's sexual needs.
18. If my sexual partner performed a sexual request for me, I wouldn't feel that I'd have to repay him/her later on. (R)
19. I'm not the sort of person who would help a partner with a sexual problem.
20. If my sexual partner wanted something special from me, s/he would have to do something sexual for me.
21. If I were feeling sexually needy, I'd ask my sexual partner for help.
22. If my sexual partner became emotionally upset, I would try to avoid him/her.
23. People should keep their sexual problems to themselves.
24. If a sexual partner were to ignore my sexual needs, I'd feel hurt.

Source. This scale is reprinted with permission of the author.

Note. (R) = reverse scored.

Index of Sexual Satisfaction

Walter W. Hudson,[1] WALMYR Publishing Co.

The Index of Sexual Satisfaction (ISS) is a short-form scale designed to measure the degree of dissatisfaction in the sexual component of a dyadic relationship.

Description

The ISS contains 25 category-partition (Likert-type) items some of which are worded negatively to partially offset the potential for response set bias. Each item is scored on a relative frequency scale as shown in the scoring key of the instrument. Obtained scores range from 0 to 100, with higher scores indicating greater degrees of sexual discord. The ISS has a clinical cutting score of 30 such that scores above that value indicate the presence of a clinically significant degree of sexual discord in the relationship. The ISS can be used with all English-speaking populations aged 12 or older.

The readability statistics for the ISS are as follows: Flesch Reading Ease: 79; Gunning's Fog Index: 8; and Flesch-Kincaid Grade Level: 5.

Response Mode and Timing

The ISS is a self-report scale that is normally completed in 5-7 minutes.

Scoring

Items noted below the copyright notation on the scale must first be reverse scored by subtracting the item response from $K + 1$, where K is the number of response categories in the scoring key. After making all appropriate item reversals, compute the total score as $S = (\Sigma X_i - N)(100) / [(K - 1)N]$, where X is an item response, i is item, K is the number of response categories, and N is the number of properly completed items. Total scores remain valid in the face of

missing values (omitted items) provided the respondent completes at least 80% of the items. The effect of the scoring formula is to replace missing values with the mean item response value so that scores range from 0 to 100 regardless of the value of N.

Reliability

Cronbach's alpha = .92, and *SEM* = 4.24. Test-retest reliability is not available.

Validity

The known-groups validity coefficient is .76 as determined by the point biserial correlation between group status (troubled vs. untroubled criterion groups) and the ISS scores. Detailed information about content, factorial, and construct validity are reported in the *WALMYR Assessment Scale Scoring Manual*, which is available from the publisher.

Other Information

The ISS is a copyrighted, commercial assessment scale and may not be copied, reproduced, altered, or translated into other languages. It may be obtained in tear-off pads of 50 copies per pad at $0.30 per copy ($15.00 per pad) by writing the WALMYR Publishing Co., P.O. Box 6229, Tallahassee, FL 32314-6229; phone and fax: (850) 656-2787; email: walmyr@syspak.com.

References

Hudson, W. W., Harrison, D. F., & Crosscup, P. C. (1981). A short-form scale to measure sexual discord in dyadic relationships. *The Journal of Sex Research, 17,* 157-174.

Murphy, G. J. (1978). *The family in later life: A cross-ethnic study in marital and sexual satisfaction.* Unpublished doctoral dissertation, Tulane University, New Orleans, LA.

Murphy, G. J., Hudson, W. W., & Cheung, P. P. L. (1980). Marital and sexual discord among older couples. *Social Work Research & Abstracts, 16*(1), 11-16.

Nurius, P. S., & Hudson, W. W. (1993). *Human services practice, evaluation & computers.* Pacific Grove, CA: Brooks/Cole.

---

[1]Address correspondence to Walter W. Hudson, WALMYR Publishing Co., P.O. Box 6229, Tallahassee, FL 32314-6229; email: walmyr@syspac.com.

Exhibit

 INDEX OF SEXUAL SATISFACTION (ISS)

Name: _____ Today's Date: _____

This questionnaire is designed to measure the degree of satisfaction you have in the sexual relationship with your partner. It is not a test, so there are no right or wrong answers. Answer each item as carefully and as accurately as you can by placing a number beside each one as follows.

    1 = None of the time
    2 = Very rarely
    3 = A little of the time
    4 = Some of the time
    5 = A good part of the time
    6 = Most of the time
    7 = All of the time

___

1. _____ I feel that my partner enjoys our sex life.
2. _____ Our sex life is very exciting.
3. _____ Sex is fun for my partner and me.
4. _____ Sex with my partner has become a chore for me.
5. _____ I feel that our sex is dirty and disgusting.
6. _____ Our sex life is monotonous.
7. _____ When we have sex it is too rushed and hurriedly completed.
8. _____ I feel that my sex life is lacking in quality.
9. _____ My partner is sexually very exciting.
10. _____ I enjoy the sex techniques that my partner likes or uses.
11. _____ I feel that my partner wants too much sex from me.
12. _____ I think that our sex is wonderful.
13. _____ My partner dwells on sex too much.
14. _____ I try to avoid sexual contact with my partner.
15. _____ My partner is too rough or brutal when we have sex.
16. _____ My partner is a wonderful sex mate.
17. _____ I feel that sex is a normal function of our relationship.
18. _____ My partner does not want sex when I do.
19. _____ I feel that our sex life really adds a lot to our relationship.
20. _____ My partner seems to avoid sexual contact with me.
21. _____ It is easy for me to get sexually excited by my partner.
22. _____ I feel that my partner is sexually pleased with me.
23. _____ My partner is very sensitive to my sexual needs and desires.
24. _____ My partner does not satisfy me sexually.
25. _____ I feel that my sex life is boring.

Source. This scale is reprinted with permission of WALMYR Publishing Co.

Interpersonal Exchange Model of Sexual Satisfaction Questionnaire

Kelli-an Lawrance, *Windsor-Essex County Health Unit*
E. Sandra Byers,[1] *University of New Brunswick*

The study of sexual satisfaction has been hampered by poor conceptualization of the construct. Measurement of sexual satisfaction has been similarly weak. For example, there are a number of sexual satisfaction scales that include items that are contemporaneously used as predictors of sexual satisfaction. Including the same items (e.g., frequency of sexual activities; orgasmic consistency) in both the predictor and criterion measures impedes the interpretation of the relationship between the variables. As well, the psychometric properties of many sexual satisfaction scales are poor or unknown. Therefore, the Interpersonal Exchange Model of Sexual Satisfaction questionnaire (IEMSS) was developed within the tradition of social exchange models to provide a conceptual framework for studying sexual satisfaction and to overcome some of the methodological weaknesses in previous research (see Lawrance & Byers, 1995, for a full description of the IEMSS). For the purpose of developing the IEMSS, we defined *sexual satisfaction* as an affective response arising from one's subjective evaluation of the positive and negative dimensions associated with one's sexual relationship.

The IEMSS proposes that satisfaction with the sexual relationship will be greater to the extent that (a) the level of rewards exceeds level of costs; (b) the level of *relative rewards* or comparison level for rewards (i.e., the level of rewards received compared to the level of rewards one expects to experience in the sexual relationship) exceeds the level of relative costs (i.e., the level of costs received compared to the level of costs one expects to receive); (c) equality is perceived to exist between own and partner's levels of rewards, and between own and partner's levels of costs in the sexual relationship; and (d) based on the findings of Lawrance and Byers (1995), relationship satisfaction is high. Finally, because sexual satisfaction is probably influenced by the *history* of exchanges in the sexual relationship, multiple assessments of the levels/equality of exchanges provide a better prediction of sexual satisfaction than a one-time measure of these variables.

Description and Scoring

The IEMSS is a self-report instrument that measures the various components contained in the IEMSS in three separate scales. It also contains a checklist of specific sexual rewards and costs that might occur in a relationship.

A background questionnaire (Q-1 to Q-6 and Q-17 to Q-20 in the exhibit) is used to collect demographic information that is not part of the model, including frequency of affectionate behavior, frequency of sexual activities, and sexual concerns.

The Global Measure of Sexual Satisfaction (GMSEX, Q-16) assesses global satisfaction with the sexual relationship. Respondents rate their sexual relationship on five 7-point bipolar scales: *good-bad, pleasant-unpleasant, positive-negative, satisfying-unsatisfying, valuable-worthless.* Possible scores on the GMSEX range from 5 to 35, with lower scores indicating less sexual satisfaction. The Global Measure of Relationship Satisfaction (GMREL, Q-7) is identical to the GMSEX except that participants rate their overall relationship. The Exchanges Questionnaire is a six-item measure (Q-10 to Q-15) that assesses levels of rewards and costs in a sexual relationship with a partner. Three items require respondents to think of their sexual relationship over the previous 3 months and indicate (a) how rewarding their sexual relationship is, (b) how their level of rewards compares to their own expectations about how rewarding their sexual relationship "should" be, and (c) how their level of rewards compares with the level of rewards their partner receives in the sexual relationship. The other three items assess costs using the same format. Level of rewards (REW) and level of costs (CST) are rated on 9-point scales with endpoints of *not at all rewarding (costly)* (1) and *extremely rewarding (costly)* (9). Relative reward level (CLrew) and relative cost level (CLcst) are also rated on 9-point scales with anchors of *much less rewarding (costly) in comparison* (1) and *much more rewarding (costly) in comparison* (9). Perceived equality of rewards (EQrew) and perceived equality of costs (EQcst) are rated on 9-point scales with anchors of *my rewards [costs] are much higher* and *my partner's rewards (costs) are much higher.* The equality items are recoded such that the midpoint, representing perfect equality, is assigned a score of 4, and both endpoints are assigned scores of 0. REW-CST and CLrew-CLcst scores are calculated by subtracting the cost score from the reward score so that the possible range of scores for both of these measures is –8 to 8.

The Rewards/Costs Checklist (Q-9) was developed based on the open-ended responses of university students (Lawrance & Byers, 1992b). It includes 46 items representing either rewards or costs in a sexual relationship. Examples of these items are the following: *level of affection*

---

[1]Address correspondence to E. Sandra Byers, Department of Psychology, University of New Brunswick, Fredericton, New Brunswick E3B 6E4, Canada; email: byers@unb.ca.

expressed during sexual activities, amount of spontaneity in your sex life, degree of privacy you and your partner have for sexual activities, and *engaging in sexual acts that you dislike but your partner enjoys.* For each item, respondents indicate whether it is generally a reward in their sexual relationship, generally a cost, both a reward and a cost, or neither a reward nor a cost. The total number of rewards and costs are determined by counting the number of items endorsed. Responses to individual items are used to determine the types of rewards and costs experienced by the participants.

Response Mode and Timing

The IEMSS takes approximately 10 minutes to complete. All items are objective, requiring respondents to either circle a number or check an item on a checklist.

Reliability and Validity

Evidence for the reliability and validity of the IEMSS comes from a study using university students who had been dating and cohabiting for more than 1 year (Lawrance & Byers, 1992b) and a study using a community sample of married and cohabiting individuals (Lawrance & Byers, 1995). Good 2-week and 3-month test-retest reliability were demonstrated for the GMSEX, $r = .84$ and $.78$, $p < .001$, respectively. Furthermore, internal consistency of the GMSEX was high for both the student sample ($\alpha = .90$) and the community sample ($\alpha = .96$). Evidence for the validity of the GMSEX comes from its significant correlations with scores on the Index of Sexual Satisfaction (ISS; Hudson, Harrison, & Crosscup, 1981), $r = .65$, $p < .001$, and with the single-item measure of sexual satisfaction, $r = .70$, $p < .001$ (Lawrance & Byers, 1992b).

Two-week and 3-month test-retest reliability of the GMREL is good, $r = .81$ and $.70$, $p < .001$, respectively.

Internal consistency was high for the student sample ($\alpha = .91$) and the community sample ($\alpha = .96$). Based on the student sample, the GMREL correlated significantly with the Dyadic Adjustment Scale (Spanier, 1976), $r = .69$, $p < .001$, supporting its validity.

Three-month test-retest reliabilities based on the community sample for REW, CST, CLrew, CLcst, REW-CST, and CLrew-CLcst were moderate, as expected, ranging from .43 to .67. Evidence for the validity of levels of rewards and costs comes from the student sample (Lawrance & Byers, 1992b). Level of rewards was significantly correlated with the ISS (Hudson et al., 1981) as well as with a single-item measure of sexual satisfaction, $rs = -.66$ and $.64$, $p < .001$. Level of costs was significantly correlated with the ISS but not with the single-item measure, $r = .30$, $p < .01$, and $r = -.15$, *ns,* respectively. As further evidence of their validity, the items on the Exchanges Questionnaire and the components of the model also are all significantly correlated with GMSEX (Lawrance & Byers, 1995).

References

Hudson, W., Harrison, D., & Crosscup, P. (1981). A short-form scale to measure sexual discord in dyadic relationships. *The Journal of Sex Research, 17,* 157-174.

Lawrance, K., & Byers, E. S. (1992a). Development of the Interpersonal Exchange Model of Sexual Satisfaction in long term relationships. *Canadian Journal of Human Sexuality, 1,* 123-128.

Lawrance, K., & Byers, E. S. (1992b, May). *Sexual satisfaction: A social exchange perspective.* Paper presented at the annual meeting of the Canadian Psychological Association, Quebec.

Lawrance, K., & Byers, E.S. (1995). Sexual satisfaction in long-term heterosexual relationships: The Interpersonal Exchange Model of Sexual Satisfaction. *Personal Relationships, 2,* 267-285.

Spanier, G. (1976). Measuring dyadic adjustment: New scales for assessing the quality of marriage and similar dyads. *Journal of Marriage and the Family, 38,* 15-28.

Exhibit

Sexual Relationship Study

No two relationships are alike. Therefore, we would like you to describe *your* overall relationship with your partner by answering the following questions. Please answer the questions in the order they are presented. There are no right or wrong answers.

Remember, *all* the information you provide is confidential and anonymous.

Q-1   Sex (Circle one):   1 male   2 female
Q-2   a. How old are you? _____ years old
       b. How old is your partner? _____ years old
Q-3   What type of relationship do you and your partner have?
       (Circle one)
           1   married   2   cohabiting   3   other (please specify:_____)
Q-4   How long have you and your partner been living together? _____ years
Q-5   Before your relationship with your present partner, were you ever seriously involved with someone else?
       (Circle one)
           1 no   2 yes

Q-6 Do you or your partner have any children?
    (Circle one)
    1 no   2 yes → *If yes,* how many children in each of the following age groups live with you? (fill in each space;
           write "0" if you have no children that age living with you)
    _____ under 5 years of age
    _____ 6 to 13 years of age
    _____ 14 to 19 years of age
    _____ 20 years of age or older

Q-7 In general, how would you describe your *overall* relationship with your partner? For *each* pair of words below, circle
the number which best describes your relationship, as a whole.

Very good						Very bad
7	6	5	4	3	2	1
Very pleasant						Very unpleasant
7	6	5	4	3	2	1
Very positive						Very negative
7	6	5	4	3	2	1
Very satisfying						Very unsatisfying
7	6	5	4	3	2	1
Very valuable						Worthless
7	6	5	4	3	2	1

Q-8 In the last 3 months, how often have you and your partner affectionately kissed, hugged, or cuddled with each
other?
    (Circle one)
    1   rarely, or never
    2   once a month
    3   2 or 3 times a month
    4   once or twice a week
    5   3 or 4 times a week
    6   once a day, or more

On the next few pages are some questions about your SEXUAL relationship with your partner. Before answering them, it is
important that you carefully read the information on this page.

Think about your *job.*

If you're like most people, you can give concrete examples of positive, pleasing things you like about your job. These are
"rewards."

Most people can also give concrete examples of negative, displeasing things they don't like about their job. These are
"costs."

Below are some rewards and costs that could be associated with a job.

        rate of pay
        level of responsibility
        interactions with your boss
        the hour at which you start work
        opportunity for advancement

"Rate of pay" would be a reward if you felt that you were being *paid well* . . . but it would be a *cost* if you felt that you
were being *underpaid.*

"Level of responsibility" would be a reward if you had *just enough* responsibility at work . . . but it would be a cost if
you had either *too much* or *too little* responsibility.

"Interactions with your boss" would be neither a reward nor a cost if you really didn't interact much with your boss.

"The hour you start work" would be both a reward and a cost if you liked starting work at that time, but disliked the
rush-hour traffic at that time.

Now, instead of thinking about your job, *think about the rewards and costs associated with your sexual relationship with
your partner,* and answer the questions below.

Q-9 Below is a list of rewards and costs that many people experience in their sexual relationships. Please indicate the
rewards and costs associated with *your* sexual relationship with your partner.
If the item is usually a *reward* in your sexual relationship, *check REW.*

If the item is usually a *cost* in your sexual relationship, *check CST.*
If the item is *neither* a reward nor a cost, *leave both spaces blank.*
A few items might be both a reward and a cost at the same time.
  If the item is *both* a reward and a cost, *check REW and CST.*
Remember, things that are positive, pleasing, *"just right"* are *rewards.*
Things that are negative, displeasing, *"too little/too much"* are *costs.*

REW   CST

_____   _____   level of affection expressed during sexual activities
_____   _____   degree of emotional intimacy (feeling close; sharing feelings)
_____   _____   extent to which you and partner communicate about sex
_____   _____   amount of variety in sexual activities; locations; times
_____   _____   amount/type of foreplay (before intercourse or orgasm)
_____   _____   how often you experience orgasm (climax)
_____   _____   amount/type of afterplay (after intercourse or orgasm)
_____   _____   frequency of sexual activities
_____   _____   degree of privacy you and partner have for sex
_____   _____   oral sex: your partner stimulates you
_____   _____   oral sex: you stimulate your partner
_____   _____   physical sensations from touching, caressing, hugging
_____   _____   feelings of physical discomfort during/after sex
_____   _____   amount of fun experienced during sexual interactions
_____   _____   who initiates sexual activities
_____   _____   level of stress/relaxation felt during sexual activities
_____   _____   telling your partner you enjoyed your sexual interaction
_____   _____   partner telling you that she/he enjoyed your sexual interaction
_____   _____   conceiving a child
_____   _____   how you feel about yourself during/after sexual activities
_____   _____   degree of consideration partner shows for your feelings
_____   _____   how partner physically treats you when you have sex
_____   _____   having sex when you're not in the mood
_____   _____   having sex when your partner is not in the mood
_____   _____   extent to which you "let your guard down"
_____   _____   extent to which your partner "lets her/his guard down"
_____   _____   method of birth control used by you/your partner
_____   _____   how comfortable you feel with your partner
_____   _____   how partner influences/forces you to engage in sex acts
_____   _____   extent to which you and partner argue after sex
_____   _____   being with the same partner each time you have sex
_____   _____   amount of time that is spent engaging in sexual activities
_____   _____   how easily you reach orgasm (climax)
_____   _____   how your partner responds to your sexual advances
_____   _____   being naked/your partner seeing you naked
_____   _____   partner being naked/seeing your partner naked
_____   _____   extent to which partner tells others about your sex life
_____   _____   pleasing/trying to please your partner sexually
_____   _____   extent to which sexual interactions make you feel secure about your total relationship with
                your partner
_____   _____   degree to which you feel sexually aroused/excited
_____   _____   amount of spontaneity in your sex life
_____   _____   level of power/control you feel during/after sex
_____   _____   engaging in activities you dislike, but partner enjoys
_____   _____   engaging in activities partner dislikes, but you enjoy
_____   _____   risk of getting sexually transmitted disease from partner
_____   _____   degree to which current sexual relationship interferes with other possible relationships
_____   _____   other: _____
_____   _____   other: _____
_____   _____   other: _____

Q-10   Think about the *rewards* that you have received in *your sexual relationship with your partner* within the past 3 months. How rewarding is your sexual relationship with your partner? (Circle a number)

Not at all   Extremely
rewarding   rewarding
     1   2   3   4   5   6   7   8   9

Q-11   Most people have a general *expectation* about *how rewarding* their sexual relationship "should be." Compared to this general expectation, they may feel that their sexual relationship is more rewarding, less rewarding, or as rewarding as it "should be."

Based on your *own* expectation about how rewarding *your sexual relationship with your partner* "should be," how does your level of rewards compare to that expectation? (Circle a number)

Much less   Much more
rewarding in   rewarding in
comparison   comparison
     1   2   3   4   5   6   7   8   9

Q-12   How does the level of *rewards* that you get from your sexual relationship with your partner compare to the level of rewards that your partner seems to get from the relationship? (Circle a number)

My rewards are   Partner's rewards
much higher   are much higher
     1   2   3   4   5   6   7   8   9

Q-13   Think about the *costs* that you have incurred in your sexual relationship with your partner within the past 3 months. How costly is your sexual relationship with your partner? (Circle a number)

Not at all costly   Extremely costly
     1   2   3   4   5   6   7   8   9

Q-14   Most people have a general *expectation* about *how costly* their sexual relationship "should be." Compared to this general expectation, they may feel that their sexual relationship is more costly, less costly, or as costly as it "should be."

Based on your *own* expectation about how costly your sexual relationship with your partner "should be," how does your level of costs compare to that expectation? (Circle a number)

Much less costly   Much more costly
in comparison   in comparison
     1   2   3   4   5   6   7   8   9

Q-15   How does the level of *costs* that you incur in your sexual relationship with your partner compare to the level of costs that your partner seems to incur in the relationship? (Circle a number)

My costs are   Partner's costs are
much higher   much higher
     1   2   3   4   5   6   7   8   9

Q-16   Overall, how would you describe your *sexual* relationship with your partner? For each pair of words, circle the number which best describes your sexual relationship.

Very good   Very bad
     7   6   5   4   3   2   1
Very pleasant   Very unpleasant
     7   6   5   4   3   2   1
Very positive   Very negative
     7   6   5   4   3   2   1
Very satisfying   Very unsatisfying
     7   6   5   4   3   2   1
Very valuable   Worthless
     7   6   5   4   3   2   1

Q-17   In the last 3 months, how often have you and your partner engaged in sexual activities (of any type) with each other?

(Circle one)
1   rarely, or never
2   once a month
3   2 or 3 times a month
4   once or twice a week
5   3 or 4 times a week
6   once a day, or more

Sometimes, couples experience difficulties in their sexual relationship. The following questions ask about some common concerns that couples often encounter.

Q-18   Have *you* experienced any of the following concerns in the past 3 months?
(Circle all that apply)
1 My partner chooses inconvenient times for sex
2 I am unable to relax
3 I am not interested in sex
4 I like to do things that my partner does not like to do
5 My partner asks me to do things I don't like to do
6 I feel "turned off"
7 There is too little foreplay before intercourse
8 There is too little "tenderness" after intercourse
9 I am attracted to someone other than my partner

Q-19   Have *you* or *your partner* experienced any of the following difficulties in the past 3 months? (Circle all that apply for you, then for your partner)

I have:	My partner has:	
1	1	trouble getting sexually excited
2	2	trouble maintaining sexual excitement
3	3	premature orgasm (orgasm occurs too quickly)
4	4	inhibited orgasm (takes too long to reach orgasm)
5	5	anorgasmia (unable to reach orgasm)
6	6	medication(s) that interfere with sex
7	7	an illness that interferes with sexual response

My partner is _____ male _____ female.

Q-20   In the last 3 months, have you and/or your partner sought counseling from a professional?
1 no
2 yes *If yes→* what were you seeking help for?
1 sexual problems
2 marital problems
3 personal problems

Please feel free to expand upon any answers you've given, to add any information that you feel we've overlooked, or to comment on any aspect of this survey!

Sexual Satisfaction Inventory

Marilyn Peddicord Whitley,[1] *Portland Veterans Administration Medical Center*

The Sexual Satisfaction Inventory was initially designed to assess sexual satisfaction in married professional women as a correlate of the personality trait of assertiveness (Whitley, 1974; Whitley & Paulsen, 1975). The current version of the inventory can be used to assess overall sexual satisfaction in women, as well as sexual satisfaction in several specific areas.

[1]Address correspondence to Marilyn Peddicord Whitley, Oregon Health Sciences University School of Nursing, P.O. Box 1034, Portland, OR 97207.
[2]Additional details may be obtained from the author.

Description

The original instrument contained 31 Likert-type items designed to allow individuals to rate the level of sexual satisfaction they received from various sexual activities. Factor analysis of the original data set resulted in a reduction of the inventory to 23 items.[2] Additional items dealing with breast/chest stimulation were added to produce the current 32-item instrument. Factor analysis of data obtained from a sample of 52 women volunteers revealed eight factors with eigenvalues greater than 1, accounting for 95% of the variance. The loadings of each item on these factors are available from the author.

Response Mode and Timing

Respondents were asked to indicate their degree of satisfaction with each activity on a 5-point scale from *no satisfaction* to *maximum satisfaction*. A *not applicable* option is also provided. The scale requires approximately 7 minutes to complete.

Scoring

A total can be computed by adding the scores for the 32 items. Because some items will not be applicable to some women, a mean score may also be computed, based only on the applicable items. Scores for each of the factors may also be computed, using the items loading on each factor.

Reliability and Validity

The Cronbach alpha coefficient for the 32-item inventory is .78. The scale has face validity but has not been used in research designed to assess its construct validity.

Other Information

The original study was supported by Grant 67-0381 from the National Institute of Mental Health, U.S. Public Health Service. The secondary study was supported by a Biomedical Research Support Grant RR-057-58, Division of Resource Research.

References

Whitley, M. P. (1974). *A correlational survey comparing the levels of assertiveness with levels of sexual satisfaction in employed sexually active professional women.* Unpublished master's thesis, University of Washington, Seattle.

Whitley, M. P., & Paulsen, S. B. (1975). Assertiveness and sexual satisfaction in employed professional women. *Journal of Marriage and the Family, 37,* 573-581.

Exhibit

Sexual Satisfaction Inventory

The following is a list of activities often engaged in before, during, and directly after the time of sexual activity. Please rate the average level of sexual satisfaction you feel you derive from each activity. Include activities you might engage in during the time immediately prior to, during, and after sexual intercourse. Check the *not applicable* column for any activities you do not engage in during this time.

To rate: Circle the number you feel best describes the usual level of satisfaction you get from each activity listed. Number 1 represents no satisfaction; number 5 represents maximum satisfaction.

1. Kissing your partner[a]
2. Stroking your partner
3. French (open mouth) kissing your partner
4. Drinking alcoholic beverages
5. Holding hands
6. Smelling scents you consider erotic
7. Eating with your partner
8. Oral-genital stimulation of you by your partner
9. Using drugs other than alcohol
10. Undressing in front of your partner
11. Having your breast/chest stimulated by your partner
12. Sexual intercourse with your partner
13. Hugging your partner
14. Oral-genital stimulation of your partner by you
15. Talking with your partner
16. Stimulating your partner's breasts/chest
17. Watching your partner undress
18. Manual stimulation by your partner of your genital area
19. Being held by your partner
20. Sexual activity with your partner without experiencing orgasm (climax of any kind)
21. Self-stimulation of your genital area
22. You and your partner undressing each other
23. Bathing with your partner
24. Dancing with your partner
25. Orgasm experienced more than once during a single sexual encounter

If you experience orgasms by any of the following means, please rate the degree of satisfaction you achieve from each of them.

26. Orgasm with vaginal intercourse only
27. Orgasm with combination of vaginal intercourse and clitoral stimulation
28. Orgasm with clitoral manipulation by your partner
29. Orgasms with clitoral manipulation by yourself
30. Orgasms by fantasy and daydreams
31. Orgasm with oral-genital contact
32. Orgasm with anal entry

Source. This scale was originally published in *Journal of Marriage and the Family.* Reprinted with permission.

a. Each item is followed by a 5-point scale labeled from *no satisfaction* to *maximum satisfaction.* A *not applicable* option is also provided.

The Multidimensional Sexual Self-Concept Questionnaire

William E. Snell, Jr.,[1] *Southeast Missouri State University*

The Multidimensional Sexual Self-Concept Questionnaire (MSSCQ; Snell, 1995) is an objective self-report instrument designed to measure the following 20 psychological aspects of human sexuality: (1) *sexual anxiety,* defined as the tendency to feel tension, discomfort, and anxiety about the sexual aspects of one's life; (2) *sexual self-efficacy,* defined as the belief that one has the ability to deal effectively with the sexual aspects of oneself; (3) *sexual consciousness,* defined as the tendency to think and reflect about the nature of one's own sexuality; (4) *motivation to avoid risky sex,* defined as the motivation and desire to avoid unhealthy patterns of risky sexual behaviors (e.g., unprotected sexual behavior); (5) *chance/luck sexual control,* defined as the belief that the sexual aspects of one's life are determined by chance and luck considerations; (6) *sexual preoccupation,* defined as the tendency to think about sex to an excessive degree; (7) *sexual assertiveness,* defined as

the tendency to be assertive about the sexual aspects of one's life; (8) *sexual optimism,* defined as the expectation that the sexual aspects of one's life will be positive and rewarding in the future; (9) *sexual problem self-blame,* defined as the tendency to blame oneself when the sexual aspects of one's life are unhealthy, negative, or undesirable in nature; (10) *sexual monitoring,* defined as the tendency to be aware of the public impression that one's sexuality makes on others; (11) *sexual motivation,* defined as the motivation and desire to be involved in a sexual relationship; (12) *sexual problem management,* defined as the tendency to believe that one has the capacity/skills to effectively manage and handle any sexual problems that one might develop or encounter; (13) *sexual esteem,* defined as a generalized tendency to positively evaluate one's own capacity to engage in healthy sexual behaviors and to experience one's sexuality in a satisfying and enjoyable way; (14) *sexual satisfaction,* defined as the tendency to be highly satisfied with the sexual aspects of one's life; (15) *power-other sexual control,* defined as the belief that the sexual aspects of one's life are controlled by others who are more powerful and influential than oneself; (16) *sexual*

[1]Address correspondence to William E. Snell, Jr., Department of Psychology, One University Plaza, Southeast Missouri State University, Cape Girardeau, MO 63701; email: wesnell@semovm.semo.edu.

self-schemata, defined as a cognitive framework that organizes and guides the processing of information about the sexual-related aspects of oneself; (17) *fear of sex,* defined as a fear of engaging in sexual relations with another individual; (18) *sexual problem prevention,* defined as the belief that one has the ability to prevent oneself from developing any sexual problems or disorders; (19) *sexual depression,* defined as the experience of feelings of sadness, unhappiness, and depression regarding one's sex life; and (20) *internal sexual control,* defined as the belief that the sexual aspects of one's life are determined by one's own personal control.

The MSSCQ (Snell, 1995) was based on previous work by Snell and Papini (1989), Snell, Fisher, and Schuh (1992), Snell, Fisher, and Miller (1991), and Snell, Fisher, and Walters (1993). Scores on the MSSCQ can be treated as individual difference measures of the 20 sexuality-related constructs measured by this instrument or as dependent variables when examining predictive correlates of these concepts.

Description

The MSSCQ consists of 100 items arranged in a format in which respondents indicate how characteristic of them each statement is. A 5-point Likert-type scale is used to collect data on people's responses, with each item scored from 0 to 4: *not at all characteristic of me* (0), *slightly characteristic of me* (1), *somewhat characteristic of me* (2), *moderately characteristic of me* (3), and *very characteristic of me* (4). To create subscale scores (discussed below), the items on each subscale are averaged. Higher scores thus correspond to greater amounts of the relevant MSSCQ tendency.

Response Mode and Timing

People respond to the 100 items on the MSSCQ by marking their answers on separate machine-scorable answer sheets. In most instances, the scale usually requires about 45-60 minutes to complete.

Scoring

After several items are reverse coded (Items 27, 47, 68, 77, 88, and 97, designated with an R), the relevant items on each subscale are then coded so that A = 0, B = 1, C = 2, D = 3, and E = 4. Next, the items on each subscale are averaged, so that higher scores correspond to greater amounts of each tendency. Scores on the 20 subscales can thus range from 0 to 4. The items on the MSSCQ subscales alternate in ascending numerical order for each subscale (e.g., Subscale 1 consists of Items 1, 21, 41, 61, and 81; Subscale 2 consists of Items 2, 22, 42, 62, and 82).

Reliability

The internal consistency of the 20 subscales on the MSSCQ was determined by calculating Cronbach alpha coefficients, using 473 participants (302 females; 170 males; 1 gender unspecified) drawn from lower division psychology courses at a small midwestern university (Snell, 1995). Most of the sample (85%) was between 16 and 25 years of age. Based on five items per subscale, the alphas for all subjects on the 20 subscales were as follows: .84, .85, .78, .72, .88, .94, .84, .78, .84, .84, .89, .84, .88, .91, .85, .87, .85, .85, .85, and .76 (respectively). In brief, the 20 MSSCQ subscales have more than adequate internal consistency.

Validity

Evidence for the validity of the MSSCQ comes from a recent research investigation (Snell, 1995). Snell found that among university students, the MSSCQ subscales were related in predictable ways to men's and women's contraceptive use. Among males, a history of reliable, effective contraception was negatively associated with (1) sexual anxiety, (5) chance/luck sexual control, (17) sexual fear, and (19) sexual depression, and positively associated with (2) sexual self-efficacy, (8) sexual optimism, (11) sexual motivation, (13) sexual esteem, (14) sexual satisfaction, and (16) sexual self-schemata. By contrast, among females, long-term effective contraception use was negatively associated with (17) sexual fear, (19) sexual depression, and (20) internal sexual control, and positively associated with (2) sexual self-efficacy, (7) sexual assertiveness, (11) sexual motivation, (14) sexual satisfaction, and (16) sexual self-schemata.

Additional findings indicated that males reported higher levels of (5) chance/luck sexual control, (6) sexual preoccupation, (9) sexual problems self-blame, and (11) motivation to be sexually active than did females. By contrast, females reported greater (4) motivation to avoid risky sexual behavior and (17) fear of sexual relations than did males.

References

Fisher, T. D., & Snell, W. E., Jr. (1995). *Validation of the Multidimensional Sexuality Questionnaire.* Unpublished manuscript, Ohio University at Mansfield.

Snell, W. E., Jr. (1995, April). *The Extended Multidimensional Sexuality Questionnaire: Measuring psychological tendencies associated with human sexuality.* Paper presented at the annual meeting of the Southwestern Psychological Association, Houston, TX.

Snell, W. E., Jr., Fisher, T. D., & Miller, R. S. (1991). Development of the Sexual Awareness Questionnaire: Components, reliability, and validity. *Annals of Sex Research, 4,* 65-92.

Snell, W. E., Jr., Fisher, T. D., & Schuh, T. (1992). Reliability and validity of the Sexuality Scale: A measure of sexual-esteem, sexual-depression, and sexual-preoccupation. *The Journal of Sex Research, 29,* 261-273.

Snell, W. E., Jr., Fisher, T. D., & Walters, A. S. (1993). The Multidimensional Sexuality Questionnaire: An objective self-report measure of psychological tendencies associated with human sexuality. *Annals of Sex Research, 6,* 27-55.

Snell, W. E., Jr., & Papini, D. R. (1989). The Sexuality Scale: An instrument to measure sexual-esteem, sexual-depression, and sexual-preoccupation. *The Journal of Sex Research, 26,* 256-263.

Exhibit

The Multidimensional Sexual Self-Concept Questionnaire

Instructions: The items in this questionnaire refer to people's sexuality. Please read each item carefully and decide to what extent it is characteristic of you. Give each item a rating of how much it applies to you by using the following scale:

A	=	*Not at all* characteristic of me.
B	=	*Slightly* characteristic of me.
C	=	*Somewhat* characteristic of me.
D	=	*Moderately* characteristic of me.
E	=	*Very* characteristic of me.

Note: Remember to respond to all items, even if you are not completely sure. Your answers will be kept in the strictest confidence. Also, please be honest in responding to these statements.

1. I feel anxious when I think about the sexual aspects of my life.
2. I have the ability to take care of any sexual needs and desires that I may have.
3. I am very aware of my sexual feelings and needs.
4. I am motivated to avoid engaging in "risky" (i.e., unprotected) sexual behavior.
5. The sexual aspects of my life are determined mostly by chance happenings.
6. I think about sex "all the time."
7. I'm very assertive about the sexual aspects of my life.
8. I expect that the sexual aspects of my life will be positive and rewarding in the future.
9. I would be to blame if the sexual aspects of my life were not going very well.
10. I notice how others perceive and react to the sexual aspects of my life.
11. I'm motivated to be sexually active.
12. If I were to experience a sexual problem, I myself would be in control of whether this improved.
13. I derive a sense of self-pride from the way I handle my own sexual needs and desires.
14. I am satisfied with the way my sexual needs are currently being met.
15. My sexual behaviors are determined largely by other more powerful and influential people.
16. Not only would I be a good sexual partner, but it's quite important to me that I be a good sexual partner.
17. I am afraid of becoming sexually involved with another person.
18. If I am careful, then I will be able to prevent myself from having any sexual problems.
19. I am depressed about the sexual aspects of my life.
20. My sexuality is something that I am largely responsible for.
21. I worry about the sexual aspects of my life.
22. I am competent enough to make sure that my sexual needs are fulfilled.
23. I am very aware of my sexual motivations and desires.
24. I am motivated to keep myself from having any "risky" sexual behavior (e.g., exposure to sexual diseases).
25. Most things that affect the sexual aspects of my life happen to me by accident.
26. I think about sex more than anything else.
27. I'm not very direct about voicing my sexual needs and preferences. (R)
28. I believe that in the future the sexual aspects of my life will be healthy and positive.
29. If the sexual aspects of my life were to go wrong, I would be the person to blame.
30. I'm concerned with how others evaluate my own sexual beliefs and behaviors.
31. I'm motivated to devote time and effort to sex.
32. If I were to experience a sexual problem, my own behavior would determine whether I improved.
33. I am proud of the way I deal with and handle my own sexual desires and needs.
34. I am satisfied with the status of my own sexual fulfillment.
35. My sexual behaviors are largely controlled by people other than myself (e.g., my partner, friends, family).
36. Not only would I be a skilled sexual partner, but it's very important to me that I be a skilled sexual partner.
37. I have a fear of sexual relationships.
38. I can pretty much prevent myself from developing sexual problems by taking good care of myself.
39. I am disappointed about the quality of my sex life.
40. The sexual aspects of my life are determined in large part by my own behavior.
41. Thinking about the sexual aspects of my life often leaves me with an uneasy feeling.
42. I have the skills and ability to ensure rewarding sexual behaviors for myself.
43. I tend to think about my own sexual beliefs and attitudes.
44. I want to avoid engaging in sex where I might be exposed to sexual diseases.

45. Luck plays a big part in influencing the sexual aspects of my life.
46. I tend to be preoccupied with sex.
47. I am somewhat passive about expressing my own sexual desires. (R)
48. I do not expect to suffer any sexual problems or frustrations in the future.
49. If I were to develop a sexual disorder, then I would be to blame for not taking good care of myself.
50. I am quick to notice other people's reactions to the sexual aspects of my own life.
51. I have a desire to be sexually active.
52. If I were to become sexually maladjusted, I myself would be responsible for making myself better.
53. I am pleased with how I handle my own sexual tendencies and behaviors.
54. The sexual aspects of my life are personally gratifying to me.
55. My sexual behavior is determined by the actions of powerful others (e.g., my partner, friends, family).
56. Not only could I relate well to a sexual partner, but it's important to me that I be able to do so.
57. I am fearful of engaging in sexual activity.
58. If just I look out for myself, then I will be able to avoid any sexual problems in the future.
59. I feel discouraged about my sex life.
60. I am in control of and am responsible for the sexual aspects of my life.
61. I worry about the sexual aspects of my life.
62. I am able to cope with and to handle my own sexual needs and wants.
63. I'm very alert to changes in my sexual thoughts, feelings, and desires.
64. I really want to prevent myself from being exposed to sexual diseases.
65. The sexual aspects of my life are largely a matter of (good or bad) fortune.
66. I'm constantly thinking about having sex.
67. I do not hesitate to ask for what I want in a sexual relationship.
68. I will probably experience some sexual problems in the future. (R)
69. If I were to develop a sexual problem, then it would be my own fault for letting it happen.
70. I'm concerned about how the sexual aspects of my life appear to others.
71. It's important to me that I involve myself in sexual activity.
72. If I developed any sexual problems, my recovery would depend in large part on what I myself would do.
73. I have positive feelings about the way I approach my own sexual needs and desires.
74. The sexual aspects of my life are satisfactory, compared to most people's.
75. In order to be sexually active, I have to conform to other, more powerful individuals.
76. I am able to "connect" well with a sexual partner, and it's important to me that I am able to do so.
77. I don't have much fear about engaging in sex. (R)
78. I will be able to avoid any sexual problems, if I just take good care of myself.
79. I feel unhappy about my sexual experiences.
80. The main thing which affects the sexual aspects of my life is what I myself do.
81. I feel nervous when I think about the sexual aspects of my life.
82. I have the capability to take care of my own sexual needs and desires.
83. I am very aware of the sexual aspects of myself (e.g., habits, thoughts, beliefs).
84. I am really motivated to avoid any sexual activity that might expose me to sexual diseases.
85. The sexual aspects of my life are a matter of fate (destiny).
86. I think about sex the majority of the time.
87. When it comes to sex, I usually ask for what I want.
88. I anticipate that in the future the sexual aspects of my life will be frustrating. (R)
89. If something went wrong with my own sexuality, then it would be my own fault.
90. I'm aware of the public impression created by my own sexual behaviors and attitudes.
91. I strive to keep myself sexually active.
92. If I developed a sexual disorder, my recovery would depend on how I myself dealt with the problem.
93. I feel good about the way I express my own sexual needs and desires.
94. I am satisfied with the sexual aspects of my life.
95. My sexual behavior is mostly determined by people who have influence and control over me.
96. Not only am I capable of relating to a sexual partner, but it's important to me that I relate very well.
97. I'm not afraid of becoming sexually active. (R)
98. If I just pay careful attention, I'll be able to prevent myself from having any sexual problems.
99. I feel sad when I think about my sexual experiences.
100. My sexuality is something that I myself am in charge of.
101. I responded to the above items based on:
     (A) A current relationship.
     (B) A past close relationship.
     (C) An imagined close relationship.

The Sexual Self-Disclosure Scale

Joseph A. Catania,[1] *University of California, San Francisco*

The Sexual Self-Disclosure Scale (SSDS) is a 19-item Likert-type scale measuring the degree of threat associated with sexuality questions. The scale items assess respondent's self-reported ease or difficulty with disclosing information in different contexts and interpersonal situations.

Description

The self-administered scale requires respondents to imagine themselves in the different situations described by each item and then rate how easy or difficult it would be to reveal sexual information under each circumstance. A short, seven-item form is also shown in the exhibit. An interviewer-administered version of the scale and English and Spanish versions are also available.

Response Mode and Timing

Ratings are made on 6-point Likert-type scales, where 1 = *extremely easy* to 6 = *extremely difficult*. All forms take approximately 3-5 minutes to complete.

Scoring

Scores are produced by summing across items. Lower scores indicate less threat.

Reliability and Validity

The SSDS has been administered to college students and a national probability sample. The scale was administered to participants recruited from introductory social science classes at a large western university ($N = 66$ males, 127 females) who were asked to participate in a study assessing response bias in self-administered questionnaires and sample bias in face-to-face interviews (Catania, McDermott, & Pollack, 1986). Respondents' mean age was 24.6 years; education, 12-19 years; 100% Caucasian, heterosexuals; 89% with prior coital experience, 65 respondents having had coitus with their current partner. Internal consistency reliability (Cronbach's alpha) was .93; Test-reset r was .92.

In terms of construct validity, the scale was also found to correlate significantly with Chelune's (1976) General Self-Disclosure Scale, $r(72) = -.51$, $p < .0001$. Note that lower SSDS scores indicate less threat, whereas higher scores on Chelune's scale indicate less threat. One item from the Chelune scale concerning sexuality was removed to eliminate redundancy between scales.

The discriminant validity of the SSDS was assessed in a separate analysis in which introductory psychology students ($n = 90$) were compared with students in a human

sexuality course ($n = 84$). We hypothesized that the human sexuality students, on the basis of self-selection for a course of that nature, would be more sexually self-disclosing than the average introductory psychology student. This hypothesis was supported: Intro. Psych. $M = 60.7, SD = 16.2$; Sex. Cour. $M = 54.6, SD = 17.1$; $t(172) = 1.66, p < .05$. Note that groups did not differ in age, $t(172) = 1.14, p > .10$; number of sex books read, $t(172) = .30, p > .10$; number of lifetime sexual partners, $t(172) = .09, p > .10$; virginity status, $\chi^2(1, N = 174) = .01, p > .10$; and sex composition, $\chi^2(1, N = 174) = .01, p > .10$. Both the number of sexuality books read and total sex partners had small but significant negative correlations with threat, $r(86) = -.24, p < .03$; $r(86) = .23, p < .05$, respectively. No differences in number of partial responders, 24% of participants who circled one or more items, were detected when comparing respondents who did versus did not receive the SSDS at baseline, $\chi^2(1, N = 193) = .06, p > .10$. This finding indicates that the SSDS did not sensitize respondents to making fewer nonresponses. Volunteers, relative to nonvolunteers, were significantly less threatened about disclosing sexual information, $t(191) = 7.22, p < .0001$. Furthermore, the order of presentation of SSDS or general self-disclosure scales had no significant effects on sexual behavior and pathology summary scores. Summary scores included variety (the total number of different sexual behaviors performed), frequency (total frequency of sexual behaviors performed), and pathology (average percentage of sexual episodes negatively influenced by sexual problems). All t values were less than 1.49, and all two-tailed p values were greater than .14.

The shortened version was administered by phone to 2,018 respondents who were randomly selected, through probability sampling using random-digit dialing of the contiguous United States, to participate in the recently completed (1995) National Survey Methods study (unpublished data; information is available from the author) (reliability = .80, Cronbach's alpha). Normative data are provided for gender and levels of education; ethnic groups were excluded because there was an insufficient number of non-White ethnic groups to pursue differences (see Table 1).

Table 1 Normative Data for the Sexual
          Self-Disclosure Scale/National Methods
          Survey Study

	N	M	SD	Range	Mdn	Alpha
National sample	2,018	21.68	.09	21.0	22.0	.80
Male—national sample	953	21.82	4.24	21.0	22.0	.82
Female—national sample	1,065	21.54	4.17	20.0	22.0	.81
Education						
< 12—national sample	144	21.35	4.62	21.0	21.65	.83
= 12—high-risk cities	642	21.65	4.34	21.0	22.0	.81
> 12—national sample	1,215	21.80	3.96	20.0	22.0	.80

[1]Address correspondence to Joseph A. Catania, Center for AIDS Prevention Studies, University of California, San Francisco, 74 New Montgomery, Suite 600, San Francisco, CA 94105.

References

Catania, J. A., McDermott, L. J., & Pollack, L. M. (1986). Questionnaire response bias and face-to-face interview sample bias in sexuality research. *The Journal of Sex Research, 22,* 210-230.

Chelune, G. (1976). Self-disclosure situations survey: A new approach to measuring self-disclosure. *Journal Supplement Abstract Service: Catalog of Selected Documents in Psychology, 6,* 11-112. (Ms. No. 1367)

Exhibit

The Sexual Self-Disclosure Scale

Instructions: The following describe different situations in which people may or may not wish to discuss sexual matters. Imagine yourself in each of the situations listed below and circle that number which best shows how easy or difficult it would be for you to reveal sexual information in that situation. Use the key below as a guide for making your answer.

Key   1   Extremely easy   4   Somewhat difficult
           2   Moderately easy   5   Moderately difficult
           3   Somewhat easy   6   Extremely difficult

1. If you were asked to complete an anonymous questionnaire containing personal questions on sexuality, the answers to which you had been told would never be publicly associated with you personally, how easy or difficult would this be in the following situation:
   a. In the privacy of your own home, with no one else present.[a]
   b. During a large (25 or more people) group meeting, where most others are also filling out the questionnaire.
2. If you were asked personal sexual questions in a private face-to-face situation (for instance, only you and an interviewer), the answers to which you had been told would never be revealed, how much difficulty or ease would you have in doing this in the following situations:
   a. With a young (20-30 years) female interviewer
   b. With a young (20-30 years) male interviewer
   c. With an older (50 years and older) female interviewer
   d. With an older (50 years and older) male interviewer
   e. With a young (25-35 years) female medical doctor
   f. With a young (25-35 years) male medical doctor
   g. With an older (50+ years) female medical doctor
   h. With an older (50+ years) male medical doctor
3. How difficult or easy would it be for you to discuss a personal sexual problem or difficulty in the following situation (assume you are in private circumstances)?
   a. With a close female friend
   b. With a close male friend
   c. With a spouse or sexual partner
   d. With a personal physician
   e. With a specialist in sexual problems
4. How easy or difficult would it be for you to openly discuss your sex life and history in a group of three to five people who are:
   a. Both female and male (mixed company) that you have known only briefly
   b. All members of your own sex that you have known only briefly
5. How easy or difficult would it be for you to discuss a personal sexual problem or difficulty with your parents, or if your parents are deceased how easy or difficult would it have been to discuss such with them? (answer for both parents separately below)
   a. With your mother
   b. With your father

Short Form

1. Do you think that talking about sex in an AIDS survey is . . .
            Very easy
            Kind of easy
            Kind of hard or very hard
            Declined to answer
            Don't know[b]
2. How easy or hard would it be to fill out an anonymous questionnaire that asked questions about your sexual behavior in the privacy of your own home with no one else present? Would it be . . .

3. How easy or hard would it be for you to fill out an anonymous questionnaire that asked questions about your sexual behavior in the waiting room of a medical clinic with other patients present, who could not see what you were writing? Would it be . . .
4. How easy or hard would it be for you to answer questions about your sexual behavior if they were asked by a medical doctor in the privacy of his/her own office? Would it be . . .
5. How easy or hard would it be to answer sexual questions about your sexual behavior if they were asked by a marriage counselor in the privacy of his/her office? Would it be . . .
6. How easy would it be for you to discuss a sexual problem (read each) With a good friend? Would it be . . .
7. With a spouse or sexual partner? Would it be . . .

a. The 1-6 scale is repeated after each item.
b. These response options follow each item.

Sexual Self-Disclosure Scale

Edward S. Herold[1] and Leslie Way, *University of Guelph*

Although there has been considerable research about self-disclosure, there has been little research regarding disclosure of sexual topics. In particular, researchers have not differentiated disclosure about specific sexual topics. This differentiation is important because sexuality covers a wide range of attitudinal and behavioral areas.

Our first objective was to construct a scale consisting of sexual topics and to determine the extent of disclosure for each. The question of whether individuals vary in their disclosure to different target persons has been examined extensively. When disclosing information on sexual topics, adolescents and young adults prefer to disclose to friends and dating partner than to parents (Herold, 1984).

Our second objective was to analyze sexual self-disclosure separately for each of the target groups of mother, father, close friend of the same sex, and dating partner.

Description and Response Mode

The Sexual Self-Disclosure Scale (SSDS) was based on Jourard's Self-Disclosure Questionnaire (Jourard, 1971). The SSDS differs from Jourard's in three respects. The SSDS measures only sexual topics. The SSDS measures disclosure to the target groups of mother, father, close friend of the same sex, and dating partner. Unlike Jourard, we did not measure self-disclosure to a close friend of the opposite sex because we believed some people might have difficulty in distinguishing between close friend of the opposite sex and dating partner.

Timing and Scoring

The scale requires about 5 minutes for completion. Self-disclosure scores are obtained separately for each of the target groups. Items scores for each target group are summed and mean scores are obtained.

Reliability and Validity

Data were obtained from 203 unmarried university females aged 18-22 (Herold & Way, 1988). The respective scale means and Cronbach alpha coefficients were as follows: disclosure to mother ($M = 13.2$, alpha = .84); disclosure to father ($M = 10.1$, alpha = .71); disclosure to friend ($M = 19.7$, alpha = .89); and disclosure to dating partner ($M = 21.9$, alpha = .94). Validity for the scale is indicated by the fact that the mean scores are consistent with previous research that has found greater disclosure to friends and dating partner than to parents and the least amount of disclosure to father (Herold, 1984).

References

Herold, E. S. (1984). *The sexual behavior of Canadian young people.* Markham, Ontario: Fitzhenry & Whiteside.

Herold, E. S., & Way, L. (1988). Sexual self-disclosure among university women. *The Journal of Sex Research, 24,* 1-14.

Jourard, S. (1971). *Self-disclosure: An experimental analysis of the transparent self.* New York: Wiley.

[1]Address correspondence to Edward S. Herold, Department of Family Studies, University of Guelph, Guelph, Ontario N1G 2W1, Canada; email: eherold@facs.uoguelph.ca.

Exhibit

Sexual Self-Disclosure Scale

You are to read each item in the next section of the questionnaire and then indicate the extent that you have talked about that item to each person (i.e., the extent to which you have made your attitudes and/or behaviors known to that person). Use the rating scale below to describe the extent that you have talked about each item.

The rating scale is:

(1) Have told the person *nothing* about this aspect of me.
(2) Have talked only in *general terms* about this item.
(3) Have talked in *some detail* about this item but have not fully discussed my own attitudes or behaviors.
(4) Have talked in *complete detail* about this item to the other person. He or she knows me fully in this respect.

Choose one number in the row which corresponds to the amount of your disclosure. For example, if you have talked in general terms to your mother about your attitudes and/or behaviors regarding masturbation, you would place a 2 in column 6 of the computer card.

Items: Disclosure to mother	No Disclosure	Only General Terms	Some Detail	Complete Detail
1. My personal views on sexual morality.	1	2	3	4
2. Premarital sexual intercourse.	1	2	3	4
3. Oral sex.	1	2	3	4
4. Masturbation.	1	2	3	4
5. My sexual thoughts or fantasies.	1	2	3	4
6. Sexual techniques I find or would find pleasurable.	1	2	3	4
7. Use of contraception.	1	2	3	4
8. Sexual problems or difficulties I might have.	1	2	3	4

The Sexual Self-Disclosure Scale

William E. Snell, Jr.,[1] *Southeast Missouri State University*

The literature on human sexuality emphasizes the need for people to discuss the sexual aspects of themselves with others. Snell, Belk, Papini, and Clark (1989) examined women's and men's willingness to discuss a variety of sexual topics with parents and friends by developing an objective self-report instrument, the Sexual Self-Disclosure Scale (SSDS). The first version of the SSDS consists of 12 subscales that measure the following sexual topics (Snell & Belk, 1987): sexual behavior, sexual sensations, sexual fantasies, sexual attitudes, the meaning of sex, negative sexual affect, positive sexual affect, sexual concerns, birth control, sexual responsibility, sexual dishonesty, and rape. In another study, reported by Snell et al. (1989), women's and men's willingness to discuss a variety of sexual topics with an intimate partner was examined by extending the SSDS to include a greater variety of sexual topics. The Revised Sexual Self-Disclosure Scale (SSDS-R) consists of 24 three-item subscales measuring people's willingness to discuss the following sexual topics with an intimate partner (reported in Study 3 by Snell et al., 1989): sexual behaviors, sexual sensations, sexual fantasies, sexual preferences, meaning of sex, sexual accountability, distressing sex, sex-

[1]Address correspondence to William E. Snell, Jr., Department of Psychology, Southeast Missouri State University, One University Plaza, Cape Girardeau, MO 63701; email: wesnell@semovm.semo.edu.

ual dishonesty, sexual delay preferences, abortion and pregnancy, homosexuality, rape, AIDS, sexual morality, sexual satisfaction, sexual guilt, sexual calmness, sexual depression, sexual jealousy, sexual apathy, sexual anxiety, sexual happiness, sexual anger, and sexual fear.

Description

The initial version of the SSDS consists of 120 items that form 12 separate five-item subscales for each of two disclosure targets (male and female therapists). To respond to this version of the SSDS, individuals are asked to indicate how willing they would be to discuss the SSDS sexual topics with the disclosure targets. A 5-point Likert-type scale (scored 0 to 4) is used to measure the responses: (0) *I am not at all willing to discuss this topic with this person*, (1) *I am slightly willing to discuss this topic with this person*, (2) *I am moderately willing to discuss this topic with this person*, (3) *I am almost totally willing to discuss this topic with this person*, and (4) *I am totally willing to discuss this topic with this person*. Subscale scores are created for each disclosure target person by summing the five items on each subscale. Higher scores thus indicate greater willingness to disclose a particular SSDS sexual topic with a particular person.

The SSDS-R used by Snell et al. (1989) consists of 72 items that form 24 three-item subscales for the disclosure target (i.e., an intimate partner). In responding to the SSDS-R, individuals are asked to indicate how much they are willing to discuss the SSDS-R topics with an intimate partner. A 5-point Likert-type scale is used to collected data on the responses, with each item being scored from 0 to 4: (0) *I would not be willing to discuss this topic with an intimate partner*, (1) *I would be slightly willing to discuss this topic with an intimate partner*, (2) *I would be moderately willing to discuss this topic with an intimate partner*, (3) *I would be mostly willing to discuss this topic with an intimate partner*, and (4) *I would be completely willing to discuss this topic with an intimate partner*. To create SSDS-R subscale scores, the three items on each subscale are summed (no items are reverse scored). Higher scores thus correspond to greater willingness to discuss the SSDS-R sexual topics with an intimate partner.

The sample version of the SSDS-R in the exhibit is an example of how the SSDS-R may be modified for use with different target persons (e.g., mother, father, best female friend, best male friend).

Response Mode and Timing

Respondents indicate their answers typically on a computer scan sheet by darkening in a response from A to E. Alternatively, responses to the SSDS can be written directly on the questionnaire itself. Usually, 20-30 minutes are needed to complete the SSDS.

Scoring

The SSDS consists of 12 subscales, each containing five separate items. The labels and items for each of these subscales are as follows: (a) Sexual Behavior (Items 1, 13, 25, 37, 49); (b) Sexual Sensations (Items 2, 14, 26, 38, 50); (c) Sexual Fantasies (Items 3, 15, 27, 39, 51); (d) Sexual Attitudes (Items 4, 16, 28, 40, 52); (e) Meaning of Sex (Items 5, 17, 29, 41, 53); (f) Negative Sexual Affect (Items 6, 18, 30, 42, 54); (g) Positive Sexual Affect (Items 7, 19, 31, 43, 55); (h) Sexual Concerns (Items 8, 20, 32, 44, 56); (i) Birth Control (Items 9, 21, 33, 45, 57); (j) Sexual Responsibility (Items 10, 22, 34, 46, 58); (k) Sexual Dishonesty (Items 11, 23, 35, 47, 59); and (l) Rape (Items 12, 24, 36, 48, 60). The items are coded so that A = 0, B = 1, C = 2, D = 3, and E = 4. The five items on each subscale are then summed, so that higher scores correspond to greater sexual self-disclosure.

The SSDS-R consists of 24 subscales, each containing three separate items: (a) Sexual Behaviors (Items 1, 5, 9); (b) Sexual Sensations (Items 2, 6, 10); (c) Sexual Fantasies (Items 3, 7, 11); (d) Sexual Preferences (Items 4, 8, 12); (e) Meaning of Sex (Items 13, 18, 23); (f) Sexual Accountability (Items 14, 19, 24); (g) Distressing Sex (Items 15, 20, 25); (h) Sexual Dishonesty (Items 16, 21, 26); (i) Sexual Delay Preferences (Items 17, 22, 27); (j) Abortion and Pregnancy (Items 28, 33, 38); (k) Homosexuality (Items 29, 34, 39); (l) Rape (Items 30, 35, 40); (m) AIDS (Items 31, 36, 41); (n) Sexual Morality (Items 32, 37, 42); (o) Sexual Satisfaction (Items 43, 53, 63); (p) Sexual Guilt (Items 44, 54, 64); (q) Sexual Calmness (Items 45, 55, 65); (r) Sexual Depression (Items 46, 56, 66); (s) Sexual Jealousy (Items 47, 57, 67); (t) Sexual Apathy (Items 48, 58, 68); (u) Sexual Anxiety (Items 49, 59, 69); (v) Sexual Happiness (Items 50, 60, 70); (w) Sexual Anger (Items 51, 61, 71); and (x) Sexual Fear (Items 52, 62, 72).

Reliability

The internal consistency of the 12 subscales on the original SSDS was determined by calculating Cronbach alpha coefficients. These alphas ranged from a low of .83 to a high of .93 (average = .90) for the female therapist, and from a low of .84 to a high of .94 (average = .92) for the male therapist. The reliability coefficients for the SSDS-R ranged from a low of .59 to a high of .91 (average = .81). These reliability coefficients were all sufficiently high to justify using either version of the scale in research investigations.

Validity

Snell et al. (1989) reported that women's and men's responses to the SSDS varied as a function of the disclosure recipient and the content of the sexual disclosure. Women indicated that they were more willing to discuss the topics on the SSDS with a female than a male therapist. Also, it was found that people's responses to the SSDS-R varied as a function of respondent gender and sexual topic.

References

Snell, W. E., Jr., & Belk, S. S. (1987, April). *Development of the Sexual Self-Disclosure Scale (SSDS): Sexual disclosure to female and male therapists*. Paper presented at the annual meeting of the Southwestern Psychological Association, New Orleans, LA.

Snell, W. E., Jr., Belk, S. S., Papini, D. R., & Clark, S. (1989). Development and validation of the Sexual Self-Disclosure Scale. *Annals of Sex Research, 2*, 307-334.

Exhibit

The Sexual Self-Disclosure Scale

Instructions: This survey is concerned with the extent to which you have discussed the following 60 topics about sexuality with several different people. Listed below you will notice four columns[a] which represent the following individuals: (A) your mother, (B) your father, (C) your best male friend, and (D) your best female friend. For each of these people, indicate how much you have discussed these topics with them. Use the following scale for your responses:

Have not discussed this topic:	Have slightly discussed this topic:	Have moderately discussed this topic:	Have mostly discussed this topic:	Have fully discussed this topic

    (A)   with your mother.
    (B)   with your father.
    (C)   with your best male friend
    (D)   with your best female friend.

1. My past sexual experiences
2. The things that sexually arouse me
3. My imaginary sexual encounters
4. The sexual behaviors which I think people ought to exhibit
5. What sex means to me
6. How guilty I feel about sex
7. How satisfied I feel about the sexual aspects of my life
8. Times when sex was distressing for me
9. What I think about birth control
10. My private notion of sexual responsibility
11. The times I have faked orgasm
12. My private views about rape
13. The types of sexual behaviors I've engaged in
14. The sexual activities that "feel good" to me
15. My private sexual fantasies
16. What I consider "proper" sexual behaviors
17. What it means to me to make love together with someone
18. How anxious I feel about my sex life
19. How content I feel about the sexual aspects of my life
20. Times when I had undesired sex
21. How I feel about abortions
22. The responsibility one ought to assume for one's sexuality
23. The times I have pretended to enjoy sex
24. The "truths and falsehoods" about rape
25. The number of times I have had sex
26. The behaviors that are sexually exciting to me
27. My sexually exciting imaginary thoughts
28. The sexual conduct that people ought to exhibit
29. What I think and feel about having sex with someone
30. How depressed I feel about my own sexuality
31. How happy I feel about my sexuality
32. Times when I was pressured to have sex
33. How I feel about pregnancy
34. My own ideas about sexual accountability
35. The times I have lied about sexual matters
36. What women and men really feel about rape
37. The sexual positions I've tried
38. The sensations that are sexually arousing to me
39. My "juicy" sexual thoughts
40. My attitudes about sexual behaviors
41. The meaning that sexual intercourse has for me
42. How frustrated I feel about my sex life
43. How much joy that sex gives me
44. The aspects of sex that bother me
45. My private beliefs about pregnancy prevention
46. The idea of having to answer for one's sexual conduct
47. What I think about sexual disloyalty
48. Women's and men's reactions to rape
49. The places and times-of-day when I've had sex
50. The types of sexual foreplay that feel arousing to me
51. The sexual episodes that I daydream about
52. My personal beliefs about sexual morality
53. The importance that I attach to making love with someone
54. How angry I feel about the sexual aspect of my life
55. How enjoyable I feel about my sexuality
56. Times when I wanted to leave a sexual encounter
57. The pregnancy precautions that people ought to take
58. The notion one is answerable for one's sexual behaviors
59. How I feel about sexual honesty
60. Women's and men's reactions to rape

The Revised Sexual Self-Disclosure Scale (illustrated for the "intimate partner" target only)

Instructions: This survey is concerned with the extent to which you have discussed the following topics about sexuality with an intimate partner. To respond, indicate how much you have discussed these topics with an intimate partner. Use the following scale for your responses:[b]

1. My past sexual experiences
2. The kinds of touching that sexually arouse me
3. My private sexual fantasies
4. The sexual preferences that I have
5. The types of sexual behaviors I have engaged in
6. The sensations that are sexually exciting to me
7. My "juicy" sexual thoughts
8. What I would desire in a sexual encounter
9. The sexual positions I have tried
10. The types of sexual foreplay that feel arousing to me
11. The sexual episodes that I daydream about
12. The things I enjoy most about sex
13. What sex in an intimate relationship means to me
14. My private beliefs about sexual responsibility

15. Times when sex was distressing for me
16. The times I have pretended to enjoy sex
17. Times when I prefer to refrain from sexual activity
18. What it means to me to have sex with my partner
19. My own ideas about sexual accountability
20. Times when I was pressured to have sex
21. The times I have lied about sexual matters
22. The times when I might not want to have sex
23. What I think and feel about having sex with my partner
24. The notion that one is accountable for one's sexual behaviors
25. The aspects of sex that bother me
26. How I would feel about sexual dishonesty
27. My ideas about not having sex unless I want to
28. How I feel about abortions
29. My personal views about homosexuals
30. My own ideas about why rapes occur
31. My personal views about people with AIDS
32. What I consider "proper" sexual behavior
33. My beliefs about pregnancy prevention
34. Opinions I have about homosexual relationships
35. What I really feel about rape
36. Concerns that I have about the disease AIDS
37. The sexual behaviors that I consider appropriate
38. How I feel about pregnancy at this time
39. My reactions to working with a homosexual
40. My reactions to rape
41. My feelings about working with someone who has AIDS
42. My personal beliefs about sexual morality
43. How satisfied I feel about the sexual aspects of my life

44. How guilty I feel about the sexual aspects of my life
45. How calm I feel about the sexual aspects of my life
46. How depressed I feel about the sexual aspects of my life
47. How jealous I feel about the sexual aspects of my life
48. How apathetic I feel about the sexual aspects of my life
49. How anxious I feel about the sexual aspects of my life
50. How happy I feel about the sexual aspects of my life
51. How angry I feel about the sexual aspects of my life
52. How afraid I feel about the sexual aspects of my life
53. How pleased I feel about the sexual aspects of my life
54. How shameful I feel about the sexual aspects of my life
55. How serene I feel about the sexual aspects of my life
56. How sad I feel about the sexual aspects of my life
57. How possessive I feel about the sexual aspects of my life
58. How indifferent I feel about the sexual aspects of my life
59. How troubled I feel about the sexual aspects of my life
60. How cheerful I feel about the sexual aspects of my life
61. How mad I feel about the sexual aspect of my life
62. How fearful I feel about the sexual aspects of my life
63. How delighted I feel about the sexual aspects of my life
64. How embarrassed I feel about the sexual aspects of my life
65. How relaxed I feel about the sexual aspects of my life
66. How unhappy I feel about the sexual aspects of my life
67. How suspicious I feel about the sexual aspects of my life
68. How detached I feel about the sexual aspects of my life
69. How worried I feel about the sexual aspects of my life
70. How joyful I feel about the sexual aspects of my life
71. How irritated I feel about the sexual aspects of my life
72. How frightened I feel about the sexual aspects of my life

Source. This scale is reprinted with permission of the author.

a. The columns are not shown here to save space.

b. The scale is the same as that for the SSDS except that "with an intimate partner" follows each descriptor.

Sexual Self-Efficacy Scale for Female Functioning

Sally Bailes[1] and Laura Creti, *SMBD-Jewish General Hospital and Concordia University*

Catherine S. Fichten, *SMBD-Jewish General Hospital and Dawson College*

Eva Libman and William Brender, *SMBD-Jewish General Hospital and Concordia University*

Rhonda Amsel, *McGill University*

The Sexual Self-Efficacy Scale for Females (SSES-F) is a measure of perceived competence in the behavioral, cognitive, and affective dimensions of female sexual response (Bailes et al., 1989). Self-efficacy theory holds that expectations about how well one can perform in a given situation can significantly influence behavior in that situation. It is thought that self-efficacy influences what tasks one will undertake and to what degree one will persist when

[1]Address correspondence to Sally Bailes, SMBD-Jewish General Hospital, 8755 Chemin de la Cote Ste. Catherine, Montreal, Quebec H3T 1E2, Canada.

challenged (Bandura, 1982). Therefore, the evaluation and alteration of self-efficacy expectations is important in the cognitive-behavioral treatment of a number of psychosexual problems. Although self-efficacy measures have been developed to assess competency expectations for a number of behaviors, little attention has been given to female sexuality. Although Bogat, Hamernik, and Brooks (1987) developed a scale to evaluate women's orgasmic expectation and comfort in the context of Barbach's behavioral treatment program for anorgasmic women, the authors provided neither normative data nor the psychometric properties of the measure.

Fichten, Libman, and Rothenberg (1988) reported on the SSES-E, a measure of sexual self-efficacy for males focusing on erectile ability. The SSES-F was developed as a multidimensional counterpart to the SSES-E for use as a screening, assessment, and research instrument in our sex therapy practice.

Description

The SSES-F has 37 items, sampling capabilities in four phases of sexual response: interest, desire, arousal, and orgasm. In addition, the measure samples diverse aspects of female individual and interpersonal sexual expression (e.g., communication, body comfort and acceptance, and enjoyment of various sexual activities). The instrument includes the following subscales (items in parentheses): Interpersonal Orgasm (37, 29, 34, 36, 33, 32, 4, 28, 30), Interpersonal Interest/Desire (6, 5, 7, 22, 1, 9), Sensuality (19, 18, 17, 21, 20, 27), Individual Arousal (25, 31, 24, 26), Affection (15, 8, 16), Communication (14, 12, 13, 23, 35), Body Acceptance (3, 2), and Refusal (10, 11).

Female respondents indicate those activities they can do and, for each of these, rate their confidence level. An additional feature of the SSES-F is that male partners can rate how they perceive the capabilities and confidence levels of their female partners.

The SSES-F is appropriate for use with clinical and nonclinical populations, for both research and clinical purposes. It may be used by women of all ages, whether they are in relationships or unpartnered.

Response Mode and Timing

For each item, respondents check whether the female can do the described activity and rate the female's confidence in being able to engage in the activity. Confidence ratings range from 10 (*quite uncertain*) to 100 (*quite certain*). If an item is unchecked, the corresponding confidence rating is assumed to be zero. The measure takes about 10 to 15 minutes to complete.

Scoring

The SSES-F yields an overall self-efficacy strength score, as well as eight subscale scores. The total strength score is given by the average of the confidence ratings; items not checked in the "can do" column are scored as zero. The strength scores for the separate subscales are given by the average of the confidence ratings for that subscale.

Reliability

The SSES-F was administered to a nonclinical sample of 131 women (age range = 25 to 68 years). The sample included 51 married or cohabiting women and 80 single women. Thirty-six of the women completed the SSES-F a second time, after an interval of 4 weeks. The male partners of the 51 married or cohabiting women also completed the SSES-F.

Evaluation of the women's confidence ratings ($n = 131$) included a factor analysis to identify subscales and analyses to assess test-retest reliability and internal consistency. Item analysis demonstrated a high degree of internal consistency (Cronbach's alpha = .93) for the overall test. A factor analysis, using a varimax rotation, yielded eight significant factors, accounting for 68% of the total variance. Internal consistency coefficients for the separate subscales ranged from $\alpha = .70$ to $\alpha = .87$. Subscale-total and intersubscale correlations, carried out on the mean confidence score for each subscale, indicated reasonably high subscale-total correlations (range = .31 to .85) and moderate intersubscale correlations (range = .08 to .63).

Test-retest correlations for the total scores ($r = .83$, $p < .001$) and for the subscales (range = .50 to .93) indicate good stability over time. For the married or cohabiting couples, the correlation between the partners' total SSES-F scores was $r = .46$, $p < .001$.

Validity

Creti et al. (1989) reported on a preliminary validity analysis for the SSES-F. Both nonclinical and clinical samples were administered the SSES-F along with a test battery including measures of psychological, marital, and sexual adjustment and functioning. The overall strength score of the SSES-F was found to correlate significantly with other measures of sexual functioning, such as the Sexual History Form (Nowinski & LoPiccolo, 1979), the Golombok Rust Inventory of Sexual Satisfaction (Rust & Golombok, 1985), the Sexual Interaction Inventory (LoPiccolo & Steger, 1974), and with marital satisfaction (Locke Wallace Marital Adjustment Scale; Kimmel & Van der Veen, 1974). In addition, the overall strength scores of the SSES-F were significantly lower for sexually dysfunctional women who presented for sex therapy at our clinic than for those of a sample of women from the community who reported no sexual dysfunction. Sexually dysfunctional women also showed significantly lower scores than the community sample on the Interpersonal Orgasm, Interpersonal Interest/Desire, Sensuality, and Communication subscales. Finally, Creti et al. (1989) found that older women (age > 50) had significantly lower total strength scores than younger women (age < 50).

Other Information

Further validation of the measure is in progress. In addition, the SSES-F is presently being translated into French and will shortly be ready for psychometric evaluation. The authors thank Nettie Weinstein and Gloria Liederman for their assistance in collecting and entering much of the data.

References

Bailes, S., Creti, L., Fichten, C., Libman, E., Amsel, R., Liederman, G., & Brender, W. (1989, August). *The SSES-F: A multidimensional measure of sexual self-efficacy for women.* Poster presented at the annual convention of the American Psychological Association, New Orleans, LA.

Bandura, A. (1982). Self-efficacy mechanism in human agency. *American Psychologist, 37,* 122-147.

Bogat, G. A., Hamernik, K., & Brooks, L. A. (1987). The influence of self-efficacy expectations on the treatment of preorgasmic women. *Journal of Sex and Marital Therapy, 13,* 128-136.

Creti, L., Bailes, S., Fichten, C., Libman, E., Amsel, R., Liederman, G., & Brender, W. (1989, August). *Validation of the Sexual Self-Efficacy Scale for Females.* Poster presented at the annual convention of the American Psychological Association, New Orleans, LA.

Fichten, C. S., Libman, E., & Rothenberg, I. (1988). Sexual Self-Efficacy Scale–Erectile Functioning. In C. M. Davis, W. L. Yarber, & S. L. Davis (Eds.), *Sexuality-related measures: A compendium* (pp. 129-131). Lake Mills, IA: Davis, Yarber, and Davis.

Kimmel, D., & Van der Veen, F. (1974). Factors of marital adjustment. *Journal of Marriage and the Family, 36,* 57.

Libman, E., Rothenberg, I., Fichten, C. S., & Amsel, R. (1985). The SSES-E: A measure of sexual self-efficacy in erectile functioning. *Journal of Sex and Marital Therapy, 11,* 233-244.

LoPiccolo, J., & Steger, J. C. (1974). The Sexual Interaction Inventory: A new instrument for assessment of sexual dysfunction. *Archives of Sexual Behavior, 3,* 585-595.

Nowinski, J. K., & LoPiccolo, J. (1979). Assessing sexual behavior in couples. *Journal of Sex and Marital Therapy, 5,* 225-243.

Rust, J., & Golombok, S. (1985). The Golombok Rust Inventory of Sexual Satisfaction (GRISS). *British Journal of Clinical Psychology, 24,* 63-64.

Exhibit

Sexual Self-Efficacy Scale for Females

Instructions: The attached form lists sexual activities that women engage in. *For women respondents only:* Under column I *(Can Do)*, check (✔) the activities you think you could do if you were asked to do them today. For only those activities you checked in column I, rate your degree of confidence that you could do them by selecting a number from 10 to 100 using the scale given below. Write this number in column II *(Confidence)*. *For male partners only:* Under column I *(Can Do)*, check (✔) the activities you think your female partner could do if she were asked to do them today. For only those activities you checked in column I, rate your degree of confidence that your female partner could do them by selecting a number from 10 to 100 using the scale given below. Write this number in column II *(Confidence)*. If you think your partner is not able to do a particular activity, leave columns I and II blank for that activity.

										I	II
										Check if can do	Rate confidence 10-100

10   20   30   40   50   60   70   80   90   100

Quite uncertain   *Moderately certain*   *Quite certain*

Text items

1. Anticipate (think about) sexual relations without fear or anxiety.
2. Feel comfortable being nude with the partner.
3. Feel comfortable with your body.
4. In general, feel good about your ability to respond sexually.
5. Be interested in sex.
6. Feel sexual desire for the partner.
7. Feel sexually desirable to the partner.
8. Initiate an exchange of affection without feeling obliged to have sexual relations.
9. Initiate sexual activities.
10. Refuse a sexual advance by the partner.
11. Cope with the partner's refusal of your sexual advance.
12. Ask the partner to provide the type and amount of sexual stimulation needed.
13. Provide the partner with the type and amount of sexual stimulation requested.
14. Deal with discrepancies in sexual preference between you and your partner.
15. Enjoy an exchange of affection without having sexual relations.
16. Enjoy a sexual encounter with a partner without having intercourse.
17. Enjoy having your body caressed by the partner (excluding genitals and breasts).
18. Enjoy having your genitals caressed by the partner.
19. Enjoy having your breasts caressed by the partner.
20. Enjoy caressing the partner's body (excluding genitals).
21. Enjoy caressing the partner's genitals.

22. Enjoy intercourse.
23. Enjoy a lovemaking encounter in which you do not reach orgasm.
24. Feel sexually aroused in response to erotica (pictures
25. Become sexually aroused by masturbating when alone.
26. Become sexually aroused during foreplay when both partners are clothed.
27. Become sexually aroused during foreplay when both partners are nude.
28. Maintain sexual arousal throughout a sexual encounter.
29. Become sufficiently lubricated to engage in intercourse.
30. Engage in intercourse without pain or discomfort.
31. Have an orgasm while masturbating when alone.
32. Have an orgasm while the partner stimulates you by means other than intercourse.
33. Have an orgasm during intercourse with concurrent stimulation of the clitoris.
34. Have an orgasm during intercourse without concurrent stimulation of the clitoris.
35. Stimulate a partner to orgasm by means other than intercourse.
36. Stimulate a partner to orgasm by means of intercourse.
37. Reach orgasm within a reasonable period of time.

Sexual Self-Efficacy Scale–Erectile Functioning

Catherine S. Fichten,[1] *SMBD-Jewish General Hospital and Douglas Hospital*
Ilana Spector, *Douglas Hospital and McGill University*
Rhonda Amsel, *McGill University*
Laura Creti, William Brender, and Eva Libman, *SMBD-Jewish General Hospital and Concordia University*

The Sexual Self-Efficacy Scale–Erectile Functioning (SSES-E) is a measure of the cognitive dimension of erectile functioning and adjustment in men. Specifically, it evaluates a man's beliefs about his sexual and erectile competence in a variety of sexual situations. The scale may be completed by a male to obtain self-ratings or by his partner to obtain corroboration.

Self-efficacy—confidence in the belief that one can perform a certain task or behave adequately in a given situation (Bandura, 1982)—is important in sexual relationships, where it is believed that negative thinking about sexual behaviors may lead to increased performance anxiety, poorer sexual function, and perhaps, avoidance of sexual activity. The SSES-E was developed to measure sexual self-efficacy with respect to erectile functioning.

The SSES-E can be used in the clinical assessment of sexual dysfunction (e.g., Carey, Wincze, & Meisler, 1993). It can also be used to measure sexual self-efficacy as it relates

to other cognitive, affective, behavioral, or physiological variables. The measure can differentiate functional from dysfunctional groups, as well as other groups that are hypothesized to have varying levels of erectile confidence (e.g., older and younger men). The SSES-E has also been shown to be useful in evaluating how self-efficacy changes in relation to biological events, such as surgery, as well as in relation to biological interventions for erectile problems, such as injection therapy. Finally, the SSES-E is appropriate as a measure of treatment outcome for sex therapy, where the goal is not only improved sexual behavior but also more adaptive cognitions and positive affect.

Description

The SSES-E is a 25-item measure designed to follow Bandura, Adams, and Beyer's (1977) format. Item content is based on the Goals for Sex Therapy questionnaire (Lobitz & Baker, 1979) and the Erectile Difficulty Questionnaire (Reynolds, 1978).

Respondents first indicate which sexual activities they expect they (or their partner) can complete. For each of these activities, they then rate their confidence level on a

[1]Address correspondence to Catherine S. Fichten, Department of Psychology, Dawson College, 3040 Sherbrooke Street West, Montreal, Quebec H3Z 1A4, Canada.

10-point interval scale ranging from 10-100. The questionnaire can be completed by both the male respondent and by his partner.

Response Mode and Timing

The respondent places a check mark in the "Can Do" column next to each sexual activity that he expects he could do if he tried it today. For each activity checked, he also selects a number from 10 to 100 indicating confidence in his ability to perform the given activity. The reference scale labels a confidence rating of 10 as *quite uncertain,* a rating of 50-60 as *moderately certain,* and a rating of 100 as *quite certain.* Instructions allow partners to rate sexual functioning according to the same format. The scale takes an average of 10 minutes to complete.

Scoring

The SSES-E yields a self-efficacy strength score. This is obtained by summing the values in the Confidence column and dividing by 25 (the number of activities rated). Any activity that the respondent does not check off in the Can Do column is presumed to have a zero confidence rating. Higher scores indicate greater confidence in the man's erectile competence.

Reliability

A group of dysfunctional men and a control group were examined. The dysfunctional sample consisted of 17 men presenting with sexual dysfunctions (13 with male erectile disorder, 2 with hypoactive sexual desire, and 2 with premature ejaculation) at the sex therapy service of a large metropolitan hospital (Libman, Rothenberg, Fichten, & Amsel, 1985). Nine of these men presented with their female sexual partners. The control group consisted of 15 married couples with nonproblematic sexual functioning who were matched to the dysfunctional group on demographic variables: The entire sample was composed of middle-class Caucasians with a mean age of 34.

Alpha coefficients were calculated for the dysfunctional and control males and females separately. The following estimates were obtained: .92 for dysfunctional males and .94 for their female partners' ratings of their male partners, .92 for control males and .86 for their female partners.

Test-retest reliability, using the control group, was calculated over a 1-month period. Results showed a reliability coefficient of .98 for males and .97 for females.

Validity

Using the same sample, concurrent validity estimates were obtained by correlating the dysfunctional men's SSES-E scores with selected items on the Sexual History Form (Nowinski & LoPiccolo, 1979). Correlations ranged from .47 to .68 for those items asking about quality of erections and feelings of sexual arousal. These findings were replicated and/or extended by Kalogeropoulos (1991), Creti and Libman (1989), and by Libman, Fichten, and Brender (1987), who found that SSES-E scores were logically and significantly related to age, couple sexual adjustment, frequency and breadth of sexual repertoire, and global male sexual functioning, in a sample of middle-aged and older men. Also, results reported by McPhee and colleagues (McPhee, 1985; McPhee, Sullivan, & Brender, 1986) indicate that men with lower SSES-E scores have more negative cognitive schemata about sexual functioning.

Evidence for known-groups validity has also been collected. In our sample of 17 dysfunctional men and 15 controls (Libman et al., 1985), dysfunctional men ($M = 53.6, SD = 21.1$) and their partners ($M = 47.2, SD = 26.7$) scored significantly ($p < .001$) lower on the SSES-E than did functional men ($M = 88.0, SD = 10.0$) and their partners ($M = 89.5, SD = 10.4$). Moreover, a stepwise discriminant analysis indicated that SSES-E scores were able to classify dysfunctional and nondysfunctional men with 88% accuracy. In addition, data indicate that older married men (age = 65+) had significantly lower self-efficacy scores ($M = 54.10$) than their middle-aged (age = 50-64) counterparts ($M = 70.03$) (Libman et al., 1989). Also, men who underwent a transurethral prostatectomy were found to rate their postsurgery sexual self-efficacy as lower ($M = 59.3, SD = 20.3$) than presurgery ($M = 64.3, SD = 18.8$) (Libman et al., 1989; Libman et al., 1991).

The SSES-E is also sensitive to changes with therapy. Kalogeropoulos (1991) found that scores significantly improved in a sample of 53 males who had undergone vasoactive intracavernous pharmacotherapy for erectile dysfunction.

Other Information

The SSES-E is also available in French (Échelle d'Efficacité Sexuelle–Le Fonctionnement Érectile, Version E). A validation study currently in progress (Fichten, Wright, Spector, Sabourin, Brender, & Libman, 1995) shows promising results. This measure was developed with research funding from the Conseil Québécois de la Recherche Sociale. We would like to thank Ian Rothenberg for assistance with various stages of this investigation.

References

Bandura, A. (1982). Self-efficacy mechanism in human agency. *American Psychologist, 37,* 122-147.

Bandura, A., Adams, N. E., Beyer, J. (1977). Cognitive processes mediating behavioral change. *Journal of Personality and Social Psychology, 35,* 125-139.

Carey, M. P., Wincze, J. P., & Meisler, A. W. (1993). Sexual dysfunction: Male erectile disorder. In D. H. Barlow (Ed.), *Clinical handbook of psychological disorders* (2nd ed., pp. 442-480). New York: Guilford.

Creti, L., & Libman, E. (1989). Cognitions and sexual expression in the aging. *Journal of Sex & Marital Therapy, 15,* 83-101.

Fichten C. S., Libman, E., Amsel, R., Creti, L., Weinstein, N., Rothenberg, P., Liederman, G., & Brender, W. (1991). Evaluation of the sexual consequences of surgery: Retrospective and prospective strategies. *Journal of Behavioral Medicine, 14,* 267-285.

Fichten, C. S., Wright, J., Spector, I., Sabourin, S., Brender, W., & Libman, E. (1995). *Validation de l'Échelle d'Efficacité Sexuelle–Le Fonctionnement Érectile (Version E).* Manuscript in preparation.

Kalogeropoulos, D. (1991). *Vasoactive intracavernous pharmacotherapy for erectile dysfunction: Its effects on sexual, interpersonal, and psychological functioning.* Unpublished doctoral dissertation, Concordia University, Montreal, Quebec.

Libman, E., Fichten, C. S., Creti, L., Weinstein, N., Amsel, R., & Brender, W. (1989). Transurethral prostatectomy: Differential effects of age category and presurgery sexual functioning on post prostatectomy sexual adjustment. *Journal of Behavioral Medicine, 12,* 469-485.

Libman, E., Fichten, C. S., & Brender, W. (1987). *Prostatectomy and sexual functioning in the aging male: Final report to the Conseil Québécois de la Recherche Sociale.* Montreal, Quebec: Sir Mortimer B. Davis-Jewish General Hospital.

Libman E., Fichten, C. S., Rothenberg, P., Creti, L., Weinstein, N., Amsel, R., Liederman, G., & Brender, W. (1991). Prostatectomy and inguinal hernia repair: A comparison of the sexual consequences. *Journal of Sex & Marital Therapy, 17,* 27-34.

Libman, E., Rothenberg, I., Fichten, C. S., & Amsel, R. (1985). The SSES-E: A measure of sexual self-efficacy in erectile functioning. *Journal of Sex & Marital Therapy, 11,* 233-244.

Lobitz, W. C., & Baker, E. C. (1979). Group treatment of single males with erectile dysfunction. *Archives of Sexual Behavior, 8,* 127-138.

McPhee, D. C. (1985). *An investigation of cognitive patterns associated with erectile dysfunctional males.* Unpublished honor's thesis, Concordia University, Montreal, Quebec.

McPhee, D. C., Sullivan, M., & Brender, W. (1986). *Perceptions of females as associated with low erectile confidence in males.* Presentation at the Canadian Psychological Association annual conference. Abstracted in *Canadian Psychology, 21,* 370.

Nowinski, J. K., & LoPiccolo, J. (1979). Assessing sexual behavior in couples. *Journal of Sex & Marital Therapy, 5,* 225-243.

Reynolds, B. S., (1978). *Erectile Difficulty Questionnaire.* Unpublished manuscript, Human Sexuality Program, University of California, Los Angeles.

Rosen, R. C., Leiblum, S. R., & Spector, I. P. (1994). Psychologically based treatment for male erectile disorder: A cognitive-interpersonal model. *Journal of Sex & Marital Therapy, 20,* 67-85.

Spector, I. P., & Carey, M. P. (1990). Incidence and prevalence of the sexual dysfunctions: A critical review of the empirical literature. *Archives of Sexual Behavior, 19,* 389-408.

Exhibit

Sexual Self-Efficacy Scale-E

Name:_____

Date:_____

The following form lists sexual activities that men engage in.

For male respondents only:

Under column I (*Can Do*), check (✓) the activities *you expect you could do* if you were asked to do them today.

For *only* those activities you checked in column I, rate your *degree of confidence* in being able to perform them by selecting a number from 10 to 100 using the scale given below. Each activity is independent of the others. Write this number in column II (*Confidence*).

Remember, check (✓) what you *can do*. Then, rate your *confidence* in being able to do each activity if you tried to do it today. Each activity is independent of the others.

For (female) partners only:

Under column I (*Can Do*), check (✓) the activities you think *your male partner could do* if he were asked to do them today.

For only those activities you checked in column I, rate your *degree of confidence* that your male partner could do them by selecting a number from 10 to 100 using the scale given below. Write this number in column II (*Confidence*).

Remember, check (✓) what you expect your male partner *can do*. Then rate your *confidence* in your partner's ability to do each activity if he tried to do it today. Each activity is independent of the others.

										I	II
										Check if male can do	Rate confidence 10-100

10	20	30	40	50	60	70	80	90	100

Quite uncertain   *Moderately certain*   *Quite certain*

1. Anticipate (think about) having intercourse without fear or anxiety.
2. Get an erection by masturbating when alone.
3. Get an erection during foreplay when both partners are clothed.
4. Get an erection during foreplay while both partners are nude.
5. Regain an erection if it is lost during foreplay.
6. Get an erection sufficient to begin intercourse.
7. Keep an erection during intercourse until orgasm is reached.
8. Regain an erection if it is lost during intercourse.
9. Get an erection sufficient for intercourse within a reasonable period of time.
10. Engage in intercourse for as long as desired without ejaculating.
11. Stimulate the partner to orgasm by means other than intercourse.
12. Feel sexually desirable to the partner.
13. Feel comfortable about one's sexuality.
14. Enjoy a sexual encounter with the partner without having intercourse.
15. Anticipate a sexual encounter without feeling obliged to have intercourse.
16. Be interested in sex.
17. Initiate sexual activities.
18. Refuse a sexual advance by the partner.
19. Ask the partner to provide the type and amount of sexual stimulation needed.
20. Get at least a partial erection when with the partner.
21. Get a firm erection when with the partner.
22. Have an orgasm while the partner is stimulating the penis with hand or mouth.
23. Have an orgasm while penetrating (whether there is a firm erection or not).
24. Have an orgasm by masturbation when alone (whether there is a firm erection or not).
25. Get a morning erection.

Age, Gender, and Sexual Motivation Inventory

David Quadagno,[1] *Florida State University*

The Age, Gender, and Sexual Motivation Inventory (AG-SMI) was originally developed to measure the relationships between gender and age and motivations for engaging in sexual activities, favored part of a sexual experience (foreplay, intercourse, and afterplay), ideal benefit to be gained from engaging in sexual activities, and other aspects

[1]Address correspondence to David Quadagno, Department of Biological Science, Florida State University, Tallahassee, FL 32306-2043.

of sexual behavior and satisfaction (Sprague & Quadagno, 1989). The literature on sexual motivation consistently indicates that males are primarily motivated by physical and women by emotional factors when college-aged individuals are the respondents (e.g., see Bardwick, 1971; Carroll, Volk, & Hyde, 1985; Denney, Field, & Quadagno, 1984). When a diverse age group was sampled, the results from AGSMI indicated very clearly that inferences about sexual motivations for the whole population cannot be drawn from studies of a very limited and relatively inexperienced segment of it. In addition, in using the AGSMI, we found only a moderate relationship between usual motive for engaging in sexual intercourse and the respondent's assessment of its most important benefit. The AGSMI can be used to examine gender differences in many aspects of sexual behaviors, satisfaction, and motivations in a similar age group, or changes in sexuality in men and women at varying ages.

Description

The AGSMI begins with a demographic section in which the respondents record information including, but not limited to, age, gender, marital status, employment status, sexual orientation, and combined family income. The demographic section is followed by 25 questions, 23 of which are multiple choice and 2 of which call for short answers. The sample used in the development of the instrument included 95 women and 84 men ranging in age from 22 to 57 years of age; mean age for the women was 31.2 and for the men, 31.7 years.

Response Mode and Timing

Respondents can circle the letter of choice for each question on the instrument and can also write their responses to the short-answer items on the instrument. As an alternative, if it is administered to a large group at the same time, a separate answer sheet can be used to record responses. The majority of the test items have three to five response choices. The inventory requires approximately 5 to 8 minutes to complete.

Scoring

The instrument is not designed to produce any combined or total scores for groups of items. Comparisons between individuals or between groups on individual items can be made.

Reliability

A rough indication of the reliability of responses to the instrument can be gained from a comparison of the answers

of male and female respondents to three items that asked average frequency of sexual intercourse per week, usual time spent in foreplay, and usual time spent in afterplay. Assuming the respondents and their sex partners are all from the same heterosexual population, there should be no aggregate gender differences on any of these items (i.e., if men in the population are averaging sexual intercourse 3 nights per week then females in the population should also have this average frequency). In addition, if men or women have a tendency to overstate or understate the time spent in foreplay or afterplay, this response bias would be reflected in differences between their means in the sample. No significant gender differences in responses to these questions were found, suggesting that whatever response biases may be operating in these data are not strongly associated with gender.

In addition, two differently phrased questions (Questions 16 and 23) probed the favored part of a sexual encounter and found agreement for both male and female respondents.

Validity

The results reported in the questionnaire responses of the younger age groups (22-25, 26-30, and 31-35 years of age) were in perfect agreement with previously published studies of college-aged individuals (Bardwick, 1971; Carroll et al., 1985; Denney et al., 1984). The findings from our older age groups (36-57 years of age) do not have a comparable sample because of the lack of studies of this type using older individuals.

References

Bardwick, J. (1971). *The psychology of women.* New York: Harper and Row.

Carroll, J., Volk, K., & Hyde, J. (1985). Differences between males and females in motives for engaging in sexual intercourse. *Archives of Sexual Behavior, 14,* 131-139.

Denney, N., Field, J., & Quadagno, D. (1984). Sex differences in sexual needs and desires. *Archives of Sexual Behavior, 13,* 233-245.

Sprague, J., & Quadagno, D. (1989). Gender and sexual motivation: An exploration of two assumptions. *Journal of Psychology & Human Sexuality, 2,* 57-76.

Exhibit

Age, Gender, and Sexual Motivation Inventory

1. Age _____
2. Sex _____ ; *For women only:* Past menopause? Yes _____ No _____
3. What is your marital status? (Check one)
   _____ Never married
   _____ Separated
   _____ Married
   _____ Divorced
   _____ Widowed
4. If married, how long in current marriage? _____
5. Age of current spouse _____

6. What is your employment status? (Check one)
   _____ Full-time homemaker
   _____ Employed part-time outside the home
   _____ Employed full-time outside the home
   _____ Student
7. What is your approximate yearly household income? (Check one)
   _____ Below $20,000
   _____ $20,001-$30,000
   _____ $30,001-$40,000
   _____ $40,001-$50,000
   _____ $50,001-$60,000
   _____ $60,001-$80,000
   _____ Over $80,000
8. Sexual orientation (Check one)
   _____ Heterosexual _____ Bisexual _____ Homosexual
9. How religious do you think you are? (Check one)
   _____ Very religious
   _____ Moderately religious
   _____ Not religious

For the remainder of the questions please circle the best answer.

10. How many individuals have you had sexual intercourse with?
    a. None
    b. Only one
    c. Between two and five
    d. Between six and ten
    e. Between eleven and twenty
    f. Over twenty
11. How many times per week do you usually engage in sexual intercourse?
    a. Less than once
    b. Between one and two
    c. Between three and four
    d. Between five and seven
    e. More than seven
12. How often do you experience orgasm during your sexual encounters (does not have to be sexual intercourse)?
    a. Never
    b. 1-25% of the time
    c. 26-50% of the time
    d. 51-75% of the time
    e. 76-99% of the time
    f. 100% of the time

Foreplay is a word that has been used to refer to sexual activity that occurs before intercourse. *Afterplay* refers to interactions such as hugging, holding, talking, etc., that occur after intercourse. Not all sexual encounters involve sexual intercourse, but foreplay and afterplay are defined here because many of the following questions will refer to them.

13. During which of the following phases of a sexual encounter are you most likely to experience an orgasm?
    a. Foreplay
    b. Sexual intercourse
    c. Afterplay
    d. Equally in foreplay, intercourse, or afterplay
    e. I don't experience orgasms in my sexual encounters
14. *For women only:* If you experience orgasm during foreplay do you usually like to then have intercourse?
    a. Yes
    b. No
15. When you engage in sexual intercourse or other intimate sexual acts, which of the following reasons best describes your motivation on most occasions?
    a. I want the physical release
    b. I want to show my love for my partner
    c. I am afraid my partner will leave me if I don't
16. Which aspect of a sexual experience do you enjoy the most?
    a. Foreplay
    b. Intercourse
    c. Afterplay
17. Which of the following is the most important thing that you could get from a sexual experience?
    a. A feeling of being emotionally close to my partner
    b. The physical release and/or orgasm
    c. A feeling that I am in control of my partner
18. Do you usually want to spend more or less time in foreplay than your partner(s)?
    a. I want to spend more time
    b. I want to spend less time
    c. We want to spend about the same amount of time
19. Do you usually want to spend more or less time in afterplay than your partner(s)?
    a. I want to spend more time
    b. I want to spend less time
    c. We want to spend about the same amount of time

20. When you and your partner(s) disagree on the amount of time that should be spent in foreplay, who is more likely to get his/her way?
    a. I am more likely to get my way
    b. My partner is more likely to get his/her way
    c. We are each likely to get our way half of the time
    d. We don't disagree

21. When you and your partner(s) disagree on the amount of time that should be spent in afterplay, who is more likely to get his/her way?
    a. I am more likely to get my way
    b. My partner is more likely to get his/her way
    c. We are each likely to get our way half of the time
    d. We don't disagree

22. When you and your partner(s) disagree on the amount of time that should be spent in foreplay or afterplay do you discuss the problem?
    a. We do communicate our disagreements
    b. We do not communicate our disagreements
    c. We do not disagree on this

23. Which of the following rank orders best describes the importance of the various parts of a sexual encounter to you (the first listed part should be the most important and the last the least important to you)?
    a. Foreplay, intercourse, afterplay
    b. Intercourse, foreplay, afterplay
    c. Afterplay, intercourse, foreplay
    d. Foreplay, afterplay, intercourse
    e. Intercourse, afterplay, foreplay
    f. Afterplay, foreplay, intercourse

24. How often do you initiate your sexual encounters?
    a. Never
    b. 1-25% of the time
    c. 26-50% of the time
    d. 51-75% of the time
    e. 76-99% of the time
    f. 100% of the time

25. Would you prefer your partner(s) to initiate sexual encounters?
    a. More than she/he does
    b. Less than she/he does
    c. The same as she/he does

26. In most cases, do you get more sexually aroused by initiating or being pursued during a sexual encounter?
    a. Initiating the encounter
    b. Being pursued by my partner

27. What percentage of your sexual encounters would you say you find to be satisfying?
    a. None
    b. 1-25%
    c. 26-50%
    d. 51-75%
    e. 76-99%
    f. 100%

28. How satisfied are you with your typical sexual encounter?
    a. Extremely satisfied
    b. Moderately satisfied
    c. Slightly satisfied
    d. Not at all satisfied

29. During which of the three phases (foreplay, intercourse, afterplay) of a sexual encounter are you usually most dissatisfied with how your partner responds?
    a. Foreplay
    b. Intercourse
    c. Afterplay
    d. I am not dissatisfied with any part

30. Have you ever communicated your dissatisfaction to your partner(s)?
    a. Yes
    b. No

31. If you are dissatisfied, why are you dissatisfied? _____

32. With which of the three phases (foreplay, intercourse, afterplay) are you most satisfied with how your partner responds?
    a. Foreplay
    b. Intercourse
    c. Afterplay
    d. I am not satisfied with any part

33. If you are satisfied, what do you find particularly satisfying? _____

34. Do you sometimes have sex to please your partner even though you don't want to have sex?
    a. Yes
    b. No

Sexual Risk Behavior Beliefs and Self-Efficacy Scales

Karen Basen-Engquist,[1] *University of Texas M.D. Anderson Cancer Center*

Louise C. Mâsse, *Center for Health Promotion Research and Development, University of Texas School of Public Health*

Karin Coyle and Douglas Kirby, *ETR Associates*

Guy Parcel, *Center for Health Promotion Research and Development, University of Texas School of Public Health*

Stephen Banspach, *Centers for Disease Control and Prevention*

Jesse Nodora, *Arizona Department of Health Services*

The Sexual Risk Behavior Beliefs and Self-Efficacy (SRBBS) scales were developed to measure important psychosocial variables affecting sexual risk-taking and protective behavior. It was originally a component of a larger questionnaire used in evaluating the effectiveness of a multicomponent, school-based program to prevent HIV, sexually transmitted disease (STD), and pregnancy among high school students (Coyle et al., 1996). The variables measured by the SRBBS scales are attitudes, norms, self-efficacy, and barriers to condom use. These variables were derived from the theory of reasoned action (Fishbein & Ajzen, 1975), Bandura's (1986) social learning theory, and the health belief model (Rosenstock, 1974).

Description

The instrument development process for the SRBBS scales involved four stages: (a) identifying the psychosocial constructs relevant to risk behavior for HIV, STD, and pregnancy; (b) generating questionnaire items by a team of investigators, based on the theories and models described above, empirical research, and other instruments that measured these constructs; (c) pretesting the draft instrument with focus groups of high school students; and (d) revising the instrument and testing it with additional focus groups.

The scales consists of 22 items with a 3- or 4-point Likert-type response format. Three of the scales address sexual risk-taking behavior: attitudes about sexual intercourse (ASI), norms about sexual intercourse (NSI), and self-efficacy in refusing sex (SER). Five scales address protective behavior: attitudes about condom use (ACU), norms about condom use (NCU), self-efficacy in communication about condoms (SECM), self-efficacy in using and buying condoms (SECU), and barriers to condom use (BCU). These scales have been used with students of various ethnic groups and have been translated into Spanish. In our research we have used the SRBBS scales with high school students (aged

14 to 18). They are also being used with middle school students (Grades 7 and 8) in another study; however, data from this research are not yet available.

Response Mode and Timing

The SRBBS scales have been used as part of a larger, 110-item, self-administered questionnaire that takes approximately 30-45 minutes to complete. The scales were originally printed on a form that can be optically scanned. In that form, respondents marked the circle corresponding to their response (the form did not include a numeric value for the responses). The scales can be adapted so that respondents circle or mark the appropriate response on a form that cannot be optically scanned.

Scoring

The items that belong in each scale are identified in the exhibit, along with values for the responses. Two items (ASI2 and NSI2) should be scored in reverse. Scores on individual items in a scale are totaled and then divided by the number of items in the scale. This gives the scale scores the same range as the response values, enabling the user to compare the scale scores to the original response categories with ease. The range of the ASI, ACU, NSI, NCU, and BCU is 1 to 4, and the range of SER, SECM, and SECU is 1 to 3.

Reliability and Validity

An analysis of data from a multiethnic sample of 6,213 high school students from Texas and California provides all information on reliability and validity (Basen-Engquist et al., 1996).

Reliability. In a sample of 6,213 high school students from Texas and California (Basen-Engquist, et al., 1996) the Cronbach alpha measuring internal consistency reliability for the each of the scales was as follows: attitudes about sexual intercourse, .78; norms about sexual intercourse, .78; self-efficacy for refusing sex, .70; attitudes about condom use, .87; norms about condom use, .84; self-efficacy in

[1]Address correspondence to Karen Basen-Engquist, Department of Behavioral Science—Box 243, University of Texas M.D. Anderson Cancer Center, 1515 Holcombe, Houston, TX 77030; email: karen_b-e@isqu.mda.uth.tmd.edu.

communicating about condoms, .66; self-efficacy in buying and using condoms, .61; and barriers to condom use, .73.

Construct validity. Confirmatory factor analysis was used to assess construct validity. Two models were evaluated, one with items relating to sexual risk-taking behavior, the other with items relating to protective behavior. The sexual risk behavior model included three scales: ASI, NSI, and SER. In the development of the model, we discovered that correlated error terms were required between norm and attitude items that were grammatically similar to obtain a model that fit the data. The fit indexes indicated that the final data fit the model well (i.e., the χ^2 was not significant, the residuals were normally distributed, and root mean square error of approximation was < .05).

The final protective behavior model included five scales: ACU, NCU, SECM, SECU, and BCU. The fit indexes indicated a good fit for this model as well, once paths for correlated error terms between grammatically similar attitude and norm items were added.

Concurrent validity. Concurrent validity was assessed by examining specific relationships between the scales and sexual experience in the high school sample. The sexual risk behavior scales differentiated between sexually experienced and those who have never had sexual intercourse. The results indicated that attitudes and perceived norms of students who had never had sexual intercourse were less supportive of having sexual intercourse than were those of sexually experienced respondents (Effect size$_{ASI}$ = 1.09; Effect size$_{NSI}$ = .90).[2] In addition, students who were sexually experienced had lower self-efficacy for refusing sex than did students who were not (Effect size$_{SER}$ = .57). Similar findings were observed in comparisons of students who had sexual intercourse in the past 3 months with those who did not.

We also examined students' condom use and their related attitudes and norms. Protective behavior scales differentiated sexually active students who were consistent condom users from those who were not. Consistent condom users had more positive attitudes toward condom use and more favorable perceived norms about condom use than

---

[2]Effect size = | Mean$_1$ – Mean$_2$ | / Pooled standard deviation.

inconsistent users (Effect size$_{ACU}$ = .78; Effect size$_{NCU}$ = .56). Self-efficacy for using and buying condoms and communicating about condom use with partners also were higher for the consistent condom users (Effect size$_{SECM}$ = .47; Effect size$_{SECU}$ = .23; Effect size$_{BCU}$ = .20). In addition, the consistent users found carrying or buying condoms to be less of a barrier than did the inconsistent users.

Concurrent validity also was assessed by hypothesizing specific relationships between the scales and age and gender, and then testing these hypotheses in the high school sample. We hypothesized that girls would have higher scores on norms about sexual intercourse, attitudes about sexual intercourse, self-efficacy for refusing sexual intercourse, attitudes about condom use, norms about condom use, and self-efficacy in communicating about condoms, but lower scores on condom use self-efficacy. These hypotheses were confirmed. We also hypothesized that age would be positively related to all three self-efficacy scales and negatively related to norms and attitudes. These hypotheses were also confirmed, with one exception. Younger students reported higher self-efficacy in refusing sex than older students (Basen-Engquist et al., 1996).

Other Information

This work was conducted under Contract 200-91-0938 with the Centers for Disease Control and Prevention.

References

Bandura A. (1986). *Social foundations of thought and action.* Englewood Cliffs, NJ: Prentice Hall.

Basen-Engquist, K., Masse, L., Coyle, K., Parcel, G. S., Banspach, S., Kirby, D., & Nodora, J. (1996). *Validity of scales measuring the psychosocial determinants of HIV/STD-related risk behavior in adolescents.* Unpublished manuscript.

Coyle, K., Kirby, D., Parcel, G., Basen-Engquist, K., Banspach, S., Rugg, D., & Weil, M. (1996). A multi-component school-based HIV/STD and pregnancy prevention program for adolescents: The Safer Choices project. *Journal of School Health, 66,* 89-94.

Fishbein, M., & Ajzen, I.(1975). *Beliefs, attitudes, intentions, and behavior: An introduction to theory and research.* Reading, MA: Addison-Wesley.

Rosenstock, I. M. (1974). Historical origins of the health belief model. In M. H. Becker (Ed.), *The health belief model and personal health behavior* (Vol. 2, pp. 328-335). Thorofare, NJ: Charles B. Slack.

Exhibit

Student Health Questionnaire

Your beliefs

| Please fill in the answer for each question that best describes how *you* feel. |

ASI1. *I believe* people my age should wait until they are older before they have sex.
*ASI2. *I believe* it's OK for people my age to have sex with a steady boyfriend or girlfriend.
ACU1. *I believe* condoms (rubbers) should always be used if a person my age has sex.

ACU2.   *I believe* condoms (rubbers) should always be used if a person my age has sex, *even if the girl uses birth control pills.*

ACU3.   *I believe* condoms (rubbers) should always be used if a person my age has sex, *even if the two people know each other very well.*

What do your friends believe?

> The following questions ask you about your FRIENDS and what they think. Even if you're not sure, mark the answer that you think best describes what they think.

NSI1.   Most of *my friends* believe people my age should wait until they are older before they have sex.

*NSI2.   Most of *my friends* believe it's OK for people my age to have sex with a steady boyfriend or girlfriend.

NCU1.   Most of *my friends* believe condoms (rubbers) should always be used if a person my age has sex.

NCU2.   Most of *my friends* believe condoms (rubbers) should always be used if a person my age has sex, *even if the girl uses birth control pills.*

NCU3.   Most of *my friends* believe condoms (rubbers) should always be used if a person my age has sex, *even if the two people know each other very well.*

How sure are you?

> What if the following things happened to you? Imagine that these situations were to happen to you. Then tell us how sure you are that you could do what is described.

SER1.   Imagine that you met someone at a party. He or she wants to have sex with you. Even though you are very attracted to each other, you're not ready to have sex. How sure are you that you could *keep from having sex?*

SER2.   Imagine that you and your boyfriend or girlfriend have been going together, but you have not had sex. He or she really wants to have sex. Still, you don't feel ready. How sure are you that you could *keep from having sex until you feel ready?*

SER3.   Imagine that you and your boyfriend or girlfriend decide to have sex, but he or she will not use a condom (rubber). You do not want to have sex without a condom (rubber). How sure are you that you *could keep from having sex, until your partner agrees it is OK to use a condom (rubber)?*

SECM1. Imagine that you and your boyfriend or girlfriend have been having sex but have not used condoms (rubbers). You really want to start using condoms (rubbers). How sure are you that you could *tell your partner you want to start using condoms (rubbers)?*

SECM2. Imagine that you are having sex with someone you just met. You feel it is important to use condoms (rubbers). How sure are you that you could *tell that person that you want to use condoms (rubbers)?*

SECM3. Imagine that you or your partner use birth control pills to prevent pregnancy. You want to use condoms (rubbers) to keep from getting STD or HIV. How sure are you that you could *convince your partner that you also need to use condoms (rubbers)?*

SECU1. How sure are you that you could use a condom (rubber) correctly or explain to your partner how to use a condom (rubber) correctly?

SECU2. If you wanted to get a condom (rubber), how sure are you that you could go to the store and buy one?

SECU3. If you decided to have sex, how sure are you that you could have a condom (rubber) with you when you needed it?

What do you think about condoms?

> Please tell us how much you agree or disagree with the following statements.

BCU1.   It would be embarrassing to buy condoms (rubbers) in a store.

BCU2.   I would feel uncomfortable carrying condoms (rubbers) with me.

BCU3.   It would be wrong to carry a condom (rubber) with me because it would mean that I'm planning to have sex.

Key to identification of scale items and description of response formats:

ASI   =   Attitudes about sexual intercourse
ACU   =   Attitudes about condom use
NSI   =   Norms about sexual intercourse
NCU   =   Norms about condom use

Response format for attitude and norm items:

    4 = Definitely yes
    3 = Probably yes
    2 = Probably no
    1 = Definitely no

SER   = Self-efficacy for refusing sexual intercourse
SECM = Self-efficacy for communicating about condom use
SECU = Self-efficacy for buying and using condoms

Response format for self-efficacy items:

    3 = Totally sure
    2 = Kind of sure
    1 = Not sure at all

BCU = Barriers to condom use

Response format for barrier items:

    4 = I strongly agree
    3 = I kind of agree
    2 = I kind of disagree
    1 = I strongly disagree

*Item should be scored in reverse.

Health Protective Sexual Communication Scale

Joseph A. Catania,[1] *University of California, San Francisco*

The Health Protective Sexual Communication (HPSC) scale is a self-report scale that assesses how often respondents discuss health protective topics while interacting with a new, first-time sexual partner. Items address health protective concerns related to safer sex, sexual histories, and contraceptive use. Moreover, the scale assesses communication that has health protective consequences as distinct from sexual communication that may be related to enhancement of sexual pleasure. The expanded 10-item scale was based on an extension of two brief scales that have been used in two national survey studies to assess the ability to discuss sexual histories and condom use with prospective sexual partners. Findings indicate both the brief and expanded HPSC scales to be strongly linked to high-risk sexual behaviors that include multiple partners, condom use, and alcohol use before sex (Catania,

1995; Catania, Coates, & Kegeles, 1994; Dolcini, Coates, Catania, Kegeles, & Hauck, 1995).[2]

Description

The original self- or interviewer-administered scale is composed of three items (1, happened with all partners; 2, happened with some partner; 3, didn't happen) rated on a 4-point scale. The revised, expanded scale is a 12-item Likert-type scale with two questions that need to be excluded when administering the scale to gay individuals. Each item is rated on a 4-point scale (4 = *always*, 1 = *never*).

Response Mode and Timing

The scales are available in Spanish and English. Both the short and the expanded forms are self- or interviewer

[1]Address correspondence to Joseph A. Catania, Center for AIDS Prevention Studies, University of California, San Francisco, 74 New Montgomery, Suite 600, San Francisco, CA 94105.

[2]Portions of the NABS survey data collected from the NABS cohort study used to report indexes of reliability and validity are available on request from the author.

administered and take approximately 1-2 minutes to complete.

Scoring

Total scores on the brief three-item HPSC scale are produced by reverse scoring and summing across items for a total scale score. Total scores on the expanded HPSC scale are obtained by summing across items.

Reliability and Validity

The HPSC scale has been administered to varied populations, including adolescents and national urban probability samples constructed to adequately represent White, Black, and Hispanic ethnic groups, as well as high HIV-risk groups (Catania, Coates, & Kegeles, 1994; Catania, Kegeles, & Coates, 1990; Dolcini et al., 1995). The original brief version of the HPSC scale was used on a population of 114 adolescent females who participated in a study (Catania et al., 1990) that examined psychosocial correlates of condom use and multiple-partner sex. Respondents, recruited from a family planning clinic in California, were White (92%), Hispanic (4%), and other (4%) and ranged in age from 12 to 18 years. The majority of respondents were heterosexual, unmarried, and sexually active. Reliability was good (Cronbach's alpha = .67). A hierarchical multiple regression model, in which several predictor variables known to be related to sexual risk were examined, revealed that a greater willingness to request partners to use condoms as indicated by HPSC scores was associated with more frequent condom use and multiple partners (Catania et al., 1990).

The original three-item Health Communication Sexual Scale was also administered to respondents who participated in a study (Catania, Coates, & Kegeles, 1994) examining the incidence of multiple partners and related psychosocial correlates, as part of the AIDS in Multi-Ethnic Neighborhoods (AMEN)[3] study (Catania, Coates, Kegeles, et al., 1992). The AMEN study is a longitudinal study (three waves) examining the distribution of HIV, sexually transmitted diseases (STDs), related risk behaviors, and their correlates across social strata. The multiple-partner study sample, which used data generated from Wave 2, restricted inclusion criteria to unmarried heterosexuals who revealed an HIV-related risk marker at Wave 2, and being sexually active between Wave 1 and 2. Respondents ranged from 20 to 44 years of age. Reliability was excellent (Cronbach's alpha = .84). The mean, standard deviation, median, range, and reliabilities of ethnic groups, gender, and levels of education are provided in Table 1.

In earlier analysis with the HPSC scale, we examined whether its relationship to condom use was continuous across all scale values (Catania, Coates, Kegeles, et al., 1992). The scale was found to have a significant relationship to condom use primarily for those respondents scoring in the upper one third of the scale, indicating that people

[3] For further details on sampling methods for the AMEN cohort study, see Catania, Coates, Kegeles, et al. (1992).

Table 1 Normative Data for the Health Protective Sexual Communication Scale

	n	*Mean*	*SD*	*Range*	*Mdn*	*Alpha*
NABS[a] study						
National sample	155	23.82	8.21	30.0	24.0	.88
High-risk cities	810	22.93	7.32	30.0	22.0	.84
Ethnicity						
White						
National sample	101	23.06	8.19	30.0	22.28	.88
High-risk cities	342	22.53	7.02	30.0	21.93	.83
Black						
National sample	47	25.62	8.13	29.0	28.05	.87
High-risk cities	329	24.35	7.33	30.0	24.0	.83
Hispanic						
National sample	8	23.01	3.30	15.0	24.0	.60
High-risk cities	125	21.90	8.12	30.0	21.0	.87
Gender						
Male						
National sample	81	22.57	8.22	29.0	22.06	.90
High-risk cities	414	21.22	6.72	29.0	20.0	.64
Female						
National sample	68	25.88	7.85	30.0	27.23	.84
High-risk cities	379	25.30	7.46	30.0	25.0	.82
Education						
< 12 years						
National sample	14	22.24	6.01	17.0	24.0	.76
High-risk cities	97	24.78	7.89	30.0	24.0	.55
= 12 years						
National sample	49	23.67	8.5	29.0	22.9	.88
High-risk cities	196	22.36	7.53	30.0	22.0	.85
> 12 years						
National sample	91	24.53	8.48	30.0	25.0	.88
High-risk cities	517	22.74	7.02	30.0	22.0	.83
AMEN[b] study						
Total	320	22.82	7.81	30.0	22.0	.84
Ethnicity						
White	146	23.05	7.86	30.0	22.08	.86
Black	72	23.69	7.79	30.0	23.05	.83
Hispanic	85	21.57	7.65	30,0	20.0	.84
Gender						
Male	155	20.64	7.34	30.0	19.0	.84
Female	165	24.86	7.71	30.0	24.03	.83
Education						
< 12 years	41	20.32	7.30	24.0	21.0	.83
= 12 years	65	23.34	8.34	30.0	22.0	.87
> 12 years	212	23.11	7.72	30.0	22.0	.84

a. National AIDS Behavior Survey.
b. AIDS in Multi-Ethnic Neighborhoods.

who consistently communicate about sexual matters across sexual encounters and partners are significantly more likely to use condoms. Thus, the HPSC scale was scored by dichotomizing the measure so that high scores included the upper one third of scores and low scores were composed of the lower two thirds of scores. Findings from the AMEN study revealed that high levels of health protective sexual communication were significantly correlated with high levels of health protective sexual communication (high communication: condom use high = 14%, condom use low = 4%).

In a another AMEN cohort analysis, the original HPSC scale was examined in relationship to incidence of multiple partners (Dolcini et al., 1995). Reliability was fair (Cronbach's alpha = .50) for respondents who also reported two or more sex partners in the past year. A regression model for all respondents with a primary sexual partner revealed that those who also had a new sexual partner in the past year (*n* = 201) and low health protective communication (odds ratio = 1.3 per unit decrease in health protective communication, 95% confidence interval = 1.05, 1.5) were associated with having multiple partners.

We conducted further analyses on the expanded Health Communication Scale Measure used in the 1990-1991 National AIDS Behavior Survey (NABS)[4] longitudinal study (Wave 2), which was composed of three interlaced samples designed to oversample African Americans and Hispanics for adequate representation. The interlaced samples included a national sample, an urban sample of 23 cities with high prevalences of AIDS cases, and a special Hispanic urban sample. In our analyses of the expanded HPSC scale, we limited our sample to respondents who reported having at least one partner in the past 12 months, were heterosexual (defined as respondents who had only sexual partners of the opposite gender in the past 5 years), aged 18-49, and completed the HPSC scale. Respondents who described themselves as Asians, Native Americans, and Pacific Islanders were excluded because they were not adequately represented for analysis purposes (*n* = 24). Because the intent of our analyses was to examine relationships between variables, sample segments were combined without the use of poststratification weights. The resulting increase in power allowed for the detection of even very small relationships. Internal reliability was excellent (Cronbach's alpha = .85). Means, standard deviations, range, median, and reliability are given for White, Black, and Hispanic ethnic groups; male and females; and levels of education in Table 1.

A factor analysis of the expanded HPSC scale obtained a single, large eigenvalue (4.3), with an additional value falling near 1 (1.15), suggesting that there may be an additional factor, but it is not a strong element in the expanded scale. The second factor that may exist consists of items asking specifically about condom use. Given the small amount of variance accounted for by the second (6%) versus the first (37%) factor, we opted for a single-factor scale. We recommend further work that would expand the number of condom items in the scale to examine additional factors.

We examined an array of psychosocial and experiential factors that previous models and studies have indicated are important determinants of sexual communication and negotiation. From a multiple regression in which we analyzed primary antecedents, background, and demographic variables, we found respondents with higher HPSC expanded scale scores to be more likely to have greater sexual and condom relations skills, to be sexually assertive, to have ever used a condom, to be committed to using condoms in the future, to have been tested for HIV, and to be 18-29 years old (unpublished data, available from author). Respondents with high HPSC scores were also less likely to feel susceptible to STDs and less likely to report having used alcohol before sex.

We also examined a number of hypothesized gender and race interactions. An inverse relationship between sexual guilt and HPSC among Hispanic women was revealed. In contrast, Hispanic men who scored higher on sexual guilt also scored higher in HPSC. Higher communicators were also somewhat more likely to be Black than Hispanic, and were almost 3 times more likely to be women than men.

References

Catania, J. (1995). [NABS data]. Unpublished raw data.

Catania J., Coates, T., Golden, E., Dolcini, M., Peterson, J., Kegeles, S., Siegel, D., & Fullilove, M. (1994). Correlates of condom use among Black, Hispanic, and White heterosexuals in San Francisco: The AMEN longitudinal survey. *AIDS Education and Prevention, 6,* 12-26.

Catania, J., Coates, T., & Kegeles, S. (1994). A test of the AIDS risk reduction model: Psychosocial correlates of condom use in the AMEN cohort survey. *Health Psychology, 13,* 1-8.

Catania, J., Coates, T., Kegeles, S., Thompson-Fullilove, M., Peterson, J., Marin, B., Siegel, D., & Hulley, S. (1992). Condom use in multi-ethnic neighborhoods of San Francisco: The population-based AMEN (AIDS in Multi-Ethnic Neighborhoods) study. *American Journal of Public Health, 82,* 284-287.

Catania, J., Coates, T. J., Stall, R., Turner, H., Peterson, J., Hearst, N., Dolcini, M., Hudes, E., Gagnon, J., Wiley, J., & Groves, R. (1992). Prevalence of AIDS-related risk factors and condom use in the United States. *Science, 258,* 1101-1106.

Catania, J., Kegeles, S., & Coates, T. (1990). Towards an understanding of risk behavior: An AIDS risk reduction model (ARRM). *Health Education Quarterly, 17,* 53-72.

Dolcini, M. M., Coates, T. J., Catania, J. A., Kegeles, S. M., & Hauck, W. W. (1995). Multiple sexual partners and their psychosocial correlates: The population-based AIDS in Multiethnic Neighborhoods (AMEN) study. *Health Psychology, 14,* 1-10.

---

[4]For further details on sample construction and weighting of the NABS cohort study, see Catania, Coates, Stall, et al. (1992).

Exhibit

Health Protective Sexual Communication Scale

Instructions: Now I am going to read a list of things that people talk about before they have sex with each other for the first time. How often in the past 12 mos. have you . . . (read each). Would you say *always, almost always, sometimes,* or *never?*

1 = Always   2 = Almost always   3 = Sometimes   4 = Never   6 = Don't know   7 = Declined to answer

1. Asked a new sex partner how (he/she) felt about using condoms before you had intercourse.
2. Asked a new sex partner about the number of past sex partners (he/she) had.
3. Told a new sex partner about the number of sex partners you have had.
4. Told a new sex partner that you won't have sex unless a condom is used.
5. Discussed with a new sex partner the need for both of you to get tested for the AIDS virus before having sex.
6. Talked with a new sex partner about not having sex until you have known each other longer.
7. Asked a new sex partner if (he/she) has ever had some type of VD, like herpes, clap, syphilis, gonorrhea.
8. Asked a new sex partner if (he/she) ever shot drugs like heroin, cocaine, or speed.
9. Talked about whether you or a new sex partner ever had homosexual experiences.
10. Talked with a new sex partner about birth control before having sex for the first time.

Note. Items 1, 2, and 4 were used in the original short version. Items 9 and 10 are excluded for gay men and lesbians.

The Coping and Change Sexual Behavior and Behavior Change Questionnaire

David G. Ostrow,[1] Wayne DiFranceisco, and David Wagstaff, *Center for AIDS Intervention Research, Medical College of Wisconsin*

The Coping and Change Sexual Behavior and Behavior Change Questionnaire (CCS SBBCQ) assesses sexual behaviors that confer risk for HIV transmission among gay and bisexual men. It was developed as part of the Chicago component of the Multicenter AIDS Cohort Study (MACS) and the Coping & Change Study (CCS). The aims, organization, populations, and behavioral measures for both studies have been described in detail elsewhere (Chmiel et al., 1987; Joseph et al., 1987; Kaslow et al., 1987).

Description

The CCS SBBCQ has been used to develop a sexual risk index that considers the number of various types of partners as well as the number of acts performed with each of these partners (Ostrow, 1989). The four levels are no risk, low risk, modified high risk, and high risk (see Scoring section). The instrument consists of 18 items; 8 items contain sub-

[1] Address correspondence to David G. Ostrow, Center for AIDS Intervention Research, Medical College of Wisconsin, 8701 Watertown Plank Road, P.O. Box 26509, Milwaukee, WI 53226-0509; email: dostrow@post.its.mcw.edu.

parts that gather additional information if the respondent reports that he has engaged in the specific sexual behavior identified in the main question. Two items are used to assess the number of partners that the respondent thought of as steady partners, friends, casual acquaintances, or anonymous sexual partners. The remaining items are used to determine (a) how many times the respondent engaged in specific sexual behaviors during the recall period with each of the four kinds of sexual partners, and (b) how often condoms were used (*every time, sometimes, never*).

Minor variations in this questionnaire have occurred during the 10 years of study. The questionnaire included herein is from visit 12 (collected between August 1989 and September 1990), at which time the CCS SBBCQ was most extensive.

Response Mode and Timing

Respondents are asked to write the number of partners and the number of acts in the appropriate space. They are asked to place a check mark by the box that best reflects condom usage when they engaged in each specific sexual behavior with each type of partner. Because this instrument is part of a self-administered questionnaire, respondents are allowed to take as much time as they need to complete each item. Most individuals can complete these items in under 10 minutes.

Scoring

Responses to Questions 5 and 10 are used to determine an individual's score on the sexual risk index. If the respondent reported that he had no sexual partners in the past month (i.e., to Q 5 he indicates zero partners), he was at *no risk*. If he was monogamous (Q 5 indicates one partner of any type) and condoms were always used during receptive anal sex with that partner (Q 11 indicates that condoms were used *every time*), or if he had multiple partners (Q 5 indicates more than one partner) but did not engage in receptive anal sex (i.e., Q 11 indicates no receptive anal intercourse partners), he was at *low risk*. If he was monogamous and condoms were *never* used during receptive anal sex, or if he had multiple partners and condoms were not used *every time*, he was at *modified high risk*. Finally, if he had multiple partners and condoms were not used *every time* he had receptive anal sex, he was at *high risk*.

Reliability

To evaluate the extent of agreement between the MACS interview data and the self-administered CCS data, we calculated Cohen's kappa (Cohen, 1960) for each of the 18 CCS assessments. Values between .40 and .75 represent fair to good agreement (Landis & Koch, 1977). In addition, we calculated the sensitivity and specificity for the CCS sexual risk index at each MACS visit. To calculate these indexes, MACS data were assumed to reflect the true state of nature: With its longer recall period, the MACS was more likely to capture any sexual behavior that conferred risk for HIV transmission. In the present context, sensitivity is the probability that a respondent was identified as high risk by the CCS risk index given that he was so identified by the MACS risk index; specificity is the probability that a respondent was identified as low risk by the CCS risk index given that he was so identified by the MACS risk index (Fleiss, 1981).

For the measure(s) of receptive anal intercourse, Cohen's kappa had a mean of .53 ($SD = .11$); the 18 values ranged from .26 to .65. The sensitivity had a mean of .59 ($SD = .13$) and ranged from .23 to .71; the specificity had a mean of .94 ($SD = .04$) and ranged from .80 to .99. This was to be expected because men who engaged rarely (e.g., less than monthly) in unprotected anal receptive intercourse were unlikely to be identified as being at high risk on the CCS SBBCQ.

Validity

No formal psychometric studies were conducted because the sexually transmitted disease risk is directly related to the number of partners, the number of acts, and the correct and consistent use of condoms (Anderson & May, 1992; Feldblum & Fortney, 1988; Reiss & Leik, 1989; Stone, 1990). Nonetheless, the sexual risk index has been shown repeatedly to predict seroconversion for CCS participants (Joseph et al., 1987; Ostrow et al., 1993; Ostrow et al.,

1989) and to be associated with a number of psychosocial and behavioral factors known to be correlated with risky sex among gay/bisexual men, such as recreational substance use (Ostrow, 1994; Ostrow et al., 1993).

Other Information

Data from the CCS SBBCQ, as well as the other behavioral, psychosocial, and mental health sections of the questionnaire, are available for research use. The data for each wave and for various indexes are maintained at the Center for AIDS Intervention Research (CAIR) in SPSS portable files on an IBM server. Documentation consists of the questionnaires, data dictionaries, and published articles. To request use of the data, researchers can contact the first author.

It is expected that researchers seeking use of the CCS data will have specific questions and a specific data analytical proposal. In addition, it is expected that researchers will have resources to support their proposed work, as well as funds to cover the costs of copying questionnaires/data dictionaries, preparing selected data files, and any work or other materials required from CAIR personnel. Specifically, CAIR personnel could create the necessary SPSSX portable files, analyze data, and/or forward an existing file under collaborative arrangements with qualified investigators.

CAIR is supported by NIMH HIV Research Center Grant P30-MH52776. The Coping & Change Study of Men at Risk of AIDS is supported by NIMH Grant RO1-39346. The authors wish to acknowledge the collaboration and assistance of the Chicago MACS investigators (Drs. John Phair and Joan Chmiel, PIs), staff, and participants throughout the 10 years of this long-term behavioral and medical natural history study.

References

Anderson, R. M., & May, R. M. (1992). *Infectious diseases of humans: Dynamics and control*. Oxford, UK: Oxford University Press.

Chmiel, J. S., Detels, R., Kaslow, R. A., VanRaden, M., Kingsley, L. A., & Brookmeyer, R. (1987). Factors associated with prevalent human immunodeficiency virus (HIV) infection in the Multicenter AIDS Cohort Study (MACS). *American Journal of Epidemiology, 126*, 568-575.

Cohen, J. (1960). A coefficient of agreement for nominal scales. *Educational and Psychological Measurement, 20*, 37-46.

Feldblum, P. J., & Fortney, J. A. (1988). Condoms, spermicides, and the transmission of human immunodeficiency virus: A review of the literature. *American Journal of Public Health, 78*, 52-54.

Fleiss, J. L. (1981). *Statistical methods for rates and proportions* (2nd ed.). New York: Wiley.

Joseph, J. G., Montgomery, S. B., Emmons, C. A., Kessler, R. C., Ostrow, D. G., Wortman, C. G., O'Brien, K., Eller, M., & Eshleman, S. (1987). Magnitude and determinants of behavioral risk reduction: Longitudinal analysis of a cohort at risk for AIDS. *Psychology and Health, 1*, 73-96.

Kaslow, R. A., Ostrow, D. G., Detels, R., Phair, J. P., Polk, B. F., & Rinaldo, C. R., Jr. (1987). The Multicenter AIDS Cohort Study: Rationale, organization, and selected characteristics of the participants. *American Journal of Epidemiology, 126*, 310-318.

Landis, J. R., & Koch, G. G. (1977). The measurement of observer agreement for categorical data. *Biometrics, 33*, 159-174.

Ostrow, D. G. (1989). Risk reduction for transmission of human immunodeficiency virus in high-risk communities. *Psychiatric Medicine, 7,* 79-95.

Ostrow, D. G. (1994). Substance abuse and HIV infection. *Psychiatric Clinics of North America, 17,* 69-89.

Ostrow, D. G., Beltran, E. D., Joseph, J. G., DiFranceisco, W., Wesch, J., & Chmiel, J. S. (1993). Recreational drugs and sexual behavior in the Chicago MACS/CCS cohort of homosexually active men. *Journal of Substance Abuse, 5,* 311-325.

Ostrow, D. G., Joseph, J. G., Kessler, R. C., Soucy, J., Tal, M., Eller, M., & Chmiel, J. (1989). Disclosure of HIV antibody status: Behavioral and mental health correlates. *AIDS Education and Prevention, 1,* 1-11.

Reiss, I. L., & Leik, R. K. (1989). Evaluating strategies to avoid AIDS: Number of partners vs. use of condoms. *The Journal of Sex Research, 26,* 411-433.

Stone, K. M. (1990). Avoiding sexually transmitted diseases. *Obstetrics and Gynecology Clinics of North America, 17,* 789-799.

Exhibit

The Coping and Change Sexual Behavior and Behavior Change Questionnaire

An important note . . .

This questionnaire is designed to describe what men feel and believe about AIDS. It is *not* intended to provide medical advice. *None* of the statements or responses you read in this questionnaire should be taken as recommendations. A pamphlet with recommendations for safer sex should have been given to you when you enrolled in the Immune Function Study. Please consult that pamphlet, clinic staff, or your own physician in order to develop safe sexual practices.

Section A: Behavior and Behavior Change

In this section we would like to learn more about your sexual practices and how these may have changed because of the threat of AIDS. As with the rest of the questionnaire, there are no "right" or "wrong" answers here. We need, instead, your honest responses. First, we have some general questions.

1. Considering all of the different factors that may contribute to AIDS (including your own past and present behavior), what would you say are your chances of getting AIDS?

   (Circle one)

I am almost certain I will	1
A large or very large chance	2
Some chance	3
A small or very small chance	4
I am almost certain I will not	5

2. When you compare yourself to the average gay man, what would you say are your chances of getting AIDS?

   (Circle one)

Much lower	1
A little lower	2
About the same	3
A little higher	4
Much higher	5

3. Regardless of what you would say your chances are of getting AIDS, how much do you think you have been able to reduce those chances since the last time you took this questionnaire?

   (Circle one)

A lot	1
Quite a bit	2
Somewhat	3
A little bit	4
Not at all	5

4. If you did *everything* you could do to reduce your chances of getting AIDS, how much more do you think this would reduce your risk?

   (Circle one)
   Not applicable

I am already doing all I can do	0
Not at all more	1
Somewhat more	2
A lot more	3

5. We would like you to tell us, as nearly as you can, the number and types of sexual partners you had in the past month.
   a. How many *steady* sexual partners did you have in the past month? (This would include a partner in a monogamous relationship.)
      Number of partners you knew well in the past month: _____
   b. How many sexual partners did you have in the past month who, although *not steady* partners, were men you *knew well* (that is, considered friends or had known for a long time)?
      Number of partners you did not know well in the past month: _____
   c. How many sexual partners did you have in the past month who, although *not anonymous,* were men you *did not know well* (that is, considered casual acquaintances or had just met for the first time)?
      Number of partners you did not know well in the past month: _____
   d. How many sexual partners did you have in the past month whom you *did not know at all* (that is, considered anonymous)?
      Number of anonymous partners in the past month: _____
   e. How many, if any, of your sexual partners in the past month *paid you* for having sex with them?
      Number who paid you: _____
   f. How many, if any, of your sexual partners in the past month *did you pay* to have sex?
      Number who you paid: _____
6. Now we would like you to tell us *new* sexual partners you had in the past month. Count new partners who you had sex with even once.
   Number of new partners in the past month: _____
7. We are interested in learning more about your use of drugs or alcohol during sex *in the past month*. For each of the different types of partners, please indicate how frequently you drank the equivalent of 3 or more drinks or used a drug (marijuana, cocaine, MDA, LSD or other hallucinogens, "uppers," "downers") or "poppers" prior to or during sex.

Partner type	Number of times you were together for sex in the past month	Number of times you were together for sex *and*		
		Drank 3 or more drinks	Used a drug	Used poppers
Primary or steady	_____	_____	_____	_____
Regular partners	_____	_____	_____	_____
Casual partners	_____	_____	_____	_____
Anonymous partners	_____	_____	_____	_____

8. Now we would like to ask you several specific questions, all of which concern your sexual activity with other men. First, we would like to know about rimming. During the past month, have you rimmed a male sexual partner (engaged in active oral-anal sex)?
   (Circle one)
   No   5 (If no, go to Question 10)
   Yes   1
   If yes:
9. How many times last month did you rim each of these different types of sexual partners? (If you did not have any partners of a particular type, please indicate No such partners.)
   a. Primary or steady partners:
      _____ No such partners *or* _____ Number of times
   b. Partners I know well but who aren't steady or primary:
      _____ No such partners *or* _____ Number of times
   c. Casual acquaintances who are not anonymous:
      _____ No such partners *or* _____ Number of times
   d. Anonymous partners:
      _____ No such partners *or* _____ Number of times
10. Now we would like to know about *receptive* anal sex (having someone fuck you). During the past month, have you engaged in receptive anal sex?
    (Circle one)
    No   5 (If no, go to Question 12)
    Yes   1
    If yes:
11. How many times last month did you engage in receptive anal sex with each of these different types of sexual partners? (If you did not have any partners of a particular type, please indicate No such partners.)
    a. Primary or steady partners:
       _____ No such partners *or* _____ Number of times had receptive anal sex, and

b. condoms were used
_____ every time
_____ sometimes
_____ never

c. Partners I know well but who aren't steady or primary:
_____ No such partners *or* _____ Number of times had receptive anal sex, and

d. condoms were used
_____ every time
_____ sometimes
_____ never

e. Casual acquaintances who are not anonymous:
_____ No such partners *or* _____ Number of times had receptive anal sex, and

f. condoms were used
_____ every time
_____ sometimes
_____ never

g. Anonymous partners:
_____ No such partners *or* _____ Number of times had receptive anal sex, and

h. condoms were used
_____ every time
_____ sometimes
_____ never

12. Next, we would like to know about *insertive* anal sex (fucking someone). During the past month, have you engaged in insertive anal sex with any male partners?

(Circle one)

No   5 *(If no, go to Question 14)*
Yes   1

If yes:

13. How many times last month did you engage in insertive anal sex with each of these different types of sexual partners? (If you did not have any partners of a particular type, please indicate No such partners.)

a. Primary or steady partners:
_____ No such partners *or* _____ Number of times had insertive anal sex, and

b. condoms were used
_____ every time
_____ sometimes
_____ never

c. Partners I know well but who aren't steady or primary:
_____ No such partners *or* _____ Number of times had insertive anal sex, and

d. condoms were used
_____ every time
_____ sometimes
_____ never

e. Casual acquaintances who are not anonymous:
_____ No such partners *or* _____ Number of times had insertive anal sex, and

f. condoms were used
_____ every time
_____ sometimes
_____ never

g. Anonymous partners:
_____ No such partners *or* _____ Number of times had insertive anal sex, and

h. condoms were used
_____ every time
_____ sometimes
_____ never

14. Next we would like to know about *receptive* fellatio (sucking your partner's penis). During the past month, have you sucked a male sexual partner?

(Circle one)

No   5 *(If no, go to Question 16)*
Yes   1

If yes:

15. How many times last month did you perform fellatio (sucking) for each of these different types of sexual partners? (If you did not have any partners of a particular type, check the box.)
    a. Primary or steady partners:
       _____ No such partners *or* _____ Number of times performed fellatio, and
    b. condoms were used
       _____ every time
       _____ sometimes
       _____ never
    c. Partners I know well but who aren't steady or primary:
       _____ No such partners *or* _____ Number of times performed fellatio, and
    d. condoms were used
       _____ every time
       _____ sometimes
       _____ never
    e. Casual acquaintances who are not anonymous:
       _____ No such partners *or* _____ Number of times performed fellatio, and
    f. condoms were used
       _____ every time
       _____ sometimes
       _____ never
    g. Anonymous partners:
       _____ No such partners *or* _____ Number of times performed fellatio, and
    h. condoms were used
       _____ every time
       _____ sometimes
       _____ never

16. Next we would like to know about *insertive* fellatio (your partner sucking your penis). During the past month, have you been sucked by a male sexual partner?
           (Circle one)
    No   5 *(If no, go to Question 18)*
    Yes   1
    If yes:

17. How many times last month did you perform fellatio (sucking) for each of these different types of sexual partners? (If you did not have any partners of a particular type, please indicate No such partners.)
    a. Primary or steady partners:
       _____ No such partners *or* _____ Number of times received fellatio, and
    b. condoms were used
       _____ every time
       _____ sometimes
       _____ never
    c. Partners I know well but who aren't steady or primary:
       _____ No such partners *or* _____ Number of times received fellatio, and
    d. condoms were used
       _____ every time
       _____ sometimes
       _____ never
    e. Casual acquaintances who are not anonymous:
       _____ No such partners *or* _____ Number of times received fellatio, and
    f. condoms were used
       _____ every time
       _____ sometimes
       _____ never
    g. Anonymous partners:
       _____ No such partners *or* _____ Number of times received fellatio, and
    h. condoms were used
       _____ every time
       _____ sometimes
       _____ never

There are many reasons for having sex and many ways to enjoy sexual activity. In this part of the questionnaire we are trying to find out how you and your partner(s) have sex, especially focusing on your use of safe sex practices designed to reduce the chances of getting AIDS. Please notice that these questions are concerned with your sex life in the past month.

18. During the past month, for each type of partner, about how many of your sexual encounters were limited to mutual masturbation ("jacking off")?

	All	Some	None	No such partner
a. Primary or steady	____	____	____	____
b. Partners you know well but who are not steady or primary	____	____	____	____
c. Casual partners who are not anonymous	____	____	____	____
d. Anonymous partners	____	____	____	____

Attitudes Toward Erotica Questionnaire

Ilsa L. Lottes,[1] *University of Maryland, Baltimore County*
Martin S. Weinberg, *Indiana University*

The Attitudes Toward Erotica Questionnaire (ATEQ) was developed by a task force on pornography. At a midwestern university, a student was arrested for showing a sexually explicit film to raise funds for his dormitory. The arrest sparked controversy and brought the issue of pornography into sharp focus among students, faculty, and administrators. Subsequently, the University Task Force on Pornography was appointed to investigate attitudes toward sexually explicit materials by the student body.

The ATEQ includes scales measuring attitudes about harmful and positive effects of erotica, as well as attitudes toward its restriction and regulation. Because of the wide variety of sexually explicit material, the questionnaire is not designed to investigate attitudes toward erotica in general. A social scientist can adapt the questionnaire to examine attitudes about the type of erotic material most appropriate for her or his research—either a specific medium (e.g., *Playboy*) or a general form (e.g., X-rated movie).

Description

For each type of erotica, nine items (numbered 1, 4, 6, 7, 9, 10, 12, 20, and 21) assess its harmful effects and form a Harmful scale; seven items (numbered 5, 11, 13, 15, 17, 18, and 19) assess its positive effects and form a Positive scale; and five items (numbered 2, 3, 8, 14, and 16) assess

its restriction and form a Restrict scale. In the study at the university in the Midwest, 663 students (52% female) responded to items about four types of sexually explicit materials: "magazines like *Playboy*," "magazines like *Hustler*," "adult bookstore magazines," and "X-rated movies and videos like 'Deep Throat' " (Lottes, Weinberg, & Weller, 1993). From a varimax factor analysis with an orthogonal rotation of the 84 responses (21 per erotic type) of these students, one major factor emerged. This factor accounted for 63% of the variance with all factor loadings having an absolute value greater than .71. Thus, although properties of the individual Harmful, Positive, and Restrict scales are presented here, analysis based on one large random student sample (70% response rate) suggests that attitudes toward erotica are organized along a simple binary good-bad dimension.

The response options to each item are one of the 5-point Likert-type choices: *strongly disagree* (1), *disagree* (2), *no opinion* (3), *agree* (4), and *strongly agree* (5). This questionnaire is designed for a college student or general adult population. Obscenity law is strongly linked to "community standards," and the ATEQ is a tool to assess such standards.

Response Mode and Timing

Respondents write the number from 1 to 5 corresponding to their degree of agreement or disagreement with each item, or if computer scoring is available, machine-scorable answer sheets can be provided for responses. Each set of 21 items for a particular type of erotica takes 8 minutes for completion.

[1]Address correspondence to Ilsa L. Lottes, Department of Sociology and Anthropology, University of Maryland, Baltimore County, 5401 Wilkens Avenue, Baltimore, MD 21228; email: lottes@umbc2.umbc.edu.

Scoring

For 11 of the items, an agree response indicates a pro-erotica attitude and for 10 items an agree response indicates an anti-erotica attitude. To decrease the probability of a response set, the 21 items of the Harmful, Positive, and Restrict scales are not grouped together but placed randomly in the questionnaire. To obtain the scale scores for the Harmful and Positive scales, the responses to the items of each respective scale are summed. For the Harmful scale, scores can range from 9 to 45, and the higher the score, the more harm has been attributed to the erotica. For the Positive scale, scores can range from 7 to 35, and the higher the score, the more positive the effect attributed to the erotica. For the Restrict scale, four of the five items (items numbered 2, 3, 8, and 16) are scored in the reverse direction. For these reverse-direction items, recoding needs to transform all 5s to 1s and 4s to 2s and vice versa before responses to the five items are summed to give the Restrict scale score. For this scale, scores can range from 5 to 25, and the higher the score, the more restrictions on erotica are supported.

Reliability

In a sample of 663 college students, Cronbach alphas for the Harmful scale associated with *Playboy, Hustler,* adult bookstore magazines, and X-rated movies or videos were .90, .85, .84, and .85, respectively. Cronbach alphas for these same materials for the Positive scale were .73, .76, .78, and .78, respectively, and Cronbach alphas for the Restrict scale were .85, .85, .84, and .85, respectively (Lottes et al., 1993).

Validity

The construct validity of the Harmful, Positive, and Restrict scales was supported by statistically significant results for predicted correlations and group differences. As expected, Lottes et al. (1993) found that respondents who were more religious, less sexually active, and viewed erotica less often evaluated all four types of sexually explicit material as being more harmful and having fewer positive effects and supported more restrictions on their availability than did respondents who were less religious, more sexually active, and viewed erotica more often. Also as expected, males and those who had seen a specific type of sexually explicit material reported higher scores on the Positive scale and lower scores on the Harmful and Restrict scales than did females and those who had not seen the erotic material.

Reference

Lottes, I. L., Weinberg, M. S., & Weller, I. (1993). Reactions to pornography on a college campus: For or against? *Sex Roles, 29,* 69-89.

Exhibit

Attitudes Toward Erotica Questionnaire

Directions: Indicate how strongly you agree or disagree with each of the following statements by writing the number corresponding to one of the five response options below in the space provided.

Strongly disagree	Disagree	No opinion	Agree	Strongly agree
1	2	3	4	5

1. The material exploits women. _____
2. The material should be publicly sold (magazines) and publicly shown (movies). _____
3. The material should be available to adults. _____
4. The availability of the material leads to a breakdown in community morals. _____
5. The material can improve sex relations among adults. _____
6. I feel the material is offensive. _____
7. The material exploits men. _____
8. The material should be available to minors (under 18). _____
9. The material increases the probability of sexual violence. _____
10. In this material, the positioning and treatment of men is degrading to men. _____
11. The material may provide an outlet for bottled-up sexual pressures. _____
12. In this material, sex and violence are often shown together. _____
13. This material can enhance the pleasure of masturbation for women. _____
14. This material should be made illegal. _____
15. The material may teach people sexual techniques. _____
16. This material should be protected by the 1st Amendment (freedom of speech and the press). _____
17. People should be made aware of the positive effects of this material. _____
18. This material serves a more positive than negative function in society. _____
19. This material can enhance the pleasure of masturbation for men. _____
20. People should be made aware of the negative effects of this material. _____
21. In this material, the positioning and treatment of women is degrading to women. _____

The Multidimensional Sexual Perfectionism Questionnaire

William E. Snell, Jr.,[1] *Southeast Missouri State University*

Previous researchers have indicated that people sometimes apply highly rigid and perfectionistic standards of personal conduct to themselves. Snell and Rigdon (1995) developed a new multidimensional self-report instrument, the Multidimensional Sexual Perfectionism Questionnaire (MSPQ), to measure five distinct psychological tendencies associated with people's standards of sexual conduct: (a) self-oriented sexual perfectionism, (b) perceived socially prescribed sexual perfectionism, (c) partner-directed sexual perfectionism, (d) partner's self-oriented sexual perfectionism, and (e) perceived self-directed sexual perfectionism from one's partner. The MSPQ can be used in a variety of ways: as a research instrument in correlational or experimental research designs; as a pretest and posttest instrument for therapy effectiveness and recovery studies; and as a predictive correlate of sexual affect, attitudes, and behaviors.

Description

The MSPQ contains five subscales: (a) self-oriented sexual perfectionism, designed to measure excessively high, rigid, and perfectionistic sexual standards that are applied to oneself; (b) socially prescribed sexual perfection, which involves the belief that society and "generalized" others are imposing perfectionistic sexual standards and expectations for oneself; (c) partner-directed sexual perfectionism, which involves the application of perfectionistic sexual standards to one's partner; (d) partner's self-oriented sexual perfectionism, designed to measure people's perception that their partners impose rigid and perfectionistic sexual standards to themselves (i.e., to the partners themselves); and (e) self-directed sexual perfectionism from one's partner, which involves people's belief that their partners are applying excessively rigid and perfectionistic sexual standards to themselves (i.e., to the respondents themselves).

Response Mode and Timing

In responding to the MSPQ, individuals are asked to indicate how characteristic each statement is of them. A 5-point Likert-type scale is used for their responses, with each item being scored from 0 to 4: *not at all characteristic of me* (0), *slightly characteristic of me* (1), *somewhat characteristic of me* (2), *moderately characteristic of me* (3), and *very characteristic of me* (4). Although the MSPQ can be

formatted so that respondents can circle a response between A and E (or 0 to 4), corresponding to how characteristic the statement is of them, the more common scoring technique is to mark the answers on a machine-scorable answer sheet. The MSPQ requires approximately 15 minutes to complete.

Scoring

The MSPQ consists of 31 statements that are assigned to five subscales. To create subscale scores for the five subscales, several statements (16 through 30) are first recoded so that A = E, B = D, C = C, D = B, and E = A. Then the items are scored so that A = 0, B = 1, C = 2, D = 3, and E = 4. Next, they are averaged for each subscale so that higher scores correspond to greater amounts of the relevant tendency: (a) self-oriented sexual perfectionism (2, 7, 12, 17R, 22R, 27R); (b) socially prescribed sexual perfectionism (3, 8, 13, 18R, 23R, 28R); (c) partner-directed sexual perfectionism (4, 9, 14, 19R, 23R, 29R); (d) partner's self-oriented sexual perfectionism (5, 10, 15, 20R, 25R, 30R); and (e) self-directed sexual perfectionism from one's partner (6, 11, 16, 21R). Statement 1 on the MSPQ is used for informational purposes only; it is not assigned to any MSPQ subscale. Statements 30 and 31 are response-consistency filler items; they too are not assigned to any MSPQ subscale.

Reliability

To provide preliminary evidence for the reliability (i.e., internal consistency) of the MSPQ, Cronbach alphas were computed for each of the MSPQ subscales (Snell & Rigdon, 1995). These results revealed the following alphas for each MSPQ subscale: (a) self-oriented sexual perfectionism, alpha = .71; (b) socially prescribed sexual perfectionism, alpha = .37; (c) partner-directed sexual perfectionism, alpha = .67; (d) partner's self-oriented sexual perfectionism, alpha = .67; and (e) self-directed sexual perfectionism from one's partner, alpha = .75. Except for MSPQ subscale 2 (socially prescribed sexual perfectionism; alpha of .51 for the three non-reversed-worded items and .40 for the reverse-coded items), these reliability indexes were sufficiently high to justify their use in research analyses.

Validity

Preliminary evidence (Snell & Rigdon, 1995) revealed that males reported greater self-oriented sexual perfectionism than did females and that males, relative to their female counterparts, also expected greater self-directed sexual perfectionism from their sexual partners and applied similar

[1]Address correspondence to William E. Snell, Jr., Department of Psychology, Southeast Missouri State University, One University Plaza, Cape Girardeau, MO 63701; email: wesnell@semovm.semo.edu.

perfectionistic standards of sexual conduct to their partners. Other findings reported by Snell and Rigdon showed a strong pattern of similarity between people's sexual perfectionism and their tendency to be aware of the public image of their sexuality. More specifically, it was found that both males and females who were characterized by higher levels of each of the components of sexual perfectionism—especially self-oriented sexual perfectionism—reported greater sexual monitoring. That is, those with greater sexual perfectionism were more likely to be highly concerned with others' scrutiny of their sexuality. A final set of results revealed that the various types of sexual perfectionism measured by the MSPQ were related in predictable ways to the four attachment styles measured by the Relationship Scales Questionnaire (Scharfe & Bartholomew, 1994). More specifically, it was found that those males and females who possessed a secure attachment style (i.e., those with a positive relational view of themselves and others) were less likely to apply perfectionistic sexual standards either to themselves or to their sexual partners, and in addition, they were less likely to expect that their partners would apply such perfectionistic sexual standards to either partner. By contrast, an almost identical *inverse* pattern of findings was discovered for the measure of fearful attachment. In particular, it was found that a fearful attachment style was characteristic of both males and females who applied an excessively rigid and perfectionistic set of sexual standards of conduct to themselves as well as expected them from their partners.

References

Scharfe, E., & Bartholomew, K. (1994). Reliability and stability of adult attachment patterns. *Personal Relationships, 1,* 23-43.

Snell, W. E., Jr., & Rigdon, K. (1995, April). *The Sexual Perfectionism Questionnaire: Preliminary evidence for reliability and validity.* Paper presented at the annual meeting of the Southwestern Psychological Association, San Antonio, TX.

Exhibit

The Multidimensional Sexual Perfectionism Questionnaire

Instructions: Listed below are several statements that concern the topic of sexual relationships. Please read each item carefully and decide to what extent it is characteristic of you. Some of the items refer to a specific sexual relationship. Whenever possible, answer the questions with your current partner in mind. If you are not currently dating anyone, answer the questions with your most recent partner in mind. If you have never had a sexual relationship, answer in terms of what you think your responses would most likely be. Then, for each statement fill in the response on the answer sheet that indicates how much it applies to you by using the following scale:

> A = *Not at all* characteristic of me.
> B = *Slightly* characteristic of me.
> C = *Somewhat* characteristic of me.
> D = *Moderately* characteristic of me.
> E = *Very* characteristic of me.

1. I will respond to the following items based on:
   (A) A current sexual relationship.
   (B) A past sexual relationship.
   (C) An imagined sexual relationship.
2. I set very high standards for myself as a sexual partner.
3. Others would consider me a good sexual partner even if I'm not responsive every time.
4. My partner sets very high standards of excellence for her/himself as a sexual partner.
5. My partner expects me to be a perfect sexual partner.
6. I expect my partner to be a top-notch and competent sexual partner.
7. I must always be successful as a sexual partner.
8. People often expect more of me as a sexual partner than I am capable of giving.
9. My partner is perfectionistic in that this person expects to sexually satisfy me each and every time.
10. My partner demands nothing less than perfection of me as a sexual partner.
11. My partner should never let me down when it comes to my sexual needs.
12. One of my goals is to be a "perfect" sexual partner.
13. Most people expect me to always be an excellent sexual partner.
14. It makes my partner uneasy for him/her to be less than a perfect sexual partner.
15. My partner always wants me to try hard to sexually please him/her.
16. I cannot stand for my partner to be less than a satisfying sexual partner.
17. I seldom feel the need to be a "perfect" sexual partner.
18. Most people would regard me as okay, even if I did not perform well sexually.
19. My partner does not set very high goals for herself (himself) as a sexual partner.

20. My partner seldom pressures me to be a perfect sexual partner.
21. I do not expect perfectionism from my sexual partner.
22. I do not have to be the best sexual partner in the world.
23. In general, people would readily accept me even if I were not the greatest sex partner in the world.
24. My partner never aims at being perfect as a sexual partner.
25. My sexual partner does not have very high goals for me as a sexual partner.
26. In general, people would readily accept me even if I were not a great sex partner.
27. I do not have very high goals for myself as a sexual partner.
28. Most people don't expect me to be perfectionistic when it comes to sex.
29. My partner does not feel that she/he has to be the best sexual partner.
30. My partner appreciates me even if I am not a perfect sexual lover. (*response consistency filler item*)
31. Most people don't expect me to be perfectionistic when it comes to sex. (*response consistency filler item*)

Venereal Disease (Gonorrhea and Syphilis) Knowledge and Attitudes

Ibtihaj Arafat,[1] *City College of the City University of New York*
Donald E. Allen, *Oklahoma State University*

The questionnaire addresses the following: (a) How knowledgeable are college students about venereal disease (VD)? (b) How does knowledge of VD relate to the student attitudes? (c) Will the student seek treatment if infected? (d) How will the infected student seek treatment for VD? and (e) Will the student take steps to prevent infection? The instrument is oriented to practical questions directly relevant to the level of understanding of the facts and realities of the potential problem of venereal disease (Arafat & Allen, 1977).

Description, Response Mode, and Timing

The questionnaire includes six background items treated as independent variables, to classify the respondent by age, ethnic category, marital status, school, and personal experience with VD. There are 25 items included in the VD knowledge test, with a maximum score of 37 points. Of these, 10 items call for multiple-choice responses detailing facts and illusions about specific categories of venereal infection and the associated symptoms carrying two or more correct responses. Ten items are factual questions about VD calling for *yes/no/don't know* responses. Items 21 through

25 are factual questions about VD requiring short fill-in answers of one to four words.

A group of six items (26-31) relates to perceived knowledge and behavioral posture toward VD. The attitude scale is a group of eight *yes/no* items, with points assigned for the more positive and more responsible responses.

Seven hundred self-administered questionnaires were distributed to random samples in four different colleges and universities in New York in 1975. There was a return of 547 complete and usable questionnaires, for a return rate of 78%. The time needed to complete the instrument was up to 15 minutes, depending on the respondent's level of information.

Scoring

In the VD knowledge portion of 25 items, 1 point is scored for each correct response, for a maximum of 46 points. Perceived knowledge is scored from Items 26 and 31. Item 31 is the only scaled item in the instrument, reverse scored from *very good* to *poor* according to the respondent's assumption about the level of his or her knowledge of VD. Elsewhere, scoring is based on 1 point for each correct or positive answer.

Reliability

Reliability estimates for the measurement of the dependent variables of demonstrated knowledge of VD, per-

[1]Address correspondence to Ibtihaj Arafat, Department of Sociology, City College of the City University of New York, New York, NY 10010.

ceived knowledge of VD, and attitudes toward VD have not been established independently for the intended population of college students. Variation in item format did not permit calculation of an internal consistency estimate. Indirect evidence of reliability of the instrument consists of the following: (a) a very large proportion of the questionnaires was fully and unambiguously answered by the several strata of college students, and (b) the results were highly consistent among the four colleges and universities in which the random samples were taken.

Validity

There have been no independent applications of this instrument reported in the *Citation Index* for the period 1978-1983. Thus, there is no basis for judging its validity. Face validity may be inferred from the definitive results of the analysis, in that 21 of 36 correlations of measures of demonstrated knowledge, perceived knowledge, and atti-

tude level were statistically significant, and 8 of 12 *t* tests for difference by age, source of knowledge of VD, effect of fear of VD on behavior, and action in response to the VD threat were statistically significant. Such results suggest that the instrument is measuring what it is intended to measure. There is some evidence of external validity in the item relating to whether the respondent has had VD. In the sample of 547 college students, 3% answered positively. This accords reasonably well with the New York City Board of Health estimates that about 4% of the general population has venereal infection, recognizing that the exposure time for the college population is considerably less than that for the general population.

Reference

Arafat, I., & Allen, D. (1977). Venereal disease: College students' knowledge and attitudes. *The Journal of Sex Research, 13,* 223-230.

Exhibit

Venereal Disease Knowledge Questionnaire

This is a questionnaire on venereal disease in which we hope to find out about the attitudes and knowledgeability of venereal disease of students on campus. If you really have no idea of an answer, please check the box that says "I don't know." Your responses will help in this study.

Background Information

Age _____ Sex _____ Have you had VD? _____

School _____

Ethnic background: Italian _____ Jewish _____ Black _____ Puerto Rican _____ Chinese _____ Other _____

Marital status: Single _____ Married _____ Divorced _____ Other _____

Check all correct answers: (Correct answers shown by x.)

Example: The Bronx is in:

                1. U.S.A.__x__   2. New York State__x__   3. New York City__x__   4. I don't know_____

1. What are the effects of untreated syphilis:
   1. __x__ Insanity   2.__x__ Loss of eyesight   3. __x__ Heart disorders
   4. __x__ Crippled   5._____ I don't know.
2. What are the effects of untreated gonorrhea?
   1. __x__ Arthritis   2.__x__ Salpingitis, peritonitis   3.__x__ Sterility
   4. _____ Chronic pelvic disability   5. _____ I don't know.
3. How does one get syphilis?
   1. _____ Kissing   2.__x__ Sexual intercourse only   3. _____ Toilet seats
   4. _____ From eating and drinking utensils   5. _____ I don't know.
4. Where does the chancre (sore) occur?
   1. __x__ Mouth   2.__x__ Penis   3. __x__ Rectum
   4. __x__ Vagina   5._____ I don't know.
5. What are the other names for syphilis?
   1. _____ Pox   2._____ Bad blood   3. __x__ Siff
   4. _____ Old Joe   5._____ I don't know.

6. What are the other names for gonorrhea?
   1. __x__ Clap 2.____ Strain 3.__x__ Morning drop
   4. ____ The whites 5.____ I don't know.
7. What are the early signs of syphilis?
   1. ____ A rash over the whole body 2.____ Itching 3.____ Lesions in the mouth
   4. __x__ Chancre or sore 5.____ I don't know.
8. What are the early symptoms or signs of gonorrhea in males?
   1. __x__ A discharge of pus from the penis 2.__x__ Painful inflammation of the urinary canal
   3. ____ Chancre or rash appears 4.____ Swelling of the thyroid gland
   5. ____ I don't know.
9. What are the early symptoms or signs of gonorrhea in females?
   1. ____ A vaginal discharge always appears 2.__x__ She may or may not notice a vaginal discharge
   3. ____ No outward signs 4.____ Swelling of thyroid 5.____ I don't know.
10. Which of the following are the less known venereal diseases?
    1. __x__ Chancroid 2.__x__ Granuloma inguinale
    3. __x__ Lymphogranuloma venereum 4.____ Nonspecific urethritis (NSU) 5.____ I don't know.

Underline the answer: either Yes, No, or Don't know: (Correct answer in italics.)

11. Can a person have an immunity to venereal disease? Yes *No* Don't know
12. Can somebody be infected with both syphilis and gonorrhea at the same time? *Yes* No Don't know
13. Can a person die from syphilis? *Yes* No Don't know
14. Is it possible to get syphilis with someone your own sex? *Yes* No Don't know
15. Can venereal disease be transmitted in pregnancy to the unborn child? *Yes* No Don't know
16. Will using a condom lower the chance of getting venereal disease? *Yes* No Don't know
17. Does a discharge from the penis or the vagina always mean gonorrhea? Yes *No* Don't know
18. Can gonorrhea be detected from a blood test? Yes *No* Don't know
19. Can you have syphilis and not know it? *Yes* No Don't know
20. Can venereal disease produce sterility? *Yes* No Don't know

Fill in the correct answer. If you don't know, please leave empty. (Correct answer in italics.)

21. What precaution is given to newborn babies against venereal disease?
    (*Silver nitrate solution in the eyes*)
22. What is the cure for venereal disease in its early stages?
    (*Antibiotics, such as penicillin*)
23. Which venereal disease kills more of its victims?
    (*Syphilis*)
24. What is the test for gonorrhea?
    (*Microscopic search for gonococci in smear of genital mucous*)
25. How serious a problem is venereal disease today?
    (*Very serious*)

Multiple choice: Circle the number of the answer that is best for you.

26. Has your education of venereal disease come from
    1. Parents 2. Personal experience 3. Friends
    4. Books 5. No education at all
27. Does the fear of venereal disease:
    1. Prevent you from having sex 2. Limit sex to a steady boy or girl
    3. Have no effect on sexual activities
28. If you have symptoms of venereal disease whom would you tell first?
    1. Close friend 2. Your sex partner 3. Doctor
    4. Parents 5. No one
29. If you had symptoms of venereal disease, would you go to:
    1. Family doctor 2. A strange doctor 3. A clinic
    4. Probably ignore the symptoms at first
30. When you engage in sex do you:
    1. Worry about the possibility of getting VD 2. Take preventive measures against VD
    3. Pass it off as "It couldn't happen to me." 4. Never think about it.
    5. Does not apply to me.

31. My knowledge of VD is:
1. Very good   2. Good
3. Fair   4. Poor

Answer Yes or No.

32. Do you feel that you know more about VD now than when you were in high school?   Yes   No
33. Would you discuss VD with your parents?   Yes   No
34. Do you know many people who have had VD?   Yes   No
35. If you had VD, has it made you less likely to engage in sex?   Yes   No
36. If a course was given at your college on VD, would you take it?   Yes   No
37. Do you think that a check for VD should be a part of a routine physical examination?   Yes   No
38. If you were a parent, would you feel it your duty to tell your child about VD?   Yes   No
39. Have you discussed VD with your friends?   Yes   No

Thank you.

STD Attitude Scale

William L. Yarber[1] and Mohammad R. Torabi, *Indiana University*
C. Harold Veenker, *Purdue University*

Recent attitude research indicates that attitudes are best described as multidimensional, having the three components of cognitive (belief), affective (feeling), and conative (intention to act). Beliefs express one's perceptions or concepts toward an attitudinal object; feelings are described as an expression of liking or disliking relative to an attitudinal object; and intention to act is an expression of what the individual says he or she would do in a given situation (Bagozzi, 1978; Kothandapani, 1971; Ostrom, 1969; Torabi & Veenker, 1986). Attitudes are one important component determining individual health risk behavior. More attention is now given by health educators to improving or maintaining health-conducive attitudes. A scale designed specifically to measure the components of attitudes toward sexually transmitted diseases (STDs) can be valuable to educators and researchers in planning STD education and determining risk correlates of individuals.

Description

The STD Attitude Scale was developed to measure young adults' beliefs, feelings, and intentions to act toward STDs.

The scale discriminates between individuals with high-risk attitudes toward STD contraction and those with low-risk attitudes. A summated rating scale using a 5-point Likert-type format and having three subscales reflecting the attitude components was constructed. Items were developed according to a table of specifications containing three conceptual areas: nature of STD, STD prevention, and STD treatment. Each subscale contained items from the three conceptual areas.

An extensive pool of items was generated from the literature, expert contribution, and via item solicitation from students. To avoid the possibility of a response set, both positive and negative items were developed. Attention was given to the readability of each item. From the item pool, three preliminary forms with 45 items each (15 items per subscale) were administered to 457 college students. Following statistical analysis, one scale containing the 45 items (15 per subscale) that best met item selection criteria of internal consistency and discrimination power was given to 100 high school students.

A further refined scale of 33 items (11 items per subscale), subjected to jury review, was given to 2,980 secondary school students. Analysis of these data produced the final scale of 27 items, 9 items for each subscale. The final scale has items with highly significant levels of internal consistency (item score vs. subscales and total scale score)

[1]Address correspondence to William L. Yarber, Department of Applied Health Science, Indiana University, HPER Building, Bloomington, IN 47405; email: yarber@ucs.indiana.edu.

and discriminating power (upper group vs. lower group for each item).

Response Mode and Timing

Respondents indicate whether they *strongly agree, agree,* are *undecided, disagree,* or *strongly disagree* with each statement. The scale takes an average of 15 minutes to complete.

Scoring

Scoring is as follows (total scale, Items 1-27; Belief subscale, Items 1-9; Feeling subscale, Items 10-18; and Intention to Act subscale, Items 19-27): Calculate total points for each subscale and total scale, using the following point values. For Items 1, 10-14, 16, and 25: *strongly agree* = 5, *agree* = 4, *undecided* = 3, *disagree* = 2, and *strongly disagree* = 1. For Items 2-9, 15, 17-24, 26, and 27: *strongly agree* = 1, *agree* = 2, *undecided* = 3, *disagree* = 4, and *strongly disagree* = 5.

Higher subscale or total scale scores are interpreted as reflecting an attitude that predisposes one toward high-risk STD behavior, and lower scores predispose the person toward low-risk STD behavior.

Reliability

Yarber, Torabi, and Veenker (1988) reported a test-retest reliability during a 5- to 7-day period to be as follows: total scale = .71, Belief subscale = .50, Feeling subscale = .57, and Intention to Act subscale = .63. Cronbach's alpha was total scale = .73, Belief subscale = .53, Feeling subscale = .48, and Intention to Act subscale = .71.

Validity

Scale items have evidence of content and face validity because they were developed according to a table of specifications reflecting the behavioral aspects of STD and the content emphasis—preventive health behavior—of an STD education school curriculum (Yarber, 1985). Furthermore, a panel of experts judged each item's merit. The scale was developed, in part, as one component of a project for assessing the efficacy of a Centers for Disease Control education program (Yarber, 1985). Evidence of construct validity is provided by the fact that secondary school students exposed to the STD curriculum, in contrast to students receiving no STD instruction, showed improvement in scores from pretest to posttest when assessed by the scale (Yarber, 1988).

Other Information

The scale development was supported in part by U.S. Public Health Service Grant Award R30/CCR500638-01.

References

Bagozzi, R. P. (1978). The construct validity of the affective, behavioral and cognitive components of attitude by using analysis of covariance of structure. *Multivariate Behavior Research, 13,* 9-31.

Kothandapani, V. (1971). *A psychological approach to the prediction of contraceptive behavior.* Chapel Hill: Carolina Population Center, University of North Carolina.

Ostrom, T. M. (1969). The relationship between the affective, behavioral and cognitive components of attitude. *Journal of Experimental Psychology, 5,* 12-30.

Torabi, M. R., & Veenker, C. H. (1986). An alcohol attitude scale for teenagers. *Journal of School Health, 56,* 96-100.

Yarber, W. L. (1985). *STD: A guide for today's young adults.* [Student and instructor's manual] Waldorf, MD: American Alliance.

Yarber, W. L. (1988). Evaluation of the health behavior approach to school STD education. *Journal of Sex Education and Therapy, 14,* 33-38.

Yarber, W. L., Torabi, M. R., & Veenker, C. H. (1988). Development of a three-component sexually transmitted diseases attitude scale. *Journal of Sex Education and Therapy, 15,* 36-49.

Exhibit

STD Attitude Scale

Directions: Please read each statement carefully. STD means sexually transmitted diseases, once called venereal diseases. Record your reaction by marking an "X" through the letter which best describes how much you agree or disagree with the idea.

Use this key: SA = Strongly agree
A = Agree
U = Undecided
D = Disagree
SD = Strongly disagree

Example: Doing things to prevent getting an STD is the job of each person.   SA X U D SD

1. How one uses his/her sexuality has nothing to do with STD.
2. It is easy to use the prevention methods that reduce one's chances of getting an STD.
3. Responsible sex is one of the best ways of reducing the risk of STD.
4. Getting early medical care is the main key to preventing harmful effects of STD.
5. Choosing the right sex partner is important in reducing the risk of getting an STD.

6. A high rate of STD should be a concern for all people.
7. People with an STD have a duty to get their sex partners to medical care.
8. The best way to get a sex partner to STD treatment is to take him/her to the doctor with you.
9. Changing one's sex habits is necessary once the presence of an STD is known.
10. I would dislike having to follow the medical steps for treating an STD.
11. If I were sexually active, I would feel uneasy doing things before and after sex to prevent getting an STD.
12. If I were sexually active, it would be insulting if a sex partner suggested we use a condom to avoid STD.
13. I dislike talking about STD with my peers.
14. I would be uncertain about going to the doctor unless I was sure I really had an STD.
15. I would feel that I should take my sex partner with me to a clinic if I thought I had an STD.
16. It would be embarrassing to discuss STD with one's partner if one were sexually active.
17. If I were to have sex, the chance of getting an STD makes me uneasy about having sex with more than one person.
18. I like the idea of sexual abstinence (not having sex) as the best way of avoiding STD.
19. If I had an STD, I would cooperate with public health persons to find the sources of STD.
20. If I had an STD, I would avoid exposing others while I was being treated.
21. I would have regular STD checkups if I were having sex with more than one person.
22. I intend to look for STD signs before deciding to have sex with anyone.
23. I will limit my sex activity to just one partner because of the chances I might get an STD.
24. I will avoid sex contact anytime I think there is even a slight chance of getting an STD.
25. The chance of getting an STD would not stop me from having sex.
26. If I had a chance, I would support community efforts toward controlling STD.
27. I would be willing to work with others to make people aware of STD problems in my town.

Source. This scale was originally published in "Evaluation of the Health Behavior Approach to School STD Education," by W. L. Yarber, 1988, *Journal of Sex Education and Therapy, 14,* 33-38. Reprinted with permission.

STD Health Behavior Knowledge Test

William L. Yarber,[1] *Indiana University*

Assessing the "minimum base of knowledge" using multiple levels of the cognitive domain of the taxonomy of educational objectives has been suggested as one approach to determining student sexually transmitted disease (STD) knowledge (Automated Services, 1976; Bloom, 1956). The minimum knowledge base is considered to be the least amount of information needed for one to understand the fundamental STD concepts. Because it is often difficult to measure actual STD behaviors, particularly in educational settings, determining the application of behaviors in STD-related situations would increase the strength of a test that measures knowledge only (Green, 1979). The STD Health Behavior Knowledge Test was developed to measure young

adults' knowledge of individual, STD preventive health behaviors.

Description

Multiple-choice items were developed according to a table of specifications containing three conceptual areas: (a) nature of STD: medical/health problem, importance as a social problem; (b) prevention of STD: risk factors, risk reduction; and (c) treatment of STD: recognition/procedure, compliance. Most items emphasize individual STD preventive health behaviors and were derived from expert contribution and the test-item pool included in a U.S. Public Health Service, Centers for Disease Control-sponsored school STD curriculum (Yarber, 1985). During the writing of the items, attention was given to the item's reading level. A preliminary form of 21 items (18 knowledge domain, 3 application domain) was administered to 100 high school

[1]Address correspondence to William L. Yarber, Department of Applied Health Science, Indiana University, HPER Building, Bloomington, IN 47405; email: yarber@ucs.indiana.edu.

students. Using internal-criterion and item-difficulty indexes to identify the most discriminating items, an 11-item test (9 knowledge domain, 2 application domain) was administered to 2,980 secondary school students. Analyses of the data produced the final, 10-item test (8 knowledge domain, 2 application domain). The final test has items with highly significant levels of internal consistency (correlation of each item score with entire scale score) and item difficulty level (acceptable percentage of respondents selecting each item alternative).

Response Mode and Timing

Respondents indicate the letter of the alternative that they believe to be the correct answer. The test takes about 10 minutes to complete.

Scoring

Scores range from 0 to 10. Correct answers are identified by an asterisk in the exhibit. Higher scores indicate greater knowledge of individual STD preventive health behaviors than do lower scores.

Reliability

Yarber (1988) reported a test-retest reliability over a 5- to 7-day period to be .56. Cronbach's alpha was .54.

Validity

Individual test items have content or face validity, because they were developed to reflect the preventive health behaviors aspects of STD using a table of specifications

(Kroger & Yarber, 1984; Yarber, 1985). Also, a jury of experts on STD and health education and young adults judged the merits of each item. The test was developed, in part, as one component of a project assessing the efficacy of a Centers for Disease Control school STD education program (Yarber, 1985). Evidence of construct validity comes from the fact that secondary school students exposed to the STD curriculum showed improvement in scores from pretest to posttest when assessed by the test (Yarber, 1988).

Other Information

The development of the test was supported in part by U.S. Public Health Service Grant R30/CCR500638-01.

References

Automated Services. (1976). *Development of a methodology to evaluate VD education in the nation's schools.* Atlanta, GA: Centers for Disease Control.

Bloom, B. S. (Ed.). (1956). *Taxonomy of educational objectives: Handbook I. Cognitive domain.* New York: David McKay.

Green, L. (1979). Toward cost-benefit evaluation of health education: Some concepts, methods, and examples. *Health Education Monograph, 2*(Suppl.), 36-64.

Kroger, F., & Yarber, W. L. (1984). STD content in school health textbooks: An evaluation using the worth assessment procedure. *Journal of School Health, 54,* 41-44.

Yarber, W. L. (1985). *STD: A guide for today's young adults* [Student and instructor's manual]. Waldorf, MD: American Alliance Publications.

Yarber, W. L. (1988). Evaluation of the health behavior approach to school STD education. *Journal of Sex Education and Therapy, 14,* 33-38.

Exhibit

STD Knowledge Test

Part I. Directions: Choose the best answer for each question.

1. STDs mainly affect
    *1. all groups of people.
    2. lower class and poor people.
    3. middle class people living in large cities.
    4. wealthy people who can buy sex.
2. Most people get an STD
    1. from objects.
    2. by the STD forming on its own, without having sex.
    3. by skin-to-skin contact not involving sex.
    *4. by genital contact (penis, vagina).
3. Which disease is now the common health effect of STD?
    1. Central nervous system disease
    2. Heart disease
    *3. Pelvic inflammatory disease (infection of internal female sex organs)
    4. Skin and eye disease
4. Which one of the methods below is the best way of getting a partner to a doctor?
    *1. Taking him/her with you to the doctor
    2. Telling the partner over the telephone that he/she might have an STD
    3. Having an STD casefinder locate the partner
    4. Sending the partner a letter

5. Which one of the statements below dealing with preventing STD is *true*?
    1. Urination (peeing) after sex works as well for females as males.
    2. The intrauterine contraceptive device (IUD) prevents STD.
    *3. The condom (rubber) is the best prevention device for persons with more than one sex partner.
    4. Looking for STD signs before sex almost always works.
6. Which one of the statements below about STD is *not true*?
    1. Pus from the penis usually means an STD.
    *2. Any moisture from the vagina usually indicates an STD.
    3. Burning pain during urination (peeing) may indicate an STD.
    4. Blisters on the genitals probably means an STD.
7. Which one of the statements below dealing with getting an STD is *not true*?
    1. A private doctor can treat the STD.
    2. Hospitals can provide STD care.
    3. STD treatment is usually easy to find.
    *4. Most birth control clinics do not provide help for STD.
8. Which one of the statements below dealing with getting an STD is *not true*?
    *1. It is easy to get an STD from objects.
    2. Persons with different sex partners have a greater chance of getting STD than those with one partner.
    3. The risk of getting STD increases with each new sex partner a person has.
    4. It is impossible to get some STDs from infected clothes, bedsheets, and similar objects.

Part II. Directions: Read the STD life-situations below and answer the questions concerning them.

Situation 1: Henry, a member of his school's soccer team, has been having sex with some girls he knows. A few days ago, he noticed some pus coming from his penis.

9. Which one of Henry's thoughts listed below about what he should do is correct?
    1. I'll get a medical book to see if I have a disease, since doctors charge more money than I have.
    2. The pus is probably the result of a soccer injury I got last week.
    3. My girlfriends don't have any signs, so I probably don't have an STD.
    *4. Even though the pus has now stopped coming from my penis, I still shouldn't have sex until the doctor checks me.

Situation 2: Mary just found out from her doctor that she has an STD. She wants her partner to see a doctor, too. But, she doesn't know what to do. She asks a friend for advice.

10. Which one of her friend's advice listed below is correct?
    1. There is no hurry to inform the partner. He will get STD signs soon, anyway.
    2. If you give your partner's name to the doctor, you are squealing on him. STD casefinders sometimes scold the partner for having sex.
    *3. Don't have sex again until your partner is cured. You could get the STD again.
    4. Don't give your partner's name to the doctor. The STD casefinder usually tells the partner who gave his name.

Sociosexual Orientation Inventory

Jeffry A. Simpson,[1] *Texas A&M University*

Nearly 50 years ago, comprehensive surveys of the sexual practices of North American men (Kinsey, Pomeroy, & Martin, 1948) and women (Kinsey, Pomeroy, Martin, & Gebhard, 1953) revealed that individuals differ substantially on a wide array of sociosexual attitudes and behaviors. Although men, as a group, tend to display greater sexual "permissiveness" than women on most sociosexual attitudes and behaviors (e.g., men have more permissive attitudes about the acceptability of casual sex, and they are more likely to have short-term sexual affairs), one of the most striking features of the Kinsey data is that much more variability exists *within* the sexes than *between* them. Some women, for example, exhibit greater sexual permissiveness than many men; conversely, some men are less permissive than many women.

The Sociosexual Orientation Inventory (SOI; Simpson & Gangestad, 1991) was developed to measure individual differences in willingness to engage in casual, uncommitted sexual relationships. In particular, the SOI assesses individuals' past sexual behavior, their anticipated (future) sexual behavior, the content of their sexual fantasies, and their attitudes toward engaging in casual sex. Individuals who score high on the SOI are said to have an *unrestricted* sociosexual orientation. These individuals report a larger number of sexual partners in the past year, they anticipate having more sexual partners in the next 5 years, they have engaged in more "one night stands," they fantasize more often about having sex with someone other than their current (or most recent) partner, and they believe that sex without love and commitment is more acceptable. Individuals who score low on the SOI have a *restricted* sociosexual orientation. These individuals report fewer sexual partners in the past year, they anticipate having fewer sexual partners in the next 5 years, they are less likely to have had a "one night stand," they rarely fantasize about having sex with someone other than their current (or most recent) partner, and they do not believe in having sex without love and commitment.

Description

The SOI consists of seven items. Two items ask respondents to report on aspects of their past sexual behavior: (a) number of sexual partners in the past year and (b) number of times they have engaged in sex with someone on only one occasion. One item assesses future sexual behavior: number of partners anticipated in the next 5 years. One item, answered on an 8-point Likert-type scale, inquires about sexual fantasies: how often they fantasize about hav-

ing sex with someone other than their current (or most recent) partner. Three items, each answered on 9-point Likert-type scales, ask about respondents' attitudes toward engaging in casual sexual relations. Principal-axis factor analyses have indicated that these seven items define a single factor (Simpson & Gangestad, 1991).

Response Mode and Timing

Three items on the SOI (those that ask about past and future sexual behavior) require respondents to write down specific numbers of sexual partners. The remaining four items (those that inquire about fantasies and attitudes toward casual sex) are answered on traditional Likert-type scales that range from 1 to 8 or 1 to 9. Given this mixed-response format, respondents cannot respond to the SOI on machine-scored answer sheets. Rather, they must respond on the instrument itself. The SOI takes 1-2 minutes to complete.

Scoring

Item 7 should be reverse keyed. Items 5, 6, and 7 should then be aggregated to form the attitudinal component of the SOI. The following weighting scheme should be used when aggregating the five components: SOI = 5X (Item 1) + 1X (Item 2) + 5X (Item 3) + 4X (Item 4) + 2X (aggregate of Items 5-7). To ensure that Item 2 does not have a disproportionate influence when constructing the inventory, the maximum value of Item 2 should be limited to 30 partners. This weighting scheme is used because it closely approximates the scores that individuals would receive if each of the five components of the SOI were transformed to *z* scores, unit weighted, and then added together. Scores derived from the current weighting scheme correlate about .90 with the latter unit-weighting system (Simpson & Gangestad, 1991).

Scores can range from 10 (a maximally restricted orientation) to approximately 1,000 (a maximally unrestricted orientation), although the normal range in college-age samples is 10-250. Because men tend to score higher on the SOI than women (Simpson & Gangestad, 1992), respondents' sex should be partialed out prior to conducting statistical analyses or analyses should be done separately on men and women.

On occasion, some respondents will report extremely high numbers for Items 1-3. In college samples, we set 30 as the maximum value for Item 2. If college-age respondents report more than 20 partners for Items 1 or 2, these individuals may be outliers who could have a disproportionate influence on the results. Outlier detection should always be done prior to conducting analyses using the SOI.

---
[1]Address correspondence to Jeffry A. Simpson, Department of Psychology, Texas A&M University, College Station, TX 77843-4235; email: jas@psyc.tamu.edu.

Reliability

In large samples, the SOI is internally consistent (average Cronbach alpha = .75; Simpson & Gangestad, 1991, 1992; Simpson, Gangestad, & Nations, 1995). Furthermore, test-retest reliability spanning 2 months is high (r = .94; Simpson & Gangestad, 1991).

Validity

Predictions regarding restricted and unrestricted sociosexual orientations have been derived from the theoretical construct of sociosexuality (Gangestad & Simpson, 1990). Both convergent and discriminant validation evidence has been marshaled for the SOI. In terms of convergent validity, Simpson and Gangestad (1991) have found that unrestricted individuals, relative to restricted ones, (a) engage in sex earlier in their romantic relationships, (b) are more likely to engage in sex with more than one partner at a time, and (c) tend to be involved in sexual relationships characterized by less reported investment, less commitment, less love, and weaker affectional ties. Unrestricted individuals also score higher on other scales that tap related constructs (e.g., sexual permissiveness, impersonal sex). Simpson and Gangestad (1992) have shown that unrestricted individuals desire, choose, and actually acquire romantic partners who have different attributes than those of restricted individuals. Specifically, unrestricted individuals prefer partners who are more physically/sexually attractive and who have higher social status/visibility; they place less emphasis on attributes such as kindness, loyalty, and stability. Restricted individuals, on the other hand, prefer partners who are kinder and more affectionate, more faithful/loyal, and more responsible; they place less weight on attributes such as attractiveness and social status. In a laboratory dating initiation study, Simpson, Gangestad, and Biek (1993) have found that unrestricted individuals—especially unrestricted men—display more nonverbal behaviors known to facilitate rapid relationship development (e.g., more smiling, laughing, maintaining direct eye contact, and engaging in flirtatious glances).

With regard to discriminant validity, Simpson and Gangestad (1991) have found that restricted individuals, relative to unrestricted ones, (a) do *not* exhibit evidence of a lower sex drive (and, therefore, variation underlying the SOI is not contaminated by individual differences in the desire for sex per se), and (b) do *not* score higher on scales that assess sexuality-based constructs that should not correlate with the SOI (e.g., sexual satisfaction, sex guilt, and sex-related anxiety).

References

Gangestad, S. W., & Simpson, J. A. (1990). Toward an evolutionary history of female sociosexual variation. *Journal of Personality, 58,* 69-96.

Kinsey, A., Pomeroy, W., & Martin, C. (1948). *Sexual behavior in the human male.* Philadelphia: Saunders.

Kinsey, A., Pomeroy, W., Martin, C., & Gebhard, P. (1953). *Sexual behavior in the human female.* Philadelphia: Saunders.

Simpson, J. A., & Gangestad, S. W. (1991). Individual differences in sociosexuality: Evidence for convergent and discriminant validity. *Journal of Personality and Social Psychology, 60,* 870-883.

Simpson, J. A., & Gangestad, S. W. (1992). Sociosexuality and romantic partner choice. *Journal of Personality, 60,* 31-51.

Simpson, J. A., Gangestad, S. W., & Biek, M. (1993). Personality and nonverbal social behavior: An ethological perspective of relationship initiation. *Journal of Experimental Social Psychology, 29,* 434-461.

Simpson, J. A., Gangestad, S. W., & Nations, C. (1995). Sociosexuality and relationship initiation: An ethological perspective of nonverbal behavior. In G. Fletcher & J. Fitness (Eds.), *Knowledge structures in close relationships: A social psychological approach* (pp. 121-146). Hillsdale, NJ: Lawrence Erlbaum.

Exhibit

Sociosexual Orientation Inventory

Please answer *all* of the following questions honestly. Your responses will be treated as confidential and anonymous. For the questions dealing with behavior, *write* your answers in the blank spaces provided. For the questions dealing with thoughts and attitudes, *circle* the appropriate number on the scales provided.

1. With how many different partners have you had sex (sexual intercourse) within the past year? _____
2. How many different partners do you foresee yourself having sex with during the next five years? (Please give a *specific, realistic* estimate) _____
3. With how many different partners have you had sex on *one and only one* occasion? _____
4. How often do you fantasize about having sex with someone other than your current dating partner? (Circle one)
    1) Never
    2) Once every two or three months
    3) Once a month
    4) Once every two weeks
    5) Once a week
    6) A few times each week
    7) Nearly every day
    8) At least once a day

5. Sex without love is OK.

      1   2   3   4   5   6   7   8   9

   I strongly disagree   I strongly agree

6. I can imagine myself being comfortable and enjoying "casual" sex with different partners.

      1   2   3   4   5   6   7   8   9

   I strongly disagree   I strongly agree

7. I would have to be closely attached to someone (both emotionally and psychologically) before I could feel comfortable and fully enjoy having sex with him or her.

      1   2   3   4   5   6   7   8   9

   I strongly disagree   I strongly agree

Source. This scale was originally published in "Individual Differences in Sociosexuality: Evidence for Convergent and Discriminant Validity," by J. A. Simpson and S. W. Gangestad, 1991, *Journal of Personality and Social Psychology, 60,* 870-883. Reprinted with permission.

Token Resistance to Sex Scale

Suzanne L. Osman,[1] *Syracuse University*

The Token Resistance to Sex Scale (TRSS; Osman, 1995) was developed to measure the predispositional belief that women use token resistance to sexual advances, that is, they say no to sexual advances but mean yes. The belief in token resistance has been recognized as an important determinant of perceptions, opinions, and outcomes of date rape (Muehlenhard, Friedman, & Thomas, 1985; Muehlenhard & Hollabaugh, 1988; Muehlenhard & Linton, 1987; Shotland & Goodstein, 1983). Although the concept of *token resistance* has been documented, this is the first scale to measure this predispositional belief by examining the situational factors known to be associated with belief in token resistance. Past researchers have measured belief in token resistance as a dependent variable by asking independent questions about whether sexual activity was desired. This scale allows the predispositional belief in token resistance to be treated as an independent variable measure.

Description

The TRSS consists of eight items arranged on a 7-point Likert-type scale ranging from *strongly agree* to *strongly disagree.* It is most appropriate for men.

Response Mode and Timing

Respondents can write the number from 1 to 7 that corresponds to their agreement with an item. The scale can be completed in less than 5 minutes.

Scoring

All eight items are keyed in the same direction with a higher score indicating a lower belief in token resistance and a lower score indicating a higher belief in token resistance. Scores can range from 8 to 56.

Reliability

In a sample of 81 college men (Osman, 1995), the Cronbach alpha reliability score for the TRSS was .86.

Validity

As expected, Osman (1995) found that the TRSS significantly correlated with Burt's (1980) Sex Role Stereotyping Scale, $r = .21$, and with Mosher and Sirkin's (1984) Hypermasculinity Inventory, including Callous Sexual Attitudes, $r = .50$, Danger as Exciting, $r = .18$, and Violence as Manly, $r = .21$. The TRSS was the best dispositional predictor of date rape perceptions, which provides evidence of construct validity for the TRSS. As belief in token resistance gets stronger, perceptions of date rape get weaker (Osman, 1995).

[1]Address correspondence to Suzanne L. Osman, 58 Buffalo Run, E. Brunswick, NJ 08816.

References

Burt, M. R. (1980). Cultural myths and supports for rape. *Journal of Personality and Social Psychology, 38,* 217-230.

Mosher, D. L., & Sirkin, M. (1984). Measuring a macho personality constellation. *Journal of Research in Personality, 18,* 150-163.

Muehlenhard, C. L., Friedman, D. E., & Thomas, C. M. (1985). Is date rape justifiable? The effects of dating activity, who initiated, who paid and men's attitudes toward women. *Psychology of Women Quarterly, 9,* 297-309.

Muehlenhard, C. L., & Hollabaugh, L. C. (1988). Do women sometimes say no when they mean yes? The prevalence and correlates of women's token resistance to sex. *Journal of Personality and Social Psychology, 54,* 872-879.

Muehlenhard, C. L., & Linton, M. A. (1987). Date rape and sexual aggression in dating situations: Incidence and risk factors. *Journal of Counseling Psychology, 34,* 186-196.

Osman, S. L. (1995, April). *Predispositional and situational factors influencing men's perceptions of date rape.* Paper presented at the Eastern Regional Meeting of the Society for the Scientific Study of Sexuality, Atlantic City, NJ.

Shotland, R. L., & Goodstein, L. (1983). Just because she doesn't want to doesn't mean it's rape: An experimental based causal model of the perception of rape in a dating situation. *Social Psychology Quarterly, 46,* 220-232.

Exhibit

Token Resistance to Sex Scale

Respond to the following statements by indicating the degree to which you agree or disagree with the statement. Respond using the following scale for each statement.

1 = Strongly agree
2 = Agree
3 = Slightly agree
4 = Undecided, neither agree nor disagree
5 = Slightly disagree
6 = Disagree
7 = Strongly disagree

_____ 1. Women usually say "no" to sex when they really mean "yes."

_____ 2. When a man only has to use a minimal amount of force on a woman to get her to have sex, it probably means she wanted him to force her.

_____ 3. When a woman waits until the very last minute to object to sex in a sexual interaction, she probably really wants to have sex.

_____ 4. A woman who initiates a date with a man probably wants to have sex.

_____ 5. Many times a woman will pretend she doesn't want to have intercourse because she doesn't want to seem too loose, but she's really hoping the man will force her.

_____ 6. A woman who allows a man to pick her up for a date probably hopes to have sex that night.

_____ 7. When a woman allows a man to treat her to an expensive dinner on a date, it usually indicates that she is willing to have sex with him.

_____ 8. Going home with a man at the end of a date is a woman's way of communicating to him that she wants to have sex.

Psychosocial Rating Format for the Evaluation of Results of Sex Reassignment Surgery

Daniel Hunt,[1] *University of Washington*

This rating scale is designed to assist in the measurement and the uniform reporting of the follow-up results of post-surgical transsexuals. Lothstein (1982) described the problems associated with comparing the outcome data across the various follow-up studies of postsurgical patients. Specifically, she noted that the different rating formats used to measure outcome make comparisons difficult. Some researchers have used terms such as *satisfactory* or *doubtful* in attempting to provide an overall measure of their outcome judgment, but they have not uniformly defined these variables. Others have reported their follow-up findings only through the case report method. Thus, it is impossible to compare findings across studies. The standardized method of collecting and analyzing follow-up information on transsexuals reported here has been successfully used for both postsurgical transsexual follow-up information on transsexuals (Lundström, 1981) and to follow up on individuals who have been denied sex reassignment surgery (Hunt & Hampson, 1980a). The development of a scale grew out of the existing literature and my contacts with transsexuals. It was then used and tested for reliability and validity in a follow-up study of 17 biological males who had received gender-reassigning surgery an average of 8.2 years prior to follow-up contact.

This rating instrument (Hunt & Hampson, 1980b) is designed to be used by the interviewer and allows the scoring of information that is obtained during face-to-face contact. For larger postsurgical surveys, Exhibit 2 has a questionnaire form of this material. The testing reported herein refers only to the rating of the live interviews. The scoring of the interview helps the researcher to quantify the transsexual's particular situation in areas of economic history and situation, interpersonal relationships, degree of psychopathology, self-adjustment, family involvement, and the appropriateness of additional surgeries beyond the initial genital reconstruction.

Description

The rating format has six sections. Each of these sections has from one to five subcomponents that are scored by the interviewer with a rating from 0 to 3 points with the highest points indicating the best adjustment. Some questions ask the rater to draw a conclusion based on a series of events since surgery (such as the stability of the individual's job history), whereas others ask the interviewer for an assess-

ment based on a present situation, such as the current ability to support oneself financially. Each of the scores is anchored by a specific description but does ask the rater to make judgments between statements such as "frequent changes of intimates, chronically unstable relationship" and "less frequent changes of intimates, some evidence of recent improvement."

In one case, the rater is asked to differentiate the degree to which the transsexual has continued to seek additional surgeries and the appropriateness of these surgeries. This rating point was deemed valuable with the finding that 24% of the follow-up group had continued to seek multiple plastic surgeries in the hope of becoming "the complete woman." The final question asks the rater to score the degree of acceptance from the family. The variable gives more points if the interviewer has contacted the family or in some other way "confirmed" the family member's relative acceptance or rejection of the transsexual's situation after surgery.

Lundström (1981) used this instrument for a follow-up study of 31 cases that were not accepted for sex reassignment. The scale can be used for this purpose by eliminating the items that have to do with the functioning nature of the vagina or the phallus, and any other specific items only relating to the postsurgical status of the individual. The original follow-up study for which the instrument was designed also used the scale to rate retroactively the presurgical status.

No question was used in this format to evaluate physical appearance or the ability to pass in the chosen gender role. This item was discussed extensively and finally omitted because of the difficulties in judging this important but very subjective variable. It was felt that if the physical appearance interfered with the adjustment, this would be picked up on other items.

Response Mode and Timing

The questionnaire is completed by writing in the response or circling the answer on the form, depending on the item. It takes approximately 25 minutes to complete. The interview requires 45 minutes.

Scoring

Although developed initially with biologic males, the rating scale is written to allow the scoring of biologic females as well. There are 15 specific rating points, each with the 0 to 3 scoring range so that the maximum possible score is 45. The six subscales (economics, relationships, psychopathology, sexual adjustment, additional surgeries, and

[1]Address correspondence to Daniel Hunt, Department of Psychiatry and Behavioral Sciences, RP-10, School of Medicine, University of Washington, Seattle, WA 98915.

family reactions) can be individually analyzed, or the overall score may be used to compare relative outcome across different studies. The area of sexual adjustment is more heavily weighted in that it has five subcomponents and thus contributes more to the overall scoring. The higher the score the more positive the overall postsurgical rating. The follow-up of the 17 biological males found them with an average score of 33.9 and a range of between 16 and 42, with 45 being the maximum score possible.

Reliability

The rating format was developed during the process of contacting and evaluating a group of transsexuals, on the average, 8 years after their sex reassignment surgeries. These biologic males were interviewed by two experienced research clinicians. The rating format was used by both to evaluate the personal interviews and information that had been accumulated over the 8-year period. This included letters from the respondents concerning progress; phone calls to family members; interviews with husbands and boyfriends, when allowed; and reports in newspapers about the individuals over the follow-up period. Following the completion of all information gathering and interviewing, both researchers independently rated the respondents using the scale. Comparisons of these ratings provided a measure of interrater reliability using the Spearman-Brown prediction formula (see Table 1).

The range of agreement for the 15 questions was from 82% to 100% with an overall average of 90% interrater reliability. Areas of least agreement were those requiring judgments about the support system, the degree to which existing psychopathology interfered with relationships or work, and the relative stability within interpersonal relationships. However, even in these areas where relative judgments were necessary, the interrater reliability was strong.

Validity

To assess the validity of the instrument, an independent psychological measure was used and compared to this rating format. The Minnesota Multiphasic Personality Inventory (MMPI) was obtained from 10 of the 17 transsexuals at the follow-up interview. A senior, independent psychologist scored these tests and ranked the respondents from 1 to 10 as "best" and "least" likely to be able to cope. The postsurgical rating format provided an overall score for these 10 that was used to form another ranking of the best to the worst. The similarity in the two rankings was measured using the Spearman-Rank difference coefficient and was found to be similar at a significant level .62, $p < .01$.

These initial findings are supportive that a standardized format for the evaluation of transsexuals following surgery can be designed and used, allowing for agreement between judges and bearing a close relationship to an independent

Table 1 Interrater Reliability Using the Spearman-Brown Prediction Formula

Question content	Interrater reliability
1. Economic	
a. Job history	0.86
b. Ability to support self	1.00
2. Interpersonal relationships	
a. History	0.82
b. Level of satisfaction from relationships	0.84
c. Current support system	0.82
3. Psychopathology	
a. Mental status	0.86
b. Drug use	0.97
c. Legal problems	0.97
4. Sexual adjustment	
a. Doubts about surgical decision	0.84
b. Experiencing self as female (male)	0.84
c. Choice of sexual partner	0.98
d. Functional nature of vagina (phallus)	1.00
e. Sexual satisfaction	0.86
5. Postsurgical procedures	0.96
6. Family acceptance	0.88

measure that is not oriented specifically to transsexualism. However, these are limitations of which the user should be aware. The reliability and validity testing was done only on biologic males. The rating format has been successfully used in subsequent studies to assess the follow-up of biologic females, but no instrument testing was carried out on the biologic females.

It is anticipated that gender dysphoria centers will use the scale to assess economics, interpersonal relationships, psychopathology, and family acceptance. This would allow for a more refined pre- and postsurgical follow-up procedure. It is also expected that as more information becomes available about this challenging group of patients, additional variables to measure postoperative status will be added to this current rating format.

References

Hunt, D. D., & Hampson, J. L. (1980a). Follow-up of 17 biologic males after sex reassignment surgery. *American Journal of Psychiatry, 137,* 432-438.

Hunt, D. D., & Hampson, J. L. (1980b). Transsexualism: A standardized psychosocial rating format for the evaluation of results of sex reassignment surgery. *Archives of Sexual Behavior, 9,* 255-263.

Lothstein, L. M. (1982). Sex reassignment surgery. *American Journal of Psychiatry, 139,* 417-426.

Lundström, B. (1981). *Gender dysphoria: A social-psychiatric follow-up study of 31 cases not accepted for sex reassignment.* Reports from the Department of Psychiatry and Neurochemistry, St. Jorgen's Hospital, University of Totenborg, Sweden.

Exhibit 1

Standardized Rating Format for Postsurgical Transsexuals

1. Economics
   a. Job history
      - 0   severely unstable job history
      - 1   moderately unstable job history
      - 2   mildly unstable job history
      - 3   stable job history
      - nia   no information available
   b. Ability to support self
      - 0   on welfare
      - 1   financially dependent—lacks skills to support self
      - 2   financially dependent—possesses skill to support self
      - 3   financially independent—employed
      - nia   no information available

2. Interpersonal relationships
   a. History
      - 0   frequent changes of intimates: chronically unstable relationships
      - 1   less frequent changes of intimates: some evidence of recent improvement
      - 2   more recently stable relationships
      - 3   long history of stable relationships
      - nia   no information available
   b. Satisfaction gained from relationships
      - 0   none (shallow relationships)
      - 1   marginal satisfaction
      - 2   some satisfaction from relationships
      - 3   considerable satisfaction
      - nia   no information available
   c. Current support system
      - 0   no significant system
      - 1   marginal support system
      - 2   some support system
      - 3   significant support system
      - nia   no information available

3. Psychopathology
   a. Mental status
      - 0   psychopathology with major impact on relationships or productivity
      - 1   psychopathology with some impact on relationships or work
      - 2   psychopathology but no impact on relationships or work
      - 3   no psychopathology
      - nia   no information available
   b. Drug use (during entire follow-up period; excludes prescribed medications)
      - 0   alcoholism or hard drugs
      - 1   heavy use of marijuana, downers, alcohol, or tranquilizers
      - 2   occasional use of marijuana, alcohol, or tranquilizers
      - 3   no drug use
      - nia   no information available
   c. Legal problems
      - 0   frequent criminal activities
      - 1   sporadic criminal activities
      - 2   no recent history of criminal activities (last 3 years)
      - 3   no criminal activity
      - nia   no information available

4. Sexual adjustment
   a. Surgical decision
      - 0   chronic doubts about surgical changes
      - 1   occasional but significant doubts about change
      - 2   occasional but not significant doubts about change
      - 3   no doubts about surgical change
      - nia   no information available
   b. Experiencing self as a female (male)
      - 0   frequently feels like an imposter
      - 1   occasionally feels like an imposter
      - 2   feels like a woman (man) almost all the time
      - 3   feels like a woman (man) all the time
      - nia   no information available

c. Choice of sexual partner

0	has no sexual partners
1	bisexual: predominantly female (male) partners
2	bisexual: predominantly male (female) partners
3	only male (female) partners
nia	no information available

d. Functional nature of vagina (phallus)

0	vagina (phallus) not existent
1	vagina (phallus) existent but nonfunctional
2	vagina (phallus) functional but either inadequate or painful
3	vagina (phallus) functional and adequate
nia	no information available

e. Sexual satisfaction

0	completely dissatisfied with sex life
1	frequently dissatisfied with sex life
2	occasionally dissatisfied with sex life
3	completely satisfied with sex life
nia	no information available

5. Additional surgeries or procedures (includes electrolysis)

0	cosmetic surgeries or procedures of no realistic necessity
1	cosmetic surgeries of questionable realistic necessity
2	cosmetic surgeries realistically necessary
3	no cosmetic surgeries
nia	no information available

6. Current family reactions

0	all members nonaccepting (either confirmed or not confirmed)
1	some members nonaccepting (either confirmed or not confirmed)
2	all members accepting (unconfirmed)
3	all members accepting (confirmed)
nia	no information available

Exhibit 2

Trinidad Follow-Up Questionnaire

1. How many jobs have you had in the past year?
   Are you now employed? (Circle one)   Yes   No
      If yes: Quarter-time _____   Half-time _____   Full-time _____
   Have you attended a school in the past year? (Circle one)   Yes   No
      If you have attended a school:
         How many academic quarter/semesters have you attended in the past year? _____
         How many credits were you enrolled for each quarter/semester? _____
   Are you receiving public assistance or some type of social security income? Yes   No
   Are you financially dependent on a partner or other family member?   Yes   No
      If so, please specify the relationship of the persons supporting you. _____
   Please describe the types of jobs you've had in the past 3 years. (If job title is not descriptive of the skills involved, please designate the skills needed to do the job.) _____
2. Do you have any friends or intimates that you believe know you well, yes or no?
      If yes, how many of these intimates do you have? _____
         How long have you known each of them? (months, years)
            1. _____   2. _____   3. _____   4. _____
   Are you living with anyone, yes or no?
      If you are living with someone, is the main purpose: (Circle one)
         intimacy and sharing or *financial*?
   On a scale of 1 to 6, if living in the female gender role, to what degree to you pass as a female?
      I rarely pass as a female   I always pass as a female
                           1   2   3   4   5   6
   Are you married?   Yes _____   How long? _____
                                 No _____
   Have you adopted children? Yes _____   How many? _____   What age? _____
                                 No _____   If no, do you anticipate this in the future? _____

How much satisfaction do you feel you find in the relationships with your intimates? (Circle one number)
1. none
2. minimal
3. some satisfaction
4. considerable satisfaction

How would you judge your current support system: (Circle one number)
1. no significant system
2. minimal support system
3. some support system
4. significant support system

3. Have you had any complications from any of the surgeries or procedures related to your gender change? _____

Have you sought therapy or counseling in the past 3 years? Yes _____ No _____

If you have been in therapy, please designate how many times, and how long (weeks, months) you were in therapy. _____

If you have been in therapy please describe what brought you to seek help. _____

Have you been hospitalized in the past year for psychiatric reasons? Yes _____ No _____

If yes, how many times? _____ For how long? _____

If you were hospitalized, please describe the reasons or circumstances of your hospitalization. _____

Number of depressed periods in the past year   0/year
                                                 1-2/year
                                                 3-6/year
                                                 7-10/year
                                                 1-2/month

(This part of the questionnaire comes from the Beck Depression Inventory.)

Please read the following groups of statements carefully. Then pick out the one statement in each group that best describes the way you have been feeling the *past week, including today!* Circle the number beside the statement you picked. If several statements in the group seem to apply equally well, circle each one. *Be sure to read all the statements in each group before making your choice.*

0   I do not feel sad.
1   I feel sad.
2   I am sad all the time and I can't snap out of it.
3   I am so sad or unhappy that I can't stand it.

0   I am not particularly discouraged about the future.
1   I feel discouraged about the future.
2   I feel I have nothing to look forward to.
3   I feel that the future is hopeless and that things cannot improve.

0   I do not feel like a failure.
1   I feel I have failed more than the average person.
2   As I look back on my life, all I can see is a lot of failure.
3   I feel I am a complete failure as a person.

0   I get as much satisfaction out of things as I used to.
1   I don't enjoy things the way I used to.
2   I don't get real satisfaction out of anything anymore.
3   I am dissatisfied or bored with everything.

0   I don't feel particularly guilty.
1   I feel guilty a good part of the time.
2   I feel guilty most of the time.
3   I feel guilty all of the time.

0   I don't feel I am being punished.
1   I feel I may be punished.
2   I expect to be punished.
3   I feel I am being punished.

0   I don't feel disappointed in myself.
1   I am disappointed in myself.
2   I am disgusted with myself.
3   I hate myself.

0   I don't feel I am any worse than anybody else.
1   I have thoughts of killing myself, but I would not carry them out.
2   I would like to kill myself.
3   I would kill myself if I had the chance.

0   I don't cry any more than usual.
1   I cry more now than I used to.
2   I cry all the time now.
3   I used to be able to cry, but now I can't cry even though I want to.

0   I am no more irritated now that I ever am.
1   I get annoyed or irritated more easily than I used to.
2   I feel irritated all the time now.
3   I don't get irritated at all by the things that used to irritate me.

0   I have not lost interest in other people.
1   I am less interested in other people than I used to be.
2   I have lost most of my interest in other people.
3   I have lost all of my interest in other people.

0   I make decisions about as well as I ever could.
1   I put off making decisions more than I used to.
2   I have greater difficulty in making decisions than before.
3   I can't make decisions at all anymore.

0   I don't feel I look any worse than I used to.
1   I am worried that I am looking old or unattractive.
2   I feel that there are permanent changes in my appearance that make me look unattractive.
3   I believe that I look ugly.

0   I can work about as well as before.
1   It takes an extra effort to get started at doing something.
2   I have to push myself very hard to do anything.
3   I can't do any work at all.

0   I can sleep as well as usual.
1   I don't sleep as well as I used to.
2   I wake up 1-2 hours earlier than usual and find it hard to get back to sleep.
3   I wake up several hours earlier than I used to and cannot get back to sleep.

0   I don't get more tired than usual.
1   I get tired more easily than I used to.
2   I get tired from doing almost anything.
3   I am too tired to do anything.

0   My appetite is no worse than usual.
1   My appetite is not as good as it used to be.
2   My appetite is much worse now.
3   I have no appetite at all any more.

0   I haven't lost much weight, if any, lately.
1   I have lost more than 5 pounds.
2   I have lost more than 10 pounds.
3   I have lost more than 15 pounds.

I am purposely trying to lose weight by eating less.   Yes _____   No _____

0   I am not more worried about my health than usual.
1   I am worried about physical problems such as aches and pains; or upset stomach or constipation.
2   I am very worried about physical problems and it's hard to think of much else.
3   I am so worried about physical problems that I cannot think about anything else.

0   I have not noticed any recent change in my interest in sex.
1   I am less interested in sex than I used to be.
2   I am much less interested in sex now.
3   I have lost interest in sex completely.

Do you have any problems with alcohol use, yes or no?
Please quantify how much of the following you use. (For example, if you drink 3 beers a day, put that in the blank.)
   Alcohol _____ on a daily basis. (If not daily, indicate how much each month.)
   Marijuana _____ daily. (If not daily, indicate how much each month.)
   Tranquilizers (Valium, barbiturates) _____ daily. (If not daily, indicate how much each month.)
   Amphetamines (speed) _____ daily. (If not daily, indicate how much each month.)
   Narcotics (cocaine, heroine)
      Type _____   Method _____   Dosage—Indicate per day or per month _____
Have you hired a lawyer or attorney in the past year? yes or no
   If yes, please describe the circumstances. _____
   Please describe any other legal problems you have had in the past year. _____
Are you currently involved in prostitution?   Yes _____   No _____
4. If you had a chance to redo your decision about the surgery, would you do anything differently?   Yes _____ No _____
   If so, what? _____
Since the surgery, how do you feel about the change? (Circle one)
   1.   I have continuous doubts about the change.
   2.   I have occasional but significant doubts about the change.
   3.   I have occasional but not significant doubts about the change.
   4.   I have no doubts about the change.
How do you experience yourself as female? (Circle one)
   1.   I frequently feel like an imposter.
   2.   I occasionally feel like an imposter.
   3.   I feel like a woman almost all of the time.
   4.   I feel like a woman all of the time.
Do you have sexual partners? (Circle one) yes or no
   If yes, number of sexual partners you have had in the past year. _____
If you have sexual partners, what type of sexual partner do you prefer? (Circle one)
   1.   I prefer only male partners.
   2.   I prefer only female partners.
   3.   I am bisexual but prefer predominantly female partners.
   4.   I am bisexual but prefer predominantly male partners.
   5.   I am bisexual, but have no preference for male or female partners.

What is the status of your vagina? (Circle one)
1. Vagina not existent.
2. Vagina existent, but not adequate for sexual intercourse.
3. Vagina functional, but painful for sex.
4. Vagina functional and adequate for sex.

How satisfied are you with your sex life? (Circle one)
1. Completely dissatisfied with sex life.
2. Frequently dissatisfied with sex life.
3. Occasionally dissatisfied with sex life.
4. Completely satisfied with sex life.

Do you reach orgasm? Yes _____ No _____

Are you satisfied with the quality or frequency of your orgasms? (Circle one)
1. Completely dissatisfied with orgasms.
2. Frequently dissatisfied with orgasms.
3. Occasionally satisfied with orgasms.
4. Completely satisfied with orgasms.

5. Please list the cosmetic surgeries you have had and estimate the amount of money each of these procedures cost you (include electrolysis). (Example: facial silicone injection, and/or surgery on neck, head, nose, eyes, lips, etc.) _____

6. What reaction have you had from your family to your change? (family members would be mother, father, stepparents, siblings, children) _____

Prior to surgery, what type of contact did you have with your family? (family members would be mother, father, stepparents, siblings, children)
0. All are deceased.
1. No contact with any of them.
2. Occasional contact but one or all of them did not accept my gender issues.
3. Occasional contact and, while all accepted gender issues, they weren't supportive of me.
4. All accepted my gender issues and they were supportive of me.

Now, *or at any time since surgery*, how would you characterize your contact with your family?
0. All are deceased.
1. No contact.
2. Occasional contact but one or all of them have not accepted my gender issues.
3. Occasional contact and, while all accept my gender issues, they haven't been supportive of me.
4. All of them accept my gender issues and they are supportive of me.

How often do you think others suspect your pre-operative sex? (Circle one)
0/year
1-2/year
3-6/year
7-10/year
1-2/month
1 or more/week

How many times in the past year have you thought of returning back to your pre-operative sex? (Circle one)
0/year
1-2/year
3-6/year
7-10/year
1-2/month
1 or more/week

Source. This scale was originally published in "Transsexualism: A Standardized Psychosocial Rating Format for the Evaluation of Results of Sex Reassignment Surgery," by D. D. Hunt and J. L. Hampson, 1980, *Archives of Sexual Behavior, 9,* 255-263. Reprinted with permission.

Transsexual Postoperative Follow-Up Questionnaire

Leslie M. Lothstein,[1] *Institute of Living*
Eva Shinar, *Ben Gurion University*

This questionnaire is designed to collect systematic data on the psychological and social functioning of postoperative transsexual patients.

Description

The questionnaire includes 59 items, or areas of inquiry, arranged in a nine-page booklet. The face sheet asks for demographic information and lists the dates and stages of all surgeries and the name of the surgeon and the patient's therapist. These items are filled out by the patient's psychotherapist or primary clinician. Because male and female patients have to be asked separate questions about their genital surgery, pages 2, 3, and 5 are different for each sex.

The first set of questions focuses on the psychological and social aspects of the patient's genital surgery, the patient's reactions to the surgery and hospitalization, the functional and aesthetic aspects of the new genitals, the patient's compliance with physician instructions regarding care of the new genitals, the patient's feelings about the amputated body parts, and the patient's expectations about the functional capability of the new genitals. The majority of the questions are framed as Likert-type items along a 7-point scale. The scaling technique is further refined by using a 100 mm line along which exact measurements of the patient's subjective appraisal of his or her status can be judged. Interspersed with these questions are open-ended questions focusing on problems with dilation (for men) and caring for the new penis (for women), what advice they would give other patients about the operation(s), and what other surgery was desired. Another set of items (also using the Likert-type scaling) focuses on the patient's feelings about obtaining additional nongenital surgery.

A second set of questions focuses solely on psychological issues. A Likert-type scaling technique is also employed, asking each patient to rate 13 personality traits along a continuum. Finally, there is a series of open-ended questions focusing on suicidal thoughts and on dreams.

A third set of questions refocuses on the issue of surgery and the patient's responses to surgery. These questions vary from employing Likert-type response options to open-ended and *yes-no* forced-choice response items. Some of the questions focus on complications that may have arisen postsurgery, fantasies about returning to the original sex, satisfaction with intercourse and genital functioning (pre- and postsurgery), orgastic functioning, fears and anxieties about the new genitals, expectations about sexual function-

ing and satisfaction, masturbation practices (and fantasies), sexual preferences and practices (including fantasies), and changes in sex partners.

A fourth set of questions focuses on social and interpersonal relationships, changes in one's social life postsurgery, dating patterns, friendships, and future plans for marriage and children. The majority of these questions are open ended, although a few questions involve Likert-type items (with the 100 mm line) and forced-choice items. Other areas of inquiry focus on family relationships and reactions to surgery and sex change, family support and acceptance, changes in the patient's attitudes toward family and friends, and specific reactions by all primary relatives and family members to his or her surgery and new sex.

The fifth and final set of questions involves a series of open-ended questions focusing on the transsexual patient's choice of vocation. These questions focus on the kind of work he or she does, any changes in employment postsurgery, changes in salary, acceptance by peers and employers at work, reactions and attitudes by co-workers, and what vocational and/or educational plans he or she has for the future.

Response Mode and Timing

In our clinic, each of the respondents is asked to fill out the questionnaire in the presence of his or her therapist. In this way, the therapist (who intimately knows the patient and has followed him or her over the course of several years and has supported the patient through surgery) could then read the patient's responses and inquire further about responses that were either incomplete or inaccurate. This type of administration overcomes some of the objections to self-administered objective tests: that is, that they can easily be distorted in the direction of social desirability. The patient's original responses to each of the questions (i.e., without the therapist's help) form one of the databases. The questionnaire is, however, designed to be self-administered. We administer the questionnaire at intervals of 3 months, 6 months, 1 year, and yearly thereafter. It takes about 1 hour to fill out the questionnaire using the above method. However, if the patient fills out the questionnaire alone the response time is considerably shorter.

Scoring

The various items of the questionnaire can be conceptualized as describing a scale to assess a transsexual's success or failure postsurgery. Indeed, the 59-item questionnaire can be viewed as defining eight domains of measurement. These domains include the sexual, psychological, environmental, economic, parental, familial, medical, and social

---

[1]Address correspondence to Leslie M. Lothstein, Department of Clinical Psychology, Institute of Living, 400 Washington Street, Hartford, CT 06016.

adjustment and functioning of the patient. The transsexual's responses to Likert-type items can be broken down into two scores, a score of 1 to 7 and a millimeter score. Currently, we have opted to use the numeric scores for comparisons over time, within and between subjects. These scores are being used for research with contrast and control groups of transsexual and nontranssexual respondents. It is anticipated that further development of this scale will include assigning values to each of the eight areas measured and obtaining scores for each domain. A total score could then be derived indicating postsurgery outcome. As we obtain additional evidence of the usefulness of the scale, we will be better able to determine which areas are crucial for predicting successful postsurgical outcome. Research from the Minnesota Gender Identity Clinic (Satterfield, 1981) suggests that bad surgical results are associated with poor postsurgical psychological adjustment. Lothstein (1980) cautioned that good social-vocational adjustment (i.e., those domains most often chosen to assess the outcome of transsexual surgery) may be misleading and that good psychological functioning is the critical factor to success or failure postoperatively.

Reliability and Validity

All the items of the scale have face validity. Many of the questions can be answered only by transsexuals who have undergone surgery. Each of the questions was chosen after reviewing all of the extant literature on postoperative follow-up studies of transsexualism and categorizing those areas that researchers have designated as critical for determining success or failure. Our preliminary findings suggest that patients tend to be poor judges of the medical aspects of their surgery for at least 1 year postsurgery. In this sense, responses to sexual questions tend to be influenced by the patient's euphoria immediately after surgery. Independent medical assessments and the patient's requests for additional surgery (usually 1 to 2 years later) suggest that the patient's initial responses to his or her sexual functioning is a poor indicator of how well or poor the patient will eventually function. The critical areas seem to focus on the psychological, medical, and parental/familial domains.

Other Information

This scale is copyrighted 1979.

References

Lothstein, L. (1980). The postsurgical transsexual: Empirical and theoretical considerations. *Archives of Sexual Behavior, 9,* 547-564.

Lothstein, L. (1982). Sex reassignment surgery: Historical, bioethical, and theoretical issues. *American Journal of Psychiatry, 139,* 417-426.

Satterfield, S. (1981). Surgical sex reassignment: A 14-year experience. *Proceedings of the 7th International Gender Dysphoria Association.* Lake Tahoe, NV.

Exhibit

Transsexual Postoperative Follow-Up Questionnaire

Page 1-MF

Name _____

Address _____

Date of surgery: _____

    Stage 1 _____

    Stage 2 _____

    Stage 3 _____

    Additional surgery _____

Primary therapist _____

Employment now _____

Social conditions: Married   Single   Divorced   Widowed

Date _____

Phone no. _____

Surgeon _____

Surgeon _____

Surgeon _____

Surgeon _____

Page 2-M

1. The overall appearance of my new genitals.
   satisfactory–unsatisfactory[a]
2. The desire to show other people my new genitals.
   strong–weak
3. The size of the new vagina.
   satisfactory–unsatisfactory
4. The removal of my penis.
   happy–unhappy
5. How well do you expect your vagina to function during intercourse?
   adequately–inadequately
6. How painful was your post-surgery experience?
   painful–painless

7. How painful was your post-hospitalization experience?
    painful–painless
8. How have your friends reacted to the appearance of your new genitals?
    liked it–disliked it
9. Have you felt a sensation that your penis still exists after surgery?
    yes _____   no _____
    If you answered yes, rate the strength of that sensation.
    strong–weak
10. Do you miss your penis?
    yes _____   no _____
11. How well have you carried out your doctor's orders regarding the use of a dilator?
    well–poorly
    Did you have any difficulties in using the dilator? Explain in detail.

Page 2-F
1. The overall appearance of my new genitals.
    satisfactory–unsatisfactory
2. The desire to show other people my new genitals.
    strong–weak
3. The size of the new penis.
    satisfactory–unsatisfactory
4. The removal of my breasts.
    happy–unhappy
5. How well do you expect your penis to function during intercourse?
    satisfactory–unsatisfactory
6. How painful was your post-surgery experience?
    painful–painless
7. How painful was your post-hospitalization experience?
    painful–painless
8. How have your friends reacted to the appearance of your new genitals?
    liked it–disliked it
9. Have you felt a sensation that your breasts still exist after surgery?
    yes _____   no _____
10. Do you miss your breasts?
    yes _____   no _____
11. How well have you carried out your doctor's orders regarding the care of your penis?
    well–poorly
11a. The removal of my ovaries and uterus.
    happy–unhappy

Page 3-M
12. How well have you carried out your doctor's orders regarding taking medication?
    well–poorly
13. How adequate was your emotional preparation for the surgery?
    adequate–inadequate
14. Would you recommend surgery to other patients?
    recommend–advise against
15. Having gone through the first (and second) phase of the surgery, what advice can you give other patients about the operation?
16. What additional parts of your body would you like to change through surgery?
17. Indicate on the scales below how strong is your desire to have additional surgery on the body parts you mentioned in question 16.
          Body Part
    (1) _____   strong–weak
    (2) _____   strong–weak
    (3) _____   strong–weak
    (4) _____   strong–weak
    (5) _____   strong–weak

Page 3-F
12. How well have you carried out your doctor's orders regarding taking medication?
    well–poorly

13. How adequate was your emotional preparation for the surgery?
    adequate–inadequate
14. Would you recommend surgery to other patients?
    recommend–advise against
15. Having gone through the first (and second) phase of the surgery, what advice can you give other patients about the operation?
16. What additional parts of your body would you like to change through surgery?
17. Indicate on the scales below how strong is your desire to have additional surgery on the body parts you mentioned in question 16.
    Body Part
    (1) _____ strong–weak
    (2) _____ strong–weak
    (3) _____ strong–weak
    (4) _____ strong–weak
    (5) _____ strong–weak

Page 4-MF
18. Mark on the following scales how you feel about yourself at the present time.
    depressed–happy
    attractive–unattractive
    anxious–relaxed
    comfortable with others–uncomfortable with others
    male–female
    happy with the way I look–unhappy with the way I look
    optimistic about the future–pessimistic about the future
    confident–insecure
    outgoing–shy
    active–passive
    assertive–submissive
    interested in sexual activity–not interested in sexual activity
    masculine–feminine
19. Have you thought about suicide since your surgery? If so, explain in detail what suicidal thoughts you have had.
20. In your dreams after the surgery, do you see yourself as a male or a female?
21. What thoughts, dreams, or feelings have made a vivid impression on you since surgery?

Page 5-M
22. Please relate one of the most vivid dreams you have had since surgery.
23. Did you have any complications during or after your surgery? If so, please describe the complications you had.
24. Do you regret the surgery?
    yes _____   no _____
25. Would you like to change back to your original sex?
    would like to change back–would not like to change back
26. Are you satisfied with the ability of your vagina to function during intercourse?
    satisfied–dissatisfied
27. What kind of fears/concerns do you have about your new genitals?
28. How satisfactory was your sex life prior to surgery?
    satisfactory–unsatisfactory
29. How often before surgery did you experience a climax in your sexual encounters with your partner?
    never _____   occasionally _____   frequently _____   always _____

Page 5-F
22. Please relate one of the most vivid dreams you have had since surgery.
23. Did you have any complications during or after your surgery? If so, please describe the complications you had.
24. Do you regret the surgery?
    yes _____   no _____
25. Would you like to change back to your original sex?
    would like to change back–would not like to change back
26. Are you satisfied with the ability of your penis to function during intercourse?
    satisfied–dissatisfied
27. What kind of fears/concerns do you have about your new genitals?
28. How satisfactory was your sex life prior to surgery?
    satisfactory–unsatisfactory

29. How often before surgery did you experience a climax in your sexual encounters with your partner?
    never _____ occasionally _____ frequently _____ always _____

Pages 6, 7, 8 and 9-MF
30. How satisfactory do you expect your sex life to be after the surgery?
    satisfactory–unsatisfactory
31. How often do you expect (or already have) orgasms after the surgery?
32. Do you achieve orgasms through your new genitals?
    yes _____   no _____
    by other means?
    yes _____   no _____
33. How often do you masturbate?
    daily _____ several times a week _____ once a week _____ less than once a week _____ never _____
34. What do you fantasize about when you masturbate?
35. How soon after surgery did you have sexual intercourse (penis-vagina) with a partner?
36. Rate the frequency of the following types of sexual relationships.
    oral sex   none _____ occasional _____ frequent _____
    anal sex   none _____ occasional _____ frequent _____
    vaginal intercourse   none _____ occasional _____ frequent _____
37. Describe your fantasies accompanying sexual intercourse.
38. Have there been changes in the number of your sex partners?
    more _____ fewer _____ same _____
39. Do your sex partners know about the surgery?
40. Are your sex partners new or have you known them before the surgery?
41. Do you have one very close friend?
42. How many friends do you have now?
43. What kind of activities do you do for recreation? Please list.
44. What changes occurred in your social life after the surgery?
45. Do you date? _____ How often?
    frequently _____ seldom _____ not at all _____
46. Do you have a steady girlfriend?
47. Are you married now?
48. Are you planning marriage in the future?
49. Are you planning to adopt children? If so, do you have a preference for a boy or girl?
50. How supportive was your family (parents, siblings) before the surgery?
    supportive–unsupportive
51. How accepting is your family now?
    accepting–rejecting
52. How does each of the following members feel about your surgery and your new gender?
    Mother:
    Father:
    Grandfather:
    Grandmother:
    Sisters:
    Brothers:
    Ex-spouse:
    Children:
53. What changes occurred in your attitudes toward your family? Explain. Do you feel closer to them now?
54. Were you employed prior to surgery? If so, where, how long, and what type of work did you do?
55. Have you changed your place of employment after the surgery? If so, where do you work now and what kind of work do you do?
56. Has there been a change in your salary or your position after the surgery?
57. Do people at your place of employment know about your surgery?
58. How have your co-workers reacted to your surgery? What attitudes do they display toward you now?
59. What vocational and/or educational plans do you have for the future?

a. Each scale is a 7-point scale, anchored by the terms indicated.

Cross-Gender Fetishism Scale

Ray Blanchard,[1] *Clarke Institute of Psychiatry*

The Cross-Gender Fetishism Scale (CGFS; Blanchard, 1985) is a measure (for males) of the erotic arousal value of putting on women's clothes, perfume, and make-up, and shaving the legs. The term *cross-gender fetishism* was coined by Freund, Steiner, and Chan (1982) to designate fetishistic activity that is accompanied by fantasies of being female and carried out with objects symbolic of femininity. It is therefore roughly equivalent to the term *transvestism* as defined in the *DSM-III* (American Psychiatric Association, 1980).

Description

The CGFS is primarily intended to discriminate fetishistic from nonfetishistic cross-dressers (e.g., gender dysphorics, transsexuals, "drag queens," self-labeled transvestites). All items, however, contain one response option appropriate for non-cross-dressing males, so that it may be administered to control samples as well.

The scale is a self-administered, multiple-choice questionnaire. It contains 11 items: 6 with three response options and 5 with two options. Scoring weights for these response options were determined with the optimal scaling procedure for multiple-choice items outlined by Nishisato (1980). This procedure directly determines the set of scoring weights that optimizes the alpha reliability of a scale for a given population. This analysis, as well as others yielding the psychometric information reported below, was carried out on 99 adult male patients of the behavioral sexology department or gender identity clinic of a psychiatric teaching hospital. All had reported that they felt like females at least when cross-dressed, if not more generally.

Response Mode and Timing

Examinees may check or circle the response option of their choice. They are instructed to endorse one and only one response option per item. Examinees are permitted to ask for clarification on the meaning of an item. The CGFS was intended to round out a larger battery of erotic preference and gender identity measures (see the chapter by Freund and Blanchard in this volume) and should not, by itself, take more than 1 or 2 minutes to complete.

Scoring

The scoring weight for each response option is shown in parentheses in the accompanying exhibit. Because empirically derived scoring weights can vary from sample to

sample, users might wish to substitute the scoring weights given here with a simple dichotomous scheme: 1 for each positive response and 0 for each negative one.

The total score is simply the (algebraic) sum of scores on the 11 individual items. Higher (i.e., more positive) scores indicate a more extensive history of cross-gender fetishism.

Reliability

Blanchard (1985), using the scoring weight presented here, found an alpha reliability coefficient of .95.

Validity

Blanchard (1985) found that two factors with eigenvalues greater than 1 emerged from principal components analysis, accounting for 68% and 9% of the total variance. The part-remainder correlations ranged from .56 to .89.

Blanchard (1985) demonstrated the expected strong association (within the clinical population previously described) between high scores on the CGFS and heterosexual partner preference. Blanchard, Clemmensen, and Steiner (1985), predicting that heterosexual male gender patients motivated to create a favorable impression at clinical assessment would tend to minimize their history of fetishistic arousal in their self-reports, found a high significant correlation of −.48 between the CGFS and the Crowne and Marlowe (1964) Social Desirability Scale. The correlation between these two measures among homosexual gender patients—who rarely or never have fetishistic histories—was virtually zero.

References

American Psychiatric Association. (1980). *Diagnostic and statistical manual of mental disorders* (3rd ed.). Washington, DC: Author.

Blanchard, R. (1985). Research methods for the typological study of gender disorders in males. In B. W. Steiner (Ed.)., *Gender dysphoria: Development, research, management* (pp. 227-257). New York: Plenum.

Blanchard, R., Clemmensen, L. H., & Steiner, B. W. (1985). Social desirability response set and systematic distortion in the self-report of adult male gender patients. *Archives of Sexual Behavior, 14,* 505-516.

Crowne, D. P., & Marlowe, D. (1964). *The approval motive: Studies in evaluative dependence.* New York: Wiley.

Freund, K., Steiner, B. W., & Chan, S. (1982). Two types of cross-gender identity. *Archives of Sexual Behavior, 11,* 49-63.

Nishisato, S. (1980). *Analysis of categorical data: Dual scaling and its applications.* Toronto: University of Toronto Press.

[1]Address correspondence to Ray Blanchard, Gender Identity Clinic, Clarke Institute of Psychiatry, 250 College Street, Toronto, Ontario M5T 1R8, Canada; email: blanchardr@cs.clarke-inst.on.ca.

Exhibit

Cross-Gender Fetishism Scale

Instructions to Subjects

The following questions ask about your experiences in dressing or making up as the opposite sex. These questions are meant to include experiences you may have had during puberty or early adolescence as well as more recent experiences.

Please circle one and only one answer to each question. If you are not sure of the meaning of a question, you may ask the person giving the questionnaire to explain it to you. There is no time limit for answering these questions.

1. Have you ever felt sexually aroused when putting on women's underwear, stockings, or a nightgown?
   a. Yes (1.0)   c. Have never put on any of these (–1.1)
   b. No (–1.1)
2. Have you ever felt sexually aroused when putting on women's shoes or boots?
   a. Yes (1.5)   c. Have never put on either of these (–0.7)
   b. No (–0.7)
3. Have you ever felt sexually aroused when putting on women's jewelry or outer garments (blouse, skirt, dress, etc.)?
   a. Yes (1.2)   c. Have never put on any of these (–1.0)
   b. No (–1.0)
4. Have you ever felt sexually aroused when putting on women's perfume or make-up, or when shaving your legs?
   a. Yes (1.3)   c. Have never done any of these (–0.8)
   b. No (–0.8)
5. Have you ever masturbated while thinking of yourself putting on (or wearing) women's underwear, stockings, or a nightgown?
   a. Yes (1.1)   b. No (–1.0)
6. Have you ever masturbated while thinking of yourself putting on (or wearing) women's shoes or boots?
   a. Yes (1.7)   b. No (–0.4)
7. Have you ever masturbated while thinking of yourself putting on (or wearing) women's jewelry or outer garments?
   a. Yes (1.4)   b. No (–0.8)
8. Have you ever masturbated while thinking of yourself putting on (or wearing) women's perfume or make-up, or while thinking of yourself shaving your legs (or having shaved legs)?
   a. Yes (1.5)   b. No (–0.7)
9. Has there ever been a period in your life of one year (or longer) during which you always or usually felt sexually aroused when putting on female underwear or clothing?
   a. Yes (1.1)   c. Have never put on female underwear or clothing (–1.0)
   b. No (–1.0)
10. Has there ever been a period in your life of one year (or longer) during which you always or usually masturbated if you put on female underwear or clothing?
    a. Yes (1.2)   c. Have never put on female underwear or clothing (–0.8)
    b. No (–0.8)
11. Have you ever put on women's clothes or make-up for the main purpose of becoming sexually excited and masturbating?
    a. Yes (1.3)   b. No (–0.4)

Source. This scale was originally published in "Research Methods for the Typological Study of Gender Disorders in Males," by R. Blanchard, 1985, in B. W. Steiner (Ed.), *Gender Dysphoria: Development, Research, Management,* 227-257. Reprinted with permission.

Locus of Control for Wives of Transvestites

Bonnie Bullough and Vern L. Bullough,[1] *Northridge, California*

The 10-item Locus of Control scale measures attitudes and feelings about personal (internal) control of reinforcements versus external control by outsider persons or forces, such as fate. In a study of the wives of transvestites, the scale was useful in predicting how well wives coped with their husbands' cross-dressing. Wives with strong feelings of internal control were happier and more satisfied with their marriage. Women who felt externally controlled were more likely to reject their husbands and fear exposure (Weinberg & Bullough, 1988).

Description

The roots of the current scale can be traced back to the work of social learning theorists Shephard Liverant, E. J. Phares, and Julian Rotter (Rotter, 1966; Rotter, Liverant, & Crowne, 1961; Seeman, 1963). They used longer scales (up to 52 items) titled Internal Versus External Control of Reinforcements to predict learning, finding that people who felt they controlled assigned tasks learned faster than those who believed the tasks or their situation was externally controlled. Melvin Seeman, a sociologist, placed the Locus of Control scale within alienation theory, calling it "powerlessness." He used it as one of five alienation constructs: powerlessness, normlessness, meaninglessness, social isolation, and self-estrangement (Seeman, 1959). The scale was shortened to 10-14 items, and although the tools were otherwise the same, the sociological literature emphasized the negative feelings that accompany a sense of control by others. In this format, it proved useful in predicting social learning in a reformatory (Seeman, 1963) and among tuberculosis patients (Seeman & Evans, 1962); Black migration out of the ghetto (Bullough, 1967); attendance in integrated schools (Bullough, 1972a); fertility control (Groat & Neal, 1967); and the use of preventive health services, particularly family planning services (Bullough, 1972b).

The two titles of the concept and the scales caused confusion, and because "powerlessness" is awkward to say, most researchers in the field have now moved back to the original title, "internal versus external control," or more commonly simply "locus of control," although the dual relationships to alienation theory as well as social learning theory remain important in the literature.

Response Mode and Scoring

The 10-item version of the scale used by Weinberg and Bullough (1988) uses a forced-choice format. The power-lessness or external control items (checked below) are counted to obtain the score.

Reliability

Neal and Rettig (1967) analyzed data from a study of manual and nonmanual workers using alternative procedures for factor analysis. By certain factorial criteria, the generality of several alienation constructs was demonstrated, whereas using other factorial criteria the separation of the powerlessness items was shown. No published figures for the internal consistency of the 10-item scale were found in the literature. Bullough (1974) calculated an alpha score of .61 for the powerlessness items and found strong intercorrelations with hopelessness and social isolation.

Validity

The validity of the scale in predicting a wide variety of social learning behaviors has been repeatedly demonstrated, as noted in the literature cited here, which is only a small fraction of the total. In literally hundreds of situations, people who feel they are controlled by others have been shown to be less able or less motivated to learn what they need to know to successfully cope with their lives.

References

Bullough, B. (1967). Alienation in the ghetto. *American Journal of Sociology, 72*, 469-478.

Bullough, B. (1972a). Alienation and school segregation. (1972a). *Integrated Education, 10*, 29-35.

Bullough, B. (1972b). Poverty, ethnic identity, and preventive health care. *Journal of Health and Social Behavior, 13*, 347-359.

Bullough, B. (1974). *The measurement of alienation as it relates to family planning behavior.* Paper presented at the Eighth World Congress on Sociology, Toronto, Canada.

Groat, H. T., & Neal, A. G. (1967). Social psychological correlates of urban fertility. *American Sociological Review, 32*, 945-959.

Neal, A. G., & Rettig, S. (1967). On the multi-dimensionality of alienation. *American Sociological Review, 32*, 54-56.

Rotter, J. B. (1966). Generalized expectancies for internal versus external control of reinforcements. *Psychological Monographs, 80*(Serial No. 609), 1-28.

Rotter, J. B., Liverant, S., & Crowne, D. P. (1961). The growth and extinction of expectancies in chance-controlled and skilled tasks. *Journal of Psychology, 12*, 161-177.

Seeman, M. (1959). On the meaning of alienation. *American Sociological Review, 24*, 783-791.

Seeman, M. (1963). Alienation and social learning in a reformatory. *American Journal of Sociology, 69*, 270-284.

Seeman, M., & Evans, J. W. (1962). Alienation and learning in a social setting. *American Sociological Review, 27*, 772-782.

Weinberg, T. S., & Bullough, V. L. (1988). Alienation, self-image, and the importance of support groups for wives of transvestites. *The Journal of Sex Research, 24*, 262-268.

[1]Address correspondence to Vern L. Bullough, 17434 Mayall Street, Northridge, CA 91325.

Exhibit

Locus of Control

Instructions: Included below are a number of statements. In each group of two, please choose the *one* that best reflects your point of view.

1. _____ The world is run by the few people in power and there is not much the little guy can do about it.
   or
   _____ The average citizen can have an influence on government decisions.

2. _____ Being a success is a matter of hard work—luck has little or nothing to do with it.
   or
   _____ Getting a good job depends mainly on being in the right place at the right time.

3. _____ In the long run people get the respect they deserve in the world.
   or
   _____ Unfortunately, people's worth often goes unnoticed no matter how hard they try.

4. _____ Most people don't realize how much their lives are the result of accidental happenings.
   or
   _____ There is really no such thing as luck.

5. _____ People are lonely because they don't try to be friendly.
   or
   _____ There's not much use in trying to please people—if they like you, they like you.

6. _____ I have usually found that what is going to happen will happen, no matter what I do.
   or
   _____ Trusting fate has never turned out as well for me as making a definite decision.

7. _____ When I make plans I am almost certain I can make them work.
   or
   _____ It is not always wise to plan too far ahead because many things turn out to be a matter of good or bad fortune anyhow.

8. _____ What happens to me is my own doing.
   or
   _____ Sometimes I feel I don't have enough control over the direction my life is taking.

9. _____ I feel helpless in the face of what's happening in the world today.
   or
   _____ I sometimes feel personally to blame for the sad state of affairs in the world.

10. _____ Even when the odds are against me, I can usually come out on top.
    or
    _____ Sometimes bad luck keeps me from succeeding.

Sexual and Marital Impact of Vasectomy

The Editors

The purpose of this instrument is to measure any problematic or traumatic effects of vasectomy surgery on marital and sexual satisfaction. Two self-administered questionnaires for both husband and wife were developed for use prior to and following vasectomy surgery. The presurgery scale contains 11 items; the follow-up questionnaire contains 4 additional items pertaining to the surgery. The answers to most questions are limited to three or four choices with room for written remarks. The questionnaires may be used to gain baseline information regarding the degree of marital and sexual satisfaction and to measure the intensity and duration of change in areas of satisfaction after the vasectomy.

Reference

Maschhoff, T. A., Fanshier, W. E., & Hansen, D. J. (1976). Vasectomy: Its effect upon marital stability. *The Journal of Sex Research, 12,* 295-314.

Index

About the Editors

Clive M. Davis, Ph.D., is Associate Professor of Psychology at Syracuse University, where he currently serves as Chair of Undergraduate Studies in the Department of Psychology. His research and teaching are focused primarily in the areas of sexuality and communications. From 1977 to 1987, he served as editor-in-chief of *The Journal of Sex Research,* and he has served as associate editor of the *Annual Review of Sex Research* since its inception in 1990. In 1985-1986, he served as President of the Society for the Scientific Study of Sexuality, during which time he was instrumental in creating the Foundation for the Scientific Study of Sexuality, a nonprofit foundation dedicated to supporting research-related activities. He continues as president of FSSS Foundation to this day. In 1987, he was granted the Distinguished Service Award by the Society for the Scientific Study of Sexuality. He has served on the Board of Directors of the Sexuality Information and Education Council of the United States and of the American Association for Sex Educators, Counselors, and Therapists.

William L. Yarber, H.S.D., is Professor of Health Education at Indiana University, Bloomington and Senior Director of the Rural Center for AIDS/STD Prevention. He has published extensively in the HIV/STD education and sexuality education areas, with more than 75 articles in professional journals. He has authored four school HIV/STD curricula including the nation's first comprehensive school AIDS curriculum. He is Chair of the Board of Directors of the Sexuality Information and Education Council of the United States and Past President of the Society for the Scientific Study of Sexuality. In 1991, he received the Association for the Advancement of Health Education Scholar Award and the Indiana University Distinguished Teaching Award. He chaired the National Guidelines Task Force, which developed the SIECUS-sponsored *Guidelines for Comprehensive Sexuality Education: Kindergarten-12th Grade.* He has also been a consultant for the World Health Organization Global Program on AIDS and the U.S. Centers for Disease Control.

Robert Bauserman completed his Ph.D. in social psychology at Syracuse University in 1994. He has authored or coauthored several publications and presentations in such areas as the effects of childhood and adolescent sexual experience on later sexual attitudes and adjustment, the development of sexual fantasy, the effects of viewing pornography on males' attitudes about sexism and rape, and the role of pornography in sexual aggression. His research outside the area of sexuality has included work on gender role orientation and health behaviors, and on social versus personal stereotypes of masculinity and femininity. He currently teaches courses in introductory and personality psychology at the University of Michigan.

George Schreer is Assistant Professor of Psychology at Plymouth State College in New Hampshire. He received his Ph.D. in social psychology from Syracuse University in 1995. His research interests include collective sexual aggression, stereotypes, and discrimination. Currently, he teaches a course on the "darker side" of human behavior, exploring such provocative issues as sexual aggression, the impact of pornography, and sexual jealousy.

Sandra L. Davis, B.A., is Administrative Assistant for a member of the New York State Assembly. From 1983 to 1988, she served as the managing editor of *The Journal of Sex Research,* and she is currently an assistant editor for the *Annual Review of Sex Research.* She has served on the Board of Directors of the Foundation for the Scientific Study of Sexuality since 1991 and is currently the Secretary. In 1995, she received the Distinguished Service Award of the Society for the Scientific Study of Sexuality. She has also served on the Board of Directors of and as Vice President for the Central New York Persons With AIDS Support Fund. She has been a longtime member of the Board of Directors of the American Heart Association, Upstate Region, New York State, and she was President of the region in 1986-1987. She has also been a member of the Board of Directors of the American Heart Association, New York State Affiliate, and chaired the Public Policy Committee. In 1988, she received the Edmund G. Fallon Gold Heart Distinguished Service Award.

Printed in the United States
R3140200001B